S. M. Griffith
National Forage Seed P
Oregon State University
3450 S.W. Campus Way
Corvallis, Oregon   97331-7102

ANTIBODY AS A TOOL
The Applications of Immunochemistry

ANTIBODY AS A TOOL
The Applications of Immunochemistry

Edited by
JOHN J. MARCHALONIS and GREGORY W. WARR

Department of Biochemistry.,
Medical University of South Carolina, USA

A Wiley–Interscience Publication

JOHN WILEY & SONS

Chichester · New York · Brisbane · Toronto · Singapore

Library of Congress Cataloging in Publication Data:
Main entry under title:

Antibody as a tool.
  A Wiley–Interscience publication.
  Includes index.
1. Immunoglobulins.   2. Immunochemistry—
Technique.   I. Marchalonis, John J., 1940–
II. Warr, Gregory W.
QR186.7.A574   616.07′9   81-14744

ISBN 0 471 10084 6   AACR2

British Library Cataloguing in Publication Data:

Antibody as a tool: the applications of
  immunochemistry.
  1. Marchalonis, J. J.
  II. Warr, G. W.
  574.2′9   QR183.6

ISBN 0 471 10084 6

Printed and bound in Great Britain
at The Pitman Press, Bath

Contributors

L. BENADE   *Microbiological Associates, Bethesda, Md. 20816, USA.*

C. BUCANA   *Cancer Biology Program, NCI Frederick Cancer Research Center, P. O. Box B, Frederick, Maryland 21701, USA.*

C. A. C. CARRAWAY   *Departments of Anatomy and Cell Biology and Oncology, University of Miami School of Medicine, Miami, Florida 33101, USA.*

K. L. CARRAWAY   *Departments of Anatomy and Cell Biology and Oncology, University of Miami School of Medicine, Miami, Florida 33101, USA.*

A. CLARKE   *School of Botany, University of Melbourne, Parkville,, Victoria 3052, Australia.*

D. DeLUCA   *Department of Biochemistry, Medical University of South Carolina, Charleston, South Carolina 29425, USA.*

J. W. GODING   *Walter and Eliza Hall Institute, Post Office, Royal Melbourne Hospital, Parkville, Victoria 3050, Australia.*

R. M. HOGGART   *School of Botany, University of Melbourne, Parkville, Victoria 3052, Australia.*

L. C. HOYER   *Cancer Biology Program, NCI Frederick Cancer Research Center, P. O. Box B, Frederick, Maryland 21701, USA.*

v

L. Hudson   *Department of Immunology, St George's Hospital Medical School, London, UK.*

J. N. Ihle   *Cancer Biology Program, NCI Frederick Cancer Research Center, P. O. Box B, Frederick, Maryland 21701, USA.*

E. J. Jenkinson   *Department of Anatomy, The University of Birmingham, Medical School, Vincent Drive, Birmingham, B15 2TJ, UK.*

S. B. Kadin   *Department of Medicinal Chemistry, Pfizer Central Research, Groton, CT 06340, USA.*

F. Karush   *Department of Microbiology, School of Medicine, University of Pennsylvania, Philadelphia, PA 19104, USA.*

R. B. Knox   *School of Botany, University of Melbourne, Parkville, Victoria 3052, Australia.*

J. J. Marchalonis   *Department of Biochemsitry, Medical University of South Carolina, 171 Ashley Avenue, Charleston, South Carolina 29425, USA.*

I. Otterness   *Department of Pharmacology, Pfizer Central Research, Groton, CT 06340, USA.*

R. F. Searle   *Department of Anatomy, The Medical School, University of Newcastle upon Tyne, UK.*

D. Snary   *Department of Immunochemistry, Wellcome Research Laboratories, Beckenham,, Kent, UK.*

A.-C. Wang   *Department of Basic and Clinical Immunology and Microbiology, Medical University of South Carolina, Charleston, South Carolina 29425, USA.*

G. W. Warr   *Department of Biochemistry, Medical University of South Carolina, 171 Ashley Avenue, Charleston, South Carolina 29425, USA.*

Contents

Preface   ix

Basic Methods and Theory

1. Structure of antibodies and their usefulness to non-immunologists
   J. J. Marchalonis   3

2. Preparation of antigens and principles of immunization
   G. W. Warr   21

3. Purification of antibodies
   G. W. Warr   59

4. Principles of antibody reactions
   I. Otterness and F. Karush   97

5. Methods of immune diffusion, immunoelectrophoresis,
   precipitation, and agglutination
   A.-C. Wang 139

6. Principles of radioimmunoassays and related techniques
   L. Benade and J. N. Ihle 163

7. Immunofluroescence analysis
   D. DeLuca 189

8. Principles of immunoelectron microscopy
   L. C. Hoyer and C. Bucana 233

9. Production of monoclonal antibodies by cell fusion
   J. W. Goding 273

Specific Applications of Immunochemical and Related Techniques

10. Immunology and the study of plants
    R. B. Knox 293

11. The use of lectins in the study of glycoproteins
    A. E. Clarke and R. M. Hoggart 347

12. Immunochemical approaches in developmental and
    reproductive biology
    E. J. Jenkinson and R. F. Searle 403

13. Antibodies as pharmacologic and medicinal tools
    S. B. Kadin and I. Otterness 447

14. Immunological studies on parasites
    L. Hudson and D. Snary 485

15. Isolation and characterization of plasma membranes
    K. L. Carraway and C. A. C. Carraway 509

Index 561

Editors' Preface

Since the field of immunology is very well served by textbooks and manuals of laboratory technique, a reader would be justified in asking 'why another?' This question can best be answered by outlining what we believe to be the scope and purposes of *Antibody as a Tool*. This book is intended to serve as an introduction to the uses of immunochemical techniques for scientists who are not 'professional immunologists'. Our object is not to duplicate the detailed information available in such standard works as Weir's *Experimental Immunology* or *Methods in Immunology and Immunochemistry* by Williams and Chase, but rather to show how immunochemistry can provide powerful techniques for investigations in fields as diverse as botany, parasitology, pharmacology, and developmental biology, for example. To this end, we have assembled, as the second part of this volume, contributions that review specific areas of biological research in which immunochemical techniques have made important contributions. In these chapters, when appropriate, experimental methodology as used for particular, relevant, purposes, is also given. However, the first section of the book consists of nine chapters, in which is outlined the basic information about antibody production and use in techniques such as raising monoclonal antibody, radioimmunoassay, immunoelectron microscopy, and immunofluorescence. These chapters emphasize the practical aspects of antibody use, and every attempt has been made to include the simplest and most valuable techniques.

In two areas we stray outside the conventional definition of immunochemistry. These areas are the use of lectins, and the methods for isolating the plasma membrane. We felt it was very important that chapters on these subjects should find a place in this book, because immunochemistry is widely used in biological research for the study of plasma membrane structures. The plasma membrane is important in so many aspects of cellular differentiation and recognition that we felt a chapter on the isolation and characterization of this organelle would be useful: similarly, while lectins are not antibodies, their exquisite binding specificity for carbohydrates has led to their widespread use in studies of cell surface glycoconjugates.

We hope, therefore, that two themes are represented in *Antibody as a Tool*; first the ways in which immunochemical techniques can be used in basic biological research in areas removed from immunology as such, and, second, the convergence of much immunochemical and cell biological research upon the structure and function of the plasma membrane.

GREGORY W. WARR
JOHN J. MARCHALONIS
Charleston, SC
June 29, 1981

Basic Methods and Theory

Chapter 1

Structure of Antibodies and Their Usefulness to Non-Immunologists

JOHN J. MARCHALONIS

*Department of Biochemistry, Medical University of South Carolina,
171 Ashley Avenue, Charleston, SC 29425.*

I. INTRODUCTION

Antibodies have received considerable attention in the last 30 years. The amino acid sequence of many immunoglobulins was established, much attention was given to their functional properties, and in the last five years many fascinating features of the complex genetic system which determines antibody structure and variability have been unravelled. This work has been reviewed in enormous detail for both the specialist (Glynn and Steward, 1977; Litman and Good, 1978; Nisonoff *et al.*, 1975) and the more general reader (Gally and Edelman, 1972).It is not my intent to reiterate here aspects of antibody structure, function, evolution, and genetics which are discussed in great detail elsewhere. Rather, I hope to point out in a concise fashion the features of antibody recognition and function which make them useful probes for the detection and isolation of virtually any cell, macromolecule or small organic compound which the investigator plans to pursue. In essence, antibodies produced by us and all other vertebrates can recognize a vast array of 'non-self'molecular configurations which may be termed antigens. If, for example, a mouse is injected under the proper conditions (these will be outlined below) with human erythrocytes, or a virus, or a particular bacterium or a human serum protein such as human albumin, antibodies will be produced which react with characteristic antigenic determinants found on the particular molecule or cell injected. Although immunization is usually performed using fairly large complex structures, the antibodies recognize a small portion of the complex. The size of the actual determinant which is recognized would be of the order of approximately six amino acids or six monosaccharide units (Kabat, 1968). The antibody response is exquisitely specific as was established by pionerring work of Landsteiner many years ago (1945) who showed that

3

antibodies are capable of very fine discrimination between the substituent groups on a small molecule such as a benzene ring. Landsteiner introduced the concept of 'hapten' and 'carrier' which is a very important one to be kept in mind both in designing immuniztion schemes and in interpreting specificity of antibody reactions. Small organic molecules, such as 2,4-dinitrobenzene, by themselves will not cause antibody production. However, if a reactive form of this molecule, for example fluorodinitrobenzene, were coupled to a protein and this complex was injected into animals, antibodies would be produced which were specific for the dinitrobenzene molecule. The small organic molecule is termed a hapten, and the large protein molecule is termed a carrier. The need for separate recognition of haptenic and carrier determinants foreshadowed much of modern cellular immunology in the realm of cooperation between thymus-derived lymphocytes and bone-marrow-derived lymphocytes (Mitchison *et al.*, 1970)

I will not go into the mechanisms necessary for production of anti-hapten antibody at this time, but will emphasize that from a practical standpoint the coupling of small molecules to carriers has proven to be a very important means of generating antibody to a variety of low molecular weight molecules which by themselves would not generate antibody production. It has been possible to couple carbohydrate moieties to proteins and produce anti-carbohydrate antibody (Goebel, 1936) although polysaccharides are themselves immunogenic (Sutherland, 1977). Likewise, it has been possible to produce antibodies to purines and pyrimidines (Halloran and Parker, 1966) including cyclic nucleotides (Steiner, 1973) and other small molecules which are important to pharmacologists (Erlanger, 1973) and molecular biologists. The proven capacity to generate antibodies specific for hormones and pharmacologically important small molecules, coupled with the techniques of immunoassay described elsewhere in this volume, illustrate the tremendous possibilities for use of antibodies in other systems besides immunology. Over ten years ago, one of my biochemical colleagues commented to me that 'immunology provided tremendous tools for biochemists, endocrinologists, developmental biologists, and scientists of all persuasions, although it had no intellectual content itself'. The burst of activity and new information regarding immunoglobulin diversification, genetics, and evolution which followed his comments clearly indicated that the latter part of his comment was incorrect. There is no question, however, that the first half of his statement was of importance then and will continue to be of importance as long as investigators seek to identify, quantitate, and isolate biological molecules to which antibodies can be generated. The beauty of the antibody forming system is that it is a biological means of generating recognition molecules of desired specificity. The technology of this has recently been improved immeasurably because of the development of cell/cell hybridization techniques which allow the 'immortalization' of monoclonal antibody-forming cells (see Goding, Chapter 9), but the essential idea remains the same as it has for the last 100 years; namely, an animal is injected with a molecular configuration which is normally foreign to it. Following this immunization, the animal responds by producing an antibody protein which has a combining site complementary to a portion of the foreign antigenic moiety.

II. ANTIBODIES: GENERAL PROPERTIES

The inducible, antigen-specific molecules which occur in vertebrate serum and on the surfaces of their lymphocytes are representatives of a family of serum glycoproteins which has been termed immunoglobulins. Although there are many types of immunoglobulins now recognized (man for example, possesses five major immunoglobulin classes) they all share the same type of combining site for anitgen. Likewise, the original antigen receptors which occur on the surface of lymphocytes also possess combining sites for antigen which are structurally homologous to those of serum antibodies directed against the same antigen (Burnet, 1959; Marchalonis, 1975). Table 1 gives the general properties of human and murine immunoglobulins. It can be seen that these may differ in antigenic properties which determine the nature of their so-called class or isotype in addition to overall molecular organization. The majority antibody class in us and in other mammals is the so-called IgG class (or common gamma globulins). An IgG molecule consists of two γ heavy chains coupled covalently by disulphide bonds to each other and each is coupled to a light polypeptide chain which would be termed either κ or λ. The molecule has two combining sites for antigen which are formed by interaction between the variable portions of the light chain and the variable portion of the heavy chain. This is illustrated in Figure 1. Another major immunoglobulin class is the immune macroglobulins or IgM molecules. These molecules are characterized by having a heavy chain termed the μ chain which is larger than the γ chain, has a different amino acid sequence, and has a characteristic antigenic determinant which allows it to be distinguished from the γ chain and from the other heavy chains. This striking difference between the μ and γ heavy chain is shown in Figure 2 which presents a polyacrylamide gel electrophoresis pattern in sodium dodecylsulphate-containing buffer of μ, γ and light chains and purified μ and λ chains. All immunoglobulin classes, however, can possess the same light chains: κ light chains, for example, can be found in association with μ, γ, δ, α and ϵ heavy chains and the class of the molecule is that of the heavy chain. Another striking feature which distinguishes IgM (Figure 3) from IgG is that the IgM molecule occurs as a cyclic pentamer of the $(\kappa\mu)_2$ unit which is covalently associated through disluphide bonds and has an approximate molecular weight of 800,000 as opposed to the 150,000 molecular weight characteristic of IgG molecules. The heavy chains differ in all the properties described. The properties of the particular heavy chain determine the

Table 1. Properties of human and murine immunoglubulins

Immunoglobulin	Heavy chain	Sedimentation coefficient	Intact molecular weight	Mol. wt. heavy chain	CHO(%)	Fixes C⁻1 (classical)	Binds staphyloccal protein-A
Man							
IgG1	γ1	7S	150,000	50,000	2–3	++	+
IgG2	γ2	7S	150,000	50,000	2–3	+	+
IgG3	γ3	7S	170,000	60,000	2–3	+++	–
IgG4	γ4	7S	150,000	50,000	2–3	–	+
IgM	μ	19S	900,000	70,000	12	+++	+⁻*
IgA1	α1	7S	7–11	–	–		
IgA2	α2	7S	160,000	52,000	7–11	–	+
IgD	δ	7S	180,000	68,000	9–14	–	–
IgE	ε	8S	190,000	72,000	12	–	–
Mouse							
IgG1	γ1	7S	150,000	50,000	2–3	–	–
IgG2a	γ2a	7S	150,000	50,000	2–3	+	+
IgG2b	γ2b	7S	150,000	50,000		+	+
IgG3	γ3	7S	150,000	50,000		–	+
IgM	μ	19S	900,000	70,000	12	+++	–

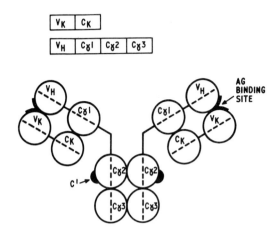

Figure 1. Schematic representation of an IgG immunoglobulin molecule. This model illustrates the domain structure of immunoglobulin light and heavy chains. Two combining sites for antigen are present and these are formed by interaction between the V_H and the V_κ portions of the molecule. The binding site for complement (C,) is shown to be located in the $C_\gamma 2$ domain. The region of the heavy chain where no domains are shown is the 'hinge' region

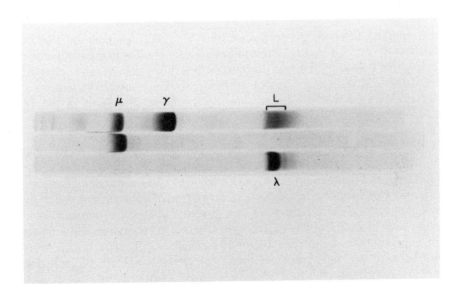

Figure 2. Resolution by polyacrylamide gel electrophoresis in sodium-dodecylsulphate-containing buffers in the presence of 2-mercaptoethanol (reducing conditions) of: (1) a mixture of IgG and IgM immunoglobulins; (2) purified μ chain of an IgM myeloma protein; and (3) the purified λ light chain of the IgM protein

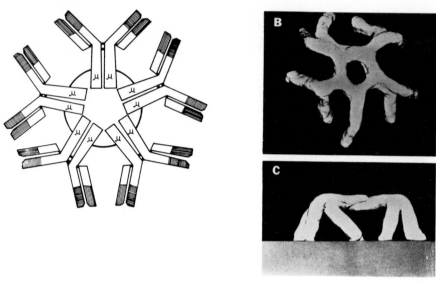

Figure 3. Planar projection model of the IgM immunoglobulin molecule showing the structure as a cyclic pentamer held together by disulphide bonds. The stippled regions represent the variable regions of the μ and light chains. Figures 3B and 3C are models representing the shape of IgM antibody bound to a flagellar antigen. (After Feinstein and Beal, 1977)

functional or effector properties of the Ig molecule. One of the best illustrations of this is that IgM antibodies are very good at fixing complement; i.e. reacting with a set of serum protein components which mediate cell lysis or destruction following reaction with antibody which is bound to an antigen. By contrast, IgA antibodies, even when of the same specificity as the IgM molecules, are very poor at fixing complement and bringing about cell lysis. Another important property which is germane to the goals of the present review is that some heavy chains bind avidly to protein-A produced by *Staphylococcus aureus* (see Table 1). This rather fortuitous event has led to important, rapid means for the purification of serum immunoglobulins of particular types and also has provided a major simplification in assays designed to isolate complexes of antibodies bound to their respective antigen. A key point which I would stress here is that members of every immunoglobulin class can express antibody specificity for a particular antigen. For this reason antibodies of any class would be useful for the development of solid phase immune adsorbents or other techniques which are dependent only upon the binding of antigen. However, not all antibodies would be equally useful in assays which involve effector functions distinct from that of antigen binding. Human IgG3 antibodies might be very useful as a solid phase immune adsorbent, but they would be useless in an assay in which the complexes are bound by a *S. aureus* protein-A. The same distinction would be made between antibodies made in rabbits where virtually all of the IgG binds protein-A and antibodies made in goats or in rats where very little of the serum IgG binds protein-A, Thus, care must be taken in deciding which class and species would be most useful for a particular system.

III. ANTIBODY DIVERSITY

The antibody forming system has provided quite a challenge to immunologists and molecular biologists for many years because it is a learning system which responds to immunization by producing large amounts of specific antibody, and, in addition, the quality of the antibody or the affinity of its binding to the particular antigen often increases with time of immunization. In addition there is the formidable problem of explaining how one individual could produce inducible proteins showing specificities for possibly millions of distinct antigenic determinants. Much of the intellectual framework underlying the search for this mechanism was laid down by the theory of clonal selection which was developed by Sir McFarlane Burnet (1959). In essence, it is now generally believed that our lymphocyte population shows a great heterogeneity inasmuch as different cells possess surface immunoglobulin receptors, each of which differs in its combining site (Figure 4). If a given antigen is introduced, only those cells which can recognize that particular antigen will be stimulated and respond. Thus the reaction is specific and large amounts of the appropriate antibody can be generated. Naturally, the story is not quite so simple and a great deal of work remains to determine precisely what cellular and biochemical mechanisms are involved in selective stimulation of cells, but the evidence for a clonal restriction of lymphocytes is compelling. Even accepting clonal restriction, there is still the problem of how the molecular and genetic mechanisms operate. The first clues to this came from studies in the middle 1960s which elucidated the amino acid sequence of homogeneous immunoglobulin light chains (Hilschmann and Craig, 1965). It was found that these light chains were unique in the sense that they possess both variable and constant sequence regions. Some sequence stretches were constant from individual to individual, a result usually observed with other proteins such as haemoglobins and cytochromes.

Immunoglobulins, however, also possess stretches of sequence which are markedly variable, not only from individual to individual, but within a given individual. Sequence analyses carried out on a large number of human and mammalian immunoglobulins established that approximately the first 110

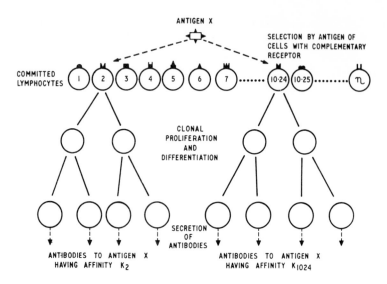

Figure 4. Illustration of the principle of clonal restriction of immunologically competent lymphocytes and specific by antigen. Based upon Marchalonis, 1977

N-terminal amino acids of heavy chains and of light chains are variable in sequence. This portion of the molecule has been termed the variable (V) region. In light chains the latter half of the molecule (approximately 100–110 amino acids) was constant from individual to individual, barring allotypic differences (genetic variation within a species). Further studies indicated that the heavy chains possessed a variable region followed by a constant region which consisted of a number of domains or regions which showed internal homology to one another. The γ chain consists of a V_H region followed by three γ chain constant region domains, whereas a μ chain has a V_H which could be exactly the same V_H as that of a γ chain but each of its four constant region domains is characteristic of the μ chain. A similar organization has been found for all the other heavy chains; moreover, heavy chains of more than one constant region type (class) can have in association with them the same heavy chain variable regions. It is the heavy chain constant regions which determine the particular class designation and the effector functions of that molecule. The Fc fragment is involved in the binding to *S. aureus* protein-A, in the fixation of complement and in the binding to the so-called Fc receptors found on lymphocytes, macrophages, and mast cells.

Statistical comparison of many variable regions (Wu and Kabat, 1970; Kehoe and Capra, 1978) showed that there are framework regions within the variable region which are relatively conserved, and there are regions termed hypervariable regions (HV) which show remarkable variability. This variability is illustrated in Figure 5 which illustrates the hypervariable regions detected

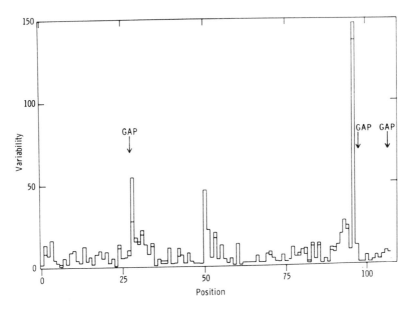

Figure 5. Diagram illustrating the frequency of variation of amino acid sequence within human myeloma light chains plotted as a function of residue position. This graph plots variability versus residue position, where variability is defined as the number of different amino acids at a given position divided by the frequency of the most common amino acid found in that position. A high frequency of amino acid interchanges occurred within three regions termed hypervariable regions. For light chains these correspond to residues 24–34, 50–56, and 89–97. (From Wu and Kabat, 1970)

in light chains by Wu and Kabat (1970). Subsequent studies documented the existence of hypervariable regions in V_H regions. Kabat predicted that the hypervariable regions most probably contributed the complementary residues involved in holding the antigen in place within the combining site. Experimental data support the essential truth of this conclusion. The antigen combining site is a cleft which is about 15 Å × 20 Å × 10 Å deep which is formed by interaction of V_H and V_L sequences, and the complementarity-determining regions are provided by the hypervariable regions of V_H and V_L (Poljak, 1978).

IV. IMMUNOGLOBULIN GENES AND ANTIBODY PRODUCTION

The organization of immunoglobulin genes is extremely complicated, with a large array of variable region genes, diversity (D) segments in the case of V_H, a small number of so-called J or joining segments and a cluster of constant region genes which arose by tandem duplication from the original constant region gene. These in man occur on the fourteenth chromosome but they are not immediately linked and recombination events are necessary to ensure synthesis of a particular immunoglobulin heavy chain. The genetic basis of clonal restriction comes from: (1) the selection and translocation of a particular variable region sequence out of all those in the heavy chains variable region pool; (2) its association with particular D, J segments; and most importantly, (3) with a constant region gene segment (Molgaard, 1980). Analogous events occur in the case of light chains, but the diversity (D) segment is lacking in these chains (Seidman *et al.*, 1979). κ chains, λ chains, and heavy chains occur on different chromosomes. In a general sense the scheme underlying antibody production then would be that during development the lymphocyte pool has undergone random translocation events such that each lymphocyte can produce a particular light chain which has a complete variable and constant region sequence and a particular heavy chain characterized by one variable region hooked to a constant region, which in the precursor of the antibody secreting lymphocyte would be the μ chain constant region. A cell would express only one surface receptor specificity as defined by the particular V_H and V_L structures exposed. If antigen which interacts with this structure with a certain binding energy (affinity) is introduced, the cell can be stimulated to become an antibody-producing cell. The production of antibodies requires the presentation of antigen in the right manner, but the elaboration of antibodies also entails the interaction of non-lymphoid cells such as macrophages with B or T cells and interactions between thymus-derived and bone-marrow-derived lymphocytes (Marchalonis, 1980). In the case of antibody production, the first antibody to be produced in the primary response is that which most generally resembles the IgM surface receptor, i.e. it is the secreted form of IgM. Following a time after immunization and secondary (booster) injection, in mice and man there is a switch to antibodies expressing the γ chain constant region rather than the μ chain constant region. Eventually, the predominant antibody class in mammals is IgG. The quality (affinity) of antibody can also improve. The first event in the process outlined here would be the translocation and fixation of a particular variable region by forming a contiguous association with D, J, and constant region gene segments. The switch from IgM to IgG or other classes consists of the translocation of this variable region to a contiguous association with constant regions distinct from μ. These events are depicted at the gene and messenger RNA levels in Figure 6. The increase in quality or capacity of the antibody to bind antigen reflects a switch to populations of variable regions which bind more avidly to the particular antigen. An interesting phenomenon is often observed here and it may be of some practical interest in the production of antibodies. It is often found that the early antibodies express lower affinity then do later antibodies but the early ones are more specific. By 'specific' it is meant that they show less cross-reaction with related or unrelated molecules than do later antibodies which are much higher affinity, but may show substantial cross-reaction with related molecules. This

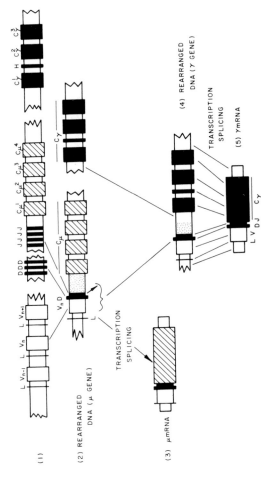

Figure 6. Recombination events leading to the formation of complete μ chain and γ chain genes. (1) This is the state of germ line DNA before rearrangement. There are more than 50 genes coding for the part of the variable (V) region, a cluster of D (diversity) gene segments coding for most of the third hypervariable region and in addition there are four J (joining) segments which complete the V region coding sequence. The Cμ gene lies at the start of the cluster containing all the heavy chain C region genes. Each domain of the μ chain has a separate coding sequence which is separated from the others by non-coding sequences. The γ chain gene also has separate coding sequences for the domains but in addition has a separate coding sequence for the hinge region (H). (2) In the first translocation event one each of the V, D, and J segments is recombined to give a complete μ chain transcription unit. This is essentially the commitment event which allows a lymphocyte to recognize specifically one antigen because it can express only one V region out of the total set which it initially possesses in the uncombined form. A similar event occurs with the combination of light chain V and C region genes, but the D region is missing. L is the short leader sequence which precedes the V region sequence. (3) Transcription of the complete, rearranged μ chain gene to produce μ chain mRNA involves a splicing mechanism in which the non-coding introns are removed. This complete μ chain mRNA can now be translated to give the μ chain. (4) This is the rearranged γ chain gene which involves deletion of the Cμ gene and translocation of the V, D, J segment and part of the J-Cμ intron to the proper juxtaposition with the Cγ gene. This is the IgM to IgG switch which occurs following prolonged time after a first injection. (5) The formation of the γ mRNA by transcription likewise involves the excision of non-coding sequences followed by the joining of the coding sequences to give a complete messenger RNA. (Based upon Molgaard (1980))

sort of phenomenon can cause problems in that many booster injections with a particular antigen may cause an animal to produce larger quantities of more active antibody, but this antibody may or may not be as useful in isolation and immunoassay as the earlier antibodies.

V. 'NON-IMMUNOLOGICAL' USES OF ANTIBODIES

As mentioned above, antibodies can be produced to protein or oligopeptide determinants, carbohydrates including individual monosaccharides, nucleic acids including individual nucleotides as well as to macromolecules and to cells, all depending upon the way the immunization is carried out. Since this chapter was intended to introduce useful features of antibodies to non-immunologists I will illustrate some of the uses to which the specificity of antibodies has been put in contexts which are generally not regarded as immunological. This is

Table 2. Uses of antibodies in 'Non-immunological' fields

Forensic pathology	Human or chicken blood on knife?
Taxonomy	Serological cross-reactions among proteins as an index of specification
Endocrinology	Hormone levels in blood
Pharmacology	Drug levels
Tumour biology	Detection and isolation of tumour cross-reacted antigens
Diagnosis	Identification of particular viral antigens

illustrated as a partial listing in Table 2. An obvious and immediate use of the properties of specificity and sensitivity which can be conferred by the use of antibodies is in the area of forensic pathology. For example, a knife found near the scene of a murder is covered with blood. Is this human blood or animal blood? Serology can be extremely useful in taxonomic studies. This type of approach has been very useful in microbiology (Sutherland, 1977) and has also found use in studies of speciation in eukaryotic systems. The degree of quantitative serological cross-reaction among molecules has generally been found to correlate very well with classifications based upon more traditional methods (Prager and Wilson, 1971). In addition, it is possible that serological studies may disclose relationships which are not obvious based upon morphological studies. A serological approach may prove quite helpful in certain areas because it is relatively inexpensive to produce and assays antibodies raised against whole cells, tissues or partially purified materials, whereas it becomes extremely laborious and expensive to isolate molecules such as cytochrome c and obtain complete amino acid sequence data. The use of antibody technology in endocrinology has been amply documented. The developments of radioimmunoassay techniques in particular, have revolutionized many of the approaches in this area. Immunoassay based upon the exquisite specificity of antibodies has also had a revolutionary effect in pharmacology. In this area, like that in endocrinology, the antibodies are most usually raised against highly purified hormone molecules or against specific drugs. For example in pharmacology, a particular drug such as penicillin would be coupled to carry proteins which would then be used in the immunization process. In principle, any organic compound of defined structure can be used as a hapten if a form of it can be synthesized which has a reactive group enabling it to be coupled covalently to a carrier protein. Antibodies can, likewise, be valuable tools in diagnosis where they are raised against either purified viral or bacterial antigens or against the intact structure and properly absorbed to render them specific for characteristic determinants.

I will use an example from the area of tumour biology to illustrate how a protocol can be constructed for the identification and isolation of antigenic proteins associated with the surface of a particular type of cancer, here murine melanoma (Gersten and Marchalonis, 1979). The overall scheme for this is illustrated in Figure 7. In the first place, it was necessary to determine whether antibodies could be raised against determinants of the murine melanoma which were characteristic of the tumour and not of mouse cells in general or of contaminating viruses with which the cell might be infected. The procedure used was to immunize goats with intact B16 melanoma cells in adjuvant and to give multiple injections in order to ensure fairly high levels of antibody. Goats were chosen because they are large animals so large quantities of serum could be obtained, and also goats are phylogenetically distinct from rodents so the possibility existed that the goat would be able to react strongly to murine melanoma determinants. Following immunization, the goats produced antibodies which reacted strongly with mouse cells. In order to remove non-specific reaction with mouse antigens in general, xenoantigens, possible alloantigens, and other adventitious determinants which might have been present on the immunizing population, the goat antiserum was exhaustively absorbed with non-melanoma cells. In our case, we used cells of the murine T cell lymphoma line EL-4 which were grown in tissue culture and contained large quantities of contaminating virus. Following this absorption, the overall titre of our goat antiserum for the B16 tumour cell was markedly diminished, but the antiserum had been rendered specific for melanoma cells. It no longer reacted with lymphoid cells, fibroblasts cells and other non-melanomas. Interestingly, in this case the antiserum was not specific for B16 melanoma alone but it apparently recognized a shared determinant found on a number of murine melanoma cell lines. The question still remains whether this antigen is a differentiation antigen which is expressed at certain phases of melanocyte development or whether it is a melanoma-specific tumour antigen. This is a

Antibody as a Tool

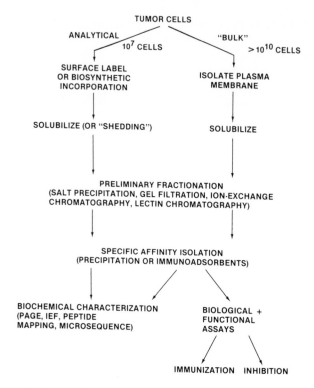

Figure 7. Schematic diagram illustrating the general approaches to be used in study of antigens associated with tumour cells. One approach to surface labelling which we have found useful is that of lactoperoxidase-catalysed radioiodination which is specific for exposed tyrosine residues (Marchalonis *et al.*, 1971). Membrane purification steps are described in Chapter 15. Abbreviations: PAGE, polyacrylamide gel electrophoresis; IEF, isoelectric focusing

difficult question to answer, but it is clear that the sort of reactivity detected here is specific only for differentiated melanoma cell tumour lines. Having established the specificity of our antiserum for melanoma cells, we next isolated the immunoglobulin and formed solid phased affinity reagents by coupling the isolated IgG antibody to a solid phase matrix consisting of Sepharose. It was then possible to use this solid phase immune adsorbent to isolate particular molecules from the surface of melanoma cells or from culture fluids in which the melanoma cells had grown (Gersten and Marchalonis, 1979). The sorts of molecules isolated are illustrated in Figure 8. This particular study is now at a branch point where a number of decisions regarding future directions can be made. I used these here to illustrate types of results and approaches which follow because, in principle, any study directed towards determining antigenic markers of particular cells follows the same general

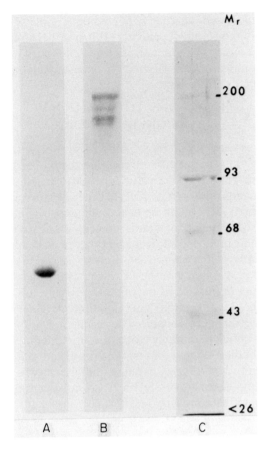

Figure 8. Affinity purified antigens of murine melanoma tumour B16 isolated using solid phase goat antiserum. Antigens were resolved by polyacrylamide gel electrophoresis in sodium-dodecylsulphate-containing buffers. (A) Reduced affinity purified B16 antigen. Sample was treated with 2-mercaptoethanol. (B) Intact B16 antigen. The numbers in (C) refer to positions at which molecular weight standards migrate. (Data of Gersten *et al.* (1981)

logic. In this particular example, now that purified antigen is available, the following avenues must be explored: (1) The biochemical structure of the molecule should be determined. (2) This antigen can be used for immunization of rats in order to produce monoclonal hybridoma antibodies directed against its particular determinants. This approach is very useful because it would provide homogeneous antibodies which could be used for diagnostic purposes and also for isolation of the molecule and possibly antigenic fragments produced by protease or chemical digestion procedures. (3) The antibodies obtained can be used in the development of diagnostic assays. The question can be addressed whether antigenic determinants characteristic of melanomas occur in this serum of patients. (4) Protocols should be designed to determine whether a mode of immunization with the purified antigen can be designed which would allow the vaccination against melanoma or the cure of animals carrying metastatic tumour.

VI. CONCLUSIONS

Antibody activity is carried out by a family of serum proteins which share combining sites for antigen, but differ in constant regions particularly of heavy chains which define classes and effector functions carried out by particular classes of antibody molecules. It is possible to generate antibodies of practically any desired specificity depending upon the manner in which the antigen is presented, i.e. the coupling of an organic molecule to a carrier and the proper immunization scheme involving adjuvants or other practical protocols, and the properties of the antigen combining site as well as those of the constant portion of the molecule, e.g. the ability of the Fc region of the γ chain to bind the A protein of *S. aureus* bacteria, can be exploited to develop schemes for the sensitive detection, quantification, and isolation of molecules bearing the characteristic antigenic determinant. The technology now exists for the production of antibodies, notably with the hybridoma technology, the detection of antibodies using radioimmunoassay and other immunoassay means and for the production of solid phase immunoadsorbents which should enable specific antibodies to be a useful tool to scientists working in many areas of modern biology and biochemistry.

ACKNOWLEDGEMENTS

This work was supported in part by grant RD-101 from the American Cancer Society and 1RO1 AI17493-01 from the National Institutes of Health. I wish to thank Ms Mary A. Jackson for typing the manuscript.

REFERENCES

Burnet, F. M. (1959). *The Clonal Selection Theory of Acquired Immunity*. Vanderbilt University Press, Nashville, Tennessee.

Erlanger, B. F. (1973). Principles and methods for the preparation of drug protein conjugates for immunological studies. *Pharm. Rev.*, **25**, 271–280.

Feinstein, A. and Beale, D. (1977). Models of immunoglobulins and antigen–antibody complexes. In L. E. Glynn and M. W. Stewart (Eds.) *Immunochemistry:An Advanced Textbook*, pp. 263–306, Wiley, New York.

Gally, J. A., and Edelman, G. M. (1972). The genetic control of immunoglobulin synthesis. *Ann. Rev. Gene.*, **6**, 1–46.

Gersten, D. M., and Marchalonis, J. J. (1979). Demonstration and isolation of murine melanoma-associated antigenic surface proteins. *Biochem. Biophys. Res. Commun.*, **90**, 1015–1024.

Gersten, D. M., Hearing, V. J., and Marchalonis, J. J. (1981). Characterization of immunologically significant unique B16 melanoma proteins produced *in vivo* and *in vitro*. *Proc. Natl. Acad. Sci. USA*, in press.

Glynn, L. E., and Steward, M. W. (Eds.) (1977). *Immunochemistry: An Advanced Textbook*. Wiley, New York.

Goebel, W. F. (1936). Chemo-immunological studies on conjugated carbohydrate-proteins. X. The immunological properties of an artificial antigen containing glucuronic acid. *J. Exp. Med.*, **64**, 29–38.

Goodman, J. W., and Wang, A. -C. (1980). Immunoglobulins: Structure, Diversity and genetics. In H. H. Fudenberg, E. P. Stites, J. L. Caldwell, and J. V. Wells (Eds), *Basic and Clinical Immunology*, pp. 28–43, Lange Medical Publications, Los Altos, California.

Halloran, M. J., and Parker, C. W. (1966). The production of antibodies to mononucleotides and DNA. *J. Immunol.*, **96**, 379–385.

Hilschmann, N., and Craig, L. C. (1965). Amino acid sequence studies with Benc-Jones proteins. *Proc. Natl. Acad. Sci. (USA)*, **53**, 1403–1409.

Kabat, E. A. (1968). *Structural Concepts in Immunology and Immunochemistry*, Holt, Rinehart and Winston, Inc.

Kehoe, J. M., and Capra, J. D. (1978). Patterns of sequence variability in immunoglobulin variable regions: Functionall, evolutionary and genetic implications. In G. W. Litman and R. A. Good (Eds.) *Comprehensive Immunology*, pp. 273–295, Plenum Medical Book Company, New York.

Landsteiner, K. (Ed.) (1945). *The Specificity of Serological Reactions*, Harvard University Press, Cambridge, Mass.

Litman, G. W., and Good, R. A. (Eds) (1978). *Comprehensive Immunology*, volume 5, *Immunoglobulins*, Plenum Medical Book Company, New York.

Marchalonis, J. J. (1975). Lymphocyte surface immunoglobulins: Molecular properties and functions as receptors for antigen. *Science*, **190**, 20–29.

Marchalonis, J. J. (1977). *Immunity in Evolution*, Harvard University Press, Cambridge, Mass.

Marchalonis, J. J. (1980). Cell interactions in immune responses. In H. H. Fudenberg, E. P. Stites, J. L. Caldwell and J. V. Wells (Eds), *Basic and Clinical Immunology*, pp. 115–128, Lange Medical Publications, Los Altos, California.

Marchalonis, J. J., Cone, R. E., and Santer, V. (1971). Enzymic iodination. A probe for accessible surface proteins of normal and neoplastic lymphocytes, *Biochem. J.*, **124**, 921–927.

Mitchison, N. A., Rajewsky, K., and Taylor, R. B. (1970). Cooperation of antigenic determinants and of cells in the induction of antibodies. In J. Sterzl and I. Riha (Eds). *Developmental Aspects of Antibody Formation and Structure*, pp. 547–561, Czechoslovak Academy of Sciences, Prague.

Molgaard, H. V. (1980). Assembly of immunoglobulin heavy chain genes. *Nature*, **286**, 657–659.

Nisonoff, A., Hopper, J. E., and Spring, S. B. (1975). *The Antibody Molecule*. Academic Press, New York.

Poljak, R. J. (1978). Studies on the three-dimensional structure of immunoglobulins. In G. W. Litman and R. A. Good. (Eds.) *Comprehensive Immunology* Volume 5. *Immunoglobulins*. pp. 1–36, Plenum Medical Book Company, New York.

Prager, E. M. and Wilson, A. C. (1971). The dependence of immunological cross-reactivity upon sequence resemblence among lysozymes. I. Microcomplement fixation studies. *J. Biochem.*, **246**, 5978–5989.

Seidman, J. G., Max, E. E., and Leder, P. (1979). A κ-immunoglobulin gene is formed by site-specific recombination without further somatic mutation. *Nature*, **280**, 370-375.

Steiner, A. L. (1973). Radioimmunoassay for the cyclic nucleotides. *Pharm. Rev.*, **25**, 309-313.

Sutherland, I. W. (1977). Immunochemical aspects of polysaccharide antigens. In L. E. Glynn and M. W. Stewart, (Eds.) *Immunochemistry: An Advanced Textbook*, pp. 399-443, Wiley, New York.

Wu, T. T. and Kabat, E. A. (1970). An analysis of the sequences of the variable regions of Benc–Jones proteins and myeloma light chain and their implications for antibody complementary. *The Antibody Molecule*. Academic Press, New York.

Antibody as a Tool
Edited by J. J. Marchalonis and G. W. Warr
© 1982 John Wiley & Sons Ltd.

Chapter 2

Preparation of Antigens and Principles of Immunization

GREGORY W. WARR

Department of Biochemistry, Medical University of South Carolina,
171 Ashley Avenue, Charleston, South Carolina 29425, USA

I. INTRODUCTION

Antibodies and the cells that secrete them recognize an antigen primarily by conformational determinants on the surface of the molecule (Atassi, 1977) and the reaction between antigen and antibody involves not only steric factors ('lock and key') but is dependent upon a variety of interactions including ionic, hydrophobic, hydrogen bonding, and Van der Waals' forces (Steward, 1977). Because of these factors it is possible to envisage an almost infinite variety of antigens, and one of the most interesting aspects of the immune system is that it appears to be capable of responding to an immense number of naturally occurring and completely synthetic antigens. As we might expect, the response of animals to antigens is not universally good. The reasons for this variability in response include intrinsic properties of the antigens (chemical and structural factors, such as whether or not the molecule is protein, carbohydrate or lipid, how large it is, and how rigid its conformation in solution is) and properties of the immune system of the responding animal. In this chapter it is not proposed to consider the underlying causes of this variability in response to antigens, except in so far as: (1) they affect the ability of the investigator to raise useful antisera; and (2) they require the use of particular techniques of immunization to overcome this problem.

As mentioned above, although the potential number of antigens is very large, it is not actually infinite. (Estimates suggest that an animal can respond to perhaps 10^6 antigenic determinants.) Even so, it would still be an impossible task to deal with the preparation of all actual or potential antigens, and thus I will only consider a limited range of topics, selected for likely relevance to a large number of investigators.

The preparation of viral or bacterial antigens will not be discussed, for the history and methodology of immunology and microbiology are so closely related that in this brief review I could say almost nothing on this topic that has not been written about previously (e.g. see Williams and Chase, 1967).

II. WHOLE ORGANISMS OR CELLS AS ANTIGENS

In this category can be included, as the most important examples, viruses, bacteria, fungi and their spores, parasites, plant pollens, nucleated cells (either derived from body tissues, or grown *in vitro*), and the enucleate erythrocytes of mammals. The collection or culture of these presents a diverse range of problems which will not be considered here. Some of these topics receive attention elsewhere in this book (Chapters 10–12), and standard methods for microbial (Norris and Ribbons, 1969) and vertebrate tissue (Willmer, 1965) culture are in widespread use.

What I will consider here is the sort of investigation for which immunization with a whole organism might be considered necessary, the methods by which the immunogen is prepared, and the bearing that the method of preparation of the immunogen might have on the quality or specificity of the antiserum produced against it.

One common reason for immunizing with a whole organism or cell is to gain insight into the antigenic 'profile' or diversity of the immunogen in question. Since any given protein molecule, for example, can be expected to bear several antigenic determinants (epitopes), a whole cell or organism will probably induce a response composed of antibodies directed to a large number of the possibly antigenic molecules. It is likely that not all the possible antigens will elicit detectable antibodies in a given animal, and it is also likely that any one molecule may elicit a variety of antibodies reacting with the varied antigenic determinants it expresses. Despite these observations, an antiserum reacting with many of the constituent antigens of a complex organism can frequently be used to monitor immunologically the purification of one of the component antigens. However, immunological criteria of purity invoke circular arguments and are subject to some other technical disadvantages, and their use as such will be considered again in a later section.

Antisera raised against a whole organism or cell are often used in a search for biological markers. Examples of these might be sera specific for bacterial strains or type-specific viral proteins, sera used for blood group or tissue typing, and sera recognizing differentiation, organ-specific or tumour-specific antigens of vertebrate cells (Ruddon, 1978).

In addition, antisera to surface markers can allow the investigator to define or manipulate the functions of cell populations. An example of functional modification is the use of antilymphocyte serum (usually raised in horses) in clinical practice to suppress the immune response of transplant recipients against their grafted organ or tissue. Similarly, antisera have been used to define cell populations. The θ or Thy-1 antigen found on the membrane of thymus lymphocytes and thymus-derived lymphocytes in mice can be used not only to identify these cells, but also to kill them (in conjunction with complement) and allow an investigator to assess their functional contributions to immune phenomena.

A. Adsorption

An antiserum raised to a whole cell or organism is likely to contain antibodies to a variety of antigens, and hence has little use in the definition of specific markers. The classical method of rendering such a serum specific has been to adsorb it with material believed to possess all the antigens present on the immunogen *except* those that are thought to be specific to the immunogen. For example, it may be desired to raise an antiserum specific for mouse liver cells. If a rabbit is immunized with mouse liver, the resulting antiserum will contain antibodies to molecules on the surface of the liver cells. Some of these molecules will occur on the cells of all mouse tissues, and some of them, it is hoped, will be specific for the liver. Thus, by adsorbing the antiserum with tissues such as kidney, brain, and blood cells, an investigator might hope to be left with a liver-specific serum.

Adsorption consists basically of incubating a serum with the material against which one desires to remove activity. Incubation is usually for about 30 minutes on ice, and then the serum is separated from the adsorbing material by centrifugation. Adsorption with soluble antigens is not usually recommended, because soluble antigen/antibody complexes remain in the serum. Soluble antigens should be covalently coupled to an insoluble, inert matrix. The use of commercially available beaded materials for this purpose is described in Chapter 3. No general recommendation can be made on the ratio of serum to adsorbent that should be used, since adsorptions should be monitored for efficacy and repeated until undesirable reactivities have been removed. However, some losses of serum unavoidably occur with every adsorption, which may be due for example, to adherence to the tubes used, and to retention in the dead volume between the particles of adsorbent after centrifugation. These losses are impossible to avoid completely, but can be reduced by diluting a serum (e.g. 1 : 1 or 1 : 2) with physiological buffer before commencing the adsorptions.

An adsorbed antiserum should always be checked carefully for specificity, whatever the purpose to which it is to be put. A useful rule is that the checks for specificity should always entail tests of a sensitivity equivalent to those that will be employed in the actual investigation. For example, if a serum will be used to define a cell-surface marker by fluorescence (Chapter 7), tests of specificity should include some carried out by the same technique of immunofluorescence. The raising of antisera to whole cells or organisms (and the process of adsorption to produce specificity) is one of the oldest operations known to serology. While it is often the most sensible starting point to an investigation of complex antigeneric structures in a cell, it is not a precise biochemical technique. The major drawback to this sort of approach is the practical difficulty in establishing absolute, or sometimes even acceptable, specificity of the reagents, which in turn results from our lack of control over the heterogeneous antibodies produced in the animal, and the enormity of the task of trying to define all the activities present in a population of antibodies (even those in an adsorbed serum). This is not to say that these methods cannot be used, because in many cases there are no alternatives. For example, purification of a mammalian cell membrane protein in amounts large enough for immunization is often very difficult, partly because a cell possesses very little membrane, in terms of mass (10^{-10} to 10^{-12}g per cell being a rough estimate), and partly because a purified molecule may not retain its native conformation (and hence antigenicity). An elegant solution to the problems of adsorption of sera and purification of antigens is to prepare hybridomas. These are hybrids between a tumour cell (of the lymphocyte line) and an antibody-producing cell from an immunized animal. The hybrid continues to produce the antibody synthesized by the cell from the immunized animal, and can be established in tissue culture. Because any antibody producing cell produces only one homogeneous antibody of a specificity that can be defined experimentally, the production of hybridomas allows one to immunize with a whole cell (or impure antigen) and select the specificity required from the hybridomas that can be produced with cells from the immunized animal. This procedure also does not require adsorption. Although the use of hybridomas (Chapter 9) is seductively simple as a concept, its application requires a considerable investment of time and effort.

B. Contamination of a Cellular Antigen

Contamination herein means the presence of antigens other than those against which it is intended to immunize. It is worth stressing that any material for immunization should be kept as sterile as possible, but aside from gross bacterial or fungal growth, contamination can take more subtle forms.

The heterogeneity of cell types found in any tissue can represent contamination. For instance, in the example of mouse liver as an antigen (see above), a crude preparation of liver cells will contain not only sessile liver cells (parenchymal, endothelial, and macrophage) but also blood cells, including lymphocytes. In addition, serum proteins may be adsorbed on to the cells, although these can usually be removed by washing them with physiological buffers. The use of cell lines grown in tissue culture can prevent contamination by uncharacterized cell types, but the adsorption of foreign proteins to the surface of cultured cells can be a significant problem. Nearly all tissue culture media are supplemented with foreign serum (usually foetal bovine) and proteins from this serum can adsorb tightly to the cells, be refractory, to removal by washing, and act as acquired cell surface antigens (Embleton and Iype, 1978).

Viruses constitute another significant problem with the use of cells as antigens, especially in the case of the mammals. Many mammals commonly used for experimental purposes suffer from widespread viral infections, which can be transmitted both vertically and horizontally (Ihle *et al.*, 1979). Cells taken from such animals may be overt producers of virus, or, even in the absence of active virus production, they may express virally encoded proteins and glycoproteins on their plasma membrane. These virally encoded molecules are highly antigenic and can easily lead to confusing reactivities in antisera raised against cells expressing them. Cultured cell lines can express and produce such viruses and their antigens, and can, in addition, become infected with viruses during the course of their laboratory use.

In order to exclude the possibility that viral antigens are responsible for observed reactivities, it may be necessary to enlist the aid of a virology laboratory. Serological tests (such as radioimmunoassay) can be used to detect viral antigens, and viral nucleic acids can be detected by the use of hybridization techniques.

C. Alteration of Cellular Antigens

It should be borne in mind that some procedures for the preparation of cells may alter their normal pattern of expression of surface antigens. The use of proteolytic enzymes to dissociate cells from solid tissues or to release them from a substratum is an obvious example requiring consideration. The treatment of cells with a fixative before immunization is not usually recommended, since this may result in the alteration or loss of antigenicity of some molecules.

III. PURIFICATION OF ANTIGENS FROM CELLS AND BIOLOGICAL FLUIDS

The reasons for attempting to purify any antigen are as varied as the reasons for raising antisera, and an investigator has to decide how pure an antigen (or specific a reagent) is necessary. Although in principle absolute purity is desirable, it is frequently difficult to obtain and, in some rather limited circumstances, may not be necessary. For example, an antiglobulin reagent is often used as second antibody in a radioimmunoassay (that is, as a reagent to precipitate the first antibody which is reacting with the primary antigen, see Chapter 6). The antigen used to raise this antiglobulin serum need not be 100% pure, as long as unwanted cross-reactivities with other components of the assay do not occur. On the other hand, if an antiglobulin reagent is to be used as a tool to study (for example, immunoglobulins either at the lymphocyte surface or under other conditions), it is highly desirable that it should be as specific as possible, i.e. that the immunizing antigen be as pure as possible. Only the investigator can judge if it is pure enough, but my own view is than an antigen should be homogeneous by a number of criteria (see below). Purity is difficult to establish unequivocally without determining the entire primary structure of the molecule, but the sort of criteria which can be used are listed below. In this section, I will refer only to proteins or glycoproteins, which comprise the vast majority of (but certainly not all) antigens of biological importance.

Because the plasma membrane is uniquely important as a site of interaction of a cell with its environment and with other cells, and also as the site to which investigators look for markers of tissue specificity, differentiation, and neoplastic transformation, the isolation and properties of the plasma membrane and its constituent molecules are dealt with in Chapter 15 of this book, and will not be discussed further here.

A. Criteria of Purity

Immunologists frequently cite immunological tests such as diffusion in agar gel or immunoelectrophoresis as evidence of purity of an antigen, meaning that a single line of precipitation is seen between a purified antigen and an antiserum raised against the starting mixture from which the antigen has been purified. An interpretation of purity based on these observations alone assumes that the antiserum in question reacts with *all* antigens present initially, and that any contaminants are at a suitable concentration to give a precipitate under the test conditions. These assumptions, particularly the former, are questionable but rarely questioned. As alternatives, but preferably as supplements, to immunological tests, physicochemical criteria of purity should be advanced. These tests consist of attempting to show that under some conditions more than one molecular species is present in the preparation. In general, techniques such as chromatography and centrifugation do not have such a high resolving power for proteins as electrophoresis, and one technique with high resolving power is polyacrylamide gel electrophoresis in the presence of the detergent sodium dodecyl sulphate (SDS) (Figure 1, Appendix IA). This technique resolves mainly on the basis of molecular size, and hence a single band on SDS–gel electrophoresis is presumptive evidence that heterogeneity in this respect does not exist. SDS–gel electrophoresis tends to obscure the influence of the native charge of a protein. This parameter can be investigated using electrophoresis without SDS at varying pH values (Chrambach and Rodbard, 1971), or more sensitively by isoelectric focusing (see Chapter 3 Figure 1 and Appendix III). Although a single band on analytical isoelectric focusing indicates homogeneity of charge, multiple bands can have causes other than impurity. Modification of charged groups on a protein, for example by deamination, can lead to apparent heterogeneity, and it should also be borne in mind that some

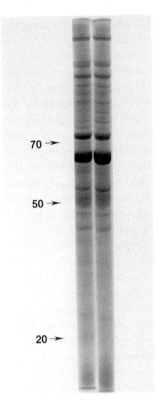

Figure 1. SDS–polyacrylamide gel electrophoresis. Membranes from two variants of the murine B16 melanoma are shown as analyzed by this technique. The gels were of 10% acrylamide, 0.25% bisacrylamide concentration and were electrophoresed (top to bottom) and stained with Coomassie Blue, as described in Appendix IA. The arrows (↓) indicate molecular weight standards ($\times 10^{-3}$).

proteins are intrinsically heterogenous, in that they possess dissimilar subunits (e.g. haemoglobins and immunoglobulins). Attempts to separate and purify subunits of a protein may be chemically successful but immunologically failures, since the conformation of the polypeptide may change on separation. An example of this can be found in the immunoglobulins, where purified heavy chains, especially from IgM, tend to aggregate once separated from their companion light chains. As a separate issue, the structure and unique variability of immunoglobulins are considered in more detail in the next chapter.

Another criterion of chemical purity, end group analysis (Gray, 1972), is also difficult to interpret if a protein consists of dissimilar subunits. In summary, as many criteria of purity as possible should be applied to an antigen preparation, but minimally, homogeneity by immunological testing and by a high-resolution technique such as polyacrylamide gel electrophoresis (under conditions of overloading to detect minor components) is frequently considered sufficient. A further immunological criterion of purification can be applied after the fact of immunization. An animal can respond to microgram quantities of antigen, and may produce antibodies to a minor contaminant in the immunizing antigen. Hence, more than one line in diffusion in agar or immunoelectrophoresis when an antiserum is reacted against the *starting mixture* from which the antigen was purified can frequently be taken to indicate impurity of the antigen. Alternatively, it may reflect a real heterogeneity of the antigen, i.e. its occurrence in more than one molecular form. Care has to be taken therefore in dissecting the evidence, which can frequently seem rather circular unless immunological assays are supplemented by biochemical ones.

Once it is decided which criteria to apply when estimating purity, these can be used to monitor steps in a purification scheme for any antigen of interest. Purification of a protein or glycoprotein antigen from any source is essentially an exercise in a variety of preparative biochemical techniques. Generally used methods are salt precipitation, centrifugation, preparative electrophoresis, gel filtration, ion exchange chromatography, and affinity chromatography. Other techniques, for example hydrophobic chromatography, can be used, but the commonest techniques are those cited above. Most of these are in such common use that knowledge and advice is widespread and easy to obtain, and excellent tests describing practical applications are available (e.g. Cooper, 1977). However, in the following chapter (Chapter 3) I will give more detailed notes on the use of these procedures for the isolation and characterization of immunoglobulins and antibodies. These have the advantage that they describe actual separations and purifications, rather than general principles, which nearly always lack experimental detail.

IV. CONJUGATED ANTIGENS AND THEIR PREPARATION

Some molecules, in native form, can react with an antibody, but are nevertheless very poor at *eliciting* its production upon injection, by themselves, into an animal. Such molecules are called haptens, and a response to them can be more readily induced by coupling them to a larger, more highly antigenic molecule, and using the conjugate for immunization.

The haptens which are frequently used by immunochemists to study the nature of antibodies raised to them, are small, chemically defined molecules such as trinitrophenol, dinitrophenol, or arsanilic acid (Nisonoff, 1967; Little and Eisen, 1967). Synthetic antigens have also been prepared (Sela and Fuchs, 1978) again, usually for the purpose of studying the immune responses of animals.

However, some haptens are naturally occurring. For example, lipids such as the Forsmann antigen, glycosphingolipids, cytolipins, and cardiolipin act as haptens (Rapport and Graf, 1967), and for this reason immunization is often carried out using crude lipid-containing fractions, or crude lipid extracts mixed with foreign proteins (Rapport and Graf, 1967). Other naturally occurring molecules of biological interest that act as haptens are nucleic acids, some antibiotics (notably penicillin), and both steroid and polypeptide hormones. For purposes of immunization, these haptens can be complexed with well-defined proteins. Nucleic acids can be complexed with methylated bovine serum albumin (Plescia, 1967), a reversible interaction based on charge, or smaller nucleosides can be covalently coupled to natural proteins or synthetic polypeptides by a variety of chemical reactions (Beiser *et al.*, 1967). Steroid hormones are also usually covalently coupled to proteins, often bovine serum albumin. Coupling is often to the ε-amino groups of lysyl residues in the protein, and takes advantage of carboxyl groups on the steroid to allow coupling by, for example, a mixed anhydride method (Erlanger *et al.*, 1967), or by carbodiimides.

Small proteins or peptides such as insulin and other peptide hormones, which are poorly immunogenic in native form, and some pharmacologically active mediators can be covalently conjugated to large protein molecules for the immunization of animals (Likhite and Sehon, 1967). The coupling compounds most commonly used are bifunctional reagents.

A. Diisocyanates

Isocyanates react with amino groups in proteins, and bifunctional diisocyanates are often used to couple protein molecules by this reaction. Tolylene diisocyanate is frequently a reagent of choice because one isocyanate group is more reactive than the other. Thus, reacting the reagent with one protein at a low temperature leads to coupling by one isocyanate group: raising the temperature and adding the second protein allows the second isocyanate group to react and bring about conjugation. Examples of coupling using isocyanates are given in Likhite and Sehon, (1967) and in Chapters 6 and 7 of this book. With diisocyanates, as with any cross-linking reaction, one is likely to get not only the desired product, but also intramolecular linkages, and coupling of molecules on a greater than 1 : 1 basis, leading to multimeric products which may contain only one species, or both species in varying proportions.

B. Carbodiimides

The reaction mechanism may be summarized in this way: these reagents react with carboxyl groups to form intermediates, which are then capable of reacting with amino groups; in this manner they are able to bring about the coupling of molecules bearing these two groups. Several carbodiimides are available commercially and an outline of methods for their use in conjugations to both proteins and solid phase matrices is given in Appendix II.

C. Diazo compounds

Treatment of most aromatic amines with nitrous acid leads to the formation of a diazonium salt, which in turn can react readily with tyrosyl, histidyl, and lysyl groups of proteins. Benzidine and anisidine have two free NH_2 groups, and upon diazotization become bifunctional reagents, which can be added to a mixture of two proteins to effect coupling (Likhite and Sehon, 1967).

D. Other Methods

A variety of reactions which can be exploited for the conjugation of molecules. Many of these are considered by Likhite and Sehon (1967), who also give considerable experimental detail.

V. IMMUNIZATION

A. Adjuvants

It is difficult to make generalizations about immunization, because most of our information comes from empirical observations made in a variety of dissimilar situations. When an animal is to be immunized with bacteria (frequently killed) or mammalian cells (frequently living at the time of injection), good antibody titres can be obtained with inoculations repeated each week for a number of weeks, or, especially in the case of bacteria, with only one or two inoculations. However, single or repeated injections with soluble antigens frequently do not produce the sustained, high-titre antibody responses that most investigators wish to see, and methods have to be employed to enhance the response of the animals to the immunogen. The main reason for the inability of many antigens to produce a sustained response is that they are rapidly cleared from the animal's body. Hence, a number of procedures can be used to prevent rapid clearance of the antigen. Use of aggregated or precipitated protein usually gives a better response than use of the soluble, undenatured form, and in fact immunization with a disaggregated protein may lead to immunological paralysis (i.e. an absence of responsiveness to the specific antigen) (Dresser, 1962). On the other hand, denaturation of a protein can lead to the alteration of antigenic determinants, which are dependent on the conformation of the molecule (Atassi, 1977). Most practical immunization schedules employ agents known as adjuvants to enhance the immune response of an animal. The preparation and use of these will be described below. Some adjuvants serve to form local antigen depots, at the immunization site, from which antigen leaks slowly. They can achieve this by adsorbing on to themselves the antigen (this usually applies in the case of inorganic adjuvant materials) or entrapping the antigen in a water-in-oil emulsion, as is the case with the Freund's-type adjuvants. In addition, many adjuvants have the ability to provoke both a local irritation at the site of injection, and a non-specific elevation of the immune response of the animal, either or both of which seem to help produce strong, sustained antibody responses. Bacteria frequently have adjuvant properties. For example, *Bordetella pertussis*, the causative organism in whooping cough, has potent effects on the antibody response (Dresser *et al.*, 1970), and it is thought that its inclusion in the triple vaccine for human use (*B. pertussis*, with the toxoids from tetanus and diphtheria) increases the magnitude of the response to the other two components. *B. pertussis* organisms have also been used to produce antibodies to immunoglobulin allotypes in mice. Allotypes in this case are the antigenic expression of genetic polymorphism (allelism) in the structural genes for the antibody molecule. Briefly, antibodies to *B. pertussis* are raised in one mouse strain, A. These antibodies are then adsorbed on to *B. pertussis* organisms by incubation in the serum taken from the immunized mouse, the organisms are washed to remove unbound and non-antibody proteins, and the *B. pertussis* with its adsorbed antibody is injected into mice of another strain, B. The B mouse not only reacts to the *B. pertussis* organisms, but to any foreign antigenic (usually allotypic) determinants on the A strain antibody molecules (Herzenberg and Herzenberg, 1978).

Complete Freund's adjuvant (see below) contains killed mycobacteria (usually *Mycobacterium butyricum*). These organisms induce a strong reaction of delayed-type hypersensitivity (Turk, 1975) and a marked inflammatory response to antigens injected with them. Other biological adjuvants have been used, for example the insoluble methylated form of bovine serum albumin, which because of its strong positve charge complexes strongly with negatively charged molecules such as nucleic acids. However, all adjuvants like methylated albumin, and especially the bacterial adjuvants, have one problem. They are themselves highly antigenic, and may contain complex and uncharacterized molecules that can give rise to antibodies of unknown specificity. In some cases this can lead to cross-reactions between adjuvant and the antigen of interest (Bucana and Hanna, 1974), but many investigators prefer to ignore this potential problem, and it would probably be true to say that practical experience bears out their judgement. These difficulties can be minimized by isolating the specific antibody from the serum (see Chapter 3).

However, if one has invested considerable time and trouble in purifying an antigen, it may be preferable, on principle, to avoid the use of antigenic adjuvants. This point can be decided by the investigator, but below are listed several alternative types of adjuvant.

1. Inorganic Colloidal Suspensions

Commonly used colloids are hydrated aluminium hydroxide (alumina) or aluminium phosphate. The adsorption of soluble proteins to these gels markedly enhances their immunogenicity, and alum precipitation is widely used in the preparation of immunizing materials for human and veterinary work. Proteins can be bound to the preformed gel (preparation described in Appendix III), or apparently with much higher efficiency, to the nascent gel, i.e. by forming the gel in the presence of the protein (Chase, 1967a).

With any batch of gel it is advisable to keep materials sterile, and also to perform tests of the protein-binding capacity. This can be carried out simply by adding different (known) amounts of the protein to a constant amount of gel, incubating the material for 30 minutes, centrifuging the precipitate with its bound protein, and estimating the amount of protein left in solution, for example by optical density at 280 nm, or by the Folin reaction (Lowry *et al.*, 1951). Gels usually have a capacity for protein that varies from 10% to over 100% of gel dry weight (Chase, 1967a). A commercially available preparation, alhydrogel (1.3% Al_2O_3 from dansk Svovlsyre, -OG. Superphospate-Fabrik, Copenhagen, Denmark) bound approximately 10% (w/w) of bovine serum albumin (James and Milne, 1972).

Water in Oil Emulsions

These adjuvants, formulated by Freund, have come to be the method of choice for immunizing animals in laboratory investigations. The oil phase consists of mineral oil and an emulsifier, usually mannide monooleate. This mixture is referred to as incomplete. If mycobacteria (usually *M. butyricum*) are added (0.05% w/v) the adjuvant is termed complete. These adjuvants can be purchased from Difco Laboratories, Detroit, Michigan, USA. They are supplied as six 10 ml ampoules of incomplete adjuvant (catalogue # 0639-60) or complete adjuvant (0638-60). These adjuvants are usully mixed with an equal volume of aqueous solution (or suspension) of the antigen, but can be used at other ratios such as 2 : 1 or 9 : 1 (Tung *et al.*, 1976). The complete adjuvant should be thoroughly mixed before use to ensure uniform dispersion of the mycobacteria.

Emulsification can be achieved by manual mixing, blending, or ultrasonication. With the latter method, heating should be avoided by using an ice bath to surround the tube containing antigen and adjuvant. The simplest, but possibly most tedious, method is to prepare the emulsion manually. This can be achieved by repeatedly drawing the mixture into a syringe through a relatively wide-gauge needle (16–19 G, for example), and expelling it. A much more satisfactory method is rapidly and repeatedly to force the mixture between two syringes, using either a needle with a hub at either end, or a stopcock. Needles with two hubs can usually be made in a workshop, and stopcocks are commercially available. I prefer to use an Ayer stopcock (catalogue # 3138, from Beckton-Dickinson, Rutherford, New Jersey) which is a three-way stopcock with two female Luer-lok tips and a male Luer-slip. The female Luer-lok tips allow for firm attachment of the two syringes (Figure 2). Considerable pressure can be produced during vigorous mixing, and to avoid

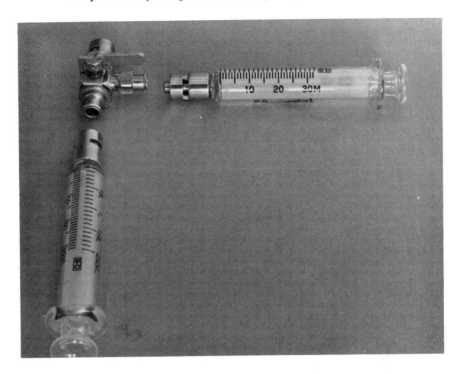

Figure 2. Syringes and stopcock for the preparation of water in oil emulsions. Two glass syringes with Luer-lok tips are shown unattached to the three-way stopcock. All items can be purchased from Beckton-Dickinson, Rutherford, New Jersey, USA

any possibility of forcing off a fitting, Luer-lok syringes are recommended. Because of mechanical strength, glass syringes are also preferred to ones made of plastic for forming emulsions. The third outlet of the stopcock allows one to test the emulsion without demounting the syringes. Emulsification can be considered to be complete when the mixture thickens to a degree such that when a drop is placed on the surface of some iced water, it does not spread out.

3. Other Adjuvants

Some proteins have been found to be better immunogens when adsorbed on to clays such as bentonite (Claman, 1963) or charcoal (Landsteiner, 1942; Chase, 1967a), than when injected in native form. The use of these substances, however, may not offer any advantages over the use of colloidal alum or Freund's adjuvants. Of potentially much greater use is the injection of proteins in polyacrylamide gel (Weintraub and Raymond, 1963). Polyacrylamide gel electrophoresis as a means of purifying an antigen offers high resolving power, but suffers from the disadvantages of having a low capacity, in terms of protein load, and difficulty of elution of material from the gel. These disadvantages can be offset, however, by immunmizing with a protein still in the gel. Injection of a few micrograms of protein in the gel slice to which it has been localized can apparently lead to a good antibody response. Considerations such as denaturation of the protein during electrophoresis in detergents such as SDS may impose some restraints.

B. Choice of Animal for Immunization

Two considerations influence this decision: (1) cost and difficulty of housing and handling an animal; and (2) the properties desired in the antibody. The cost and difficulty of housing and handling an animal are often directly proportional to its size, and have to be balanced against the increased amount of antibody than can be obtained from a larger animal. As a result, many investigators choose rabbits (typically New Zealand White) for routine immunization, since they can be kept fairly easily, are docile if handled responsibly, and can be bled frequently (up to 50 ml every 3 or 4 weeks). However, if a large amount of standardized antibody is required, it will be necessary to immunize a large animal such as a horse, donkey, goat or sheep, test trial bleedings until the required activity is present, and then bleed the animal out. Many universities or research institutes have veterinary or agricultural departments that can offer facilities, advice and help in practical matters of housing and handling the larger experimental mammals. The laboratory rodents such as rats and guinea pigs can be immunized easily, but may not be large enough to give sufficient amounts of serum. Mice are generally too small to be considered for routine immunization purposes, but a method described by Tung *et al.* (1976) allows one to produce large quantities of ascites fluid in individual mice (sometimes over 10 ml) with a very high content of antibody (5 mg per millilitre or more). This method, which works in many inbred mouse strains (Tung *et al.*, 1976), involves repeated intraperitoneal injections of antigen in Freund's adjuvant, and is described in Appendix IV.

As a broad generalization, I will offer the statement that the closer the two species are, the finer are the antigenic differences that can be detected by immunization between them. To take a rather obvious example, immunization of rabbit with imunoglobulin (Ig) from a mouse gives antibodies to this Ig (antiglobulin antibodies) which will generally react with virtually all Igs of mice, regardless of strain. Appropriate selection of immunizing antigens followed by adsorption can render these antibodies specific for an Ig class (definitions of terms and descriptions of Ig structure can be found in Chapter 1). If mice are immunized with Ig from mice of another strain, the resulting antibodies are usually against allotypic determinants (the expression of allelism in the structural genes coding each of the classes of Ig) not against the broad, class-specific determinants. Immunization of a mouse with its *own* antibodies can lead to the production of anti-idiotypic sera, that is, antibodies directed against the combining site for antigen (Capra and Kehoe, 1975). Such antisera will not recognize allotypic or class-specific determinants.

Conversely, if the genetic disparity between antigen-donating animal and immunized animal is increased, determinants that are of coarser specificity may be seen. To follow through the previous example, rabbit antibodies to mouse Ig react best with mouse Ig, and are unreactive to Ig of other species, except possibly for some cross-reactions with rat and guinea pig Ig. However, if a chicken is immunized with mouse Ig, the antibody can react well with the Ig of rodents (rats, guinea pigs), lagomorphs (rabbit), and even, on some occasions, humans (Warr *et al.*, 1978 amd unpublished observations). Presumably this antiserum is recognizing determinants common not only to Igs of rodents, but also to Igs of other mammalian orders, and this broad reactivity is probably due to the genetic disparity between the birds (believed to be evolutionary offshoots of the dinosaurs) and the mammals. This phenomenon, resulting from phylogenetic distance, should be borne in mind when selecting an animal to immunize, and when interpreting the reactivities of antibodies produced across wide genetic differences.

Another consideration when selecting an animal to be immunized is the intrinsic properties of the antibodies produced. By this I do not mean so much the binding affinity of the antibody, or its absolute amount, which are not usually problems with the endothermic vertebrates when the right immunization schedule has been found, but more that one should consider the secondary properties of the antibody molecules. This is especially relevant when one knows the sorts of assays that are going to be carried out with the antibody. Some examples of these sorts of consideration are dealt with below. Chicken antibodies do not fix mammalian complement ($C',$), so that assays depending on complement fixation or activity may not easily be carried out. They are not impossible, however, since a source of the early components of C', which bind and can bridge the gap to mammalian complement, can be added (Stolfi *et al.*, 1971).

For almost any practical immunological assay, the low molecular weight Ig classes (IgG in mammals, IgY in birds) are preferred. These classes of antibody will usually predominate automatically within a few weeks of immunization using Freund's adjuvants, and are usually excellent precipitating antibodies. One technical note on precipitation reactions with fowl IgY antibody is that for reasons unknown they usually work more efficiently at high salt concentrations (1.5 M NaCl), rather than at physiological salt levels (Benedict, 1967).

One property of certain mammalian IgG classes, which is becoming increasingly useful and widely used, is binding to the protein-A of *Staphylococcus aureus* (Goding, 1978). Assays involving protein-A binding include: alternatives to antiglobulin precipitation in a radioimmunoassay

(Jonsson and Kronvall, 1974), or radioimmune precipitation (Kessler, 1975, 1976), and use in fluorochromated or radioiodinated forms for localization of IgG (reviewed by Goding, 1978). In addition, binding to protein-A provides a very useful method for isolating IgG antibodies from serum (see Chapter 3). If it is desired to use protein-A for any of these sorts of purposes, it is necessary to choose for immunization an animal the bulk of whose IgG antibodies bind to protein-A. Such species might be the rabbit, dog, man, and mouse. Other species such as the rat, goat, and sheep do possess subclasses of protein-A binding IgG antibodies (Goudswaard et al., 1978), but in a number of cases I have found that a very variable fraction of the total antibody activity of serum from these animals would bind to protein-A. This does not necessarily preclude use of antibodies from these animals with protein-A.

C. Handling of Animals

In both Britain and the United States laws exist to regulate conditions under which animals may be kept. In addition, in Britain, investigators need Home Office licensing to enable them to carry out legally certain manipulations which are considered to be painful or detrimental to the health of an experimental animal. The onus is on an investigator to ensure that appropriate legal requirements are met in any particular case.

The husbandry of animals to be used for immunization, especially the larger mammals, is something on which the advice and preferably help of suitably qualified persons should be sought. Details of methods for restraining large animals for immunization and bleeding have been published elsewhere (Chase, 1967b; Stewart-Tull and Rowe, 1975), but information on handling and bleeding of goats is given later in this chapter (see Figure 3).

D. Immunization Procedures

The immunizing dose will depend on the intrinsic antigenicity of the immunogen, the adjuvant used, and the species immunized, and can only be determined for any individual case by trial and error and careful observation. Rabbits or larger animals are usually immunized initially with 1 mg or more of antigen in Freund's complete adjuvant. Less antigen, down to 100 μg or lower, can be successfully used if its availability is restricted.

In my experience the use of antigen in amounts greater than 5 to 10 mg for a large animal (sheep, goats, horses) has not been necessary, but this cannot be assumed to be a universally applicable observation. The use of large amounts of immunogen has inherent dangers, in that as antigen dose increases, so does that of any contaminant. Even for antigens which are apparently pure, it is difficult to exclude contamination at the level of 1% or less, but this amount of protein (i.e. 10 μg per milligram of preparation) can quite easily be

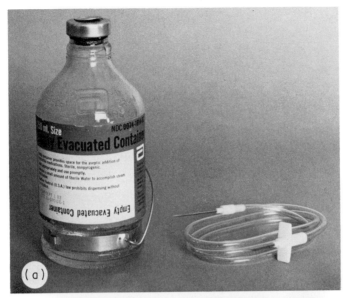

(a)

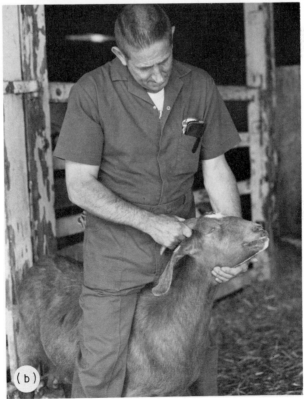

(b)

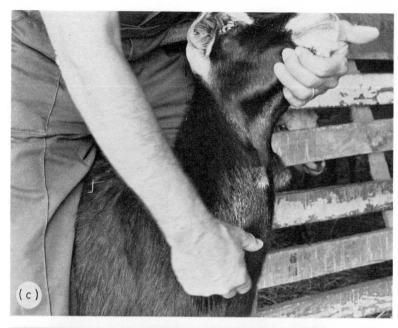

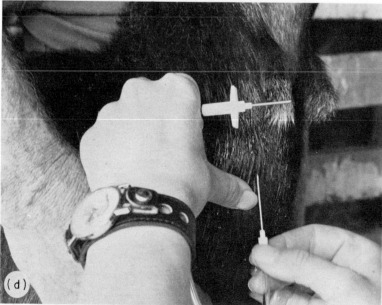

Figure 3. Restraint and bleeding of a goat. Two people are required for this operation. Figure 3(a) shows the required apparatus: an evacuated sterile container, and a bleeding set (available, for example, from Abbot Laboratories, North Chicago, Illinois, USA). Figure 3(b) shows restraint of the goat, between the handler's legs and with the head held up. If the animal can be backed up against a fence or wall it prevents its backward escape from between the handler's legs. Figure 3(c) shows the

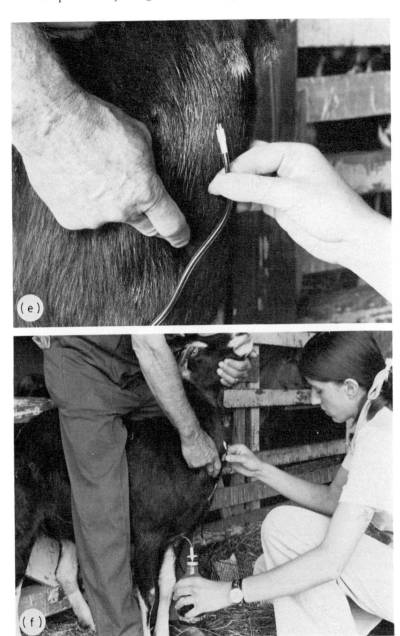

handler exerting pressure, with his middle finger, on the jugular vein at a point below which the needle is to be inserted. Figures 3(d) and 3(e) show the insertion of the needle into the jugular vein, which can be readily identified by palpation, and the needle in place. Note the continued pressure on the jugular vein by the person restraining the goat. Figure 3(f) shows the other needle of the bleeding set inserted into the evacuated container which is rapidly filling with blood immunogenic. Again, it should be emphasized that there is no substitute for careful testing of an antiserum, and an open mind in these matters is to be encouraged.

The choice of adjuvant determines to some extent the dose of antigen, route of inoculation, and the requirements for boosting. If cellular antigens are given without adjuvant, repeated weekly boosts are often given intraperitoneally (i.p.) or intravenously (i.v.). A detailed review of the effects of various immunization regimens, including the use of adjuvants, on the properties of anti-lymphocyte serum is given by James (1973).

Alum-precipitated proteins are usually administered intramuscularly (i.m.) to large animals and rabbits, or i.p. to small laboratory rodents, and administration of booster doses of the antigen (in amounts similar to or less than that of the primary dose) can be given over weeks or months depending on how the monitored response progresses.

When Freund's adjuvants are used, the complete form is generally used for the primary inoculum. In large animals, immunization is generally i.m. into the large muscles, e.g. of the thigh. The animal is usually considered to respond better if the inoculum is distributed among several sites. This practice also lessens the risk of abscess formation at the site of injection of a large volume. Rabbits are usually injected i.m. or intradermally (i.d.) with complete Freund's adjuvant, again at multiple sites. For i.d. inoculation, the rabbit is frequently injected at several sites on the flank or neck, with a total volume of 1 to 2 ml. The skin over the injection site is shaved, and the injection made into a fold of skin held between finger and thumb. A 20 or 21 G disposable needle is conveniently used. One problem with i.d. inoculation is that skin sores can develop at the injection site. These usually heal with little problem, but nevertheless may be undesirable. Injections of Freund's adjuvant (especially complete) into the feet of any animal, mammal or bird are not recommended. They can lead to considerable distress for the animal and it is unclear whether they produce better antibodies than inoculations at other sites. Fowl can be immunized i.m. with Freund's adjuvants, using the large breast or thigh muscles for this purpose. For a chicken, around 1 mg of antigen in a 1 or 2 ml total volume is usually distributed at a number of sites. Chickens have been successfully immunized using a variety of other immunization schemes, including omission of adjuvants, and i.p. and i.v. injection (Benedict, 1967). Chickens can be immunized at between 2 and 3 months of age.

When primary immunization has been carried out in complete Freund's adjuvant, boosting, if necessary, should generally be carried out using the incomplete adjuvant to avoid an intense response to the mycobacteria in the inoculum. One or more boosts with Freund's adjuvant may or may not be necessary. Some investigators routinely boost rabbits 2–3 weeks after the first immunization. This regimen, in my experience, usually leads to a good response, which can be sustained for months (or exceptionally years) without reboosting.

In those instances where antigens are infectious for man, standard safety precautions such as wearing protective clothing (gloves, laboratory coat, and a respirator) and confining the work to a ventilated cabinet should be considered. Animal studies should meet the safety standards outlined in Section IV, G. of the DHEW publication, *Guide for the Care and Use of Laboratory Animals*.

A final word on immunization is that investigators should not feel they have to follow rigidly anybody else's scheme. This is an area in which empirical observation is the only basis for decision.

VI. BLEEDING

Before an animal is immunized, a sample of blood should be taken to ensure that serum is available for comparison with the immune bleeds.

Although most experimental animals (unless gnotobiotic) have reasonable serum levels of Igs, denoting responses to various antigens (e.g. those of common infectious agents), cross-reactions between these (as seen in the pre-immune serum) and the immunizing antigen are rarely seen, unless the animal has had some prior contact with the antigen in question.

Following immunization, small test bleeds can be taken at regular intervals (1 to 2 weeks depending on circumstances) to determine when the required response has been achieved.

The quality and quantity of antibody produced can change considerably with time after immunization. The affinity of antibody produced in response to immunization with a defined hapten can increase by orders of magnitude during a response (Eisen and Siskind 1964; Siskind and Benacerraf, 1969). This process of maturation of the response, as it has been termed by some investigators, is typically seen following immunization with antigen in adjuvant. A stronger response may not always be the most desirable, however. For example, in the production of anti-lymphocyte serum early bleeds may be preferred to later ones, which are frequently very cytotoxic, and can show strong reactions with a variety of cell types befor adsorption. Again, the longer a response continues and the stronger it becomes, the greater the chance of seeing a significant response to a minor contaminant in the preparation of antigen used for immunization. This is a point on which generalizations cannot be made. I would recommend waiting long enough for the response to be predominantly of the IgG class (in mammals), which is usually the case within a few weeks of immunization in adjuvant. However, after this the decision on the quality of the antibody and whether to kill bleed will depend on the unique circumstances of the immunization and the antibody properties desired by the investigator. The activity in test bleeds can be monitored by the standard methods given in Chapter 4. When the desired activity is present, an animal can be bled out, or else be bled in moderate amounts routinely. As much as 50 ml of blood can be taken from a large rabbit every 3 weeks, and a few hundred millilitres of blood from goats, sheep, and horses every month, the exact amount depending on the size of the animal. The effect of these bleeding schedules on the animal's health should be monitored, and any necessary modifications made.

Whereas most animals can be restrained manually for immunization, for bleeding restraining devices may be preferred. In the case of rabbits, restraining cages to allow for ear bleeding (see below) are commercially available (e.g. from Hoeltge Co., 5242 Crookshank Road, Cincinnati, Ohio 45238), or can be simply made in the workshop to one's own specifications. Excellent information on the methods and apparatus required for restraining large mammals, laboratory rodents, and birds is given in the reviews by Herbert (1978) and Chase (1967b), who also provide excellent illustrated accounts of various bleeding and inoculation techniques. It is not possible in this review to give such comprehensive information as has been provided by these authors, but some information on the most commonly used techniques follows below.

A. Large Animals

These are usually test bled or bled out from the external jugular vein, into which a large gauge needle (e.g. 16 G) can readily be inserted when the animal is correctly restrained (Chase, 1967b). It is better to bleed under vacuum, rather than gravity drip, especially if large amounts of blood are required. The bleeding of a goat, and the apparatus used, are illustrated in Figure 3. Stewart-Tull and Rowe (1975) give detailed information on the bleeding (and immunization) of sheep for antiserum production.

B. Rabbits, Rodents, and Chickens

Rabbits are usually test bled from the marginal ear vein, either by making an incision with a sterile scalpel blade, or by inserting a sterile disposable needle (e.g. 22 G). In both cases blood is collected by gravity drip into a tube. The blood vessels of the rabbit ear can be induced to dilate by quickly rubbing the ear with xylene, then immediately washing it off with ethanol followed by water. Some investigators bleed from the rabbit ear by withdrawing blood directly from the central artery by use of a syringe and sterile needle (e.g. 22 G). This latter technique, although it requires a little more skill, is much quicker than bleeding from the ear vein.

It is not recommended that a vacuum be applied to a rabbit's ear to hasten bleeding from the vein, as this practice can result in damage to the middle ear. Rabbits are usually bled out by cardiac puncture under anaesthesia. Appendix V, contributed by Robert McEwan, describes this procedure as it is routinely carried out at the author's institution.

The common laboratory rodents (mice, rats, guinea pigs, and hamsters) can be test bled from the ear vein (guinea pig) as for the rabbit, by an incision made in a tail vein (mice and rats, Chase, 1967b), by cardiac puncture of an anaesthetized animal (for rats and guinea pigs: if carefully done mortality is avoidable) or by bleeding from the orbital plexus (Herbert, 1978; Chase, 1967b).

The rodents are usually kill bled by cardiac puncture under anaesthesia (Herbert, 1978; Chase, 1967b).

Chickens are readily test bled with needle and syringe from a brachial (wing) vein, with the unanesthetized bird restrained on its back (Herbert, 1978). Kill bleeding is usually done by cardiac puncture, with the bird (again usually unanesthetized) lying on its back, and the approach to the heart being made from the front of the bird, in the angle formed by the wishbone. A 2 inch needle, of relatively large gauge (18 or 19) is used, and the approach to the heart is made in a near horizontal plane (Chase, 1967b).

Other types of bleeding, including cannulation of arteries, is described for a variety of species by Chase (11967b).

C. Treatment of Test Bleeds

As with all procedures involving immunization and bleeding, attempts should be made to operate under sterile conditions. Blood is usually allowed to clot at room temperature, and if the container has not been greased it is 'ringed' to separate it from the vessel wall, and allowed to retract, usually at 4 °C overnight. Serum is then withdrawn using a Pasteur pipette, and centrifuged (e.g. 600 X g for 10 minutes) to remove any cells or debris. Chicken serum is best allowed to clot and retract at 37 °C for up to 10 or 12 hours. Because the clot does not always retract well, some authors (Chase, 1967b) recommend withdrawing chicken blood into oxalate or citrate, removing the erythrocytes, and then clotting the plasma with the addition of calcium chloride. I have never found this to be necessary, although the yield of serum from clotted chicken blood is always somewhat less than the 50% of blood volume one might expect from mammalian sources.

With any bleeding, care should be taken at all stages to avoid haemolysis, as this contaminates the serum with extraneous cellular proteins and, in some cases, proteolytic enzymes. Degradation of antibody in stored, purified IgG fractions, has been reported (James *et al.*, 1964).

Complement activity is generally destroyed by heating serum at 56 °C for 20–30 minutes.

Cloudy sera resulting from the presence of lipoproteins in blood are frequently seen. Fasting the animals before bleeding can sometimes help to avoid this problem. Although some authorities recommend throwing these lipid-containing sera away, the method for lipoprotein removal described by van Dalen *et al.* (1967) can be applied. In the author's experience, this technique, which relies on precipitation with dextran sulphate and calcium chloride, has been successfully used on chicken and rabbit sera without any gross loss of antibody activity. Its use is described in detail in Appendix VI.

Unless sera are to be used immediately, they are best stored frozen at -20 °C. If the activity is due to IgG antibodies and the freezer is not the sort that has a thaw/defrost cycle, antibody activity can be preserved for many years. It is recommended that chicken serum should not be frozen, as it can become very turbid upon thawing; instead a gamma globulin concentrate (Chapter 3) should be prepared before freezing. Because repeated freezing and thawing leads to protein denaturation and eventual loss of antibody activity, sera or fractions of them should be frozen in small aliquots of convenient size.

Further processing of serum to produce antibody preparations of varying degrees of purity is described in the next chapter (Chapter 3).

APPENDIX I. POLYACRYLAMIDE GEL ELECTROPHORESIS IN THE PRESENCE OF SODIUM-DODECYL-SULPHATE-CONTAINING BUFFERS

This procedure is modified from that described by Laemmli and Favre (1973). The use of a simpler system with less resolving power is described by Weber and Osborn (1969).

A. Glass Tubes

These are washed in chromic acid and siliconized before use to facilitate removal of the gel from the tube at the end of the run. We usually dip the tubes in a 2% solution of dichlorodimethylsilane in benzene for siliconization and allow them to air-dry before use. Tubes used can be any size to fit the available electrophoretic apparatus. We use 15 cm tubes (outside diameter 8 mm, inside diameter 6 mm) into which we pour a 12 cm running gel and a 1.5 cm stacking gel.

B. Reagents

Glass distilled water should be used for all stock solutions. Reagents should be of the highest purity available. The stock acrylamide should be kept in the dark at 4 °, but other solutions may be stored at room temperature.

1. Stock Acrylamide

This contains 20% acrylamide (w/v) plus 0.5% N,N',methylene-bisacrylamide (w/v). This stock solution should not be stored for any length of time. Fresh stock is made up after 2 weeks at 4 °.

2. Lower (Running) Gel Buffer

1.5 M Tris-HCl, pH 8.8, plus 0.4% sodium dodecyl sulphate (SDS).
90.85 g Tris (hydroxymethyl) aminomethane.
20 ml of a 10% solution (w/v) of SDS.
Water is added to 500 ml. (Final adjustment to volume is made after pH is adjusted to 8.8 with conc. HCl.)

3. Upper (Stacking) Gel Buffer

0.5 M Tris-HCl, pH 6.8, plus 0.4% SDS.
30.3 g Tris
20 ml 10% (w/v) SDS solution.
Water to 500 ml.
pH is adjusted to 6.8 with conc. HCl.

4. Reservoir Buffer for Electrophoresis (×4 concentrated)

24 g Tris.
115.2 g glycine.
Water to 2 litres.
The pH of this buffer is adjusted to 8.3 by the use of concentrated Tris or glycine solutions, not HCl or NaOH.
The concentrated stock buffer is diluted with three volumes of water before use. In addition, 10 ml of 10% (w/v) SDS solution should be present in every litre of diluted buffer to give a final SDS concentration of 0.1%.

5. Sample Buffer

15 ml glycerol.
30 ml 10% (w/v) SDS solution.
12.5 ml stock upper (stacking) gel buffer solution.
Water to 100 ml.
For the reduction of disulphide bonds, 2-mercaptoethanol is added at 5% (v/v).

6. Ammonium Persulphate

A 2% solution (w/v) should be freshly made up before use.

7. Temed

(*NNN'*,-*N'*,-tetramethyl-1,2-diaminoethane) is also required.

Antibody as a Tool

C. Pouring the Gels

The concentration of the running gel is determined by the size of the molecules it is to resolve. A 10% acrylamide (0.25% bisacrylamide) gel resolves in the range of 20,000–150,000 daltons. The following procedure is for gels of 10% and 5% acrylamide concentration, but the concentration can be varied as desired. However, it is necesary to keep the volume of the lower (running) gel buffer at one-fourth of the total volume of the gel solution. If very low acrylamide concentrations are desired, in order to resolve large or polymeric molecules, mechanical stabilization of the gel can be provided by agarose (Peacock and Dingman, 1968).

The running gel solution is prepared by mixing the following volumes (or multiples thereof). The volumes given are sufficient for 10 gels of the dimensions 15 cm length ×0.6 cm internal diameter.

Final gel concentration (acrylamide)	Water	Lower (running) gel buffer	Stock acrylamide	Ammonium persulphate (2%)
10%	6.4	7	14	0.6
5%	13.4	7	7	0.6

The solution is degassed under vacuum at room temperature, then 5 μl of TEMED are added, and mixed without shaking. The solution is poured gently into the gel tubes (using a Pasteur pipette) and care is taken to ensure that no air bubbles are trapped at the bottom or sides of the tube, which is sealed at the bottom (laboratory film, or preferably a rubber cap, can be used for this purpose). The gel solution is adjusted to the correct length in the tube, and overlaid with a few drops of isobutanol. Polymerization is generally complete within 1–2 hours.

The isobutanol and unpolymerized gel are washed away thoroughly with water, and the upper (stacking) gel is poured. This is prepared in the following manner (sufficient for 10 gels).

Water	Upper (stacking) gel buffer	Stock acrylamide	Ammonium persulphate (2%)
4.7 ml	2 ml	1.2 ml	0.1 ml

After degassing, 5μl TEMED are added, mixed, and the gel solution is poured. The height of the gel solution is adjusted, the gel is overlaid with isobutanol and allowed to polymerize. After the isobutanol and unpolymerized gel have been rized gel have been washed away with water, and the seal at the bottom of the tube removed, the gel is ready to be run.

D. Sample Preparation

A total sample volume of 200–300 μl can be accommodated on the gels described here. A minimum of 50% of the sample volume should be contributed by sample buffer. If the sample has too high a salt content (greater than about 0.2 M final) the electrophoretic run will be significantly slowed.

The sample is heated in a boiling water bath for 2 minutes, before being allowed to cool prior to application to the top of the gel.

E. Electrophoresis

The sample is carefully overlaid with reservoir buffer (which is used for both cathodic and anodic reservoirs). The gel is run vertically, with the cathode at the top, and migration is downward towards the anode. Various forms of electrophoretic tanks accommodating up to 24 tubes are available from scientific suppliers, or else can be made in a workshop. In the cathode buffer are present a few drops of a 0.05% solution of bromophenol blue dye. During the electrophoretic run, the dye will 'stack' to give a sharp blue line marking the front of the separation.

Electrophoresis is usually carried out at room temperature, with conditions of constant current. One mA per gel is used until the dye marker penetrates the running gel, and thereafter the run is continued at 2 mA per gel. A run can frequently take 5–6 hours.

F. Staining of Protein Bands

At the end of the run, gels can usually be removed by carefully injecting, with needle and syringe, water between the gel and the tube (at both ends) and then forcing the gel out with a rubber teat. Gels should not be touched with ungloved hands, as this can leave stainable fingerprints on the gel surface. Polyacrylamide gels usually have a high degree of resistance to mechanical trauma, but care should be taken to avoid damaging or breaking them. Staining is usually carried out in a tube, using a solution of 0.05% Coomassie Brilliant Blue R in acetic acid [methanol/water $(1:5:4)$]. Staining may take from 1–5 hours. Destaining is carried out in 7% (v/v) acetic acid. This method should result in the staining of bands containing as little as 1 or 2 μg protein.

APPENDIX II. CONJUGATIONS WITH CARBODIIMIDES

As generally carried out for immunological purposes, carbodiimide coupling is a simple and not very closely controlled reaction. I will describe in outline the conjugation of molecules to molecules in solution, and the conjugation of molecules to solid phase matrices bearing the appropriate —NH$_2$ or —COOH groups. Carbodiimide coupling is usually carried out in aqueous solution, at a pH of between 4.5 and 6.0. The pH is adjusted with dilute HCl or NaOH. If buffers are used they should not contain phosphate, amino groups (e.g. Tris) or carboxyl groups (e.g. acetate) because these compete with the coupling reaction. Commonly used water-soluble carbodiimides are 1-ethyl-3-(3-di-methyl-aminopropyl) carbodiimide HCl (EDC) and 1-cyclohexyl-3-(2mor-pholino-ethyl) carbodiimide methyl-*p*-toluene sulphonate (CMC). The ligand to be coupled either to the protein or the matrix should usually be present in solution at a considerable excess compared to available reactive groups. To the mixture of ligand/protein or ligand/mixture is added a further molar excess (10–100 fold) of the carbodiimide, freshly dissolved in water. The reaction can be monitored for pH changes and adjusted appropriately, especially during the first 1 or 2 hours. Reaction can be at room temperature or in the cold, and the time of reaction can be as short as 1 or 2 hours, but is more usually overnight. If necessary, it is possible to block groups on a protein molecule (e.g. by acetylation of NH$_2$ groups) to prevent intramolecular coupling by the carbodiimide. After conjugation, unreacted reagents and products can be removed by dialysis or, in the case of a solid phase matrix, simply by washing. Likhite and Sehon (1967) give a number of examples of actual coupling reactions.

APPENDIX III. PREPARATION OF ALUMINA
(AFTER CHASE, 1967a)

To 10 ml of a 10% solution of aluminium potassium sulphate or aluminium ammonium sulphate is added slowly 23 ml of 0.25 M NaOH with mixing. The precipitate which forms is left for 10 or 15 minutes, then centrifuged and washed with water. Centrifugation should not be at high speed to avoid packing the precipitate (400 × g for 5 minutes is recommended). The precipitate is ready to use when resuspended.

The solutions used should be sterile, and attempts should be made to preserve sterility, especially if the product is to be stored.

Details on the preparations of other types of inorganic colloids for use as adjuvants are given by Chase (1967a).

APPENDIX IV. PRODUCTION OF ANTIBODIES IN THE
ASCITES FLUID OF MICE

This method is based on the work of Tung *et al.* (1976).

1. Strains

Most inbred mouse strains can be expected to respond to this immunization schedule, but with differing amounts of ascites fluid and antibody concentration. Individual mice will also show differing responses dependent on age and other factors.

2. Inoculum

Mice are injected intraperitoneally with 0.2 ml of a mixture of 9 : 1 complete Freund's adjuvant to antigen solution. The antigen should be reasonably concentrated (e.g. 10 mg/ml solution or higher). For or five injections are given, with 2 weeks between the first two, and intervals of 1 week thereafter.

3. Ascites Fluid

Ascites fluid can begin to accumulate within a week or two of the second or subsequent injections. When gross ascites is present it is not necessary to reinject, unless the ascites fails to recur. The ascites fluid must be withdrawn to prevent death of the animal. A sterile 19 G 1 or 1½ inch hypodermic needle is inserted into the peritoneal cavity, and the fluid is allowed to drain through the needle into a tube. After clarification the fluid can be frozen. Fibrin clots which form in the fluid can be removed by centrifugation (e.g. at $20,000 \times g$ for 20 minutes).

This method can be used to produce ascites fluid containing specific antibody, or else to produce ascites fluid as a source of mouse IgG. In this latter case, antigen is omitted from the injected mixture, and is replaced with saline.

APPENDIX V. EXSANGUINATION OF RABBITS BY CARDIAC PUNCTURE

Rabbits are usually anaesthetized using Nembutal (pentobarbital sodium) at a dose of 30 mg per kilogram intravenously. Usually three-quarters of the calculated dose is injected at once (e.g. into the ear vein) and the rest only if needed. Anaesthesia is almost immediate, and can be checked by pinching a foot to test for absence of the withdrawal reflex. Although Nembutal used in this way is usually perfectly satisfactory, it can cause problems. The animal needs to be firmly secured for the injection, and if there are problems with underdosage or failure to make a clean injection, the animal will go through a phase of involuntary excitement. Some investigators inject rabbits intraperitoneally with Nembutal, but by this route absorption is slow, dosage is uncertain, and anaesthesia ensues slowly.

We have successfully used Vetalar[R], (ketamine hydrochloride, available from Parke-Davis and Co., Detroit, Michigan) with New Zealand White rabbits. An injection is made intramuscularly (at 30 mg per kilogram body weight) and anaesthesia ensues within minutes. With this form of anaesthesia, pedal (and other) reflexes are retained, and the eyes remain open.

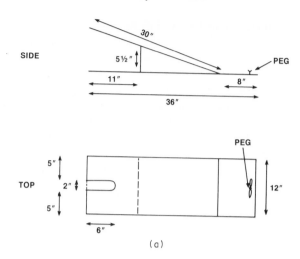

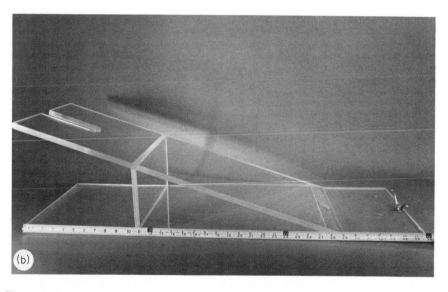

Figure 4. Board for rabbit bleeding. Figure 4(a) shows the dimensions of the board, and Figure 4(b) shows the actual apparatus

Whichever form of anaesthesia is used, the rabbit is then restrained for bleeding. We use an inclined board, as illustrated in Figure 4. The head fits under the top of the board, with the neck passing through the slot. The hind legs are tied with a loop of string which is made fast to a peg on the board. The front legs are free. The animal should be tied securely but not too tightly, as this can result in an alteration of the geometry of the thorax.

Bleeding is frequently carried out by use of a 50 ml hypodermic syringe with an attached needle (e.g. 2½ inch, 19 G). If this method is used, the syringe has to be detached from the needle when full, and reattached after being emptied. This procedure can result in dislodgement of the needle from the heart, and is also inconvenient. An alternative method which avoids these problems is to insert into the heart a needle attached to a flexible tube, in turn connected to a collection vessel on which a gentle vacuum can be applied. A suitable apparatus is illustrated in Figure 5. This utilizes a commercially available bleeding set for large animals (for example, Blood Collection Set, 36 inch, #4736 from Abbot Laboratories, North Chicago, Illinois) connected to the collecting vessel, which in turn is connected to a 50 ml syringe which is used to apply a gentle vacuum. The syringe is connected to the collecting vessel by means of a three-way stopcock (catalogue #3138, from Beckton-Dickinson) which allows the syringe to be exhausted when full of air, without dismounting the system. Using this bleeding apparatus, up to or slightly more than 100 ml of blood can be obtained from a mature rabbit.

Whichever bleeding system is used, the approach to the heart is the same. The needle is inserted at the angle formed between the last left sternal rib and the xiphoid process, but some investigators routinely use the right side equally effectively. This is illustrated in Figure 6. Normally the fur in this region is shaved, or just wetted with 70% ethanol, and the point for insertion of the needle is palpated. The needle is inserted, bevel up, at an angle of about 30° to the plane in which the rabbit lies. The beating of the heart can usually be detected before penetration is achieved, and the application of a gentle vacuum during this phase results in an immediate flow of blood once the needle is correctly positioned (Figure 6). During bleeding the operator should be prepared to adjust the position of the needle to maintain a free flow of blood.

After withdrawal of the maximum amount of blood, the operator should ensure that the animal is dead. This can be achieved by introducing a few millilitres of air into the heart (especially convenient if the apparatus described in Figure 5 is used), by severing the spinal column with bone forceps, or by breaking the neck with a blow to the back of the head.

APPENDIX VI. REMOVAL OF LIPOPROTEINS FROM SERUM

This procedure is based on that described by van Dalen *et al.* (1967) and Masseyeff *et al.* (1965).

A. Reagents

10% solution (w/v) dextran sulphate (Pharmacia Fine Chemicals).
1 M solution of calcium chloride.

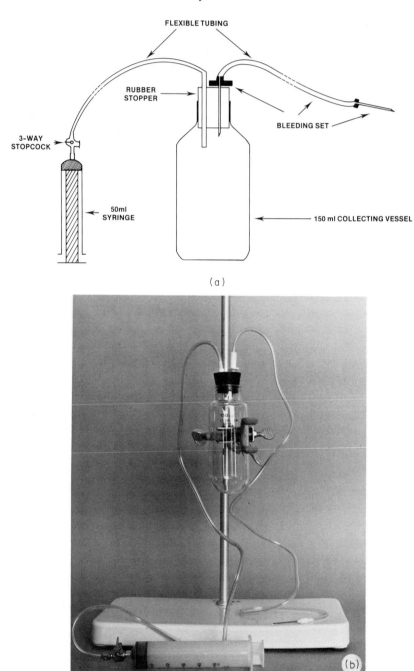

(a)

(b)

Figure 5. Rabbit bleeding apparatus. This is shown diagrammatically in Figure 5(a), and set up with a stand and clamp in Figure 5(b)

B. Procedure

To 15 ml of serum (or protein solution) is added 0.6 ml of 10% dextran sulphate with thorough mixing. 1.5 ml of 1 M calcium chloride are then added dropwise with mixing. The serum is allowed to stand at room temperature for 15 minutes and then centrifuged to remove the precipitate (10,000 × g for 30 minutes). The supernatant fluid is then dialysed against a physiological buffer or, for example, the Tris-buffered saline, pH 8.0, described in Appendix III.

Sometimes this procedure leaves the serum with residual turbidity, but a second centrifugation after the dialysis step will usually result in complete clarification of the serum.

REFERENCES

Atassi, M. Z. (1977). The complete antigenic structure of myoglobin: Approaches and conclusions for antigenic structures of proteins. In M. Z. Atassi (Ed.) *Immunochemsitry of Proteins*, Volume 2, pp. 77–176, Plenum Press, New York and London.

Beiser, S. M., Erlanger, B. F., and Tanenbaum, S. W. (1967). Preparation of purine and pyrimidine-protein conjugates. In C. A. Williams and M. W. Chase (Eds.) *Methods in Immunology and Immunochemistry* Volume 1. *Preparation of Antigens and Antibodies*, pp. 180–185, Academic Press, New York and London.

Benedict, A. A. (1967). Production and purification of chicken immunoglobulins. In C. A. Williams and M. W. Chase (Eds.) *Methods in Immunology and Immunochemistry* Volume 1, *Preparation of Antigens and Antibodies*, pp. 229–237, Academic Press, New York and London.

Bucana, C., and Hanna, M. G., Jr. (1974). Immunoelectron microscopic analysis of surface antigens common to *Mycobacterium bovis* (BCG) and tumor cells. *J. Natl. Cancer Inst.*, **53**, 1313–1323.

Capra, J. D., and Kehoe, J. M. (1975) Hypervariable regions, idiotype, and the antibody-combining site. *Adv. Immunol.*, **20**, 1–40.

Chase, M. W. (1967a). Preparation of immunogens. In C. A. Williams and M. W. Chase (Eds.) *Methods in Immunology and Immunochemistry* Volume 1. *Preparation of Antigens and Antibodies*, pp. 197–200, Academic Press, New York and London.

Chase, M. W. (1967b). Animal handling. In C. A. Williams and M. W. Chase (Eds.) *Methods in Immunology and Immunochemistry* Volume 1. *Preparation of Antigens and Antibodies*, pp. 254–306, Academic Press, New York and London.

Chrambach, A., and Rodbard, D. (1971). Polyacrylamide gel electrophoresis. *Science*, **172**, 440–451.

Claman, H. N. (1963). Tolerance to a protein antigen in adult mice and the effect of nonspecific factors. *J. Immunol.*, **91**, 833–839.

Cooper, T. G. (1977). *The Tools of Biochemistry*. Wiley, New York and London.

Dresser, D. W. (1962). Specific inhibition of antibody production. II. Paralysis induced in adult mice by small quantities of protein antigen. *Immunology*, **5**, 378–388.

Dresser, D. W., Wortis, H. H., and Anderson, H. R. (1970). The effect of pertussis vaccine on the immune response of mice to sheep red blood cells. *Clin. Exp. Immunol.*, **7**, 817–831.

Eisen, H. N., and Siskind, G. W. (1964). Variations in affinities of antibodies during the immune response. *Biochemistry*, **3**, 996–1008.

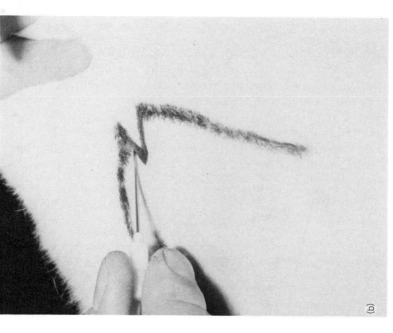

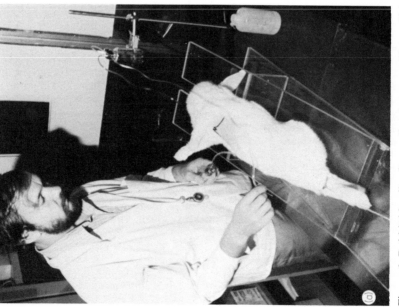

Figure 6. Rabbit bleeding by cardiac puncture. Figure 6(a) shows the anaesthetized rabbit restrained on the board shown in Figure 5, by passing the neck through the groove in the board, with the head remaining underneath the board, and by securing the legs, with a piece of cord, to the peg at the foot of the board. The area over the ribs and xiphoid process has been shaved, and the last ribs and the xiphoid process have been marked with ink. The operator is using the bleeding apparatus shown in Figure 5. Figure 6(b) shows

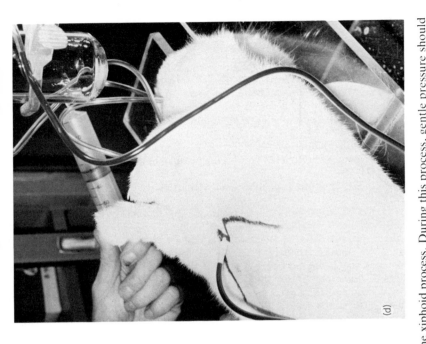

(d)

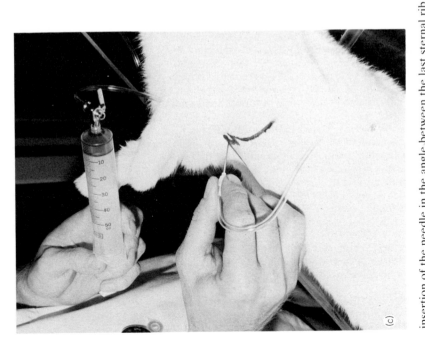

(c)

insertion of the needle in the angle between the last sternal rib and the xiphoid process. During this process, gentle pressure should be kept on the syringe, which is held in the left hand (Figure 6c), and blood will begin to flow once the heart has been penetrated (Figure 6d)

Embleton, M. J., and Iype, P. T. (1978). Surface antigens of rat liver epithelial cells grown in medium containing foetal bovine serum. *Br. J. Cancer*, **38**, 456–460.

Erlanger, B. F., Beiser, S. M., Borek, F., Edel, F., and Lieberman, S. (1967). The preparation of steroid-protein conjugates to elicit antihormonal antibodies. In C. A. Williams and M. W. Chase (Eds) *Methods in Immunology and Immunochemistry* Volume 1. *Preparation of Antigens and Antibodies*, pp. 144–150. Academic Press, New York and London.

Goding, J. W. (1978). Use of staphylococcal protein A as an immunological reagent. *J. Immunol. Methods*, **20**, 241–253.

Goudswaard, J., van der Donk., J. A., Noordzil, A., Van Dam, R. H., and Vaerman, J. P. (1978). Protein A reactivity of various mammalian immunoglobulins. *Scand. J. Immunol.*, **8**. 21–28.

Gray, W. R. (1972). End group analysis using dansyl chloride. *Methods Enzymol.*, **25**(B), 121–138.

Herbert, W. J. (1978). Laboratory animal techniques for immunology. In D. M. Weir (Ed.) *Handbook of Experimental Immunology* Volume 3. *Application of Immunological Methods*, pp. A4.1–A4.29. Blackwell, Oxford.

Herzenberg, L. A., and Herzenberg, L. A. (1978). Mouse immunoglobulin allotypes: description and special methodology. In D. M. Weir (Ed.) *Experimental Immunology* Volume 1. *Immunochemistry*, pp. 12.1–12.23. Blackwell, Oxford.

Ihle, J. N., Charman, H., and Gilden, R. V. (1979). Comparative biology of mammalian retroviruses. In J. J. Marchalonis, M. G. Hanna, Jr., and I. J. Fidler (Eds.), *Cancer Biology Reviews* Volume 1, pp. 133–219. Marcel Dekker, New York.

James, K. (1973). Preparation of anti-lymphocyte antibodies. In D. M. Weir (Ed.) *Handbook of Experimental Immunology* Volume 2. *Cellular Immunology*, pp. 31.1–31.27. Blackwell, Oxford.

James, K., Henney, C. S., and Stanworth, D. R. (1964). Structural changes in 7S γ-globulins. *Nature (Lond).*, **202**, 563–566.

James, K., and Milne, I. (1972). The effect of antilymphocytic antibody on the humoral immune response in different strains of mice. I. The response to bovine serum albumin. *Immunology*, **23**, 897–909.

Jonsson, S., and Kronvall, G. (1974). The use of protein A-containing *Staphylococcus aureus* as a solid phase anti-IgG reagent in radioimmunoassays as exemplified in the quantitation of alpha-fetoprotein in normal human adult serum. *Eur. J. Immunol.*, **4**, 29–33.

Kessler, S. W. (1975). Rapid isolation of antigens from cells with a staphylococcal protein A-antibody adsorbant: parameters of the interaction of antibody–antigen complexes with Protein A. *J. Immunol.*, **115**, 1617–1624.

Kessler, S. W. (1976). Cell membrane antigen isolation with the staphylococcal protein A–antibody adsorbent. *J. Immunol.*, **117**, 1482–1490.

Laemmli, U. K., and Favre, M. (1973). Maturation of the head of bacteriophage T4. 1. DNA packaging events. *J. Mol. Biol.*, **80**, 575–599.

Landsteiner, K. (1942). Serological reactivity of hydrolytic products from silk. *J. Exp. Med.*, **75**, 269–276.

Likhite, V., and Sehon, A. (1967). Protein–protein conjugation. In C. A. Williams and M. W. Chase (Eds.) *Methods in Immunology and Immunochemistry* Volume 1. *Preparation of Antigens and Antibodies*, pp. 150–167. Academic Press, New York and London.

Little, J. R., and Eisen, H. N. (1967). Preparation of immunogenic 2,4-dinitrophenyl and 2,4,6-trinitrophenyl proteins. In C. A. Williams and M. W. Chase *Methods in*

Immunology and Immunochemistry Volume 1. *Preparation of Antigens and Antibodies*, pp. 128–133. Academic Press, New York and London.

Lowry, O. H., Rosebrough, N. J., Farr, A. L., and Randall, R. J. (1951). Protein measurement with the Folin phenol reagent. *J. Biol. Chem.*, **193**, 265–275.

Masseyeff, R., Gombert, J., and Josselin, J. (1965). Methode de preparation de la β-2 macroglobuline du serum humain. *Immunochemistry*, **2**, 177–180.

Nisonoff, A. (1967). Conjugated and synthetic antigens. I. Coupling of diazonium compounds to proteins. In C. A. Williams and M. W. Chase (Eds.) *Methods in Immunology and Immunochemistry* Volume 1. *Preparation of Antigens and Antibodies*, pp. 120–126. Academic Press, New York and London.

Norris, J. R., and Ribbons, D. W. (1969–1973). *Methods in Microbiology* Volumes 1–9. Academic Press, London and New York.

Peacock, A. C., and Dingman, C. W. (1968). Molecular weight estimation and separation of ribonucleic acid by electrophoresis in agarose–acrylamide composite gels. *Biochemistry*, **7**, 668–674.

Plescia, O. J. (1967). Preparation of antigens for eliciting antibody with nucleoside and nucleic acid specificity. In C. A. Williams and M. W. Chase (Eds.) *Methods in Immunology and Immunochemistry* Volume 1. *Preparation of Antigens and Antibodies*, pp. 175–180. Academic Press, New York and London.

Rapport, M. M., and Graf, L. (1967). Preparation and testing of lipids for immunological study. In C. A. Williams and M. W. Chase (Eds.) *Methods in Immunology and Immunochemistry* Volume 1. *Preparation of Antigens and Antibodies*, pp. 187–196, Academic Press, New York and London.

Ruddon, R. W. (1978). *Biological markers of neoplasia: Basic and Applied Aspects*. Elsevier, New York.

Sela, M., and Fuchs, S. (1978). Preparation of synthetic antigens. In D. M. Weir (Ed.) *Handbook of Experimental Immunology* Volume 1. *Immunochemistry*, pp. 1.1–1.11, Blackwell, Oxford.

Siskind, G. W., and Benacerraf, B. (1969). Cell selection by antigen in the immune response. *Adv. Immunol.*, **10**, 1–50.

Steward, M. W. (1977). Affinity of the antibody–antigen reaction and its biological significance. In L. E. Glynn and M. W. Steward (Eds.) *Immunochemistry: An Advanced Textbook*, pp. 233–262. Wiley, London.

Stewart-Tull, D. E. S., and Rowe, R. E. C. (1975). Procedures for large-scale antiserum production in sheep. *J. Immunol. Methods*, **8**, 37–46.

Stolfi, R. L., Fugmann, R. A., Jensen, J. J., and Sigel, M. M. (1971). A C1-fixation method for the measurement of chicken anti-viral antibody. *Immunology*, **20**, 299–306.

Tung, A. S., Ju, S-T., Sato, S., and Nisonoff, A. (1976). Production of large amounts of antibodies in individual mice. *J. Immunol.*, **116**, 676–681.

Turk, J. L. (1975). *Delayed Hypersensitivity*. North Holland, Amsterdam.

van Dalen, A., Seijen, H. G., and Gruber, M. (1967). Isolation and some properties of rabbit IgM immunoglobulin. *Biochim. Biophys. Acta.*, **147**, 421–426.

Warr, G. W., Marton, G., Szenberg, A., and Marchalonis, J. J. (1978). Reactions of chicken antibodies with immunoglobulins of mouse serum and T cells. *Immunochemistry*, **15**, 615–622.

Weber, K., and Osborn, M. (1969). The reliability of molecular weight determinations by dodecyl sulfate–polyacrylamide gel electrophoresis. *J. Biol. Chem.*, **244**, 4406–4412.

Weintraub, M., and Raymond, S. (1963). Antiserums prepared with acrylamide gel used as adjuvant. *Science*, **142**, 1677–1678.

Williams, C. A., and Chase, M. W. (1967). *Methods in Immunology and Immunochemistry* Volume 1. *Preparation of Antigens and Antibodies.* Academic Press, New York and London.

Willmer, E. N. (1965). *Cells and Tissues in Culture. Methods, Biology and Physiology* Volume 3, 1965–1966. Academic Press, London and New York.

Antibody as a Tool
Edited by J.J. Marchalonis and G. W. Warr
© 1982 John Wiley & Sons Ltd

Chapter 3

Purification of Antibodies

GREGORY W. WARR

*Department of Biochemistry, Medical University of South Carolina,
171 Ashley Avenue, Charleston, South Carolina 29425, USA*

I. INTRODUCTION

The basic reason for working with a purified antibody preparation is that one has a chemically defined agent of known specificity. This property removes many of the uncertainties caused by working with whole serum, in which the presence of unwanted activities must always be suspected.

It is reasonable to ask what is meant by the term 'purified antibody'. Because the term antibody implies reactivity towards a defined antigen, it is possible to have chemically pure immunoglobulin (Ig) that is not purified antibody. Because antibodies raised in any one individual to any antigen recognize a number of determinants on that antigen, a population of purified antibody molecules showing specificity for that antigen is still not homogeneous, strictly speaking. A homogeneous antibody would by definition, be monoclonal (i.e. the product of the clone resulting from antigenic stimulation of a single lymphocyte). Such monoclonal antibodies are produced by neoplastic lymphocytes (plasmacytomas), for some of which antigen specificity has been proven (Potter *et al.*, 1977), by hybridomas between a neoplastic lymphocyte and an antibody-secreting cell from an immunized animal (Chapter 9), and unusually by some animals under particular regimens of antigenic stimulation by a certain antigen. An example of this latter case is the immunization of strain A/J mice with the azobenzenearsonate hapten (Capra *et al.*, 1975; Marchalonis *et al.*, 1979). Examples of the heterogeneity to be seen with purified Igs and specifically purified antibodies, as detected by isoelectric focusing, are shown in Figure 1.

Assuming that one has an antiserum with the desired specificities, decisions on purification of the antibody present can only be made when it has been decided to what use the antibody will be put. If antiserum is to be used in bulk for such purposes as a precipitating agent in radioimmunoassay (Chapter 5), or for use as a diagnostic agent in many applications, purification of the antibody may be either unnecessary or impossible: unnecessary because the precision of

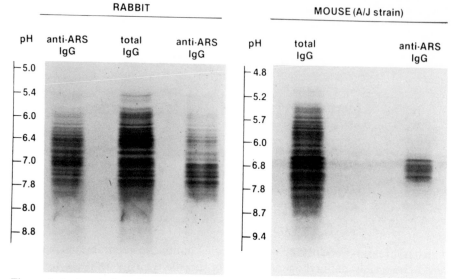

Figure 1. Isoelectric focusing of antibodies to the arsonate (ARS) hapten. Analytical thin-layer isoelectric focusing was carried out as described in Appendix IV. In the left portion of the figure are compared total normal rabbit IgG, and specific, purified antiARS IgG from two rabbits. It can be seen that the heterogeneity exhibited by the anti-ARS IgG preparations is considerable, but not as great as that of the total IgG. In contrast to this, the anti-ARS IgG produced by A/J mice (right portion of the figure) shows very restricted heterogeneity when compared with the total mouse IgG. This antibody was shown, by partial amino acid sequence analysis, to be apparently mono- (or bi-) clonal. (Marchalonis *et al.*, 1979)

the assay does not require a defined, pure reagent, the production of which is time consuming, labour intensive, and, like any other purification scheme, usually involves a net loss of antibody material; impossible because the antigens to which the antibody is directed cannot easily be isolated in the quantity and purity required for the subsequent steps of antibody purification (see below). This problem is particularly acute in the case of cell-surface antigens, and in these cases where purified antibody is required, considerable attention might be given to the preparation of antibody-producing hybridomas (Chapter 9).

It is also sometimes undesirable to prepare specific antibody when it is to undergo a subsequent modification, for example, conjugation with a fluorochrome or other labelling molecule (Chapters 6 and 7), or if it is to be coupled to a solid phase matrix for use in affinity chromatography (see below). These methods can result in a loss of antibody activity, usually by chemical coupling occurring in the antigen-binding site, and this, in turn, can result in an effective waste of the reagent. If an antibody is only available in small amounts or is precious for some other reason, many investigators will use a purified Ig preparation, which contains the specific antibodies, for these sorts of reactions.

Immunoglobulin fractions of serum are usually prepared by physicochemical methods, whereas specific antibodies nearly always have to be prepared by affinity methods (i.e. methods depending on the specificity of a biological reactivity to effect purification). There are exceptions, as will be mentioned below, particularly with reference to the use of staphylococcal protein-A to isolate certain Igs by a specific reaction with the Fc portion of the molecule [i.e. the C-terminal region distal to the antigen binding site (Chapter 1)].

In the following sections I will outline commonly used methods for the purification of Igs and antibodies by both physicochemical and affinity methods.

The purification of Igs is not only a stage in purifying antibody, but it provides an example of purification of an antigen (Chapter 2). I will only mention in passing the purification of relatively minor classes of mammalian Ig (such as IgM) since, although they are of interest to students of Igs, they are generally not the important Ig classes in experimentally produced sera. This position is occupied by the low molecular weight monomeric Igs, IgG in mammals, IgY in fowl, which on a mass basis are predominant both as serum Igs and antibodies (concentrations of around 10 mg of IgG per millilitre of serum being usual for many mammalian species).

II. PURIFICATION OF IMMUNOGLOBULINS

I will outline the commonly used methods for this purpose, giving some practical examples, and finally suggest some schemes, utilizing these methods, for practical use. Familiarity with such common techniques as dialysis, centrifugation to clarify solutions and measurement of protein concentration by absorbance at 280 nm or by the Folin-phenol reaction (Lowry *et al.* 1951, will be assumed. The removal of lipoproteins from serum (if present), which is essential before any further manipulations can be carried out, is described in Appendix VI to the preceding chapter.

A. Salt Precipitation

This technique exploits the differential solubility of proteins in the presence of different concentrations of certain ions, and is thought to induce precipitation by the effective dehydration of the proteins in solution. In the preparation of Igs, it is usually used on serum, as a first step in a purification scheme, to produce a crude fraction enriched for Igs and relatively free of albumin.

Precipitation is usually carried out using ammonium sulphate for mammalian sera (Heide and Schwick, 1978) and sodium sulphate for fowl sera (Benedict, 1967; Deutsch, 1967). To a large extent this seems to be the product of convention, but since the methods work well enough, most investigators use them in the established procedures. Some complications can arise; for example, ammonium ions can inactivate components of complement (Lachmann and Hobart, 1978) making sodium sulphate precipitation the method of choice if complement components are also being isolated. For ammonium sulphate precipitations of Igs, it is usual to use a final saturation of between 33% and 45%. This is best achieved by adding to the serum the calculated amount of a prepared saturated solution, slowly, and with constant stirring, and with all solutions at room temperature. The amount of saturated ammonium sulphate required is calculated by simple proportion, the final saturation being given (in per cent) by the formula $100x/(x + y)$, where y is the serum volume, and x is the volume of saturated ammonium sulphate required. If a protein solution already contains ammonium sulphate at a known initial saturation, and it is wished to increase this, the appropriate formula is:

$$\frac{\text{Final saturation} - \text{Initial saturation}}{100 - \text{Final saturation}} = x$$

For this purpose, saturation is expressed as a percentage, and x is the volume (in millilitres) of saturated ammonium sulphate which must be added to each millilitre of the solution to achieve the desired final saturation. To prepare a solution of saturated ammonium sulphate, an excess of the solid (800 g or slightly more) is added to 1000 ml of glass-distilled water. The dissolution of the ammonium sulphate can be speeded up by stirring and gently heating. The solution should be left at room temperature, at least overnight, and the undissolved ammonium sulphate can be left at the bottom of the vessel. The pH of the solution is best adjusted to neutrality with ammonium hydroxide and sulphuric acid. It is not recommended, as a general rule, that solid ammonium sulphate be added to serum or solutions of proteins because, unless this is carried out very slowly with adequate stirring, high local concentrations of salt occur and can result in the precipitation of unwanted proteins, especially albumin. The addition of solid ammonium sulphate is useful, however, when very large volumes are being dealt with, as a further dilution caused by addition of ammonium sulphate in solution may be undesirable.

Following the addition of ammonium sulphate, the precipitate is allowed to form, preferably overnight at room temperature, and is then harvested by centrifugation. Washing of the precipitate by ammonium sulphate solution of the same saturation is recommended by some investigators. However, the precipitate can pack tightly on centrifugation, and as an alternative to washing, repeated precipitations (up to a total of three) may be carried out. The precipitate can readily be dissolved (usually to one-half the starting volume of serum), in water or a buffer such as phosphate-buffered saline, or borate- or Tris-based buffers. Given in Appendix I is the composition of a Tris-based buffer, containing of NaCl, at pH 8.0, which we have found to be satisfactory for general use with Igs. Residual ammonium sulphate in the redissolved precipitate can be removed either by dialysis or by gel filtration using a matrix with suitable exclusion limits (see below).

For fowl serum, precipitation with sodium sulphate as described by Deutsch (1967) or Benedict (1967) is usually carried out; three sequential precipitations are performed, the first at 17% or 18% (w/v) sodium sulphate, the second two at 14% or 15% (w/v) sodium sulphate. The additions of sodium sulphate can be made with the solid or with solutions of appropriate concentration. Again, harvesting of the precipitate is carried out by centrifugation, and the redissolved precipitate has to be desalted, usually by dialysis.

Methods have been published that allow the selective isolation of some of the classes of mammalian Ig by means including salt precipitation. For example, the use of $ZnSO_4$ to precipitate human IgA in a purification scheme for IgG, IgM, and IgA has been reported by Vaerman *et al.*, (1963).

As an alternative to adding salt to bring about precipitation, salt can be removed from serum to induce precipitation. If a normal sample of mammalian serum is dialysed against water, a precipitate usually forms. With human serum this euglobulin precipitate contains both non-Ig and Ig molecules, especially IgM, which can then be further purified. Euglobulin precipitation is not always efficient and is infrequently used except as a first step in the isolation of IgM.

B. Gel Filtration

This method separates molecules according to their size (Porath, 1960; Porath and Flodin, 1959; Tiselius *et al.*, 1963) and is very easily and reproducibly applied to the separation of Igs. Strictly speaking, gel filtration separates molecules on the basis of their effective hydrodynamic radius, rather than molecular weight (Burnett *et al.*, 1976), but this consideration is not relevant to the preparative applications discussed here.

As usually carried out, gel filtration involves the application of a solution of proteins to a column packed with porous beads. Depending on the size of the pores in the beads molecules will be able to penetrate them to a variable degree during their passage through the column. Some proteins will be too large to enter the beads and will flow through the column without being retarded. Molecules of an intermediate size will enter the beads, to an extent depending on their size, and will be retarded to a degree inversely proportional to this parameter.

The volume in which totally excluded proteins are eluted is equal to the volume of buffer between the beads and is called the dead volume or void volume (V_o) of the column. The total volume of the column (V_t) is the volume included in the beads plus the void volume, and it can be measured as the volume in which a totally included small molecule or ion is eluted from the column.

The partition coefficient (K_{av}) for a molecule is calculated from the formula: $K_{av} = V_e - V_o/V_t - V_o$ where V_e is the volume in which elution of the molecule occurs. K_{av} shows an approximately linear plot against log molecular weight, as also does the value V_e (Andrews, 1964, 1965).

Columns are usually made of glass or plastic and can be made in a workshop or purchased from suppliers. Details on the preparation (and packing) of columns are included in Appendix II to this chapter.

C. Media for Gel Filtration

The most commonly used materials are the commercially available cross-linked dextran and agarose beads (trademarks Sephadex® and Sepharose®, respectively, of Pharmacia Fine Chemicals, Box 175 S-751 04 Uppsala 1, Sweden) or the polyacrylamide beads (trademark Bio-Gel P®) produced by Bio-Rad Laboratories, 2200 Wright Ave., Richmond, California 94804, USA, which also market agarose beads (Bio-gel A®). Both companies offer extensive ranges of these products, with different beads giving exclusion limits ranging from less than 1000 daltons to 150×10^6 daltons. On request these companies will also supply excellent technical information. Listed in Table 1 are the molecular weight separation ranges (for globular proteins) of the commercially available gel filtration media. The agarose gels are generally of a high porosity and are used to fractionate molecules with molecular weights of from around 100,000 up to submicroscopic particles such as viruses. In contrast, the dextran and polyacrylamide beads, depending on type chosen, separate molecules of up to approximately 500,000 molecular weight.

It is claimed that the polyacrylamide beads have a lower tendency to adsorb proteins non-specifically than do the dextrans. However, non-specific adsorption to gel filtration media has not proved a problem in my experience with preparing Igs. Both the dextran and polyacrylamide gels that fractionate at the top end of the molecular weight range (e.g. Sephadex G-200 and Bio-Gel P-300) have a tendency to compress and run slowly unless great care is taken in packing and running the column, particularly with regard to the head of hydrostatic pressure employed, which should be no more than 10 inches (about 25 cm) of water. However, the beads with the lower exclusion limits (especially the polyacrylamide beads) have high flow rates and good resistance to compression. For routine desalting of proteins by gel filtration products such as Bio-Gel P2, especially the lower mesh beads (i.e. of larger size), give very

Table 1. Media for gel filtration

Bead type	Effective molecular weight separation range for globular proteins or peptides[a]
Cross-linked dextran beads[b]	
Sephadex®	
G-10	0– 700
G-15	0– 1,500
G-25	1,000– 5,000
G-50	1,500– 20,000
G-75	5,000– 40,000
G-100	9,000–100,000
G-150	10,000–200,000
G-200	20,000–400,000
Polyacrylamide cross-linked dextran beads[b]	
Sephacryl®	
S-200	4,000–250,000
S-300	$5,000–1.5 \times 10^6$
Agarose and cross-linked agarose beads[b,c]	
Sepharose®	
6B or CL 6B	$10,000– 4 \times 10^6$
4B or CL 4B	$20,000–20 \times 10^6$
2B or CL 2B	$20,000–40 \times 10^6$
Bio-Gel®	
A - 0.5 M	$10,000–5 \times 10^5$
A - 1.5 M	$50,000–1.5 \times 10^6$
A - 5 M	$100,000–5 \times 10^6$
A - 15 M	$500,000–1.5 \times 10^7$
A - 50 M	$10^6–5 \times 10^7$
A - 150 M	$5 \times 10^6 - 5 \times 10^8$
Polyacrylamide beads[c]	
Bio-Gel®	
P-2	0– 1,800
P-4	0– 4,000
P-6	1,000– 6,000
P-10	2,000– 20,000
P-30	5,000– 40,000
P-60	10,000– 60,000
P-100	10,000–100,000
P-150	20,000–110,000
P-200	50,000–200,000
P-300	50,000–400,000

[*Table Cont.*

Table 1. *Contd.* Media for gel filtration

Bead Type	Effective molecular weight separation range for globular proteins or peptides[a]
	Polyacrylamide–agarose beads[d]
Ultrogel®	
AcA 54	6,000– 70,000
AcA 44	12,000–130,000
AcA 34	20,000–400,000
AcA 22	60,000–10^6

[a]These values are from manufacturers' information and may need revising for the separation of particular proteins.
[b]Pharmacia Fine Chemicals, 800 Centennial Avenue, Piscataway, New Jersey 08854, USA or (in UK) Prince Regent Rd., Hounslow, Middlesex TW3 1NE, UK.
[c]Bio-Rad Laboratories, 32nd and Griffen Avenue, Richmond, California 94804, USA or (in UK) Caxton Way, Watford, Herts, UK.
[d]LKB Instruments, 12221 Parklawn Drive, Rockville, Maryland 20852, USA, or (in UK) 232 Addington Road, South Croydon, Surrey CR2 8YD, UK.
See section outlining puirification schemes for recommendation of particular media for the separation and desalting of immunoglobulins.

fast and satisfactory operation. However, for the separation of proteins, a high flow rate and large bead size are not recommended. The finer the bead the better the resolution, and resolution of protein peaks is always better the slower the flow rate, simply because at high flow rates the protein species are unable to equilibrate between the excluded and included phases of the beads. Obviously there are practical limits to this principle, and flow rates from 1 ml to 10 ml per square centimetre column area per hour are usually employed; and the larger the pore size of the bead, the lower is the optimal flow rate, as far as the cross-linked dextran and polyacrylamide beads go. In preparative work with Igs, gel filtration can be used to desalt proteins and to separate Igs of different sizes (usually IgM and IgG) at any stage between or including the first and last steps of purification. Sephadex G-200 has traditionally been a medium of choice for separating Igs by gel filtration. When whole serum (human, for example) is resolved by this method, three major peaks are seen (Flodin and Killander, 1962). The first peak, at the void volume of the column, contains IgM (molecular weight 900,000) and α2-macroglobulin, both of which are excluded from the gel, and the first of the included peaks contains IgG, and the second included peak contains albumin and small globulins. IgA is found usually in the trough between the IgM and IgG peaks. None of these fractions provides a purified protein from serum, and further steps are always necessary. Filtration on Sephadex G-200 is adequate for the separation of IgG from IgM if the IgM fraction is to be discarded, but it is not entirely satisfactory if it is desired to purify IgM. The major problem is that aggregates of IgG (or any other proteins) can be large enough to be excluded

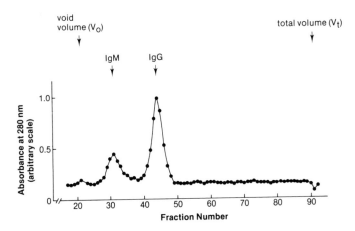

Figure 2. The separation, by gel filtration on Sepharose 6B, of canine IgM and IgG. Two major peaks are resolved when a mixture of dog IgM and IgG is fractioned on Sepaharose 6B, and these elute in almost identical positions to human IgM and IgG standards (arrowed). A peak of aggregated protein can be seen at the void volume (V_o). V_o and total volume (V_t) were estimated from the elution volumes of blue dextran and phenol red, respectively. (From the unpublished data of G. Warr and I. Hart)

from the gel, and hence, co-elute with the IgM. For this reason the use of a Sepharose 6B agarose gel might be preferred because both IgM and IgG are included (and resolved), whereas the large protein aggregates appear at the void volume of the column and can often be seen as a visibly opalescent fraction. Figure 2 illustrates the resolution that can be obtained when IgM and IgG are chromatographed on Sepharose 6B, and it shows the separation of the IgM from the aggregate peak at the void volume. IgA, if it is present, tends to chromatograph as a shoulder on the leading edge of the IgG peak. Sepharose 6B (or preferably the more stable cross-linked CL form) also has the advantage that it is resistant to compression in the columns and is, therefore, tolerant of high hydrostatic pressure, which allows a significantly faster flow rate than with Sephadex G-200. The same advantage applies to the polyacrylamide/agarose beads and the polyacrylamide cross-linked dextran beads (Table 1). These beads not only give a high flow rate, but excellent resolution also; and serious consideration should be given to using Sepharose 6B-CL, Sephacryl S-300, Biogel A 1.5 M or 5 M (Hannon *et al.*, 1975, Burgin-Wolf *et al.*, 1971) or Ultrogel AcA 22 or 34 for routine preparative gel filtration of Igs.

D. Electrophoresis

The variety and high resolution of electrophoretic techniques make them very powerful methods both for the preparation and for the analysis of proteins. The immensity of the field makes it impossible to deal adequately with it in this short section, but some of the more common applications in Ig preparation and characterization will be mentioned. A full discussion of the theory underlying the movement of charged particles in an electric field is beyond the scope of this chapter. The interested reader should refer to Cann (1968) and the whole of the excellent Chapter 6 in Williams and Chase (1968) for more detailed theoretical and experimental information.

Put simply, electrophoresis involves the separation of charged species by the application of an electric field to the solution in which they are present. The rate of migration of a particle in an electric field depends on its net charge, the strength of the electric field, the composition of the solvent, and the frictional coefficient of the particle, which in turn depends on the size and shape of the particle and the viscosity of the medium in which it is migrating. The net charge of any given molecule depends not only on such intrinsic factors as number and type of charged groups on the molecule, but also on the pH of the buffer in which the electrophoresis is being carried out. All proteins have an isoelectric point at which their net charge is zero; they are negatively charged at pHs above this point and positively charged at pHs below this point. A high ionic strength medium will tend to retard electrophoretic mobility for a number of reasons involving the interaction of the ions in the medium with the charge at the surface of the particle.

It is hoped that this brief outline will give some idea of the factors influencing the separation of proteins by electrophoresis and the rationale for the great variety of available techniques. Most investigators use well-established procedures for electrophoretic separation (or analysis) of Igs, and these generally yield satisfactory results.

The major electrophoretic methods for separation of proteins depend on: (1) electrophoretic mobility; (2) molecular sieving contributed by the matrix, e.g. polyacrylamide or starch gels in which the separation occurs; or (3) isoelectric point, in which electrophoresis occurs in a pH gradient and the proteins migrate to their isoelectric points (see Figure 1, and Williamson, 1978).

Electrophoretic Mobility

Electrophoretic mobility, as classically measured by moving-boundary electrophoresis (Tiselius, 1937) is a value which is of interest primarily to students of the physical chemistry of proteins. For preparative purposes, separation on the basis of electrophoretic mobility is more often carried out using the less precise but easier method of zone electrophoresis on supporting media. These media are usually granular and do not allow penetration of the buffer, thus effectively increasing the path migrating molecules must take. Typical media for block electrophoresis are potato starch or a copolymer of polyvinyl chloride and polyvinyl acetate (commercially available as Pevikon from Stockholms

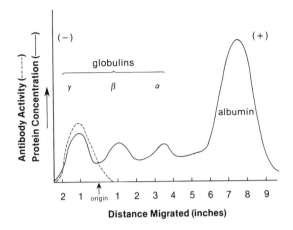

Figure 3. Starch block zone electrophoretic separation of serum. An idealized separation of human serum is shown, with albumin and α, β, and γ-globulin peaks identified. The peak of antibody activity denoted by the dotted line shows the region of the separation in which not only antibody activity, but also immunoglobulin classes, are to be found. As an alternative to antibody activity as a method of identifying immunoglobulins, techniques such as immunodiffusion (in agar gels) against antiglobulin sera can be utilized

Superfosfat Fabriks A. B., Stockholm, Sweden). In addition, the low exclusion limit Sephadex and Bio-Gel beads (Table 1) can be used, although these are porous to the buffer. Details on preparing and running a starch block are given in Appendix III. Preparative zone electrophoresis has the attraction that apparatus and methods are simple, cheap, and effective at producing a relatively purified γ-globulin fraction from whole serum, which can then be further fractionated. Figure 3 shows an idealized typical starch block electrophoretic separation of whole serum. Major peaks correspond to those seen on moving boundary electrophoresis (i.e. albumin, and α-, β- and γ-globulins, with subfractionation sometimes seen). Further details of preparative zone electrophoresis are given by Muller-Eberhard and Osterland (1968).

Molecular Sieving Effects

In this type of separation, the proteins migrate, under the influence of an electric field, through a medium which acts as a mesh, retarding the molecules according to their size. This method has great power to resolve molecules, but it is used primarily for analytical purposes. For preparative work, the major disadvantages are the capacity of the system and the difficulty of recovering proteins from within the medium in which electrophoresis has occurred. This latter problem can be overcome with somewhat complex apparatus which electrophoretically during the run. The media used have included starch gels (Smithies, 1955), polyacrylamide gels (Ornstein, 1964; Davis, 1964), and low-concentration polyacrylamide gels stabilized with agarose for the separation of large molecules (Peacock and Dingman, 1968). Buffers have been used with low pH, high pH, and in the presence or absence of denaturants such as urea (see Gordon, 1969, for a general text) or the anionic detergent sodium dodecyl sulphate (Weber and Osborn, 1969). It is impossible to do justice to all these methods here, and a fuller discussion of their use in fractionating Igs can be found in Stanworth and Turner (1978). For analytical purposes, polyacrylamide gel electrophoresis in the presence of sodium dodecyl sulphate (SDS) has exceptionally high powers of resolution. The dodecyl sulphate moieties bind to proteins (probably through both hydrophobic and ionic interactions) and denature them so that they assume an extended configuration. The dodecyl sulphate masks native charge on the molecule, and electrophoretic mobility through the gel matrix is inversely proportional to the molecular weight of the protein (Weber and Osborn, 1969). This property allows the construction of a straight line plot of relative mobility versus log molecular weight and can be used to estimate molecular weight. Glycosylation of a protein reduces the amount of dodecyl sulphate bound per unit mass and can lead to anomalous electrophoretic mobilities and incorrect molecular weight determinations (Segrest *et al.*, 1971). Because of its simplicity and high resolving power, SDS–polyacrylamide gel electrophoresis has become a widely used technique. This technique as used in the author's laboratory is described in Appendix I to Chapter 2.

Isoelectric Point

The inclusion of commercially available carrier ampholytes (e.g. from LKB Produkter, Pharmacia or Bio-Rad) in an electrophoretic medium results in the establishment of a pH gradient during electrophoresis. This arises because the ampholytes are selected for a (given) range of isoelectric points (pI), and they migrate to their respective pIs in the gradients of pH which they thereby establish. Proteins applied to the gel behave in a similar fashion, migrating to their isoelectric point in the pH gradient. Appendix IV describes analytical thin-layer isoelectric focusing as carried out in the author's laboratory (see Figure 1 for examples). Williamson (1978) descibes a range of analytical and preparative isoelectric focusing procedures.

Since charge heterogeneity is one of the characteristic properties of Igs, they exhibit a wide range of isoelectric points; and a pool of normal IgG from serum frequently resolves into 30 or more bands (Figure 1). The combined resolving power of isoelectric focusing and polyacrylamide gel electrophoresis in sodium dodecyl sulphate has been taken advantage of in various two-dimensional electrophoretic methods; one dimension being isoelectric focusing, the second being polyacrylamide gel electrophoresis in sodium dodecylsulphate-containing buffers (O'Farrell and O'Farrell, 1967). It seems unlikely that two-dimensional electrophoretic systems have any advantage over the one-dimensional methods for the routine preparation or characterization of Igs.

E. Ion Exchange Chromatography

The selective adsorption and desorption of proteins to an insolubilized matrix by charge interaction is a step frequently used in the purification of Igs. Ion exchange matrices bearing positively charged groups (anion exchangers) or negatively charged groups (cation exchangers) are commercially available. However, for Ig separation, the weak anion exchangers bearing the basic diethylaminoethyl (DEAE) functional groups are almost universally used. These can be purchased linked to different matrices: to Sephadex®, Sepharose® and cellulose beads from Pharmacia Fine Chemicals; linked to fibrous or microcrystalline cellulose from Whatman (W. and R. Balston, Ltd, Springfield Mill, Maidstone, Kent, England or H. Reeve Angel Inc., 9 Bridewell Place, Clifton, New Jersey, USA); and linked to agarose beads or fibrous cellulose from Bio-Rad Laboratories. In practice there is frequently little to choose between these various forms, although they vary in bead porosity, flow rate, and capacity, and the Sephadex-based exchangers show considerable changes in bead volume depending on pH or ionic strength of the buffer. Whichever type of support is chosen, the functional applications for Ig fractionation are very similar. The ion exchanger is precycled with acid and alkali, according to the manufacturer's instructions, usually a wash with 0.5 M HCl followed by a wash with 0.5 M NaOH (this step being unnecessary with some forms of DEAE–cellulose, and DEAE–Sephadex/Sepharose supplied by Whatman and Pharmacia). The exchanger can then be equilibrated in buffer of the pH at which it is to be used, usually at a high molar concentration and with a number of changes. This equilibration is complete when the pH of the buffer remains stable, and the exchanger can then be washed into buffer of the desired starting molarity. With the fibrous and microcrystalline celluloses, 'fines' should be removed by allowing a suspension of the exchanger to settle under gravity and then decanting and discarding the supernatant fluid with suspended fine particulate material. The exchanger is then ready for use, either for column chromatography or batch-wise procedures. An example of a batch-wise procedure used to prepare an IgG fraction of horse serum uncontaminated with IgM is given by James (1973), but in general column methods offer opportunities for improved resolution. Packing a column is essentially as described for gel filtration (Appendix II). Size of the column has to be determined on the basis of sample size and capacity of the exchanger, and it is best determined empirically for any given case. A rule of thumb is that for fibrous DEAE–cellulose ion exchangers, 1–2 g dry weight will suffice for 1 ml of serum. For the bead type (Sephadex/Sepharose) DEAE exchangers, functional capacity depends on the porosity of the bead, which limits access of proteins to the internal charged groups of bead. Some degree of temperature control is useful with ion exchange separations, which are often carried out in a cold (4-6 °C) room. For anion exchange chromatography, it is better to use a cation-based buffer (e.g. Tris) than an anion-based buffer (e.g. phosphate) to avoid participation of the buffer ions in the ion exchange process. In practice, however, this principle can, and has been, ignored, in that it is common practice to separate Igs on DEAE exchangers using phosphate buffers, at constant pH but increasing molarity, to elute proteins. For Ig separation, the column is packed in a buffer around pH 8.0, of low molarity (e.g. 0.01 M) against which the protein sample has also been dialysed. Note that during dialysis against low molarity buffers, euglobulin precipitation may occur. At pH 8.0, the gamma globulins have the lowest charge of the serum proteins, and at this or even a lower pH, IgG can often by eluted from the column as the only protein not bound in the starting buffer (Levy and Sober, 1960; Patrick and Virella, 1978). Bound proteins can be eluted by increasing the ionic strength of the buffer (either the buffering species or by adding NaCl) or by changing the pH, or both (Sober and Peterson, 1958; Tombs *et al.*, 1961; Fahey *et al.*, 1958). A gradient elution is often preferable to a stepwise elution, since it helps to prevent the tailing of a protein peak during elution. With increasing salt concentrations or declining pH, serum proteins other than the unbound IgG elute. Bound IgG subclasses (if any, and depending on species), IgA, and IgM elute, in that order, but are usually contaminated with other serum proteins (Fahey *et al.*, 1958; Fahey, 1967). The column fractions then require either recycling or alternative purification steps to yield a homogeneous preparation. Suggested buffers for Ig separation include phosphate pH 8.0, molarity 0.01 to 0.3 M, or Tris–HCl, 0.02 to 0.3 M, pH 8.0 using either Tris or NaCl to form the gradient of ionic strength.

Gradients, as mentioned before, can be stepwise (manually produced by changing the eluting buffer), linear (using two identical connected vessels), or concave (using conical and spherical vessels to generate the gradient) (Sober and Peterson, 1958). If more complex or irregular gradients are desired, these can be generated using an ultrograd gradient maker available from LKB Instruments, and a cheaper but quite versatile apparatus for constructing complex gradients is described by Sober and Peterson (1959). The elution profiles of Igs and other serum proteins from DEAE exchangers vary considerably from species to species (e.g. this method is not very satisfactory with mouse IgG; Fahey, 1967), and it will be necessary for investigators to modify conditions according to the success of their separations. A reasonable starting point for a separation on DEAE exhanger would be to use a linear gradient of molarity 0.01 or 0.02 to 0.3, using either a Tris–HCl or a phosphate buffer, pH 8.0, with a total elution volume of between 50 and 100 times the starting volume (if serum or a concentrated protein solution is to be applied to the column).

F. Centrifugation

The sedimentation of proteins in solution by high speed centrifugation is the method of choice for accurate molecular-weight determination by a number of methods (Svedberg and Pederson, 1940; Williams, 1963) and has also been used to separate, on a preparative scale, IgM (MW 900,000) from IgG (MW 150,000) (van Dalen *et al.*, 1967). However, the use of ultracentrifugation in such procedures has almost entirely been superseded by other techniques of size separation, such as gel filtration. As a preparative instrument for use with Igs, the centrifuge has been reduced to the status of a workhorse, used for such tasks as spinning out salt precipitates or clarifying protein solutions.

G. Isolation of Igs by the use of Protein-A

The A protein incorporated into the cell wall of some strains of *Staphylococcus aureus* has the property of binding strongly and specifically to the Fc portion of certain mammalian Ig classes and subclasses, especially IgG (Forsgren and Sjoquist, 1966; Kronvall and Williams, 1969; Kronvall *et al.*, 1970a, b; Goding, 1978). This property has rendered it extremely useful in such applications as visualizing antibody reactions (see Goding, 1978) replacing antiglobulin antibody as a second reagent in immune precipitation (Kessler, 1975, 1976), and radioimmunoassay (Jonsson and Kronvall, 1974). This has made the use of protein-A a method of choice in the isolation of those Igs to which it binds (Goding, 1978).

Protein-A can be prepared from the culture of mutants of *S. aureus* which fail to incorporate it into their cell walls, or alternatively, it can be purchased from Pharmacia Fine Chemicals, either as a purified protein or already covalently coupled to Sepharose® CL-4B. For the average laboratory, this latter form is probably the most satisfactory if affinity preparation of Igs is being contemplated. With care, a single column of protein-A–Sepharose can be used repeatedly for the purification of Igs from a variety of mammalian sera, an advantage which helps to offset the initial cost of this reagent.

Listed in Table 2 are those Igs, from a variety of mammalian species, which bind to protein-A. The preparation and use of a simple column for affinity chromatography with protein-A–Sepharose is described in Appendix II. The main attractions of this method are its simplicity, speed, and the purity of the product. In a single step, Igs can be prepared from serum, free of non-immunoglobulin contamination above a trace level. Protein-A followed by another preparative step (e.g. ion exchange chromatography) can ensure

Table 2. Binding of mammalian immunoglobulins to protein A

Species	Class of Ig	Notes
Mouse	IgG2a, IgG2b, IgG3	Some IgM and IgGl are bound under certain conditons. (Kronvall *et al.*, 1970a, b; Mackenzie *et al.*, 1977; Ey *et al.*, 1978)
Rat	IgGl, IgG2c	IgG2a and IgG2b not bound. Some IgM and IgA bound (Medgyesi *et al.*, 1978)
Guinea pig	IgG1, IgG2	All IgG bound (Forsgren, 1968)
Rabbit	IgG	All IgG bound, traces of IgM bound (Goding, 1976)
Sheep, cow, goat	IgG	Not all IgG bound (Kessler, 1976; Goudswaard *et al.*, 1978)
Dog	IgG, IgM, IgA	Virtually all serum, IgM, IgA, and IgG may be bound by protein-A. (Goudswaard *et al.*, 1978; Warr and Hart, 1979)
Man	IgG1, IgG2, IgG4	Some IgM and IgA also binds (Saltvedt and Harboe,, 1976; Hjelm, 1975)
Echidna	IgG1, IgG2	(Marchalonis *et al.*, 1978)

virtually 100% purity of IgG. The major drawback to the method is that not all Ig classes and subclasses bind (Table 2). For example, of the four human IgG subclasses, IgG3 does not bind (Kronvall and Williams, 1969) and of the four murine IgG subclasses, IgG1 was reported not to bind (Kronvall *et al.*, 1970a). However, it has recently been suggested that mouse IgG1 will bind to protein-A if the pH is elevated to 8.0 (Ey *et al.*, 1978). In the rabbit, protein-A reacts with all the detectable IgG antibody in the serum (Goding, 1978), and in the dog, the majority of serum IgM and IgG molecules react with protein-A and can then easily be separated by gel filtration (Warr and Hart, 1979) Both the IgG subclasses in the guinea pig react with protein-A, but in the rat, goat, sheep, and horse not all the IgG subclasses will bind (Goding, 1978; Goudswaard *et al.*, 1978), a problem which can lead to poor recovery of antibody activity.

In using protein-A–Sepharose to purify Ig from serum, the general method outlined below for affinity chromatography can be used. However, the affinity between protein-A and IgG is usually very high, and this can allow the serum to be run through the column at a faster speed than is normal for affinity chromatography (i.e. 5 ml/hour). However, if in doubt the operator should always check the efficiency of the removal of IgG from the serum by running it a second time over the column, after it has been regenerated. To elute bound

IgG from protein-A–Sepharose, it is common to use an unbuffered solution of 0.15 M NaCl, 0.58% (v/v) acetic acid in water. This has a pH around 3.5 and usually gives an efficient elution. Other eluting buffers can be used (see below) and the choice of such buffers depends not only on efficiency of elution but also on destruction of antibody activity that can occur. The latter is unpredictable and variable between different antibody preparations.

After elution of bound Ig from the protein-A–Sepharose, the column should be washed in physiological buffer (about five column volumes), after which it is ready for further use.

H. Suggested Schemes for the Purification of Igs

The following outlines are intended to be rough guides only, and any purification scheme that is satisfactory can be devised or used. My definition of a satisfactory purification scheme would be one with an acceptable yield of the desired Ig in a purified state. Depending on the purpose for which it is required, minimal criteria for purity of an Ig would usually be a single arc on immunoelectrophoresis against an antiserum made to the starting whole serum, and homogeneity by polyacrylamide gel electrophoresis in sodium do-decylsulphate-containing buffers (see Chapter 2 for criteria of purity).

I. IgG

In species where a substantial portion of IgG binds to protein-A, this method is unequivocally recommended for use directly with serum. Suitable species for this approach might be mouse, rabbit, guinea pig, dog, and man. In some species, other classes of Ig, such as IgM or IgA, bind to a greater or lesser degree to protein-A. The IgG can usually be separated from these by using gel filtration, following elution from the protein-A.

In some species, a variable proportion of IgG will not bind to protein-A. A common alternative approach to the isolation of IgG that can be used in these cases is salt precipitation (e.g. 33% saturated ammonium sulphate) followed by ion exchange chromatography on DEAE–cellulose. This method has been used for human IgG (Patrick and Virella, 1978) and can be used equally well for some other species. If necessary, a final step of gel filtration can be added. An alternative method for the preparation of IgG is to separate serum by zone electrophoresis (e.g. on starch) and follow this by gel filtration. This latter method has the advantage that IgM is one of the by-products, but it may still be necessary to purify the IgG in a further step, such as ion-exchange chromatography.

J. IgM

IgM often occurs at a low concentration in serum. If desired, its level can be raised experimentally or by choice of appropriate animals. Examples of these approaches are the use of trypanosome-infected rabbits (Maarten *et al.*, 1978) or old mice of the strain NZB, which tend to have elevated serum IgM levels. Unless substantial amounts of serum IgM bind to protein-A (e.g. as in the dog), the usual method of preparation of IgM is to take the cathodal, Ig-containing fraction from a zone electrophoretic separation and subject this to gel filtration (e.g. on Sepharose 6B).

III. PURIFICATION OF SPECIFIC ANTIBODIES: AFFINITY CHROMATOGRAPHY

For the purification of antibodies, the application of affinity chromatography involves the coupling of an antigen to an insoluble matrix, the binding of the antibody to the now insolubilized antigen, and finally its elution in a (hopefully) pure form. Each of these stages, and some of the problems involved, are considered below.

A. Choice of Matrix for Insolubilising Antigen

The first matrix widely used for the covalent coupling of antigen was cellulose (Fuchs and Sela, 1978). This material has a tendency to quite high non-specific binding of non-antibody proteins and is no longer in wide use. The commonly used matrices are the beaded agarose and polyacrylamide gel filtration media. The polyacrylamide beads have the lowest tendency to non-specific absorption but also have a low porosity which limits their capacity to bind antibody. This is because much of the antigen coupled on the internal surfaces of the bead is rendered unavailable, by steric interference, to bind antibody. The agarose matrices are probably the most commonly used supports for antigens in affinity chromatography, although in certain applications non-specific binding has been observed (Haustein and Warr, 1976). This is not usually a problem, however, in the routine preparation of antibodies by affinity chromatography. A potentially more important problem involves the use of cyanogen bromide (CNBr) to activate agarose for the coupling of antigens containing a primary amino group. The covalent linkage thus formed between the agarose and antigen is unstable, and leakage of the antigen from the column occurs continuously (Parikh *et al.*, 1974; Parikh and Cuatrecasas, 1977). This rate of leakage is often inversely proportional to the size of the coupled antigen, probably because multiple linkages occur with larger molecules (assuming availability of NH_2 groups) which then serve to stabilize the attachment. With most protein antigens the rate of leakage is generally sufficiently low so as not to prove a significant problem, but nevertheless it should always be borne in mind.

B. Reactive Groups on the Matrix

The availability of reactive groups on the antigen determines the chemical form in which the matrix is prepared. Antigens are usually coupled by means of amino, carboxyl, or hydroxyl groups; but they can also be reacted via sulphhydryl groups or through phenolic groups by means of a diazonium derivative. A given matrix is usually either directly activated by a reagent so that it is then available for immediate coupling with an appropriate antigen, or else it is substituted with, e.g. amino or carboxyl groups, so that a subsequent coupling step can be carried out simply.

C. Agarose

Activation of agarose beads by CNBr to give a derivative reactive with amino groups on an antigen is the most commonly used method, and despite the drawbacks mentioned above, it generally proves satisfactory for most immunoadsorbent work. A simple version of this method is given in Appendix V.

Agarose gels can be converted quite simply to the carboxymethyl form (Inman, 1975), giving a COOH group on the matrix which can then be coupled to NH_2 groups on an antigen using carbodiimide. Alternatively, NH_2 groups can be introduced by reacting the carboxymethyl groups (with carbodiimide) with a diamine (Inman, 1975). The resulting free amino group on the matrix can then be reacted by a variety of methods. For example, carbodiimides can be used to couple to COOH groups on antigens, and the NH_2 group is also available for reaction with isothiocyanate and diazonium derivatives of antigens. Antigens coupled to agarose by this method are bound by relatively stable covalent linkages. Agaroses can be purchased from Pharmacia or Bio-Rad already substituted with carboxyl or amino groups, although these are usually on spacer 'arms' of differing lengths, for investigators who wish to couple a small molecule at some distance from the matrix (usually to avoid problems of steric hindrance). The use of spacer groups can lead to additional problems, e.g. in terms of hydrophobic interactions between the spacer and molecules other than those it is wished to isolate (O'Carra *et al.*, 1974a,b). The Affi-gel® derivatives available from Bio-Rad are connected to the agarose matrix by the more stable ether linkages, whereas the CH— and AH—Sepharose® available from Pharmacia are derived from CNBr activated agarose and hence are more liable to suffer from significant leakage.

Both manufacturers (Pharmacia and Bio-Rad) supply agarose beads with other available reactive groups or in an activated form for immediate coupling. For the applications of coupling methods used with these agarose derivatives, readers are referred to the manufacturer's information. Inman (1975) gives methods for introducing NH_2 and COOH groupings into agarose matrices, and Appendix II of Chapter 2 gives a simple method for carbodiimide coupling which can be used with these derivatives.

D. Polyacrylamide beads

Inman and Dintzis (1969) give details on the conversion of polyacrylamide beads (Bio-Gel P® from Bio-Rad) to useful aminoethyl and hydrazide derivatives and illustrate how these can be used to couple, by stable covalent bonds, molecules containing a variety of reactive groups. Carboxylated, aminoethylated, and hydrazide derivatives of polyacrylamide beads are also available from Bio-Rad. Proteins containing free NH_2 groups can also be coupled directly to polyacrylamide beads using the bifunctional reagent glutaraldehyde (Weston and Avrameas, 1971; Ternynk and Avrameas, 1972).

E. Binding of Antibody to an Immunoadsorbent

The antigen, bound to the chosen matrix, is packed into a column. A simple column can be constructed in the laboratory (Appendix II) or purchased. Antiserum should be free of lipid (Appendix VI, Chapter 2) and suspended particulate matter. The latter can be removed by centrifugation or filtration. Before the antiserum is passed over the column, the column should be prewashed with the chosen eluting buffer (see below) to remove any antigen not bound in a stable manner, and then washed again in physiological buffer. As a general principle, the rate of flow of antiserum through an immunoadsorbent column should not exceeed 5 ml per hour. After the antiserum has been passed over the immunoadsorbent, washing of the column is carried out with buffer (e.g. Tris-buffered saline, Appendix I), until protein is no longer detectable in the effluent. The easiest way to determine protein concentration in the effluent is to measure optical density at 280 nm.

F. Elution of Antibody from an Immunoadsorbent

Elution can in principle be specific (i.e. by competition with homologous antigen) or non-specific (i.e. by interference with the antigen/antibody reaction). Specific elution is usually only possible with small antigens (e.g. haptens) which can then be separated from the eluted antibody by dialysis. However, elution by non-specific means is usually resorted to, and is generally accomplished by alteration of the pH (most frequently downwards) or by the use of chaotropic ('chaos inducing') ions such as (sodium) thiocyanate at 3.5 M, or denaturants such as urea at 4-6 M. The composition of some eluting buffers is given in Appendix VI. The choice of buffer depends frequently on empirical observation. Any of the eluting buffers described denature the antibody and can result in loss of activity when the antibody is renatured (generally by dialysis against physiological buffers). Urea can chemically modify Igs, in that cyanate (formed in the urea solution) can cause carbamylation of amino groups. This is not usually a problem unless amino acid sequence analysis is contemplated. Whether or not a particular buffer will irreversibly destroy the biological activity of a given antibody is unpredictable and has to be determined in each case. Klein (1972) has reported on the relative efficiencies of a number of eluting buffers, in terms of recovery both of protein and activity, with rabbit anti-human IgG antibodies. Whatever the eluting buffer used, it is generally recommended that the antibody spend the least possible time in the potentially denaturing conditions of the eluant. If elution is carried out at extremes of pH, adjustment of pH to physiological values can readily by achieved. However, thiocyanate and urea are usually removed by gel filtration or dialysis.

The quantitative recovery of protein from an immunoadsorbent column can vary. Some adsorbed antibody becomes bound very tightly, presumably by secondary interactions with the column matrix, and is difficult to elute; but with subsequent use, these high affinity sites become more fully occupied, and recovery from the column improves. The presence of residual bound antibody on a column, coupled with potential ligand leakage, makes it important to prewash an immunoadsorbent with eluting buffer, then physiological buffer, before *every* use.

APPENDIX I. PREPARATION OF Tris–HCl BUFFER, pH 8.0

This buffer contains Tris (hydroxymethyl) amino methane at 0.05 M and NaCl at 0.15 M. The following method gives 10 litres of buffer.

A. Reagents (analytical grade)

Tris   60.57 g
Concentrated HCl, about 30 ml
NaCl   87.65g
The NaCl and Tris are dissolved in 1–2 litres distilled water and about 20 ml HCl added. The pH is then carefully titrated to 8.0 by the addition of concentrated HCl dropwise (up to 6 or 7 ml may be required). The resulting solution is made up to 10 litres with distilled water.

To preserve the buffer, 0.5 g of merthiolate (also known as thiomersal and thimerosal) can be added per 10 litres. Alternative preservatives are Hibitane (chlorhexidine) at 0.002% or sodium azide at 0.02%.

APPENDIX II. COLUMN CHROMATOGRAPHY

The three main forms of column chromatography used in the preparation of antibodies are gel filtration, ion exchange, and affinity chromatography. Gel filtration demands the greatest attention to column design, preparation and packing of matrix, and running conditions. Ion exchange and affinity chromatography frequently separate on all or none adsorbed/desorbed basis, and these procedures can often be carried out using coarser and cheaper apparatus.

A. Choice of Columns

1. Gel Filtration

This can be used for desalting proteins or for separating mixtures of proteins. For desalting, a matrix is chosen which excludes the proteins and includes the salts. Usually G-25 Sephadex® or P-2 Bio-Gel® of the coarsest mesh size and fastest flow rates are chosen. Column size depends on the matrix chosen and the volume of sample. Prepacked columns which will handle 0.5 ml or slightly larger volumes are commercially available (e.g. Quick-Sep™ columns from Isolab Inc., Akron, Ohio). For larger volumes, simple columns can be made from the barrels of disposable plastic syringes. After removing the plunger, fine-mesh nylon netting can be trapped in the bottom of the syringe barrel using either a tightly-fitting rubber 0-ring or the rubber end of the plunger (through which a hole has to be drilled). The required amount of gel can then be poured directly into the syringe barrel. A rubber stopper pierced with a needle or glass tube can be fitted into the syringe top and attached with tubing to a buffer reservoir to give continuous flow under gravity.

The separation of proteins by gel filtration requires more precise attention to column design. A column 0.5–1.0 m long and 2–3 cm in diameter is usually satisfactory for handling a few millilitres of serum or up to 100 mg protein. Commercially available columns offer not only the advantages of convenience but also have some real benefits such as fittings and flow adaptors which: (1) minimize dead volume in the column, in which mixing could occur and reduce resolution; and (2) enable one to apply sample and buffer immediately to the gel bed without disturbing it, or having to remove stoppers from the column, or pipette buffer and sample on to the surface of the gel. Whether these benefits justify the costs is a question to which no clear answer can be given. Simple columns consisting of a glass tube of appropriate diameter with a sintered glass disk (to support the gel) at the bottom, and a stopcock on the outlet, can be purchased cheaply (or made in a workshop), and with care these can be perfectly adequate. An alternative cheap column is one in which the sintered glass disk is replaced by large glass beads and glass wool to support the gel, and the stopcock is replaced by a clamp on a piece of flexible tubing. Such a column tends to have a large dead volume and can be recommended only for investigators in straitened circumstances. With these simpler sorts of columns, a head of buffer has to be maintained above the gel bed, and continuous flow is provided by placing a rubber stopper (pierced with tubing attached to a buffer reservoir) in the top of the column. For columns run under gravity, rather than by use of a pump (which is definitely the best and recommended method), a Mariotte flask is recommended, especially for the gels which have a high water regain (e.g. Sephadex G-200 or Bio-Gel P-300) and require accurate control of the low pressure head. If the pressure is too high, the column packs down and ceases flowing; if it is too low, the column will slow down or even cease to flow.

2. Ion exchange and Affinity Chromatography

For these, any of the above columns can be used as required. If subtle chromatography is to be performed by ion exchange (e.g. development of the column with starting buffer taking advantage of slight differences in the strength of interaction with the exchanger, rather than using a gradient to elute proteins more rapidly in an all or none fashion), then one of the more sophisticated columns is recommended. For affinity chromatography, a column made from the barrel of a disposable syringe can frequently be entirely satisfactory.

B. Preparation of the Column Medium

For gel filtration, some media come preswollen. These media include the agarose, agarose/acrylamide, and dextran polyacrylamide beads. These media all have the properties of high mechanical resistance to packing down, a high flow rate, and high resolution. It is recommended that they be used whenever possible. Because they are preswollen, they merely need to be washed in the appropriate buffer and degassed under vacuum before pouring the column. When hydrating the dried beads, heating them on a boiling water bath is recommended, as this hastens swelling, aids sterilization, and degasses. Vigorous stirring, which can break the beads, is not recommended. Adherence to manufacturer's recommendations is advisable.

For ion exchange chromatogaphy, some media are preswollen. The preparation of ion exchangers is briefly described in the body of the text, but the manufacturers usually supply comprehensive information.

C. Packing a Column

All media should be degassed and packed at the temperature at which the column is to be run. The following procedure can be followed for both gel filtration and ion exchange media, although the greatest care should be taken with packing columns for gel filtration to ensure even settling of the beads. The medium to be packed is made into a slurry by the addition of buffer. The slurry should not be so thick that it traps air bubbles. The bed volume of the medium should be predetermined in order to allow the desired column to be packed in one procedure. The column is run through with buffer, making sure that the dead volume spaces do not contain trapped air. The outlet is closed, and it is not necessary to leave more than a few millilitres of buffer in the column. An extension or funnel is added to the column since the volume of the slurry can be up to 150% of that of the final packed bed volume of gel. The slurry is carefully poured into the column, which should be clamped vertically, and after a few centimetres of gel have settled the column outlet is opened. The hydrostatic pressure during packing should be controlled for those high-water regain gel filtration media which pack down and cease to flow if the pressure is too high (see body of text). Once the medium has settled, three or four column volumes of buffer should be run through at operating pressure. If a flow adaptor is not used, the surface of the medium can be protected by a disk of nylon netting or filter paper.

D. Sample Application

If a flow adaptor is not used, a sample is loaded by allowing the buffer to drain into the gel bed, applying the sample (clarified by centrifugation or filtration) to the surface of the gel and allowing it to drain into the gel bed. The resolution of the run will be improved if the sides of the column are then rinsed with a small volume of buffer, which is allowed to drain into the gel before the head of buffer is re-added to the top of the column. A column should never be allowed to run dry during loading or at any other stage.

If it is wished to avoid draining the top of the column to load the sample, an alternative application procedure can be used, in which the sample is applied through the head of buffer on top of the column. For this purpose, the sample must be more dense than the buffer. If necessary, reagents which will not affect the particular separation can be added to the sample. These include glycerol, sucrose, and salts (the latter cannot be used for ion exchange). The sample is then taken up into a long-nosed pipette or a syringe with an extension of fine plastic tubing. The end of the pipette or tubing is held a few millimetres above the top of the column bed, and the sample is carefully expelled. Care not to disturb the sample/buffer interface should be taken when withdrawing the pipette or syringe.

APPENDIX III. ZONE ELECTROPHORESIS ON STARCH BLOCKS

Potato starch for block electrophoresis can be purchased from most scientific supply companies as a dry powder. This usually needs repeated washings with distilled water before it is fit to use. The starch is suspended in distilled water and allowed to settle, after which the water is decanted. This procedure is

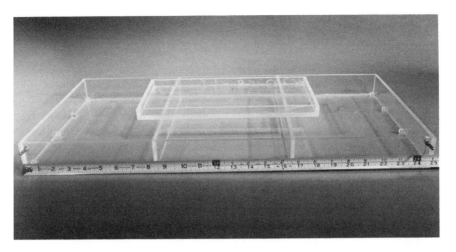

Figure 4. Apparatus for zone electrophoresis in blocks. The tray to contain starch and sample resting on top of the buffer tank, is shown in running position (but without starch, sample, or wicks). Note the electrode connections to the two outer chambers, which are to be filled with buffer for the run. All apparatus is made from plexiglass, and the electrodes from platinum wire

repeated until the surface of the settled starch and the supernatant fluid are clean. Electrophoresis is carried out in Barbital (diethyl barbiturate) buffer 0.05 M, pH 8.6 (0.63 g barbital, 4.87 g sodium barbital, 1.90 g sodium acetate, made up to 1 litre with distilled water); and after the starch has been dried on a Buchner funnel, it is resuspended in this buffer. A tray (Figure 4) constructed of perspex, plexiglass, or other suitable non-conducting material, approximately 30 cm × 20 cm × 1.5 cm, is suitable for the electrophoresis of up to 20 ml of serum. Blocks can be scaled down in size as desired.

Wicks, the width of the tray, and cut from uncoloured absorbent paper or filter paper, are soaked in buffer and pressed against each end of the tray before the starch is poured in as the thickest slurry manageable. Paper towels are gently laid on the surface of the poured starch to adsorb excess buffer as the starch settles, and these are replaced by dry ones as necessary. The block should be quite dry to the touch before loading the sample. If this drying procedure results in the level of the starch falling below the top of the tray, more may be added and dried out as before. To level the surface of the block, a ruler or similar straight edge is repeatedly moved across the entire length of the tray until all irregularities are smoothed or removed, leaving a flat surface.

The origin is positioned slightly to the cathodal side of centre. At the origin, a cut is made with a spatula across the width of the block to within 1 cm of each side and reaching to the bottom of the tray. The width of the trough is increased to about 1–2 mm by gently moving the spatula from side to side along the cut.

Before loading, the serum is clarified by centrifugation or filtration. A

Pasteur pipette is used to apply the sample slowly across the length of the trough. The trough is repeatedly filled until the whole sample is loaded.

When loading, a paper towel is placed about 1–2 cm on either side of the trough, to absorb the displaced buffer. To avoid absorbing the sample with the towels, they are moved further away from the origin as the sample penetrates the starch. Before the last of the serum is absorbed, the walls of the trough are gently pressed together, and the surface of the block is smoothed. The block is now entirely covered with thin polyethylene food wrap. The trapping of air bubbles must be avoided, and the plastic film is then securely taped to the bottom of the block.

A dye marker is provided by piercing the plastic film and starch block at the origin with a needle previously dipped into Bromophenol Blue powder. Each wick is placed in an electrophoresis tank containing barbital buffer, the tank nearest the origin being connected to the cathode. If it is not possible to use tanks such as those sold for use with, for example, immunoelectrophoresis, they can be simply constructed in a workshop from plexiglass or similar material (e.g. Figure 4).

The block is now run at 400–500 V, at 4 °C. The current is usually around 15–25 mA, depending on the dryness of the starch (the wetter the starch, the higher the current).

A block of this size with a capacity for 20 ml of serum typically takes about 60 hours to run. The run should be stopped when the Bromophenol Blue has migrated to within 5 cm of the anodal end of the block.

To elute proteins from the block, sequential 1 cm slices of starch are cut from the block starting at either end. These slices are thoroughly suspended in 10 ml of buffer (e.g. phosphate or Tris at physiological salt levels), and the starch is allowed to settle. Protein can be detected in the supernatant fluid either by optical density at 280 nm, or by the Folin method (Lowry *et al.*, 1951). Igs can be detected by immunodiffusion (Chapter 4). A typical distribution of Ig in the cathodal fractions of starch block separation is shown in Figure 3. Those fractions containing the Ig are pooled and the starch is resuspended, following which the supernatant fluid is separated from the starch by filtration under vacuum using a Buchner funnel. The starch can be washed briefly with physiological buffer to recover as much protein as possible. The filtered fluid is then ready for further fractionation, usually after concentration by any suitable method, e.g. vacuum dialysis.

APPENDIX IV. ANALYTICAL ISOELECTRICAL FOCUSING IN POLYACRYLAMIDE GELS

This can be carried out using either rod gels or a thin layer of acrylamide in the form of a slab. The former method will usually allow the loading of a larger sample, but a run with a slab gel can be completed much more quickly; and many samples can be run in the one slab gel for which it is easy to determine the pH gradient. For rod gel isoelectric focusing, one can use essentially the same apparatus as for rod SDS–polyacrylamide gels (Appendix I, Chapter 2). The method I shall describe here for isoelectric focusing on a thin slab of polyacrylamide is most easily carried out using commercially available equipment (e.g. the LKB 2117 Multiphor, from LKB Produkter AB S-161 25 Broma 1 Sweden). The technique described here involves polymerizing the gel on a thin glass plate, which then is placed on a plate cooled by flowing cold water during the run. Without such cooling, the run cannot be carried out so quickly; so if the investigator uses, designs, or builds alternative apparatus, this is a point to be considered.

A. Equipment

Unless otherwise specified, this is a part of the LKB 2117 Multiphor.

Glass Plates 26 cm × 12.5 cm × 0.3 cm, 26 × 12.5 cm × 0.1 cm.

Rubber Gasket 2 mm thick, 5 mm wide, to run around the circumference of the glass plates. This gasket is to be trapped between one thick and one thin plate for pouring the gel. It is cut at one corner to allow the gel to be poured, and the apparatus is clamped together with metal clips (binder clips or bulldog clips will suffice).

Glass Cooling Plate As supplied with the LKB 2117 Multiphor, this measures 26 × 12.5 cm, has a ground glass top, and is connected to a cold water tap or recirculating cooling apparatus.

Electrodes, Buffers and Wicks. The LKB 2117 Multiphor does not use buffer reservoirs. Instead , strips of thick absorbent paper are soaked in the electrode buffers and placed on the edges of the gel. When the apparatus is assembled, platinum wire electrodes make contact directly with these buffer-soaked wicks. There is no reason why, with alternative apparatus, more conventional buffer reservoirs and wicks should not be used.

Power Supply Any DC power supply can be used, and it should, if possible, have an output going up to 1000 V and 40 Watts. This high power output, which must be combined with efficient cooling, can allow a run to be completed in less than 2 hours.

B. Reagents

Unless otherwise stated, these should be of the highest grade of purity obtainable.

Gel Solutions A. 29.1% (w/v) acrylamide in distilled water. Filter if necessary, store for up to 2 weeks at 4 °C in the dark. B. *NN'*-methylene bisacrylamide solution at 0.9% (w/v) in distilled water. Treat as for acrylamide stock. C. Riboflavin solution, 0.004% (w/v) in distilled water. Store up to 2 weeks at 4 °C in the dark.

Ampholines® These can be purchased from LKB. Bio-Rad (2200 Wright Ave., Richmond, California, 94804), also market comparable ampholytes under the trade name Bio-Lytes®. For focusing in the full range of pH (3.5–9.5), ampholines® in the ranges 3.5–10, 4–6, 5–7, and 9–11 are required.

Glycerol Reagent grade. This is added to the gel, the intention being to help control diffusion and thermal convection. Its inclusion is optional.

Urea Reagent grade. This is added to the gel if it is necessary that the molecules, to be focused, be kept in the dissociated or denatured state.

C. Pouring and Running the Gel

The following method refers to the LKB 2117 Multiphor but can easily be modified, in terms of volume or ingredients, as desired for other apparatus or purposes.
Mix in a 100 ml vacuum flask the following solutions:
10 ml gel solution A
10 ml gel solution B
36 ml distilled water. In this can be present glycerol (3 ml) or urea to give the final required molarity, if desired
2.8 ml ampholine pH 3.5–10
0.2 ml ampholine pH 4–6
0.2 ml ampholine pH 5–7
0.4 ampholine pH 9–10
Mix and degas under vacuum. Add 0.4 ml of the 0.004% riboflavin solution and mix gently to avoid re-aerating the solution. Introduce the mixture into the gel apparatus.
   The thick and thin plates are clamped together with the rubber gasket and stood upright (Figure 5). A second, thick glass plate is usually placed behind the thin one for support. As an alternative to using the plates, gaskets, and clamps, the Bio-Rad Capillary Gel Caster (catalogue #170-4219), which is simple, reproducible in use and requires only the thin plate for gel casting, is recommended. We usually introduce the solution gently (without bubbles) by using a 50 ml syringe with an attached needle. The needle is 18 G stainless steel, 18 cm long, unbevelled and unsharpened (supplied by Popper and Sons, Inc., New Hyde Park, New York 11040). The apparatus is filled to the top, and the

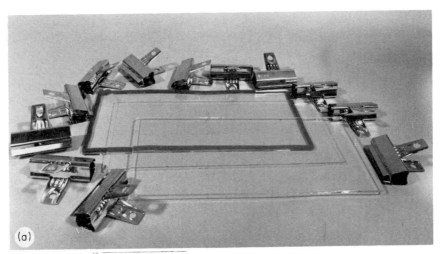

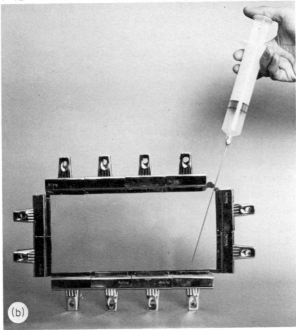

Figure 5. Apparatus for casting thin layer polyacrylamide gels for isoelectric focusing. The apparatus described here is part of that supplied for the LKB Multiphor 2117, but the principles are of general application. Figure 5(a) shows the component parts, i.e. 1 mm (thin) glass plate, 2 thick glass plates (3 mm), 1 rubber gasket, and 12 spring clamps. In Figure 5(b) is shown a way of introducing the gel solution into the assembled apparatus. After filling, the gel is polymerized by exposing the apparatus, in the position shown in Figure 5(b), to fluorescent light for a minimum of 30–60 minutes (depending on light intensity)

gasket closed. Every effort should be made to avoid trapping air bubbles anywhere in the apparatus. The gel is polymerized by fluorescent light and is usually complete within an hour.

The most difficult stage of the operation is removing the thick plate and leaving the gel adherent to the thin plate. Siliconizing the thick plate often, in our experience, leads to the anomalous adherence of the gel to the siliconized plate. One can, therefore, try siliconizing the thin glass plate (see Appendix I, Chapter 2, for siliconization), leaving the thick plate unsiliconized. Injecting water between the gel and the glass plate can lead to uneven dilution of ampholytes in the gel, and purely mechanical methods of separation are recommended. LKB recommend chilling the apparatus (4 °C, 15 minutes) as an aid to promoting the easy removal of the thick glass plate.

Once the thick plate and gasket have been removed, the samples can be applied. This is usually done by using a piece of chromatography or filter paper (e.g. Whatman 3MM) on to which is absorbed a suitable volume of the sample solution, and the paper is then placed on the surface of the gel. The size of the sample applicator depends on a number of factors such as the concentration of protein in the sample, which should usually be in the range 1–5 mg/ml. For most purposes, an applicator 0.5 cm × 1.0 cm is usually satisfactory. After loading the sample the electrode wicks are placed on the surface of the gel. For the pH 3.5–9.5 run described here, the anode solution is 1 M phosphoric acid, and the cathode solution is 1 M sodium hydroxide. The gel, still on the thin plate, is then placed on the cooling plate. To ensure good transfer of heat, the cooling plate surface is wetted with water or a dilute detergent solution before the gel plate is positioned. The run can then be started. The current is usually high at the beginning of a run and drops steadily thereafter. The rate at which the voltage can be increased to maximum depends on the efficiency of the cooling system, but the power output should be closely monitored and the voltage increased every 10–15 minutes to maintain the level the operator has decided on, until maximum voltage (1000 V) is reached. At the end of the run (suggested trial time 2 hours), the electrode wicks and pieces of sample application paper are removed. (This can be done earlier during the run in the case of the sample applicators.) The position on the gel in which the sample is applied should be in a region in which it is not expected to focus. The pH gradient should be measured immediately. This can be done most easily and accurately using a flat-surface combination pH electrode directly on the surface of the gel. An alternative but less satisfactory method is to use narrow-range pH paper on the surface of the gel. If a flat-surface electrode is unavailable, pieces of gel (away from the sample lanes) can be taken with a cork borer and mixed with distilled water for pH determination using a conventional pH electrode.

D. Staining the Gel

Ampholytes can frequently take up stain, and although methods have been described to allow the immediate staining of isoelectric focusing gels without removal of ampholytes, I have not found them to be entirely satisfactory. The following procedure, although a little more time consuming, usually gives satisfactory staining of proteins. With a little care, the gel can be kept adherent to the thin glass plate throughout the whole procedure.

E. Reagents

Fixative 17.3 sulphosalicylic acid, 57.5 g trichloroacetic acid made up to 500 ml with distilled water.

De-stain 500 ml ethanol, 160 ml glacial acetic acid made up to 2 litres with distilled water.

Stain 0.115% (w/v) Coomassie Brilliant Blue R-250 in de-stain.

F. Procedure

The gel is placed in fixing solution (minimum 1 hour at room temperature). The gel is then placed in de-stain, preferably a minimum of two washes each of 30 minutes also at room temperature. This procedure raises the pH to prevent precipitation of stain on the surface of the gel. The gel is then immersed in stain at 60 °C for 10 minutes, taken out and placed in de-stain until differentiation of the protein bands from the gel background is obtained. For further storage and de-staining, 7% acetic acid in distilled water is recommended.

APPENDIX V. CONJUGATION OF LIGANDS TO SEPHAROSE® USING CNBr

This procedure uses a method for CNBr activation of the Sepharose® which eliminates the need for titration of pH during the reaction (Parikh *et al.*, 1974).

A. Reagents

Sepharose® The cross linked (CL) or regular forms of Sepharose® 4B (supplied by Pharmacia) can both be used. Because some of the OH groups on the matrix have been utilized for the cross-linking, the capacity of the activated CL form for ligand may be up to 50% lower than that of the uncross-linked form. Against this can be set the advantages of the CL form in terms of chemical and thermal stability, especially if harsh elution conditions are to be used with the final immunoadsorbent.

Cyanogen bromide This can be kept stored at −20°C as a stock solution in water-free acetonitrile or dimethylformamide, at a concentration of 1 g per millilitre.

Activation Buffer 2 M sodium carbonate.

Washing Buffer 0.1 M sodium bicarbonate, pH 9.5.

Coupling Buffer Physiological phosphate-buffered saline (0.02 M phosphate, 0.15 MNaCl, pH 7.3) can be used perfectly satisfactorily. If the protein to be coupled shows a significant tendency to associate, the molarity of NaCl can be increased to 0.5 M to reduce the protein on protein adsorption. For most proteins, coupling proceeds rapidly at pH 7.3, but if problems occur in this regard, the pH of the phosphate buffer can be raised to 8.0.

B. Procedures

Wash the Sepharose® 4B-CL into 2 M Na_2CO_3 and pack by centrifugation in a bench centrifuge. To the packed Sepharose®, add 2 volumes of 2 M Na_2CO_3 and resuspend in a capped bottle. Add 0.2 volumes of the stock CNBr solution (i.e. 200 mg CNBr per millilitre Sepharose®), cap the bottle, and mix vigorously for 2 to 3 minutes. (*Note:* This reaction is carried out at room temperature. It is important that all procedures involving CNBr be carried out in a functioning fume hood.) Pour slurry into a sintered glass funnel, and wash under suction with: (1) 10 volumes 0.1 M $NaHCO_3$, pH 9.5; (2) 10 volumes distilled water; and (3) 10 volumes of coupling buffer. Do not allow the activated gel to dry out, but add it immediately to a solution (in coupling buffer) of the ligand to be coupled. For proteins, it is suggested that between 5 and 10 mg of protein be offered per millilitre packed gel.

Coupling should be carried out for 2–4 hours at room temperature, or overnight at 4 °C. The reactants should be mixed, preferably by end-over-end tumbling. Magnetic stirring nearly always results in breakage of the agarose beads. Coupling of most proteins occurs very quickly: unless the protein in question is unstable at room temperature, there is no compelling reason to choose one temperature rather than another.

After coupling, the efficiency of the reaction can be determined by centrifuging the gel and determining the concentration of unbound protein remaining in the supernatant fluid (by Folin reaction or adsorbance at 280 nm). Some protein will be non-covalently bound to the gel and can be washed away by three cycles of washing alternately in high pH (0.03 M sodium borate, 1 M NaCl, pH 8.5) and low pH (0.1 M sodium acetate, 1 M NaCl, pH 4.0), after which bound nitrogen on the gel can be accurately determined by the Kjeldahl method. Unless an accurate estimate of bound nitrogen is required, the washings in high and low pH buffers could well be omitted since it is recommended (see below) that the coupled gel be thoroughly washed with an eluting buffer before use. Although the remaining reactive groups on the activated Sepharose® decay quite rapidly, to make sure they are all blocked, the coupled beads can be incubated with 1 M ethanolamine, at pH 8.0, at room temperature or 4 °C, for 2 hours. If Tris-containing buffers are available, they can also be used very conveniently to block remaining reactive groups. The coupled gel can then be washed and stored in buffer containing preservative at 4 °C.

Before use, the coupled gel should be thoroughly prewashed with the eluting buffer to be used in the actual experiment. The washing should be repeated until protein is no longer detectable in the column eluate. Protein leaks from the column not only because of the inherent instability of the bond formed by the CNBr reaction, but also because non-covalently coupled proteins are often present on the gel. This is sometimes the case despite the use of high salt (0.5 M NaCl) coupling buffers, and washing with high and low pH buffers after coupling (see above).

Using the procedure outlined above, we routinely obtain coupling efficiencies in excess of 80% when offering 1gG at a ratio of 5 mg protein per millilitre of gel.

APPENDIX VI. BUFFERS FOR THE ELUTION OF ANTIBODY FROM IMMUNE-AFFINITY COLUMNS

1. Acetic acid, unbuffered.

This consists simply of a 0.15 M NaCl (8.77 g per litre) solution made 0.5% (v/v) with glacial acetic acid. The pH is usually around or just below 3.5. This buffer is frequently used for eluting Ig from protein A–Sepharose columns. It can, if wished, be adjusted more accurately to a desired pH.

2. Glycine–HCl, pH 2.5

To 25 ml of 0.2 M glycine (15.01 g per litre) is added 14 ml of 0.2 M HCl. The pH is adjusted accurately to 2.5, and the buffer is diluted to 100 ml with water. This buffer can be made 0.15 M in NaCl if desired (0.877 g per 100 ml).

3. Sodium thiocyanate (molecular weight 81.07)

This is used as a 3.5 M solution in water. The potassium salt can be used equally as well.

4. Guanidine hydrochloride (molecular weight 95.5)

This is usually used as a 4 M solution in water (382 g/litre).

5. Urea (molecular weight 60.6)

This can be used at a variety of molarities depending on circumstances: 8 M (480.48 g per litre) is a concentration convenient for use in affinity chromatography with antibodies. It can be noted that, at neutral or alkaline pH, urea in solution is in equilibrium with cyanate ions.

REFERENCES

Andrews, P. (1964). Estimation of molecular weights of proteins by Sephadex gel-filtration. *Biochem. J.*, **91** 222–233.

Andrews, P. (1965). The gel-filtration behaviour of proteins related to their molecular weight over a wide range. *Biochem. J.*, **96**, 595–606.

Benedict, A. A. (1967). Production and purification of chicken immunoglobulins. In C. A. Willams and M. W. Chase (Eds) *Methods in Immunology and Immunochemistry* volume 1. *Preparation of Antigens and Antibodies*, pp. 229–237. Academic Press, London and New York.

Burgin-Wolf, A., Hernandez, R., and Just, M. (1971). Separation of rubella IgM, IgA and IgG antibodies by gel filtration on agarose. *Lancet*, **ii**, 1278–1280.

Burnett, D., Wood, S. M., and Bradwell, A. R. (1976). Estimation of the stokes radii of serum proteins for a study of protein movement from blood to amniotic fluid. *Biochim. Biophys. Acta*, **427**, 231–237.

Cann, J. R. (1968). Factors Governing the rate of migration of charged particles in an electric field. In C. A. Williams and M. W. Chase (Eds) *Methods in Immunology and Immunochemistry*, volume 2. *Physical and Chemical Methods*, pp. 1–6. Academic Press, New York and London.

Capra, J. D., Tung, A. S., and Nisonoff, A. (1975). Structural studies on induced antibodies with defined idiotypic specificities. I. The heavy chains of anti-azopheny-larsonate antibodies from A/J mice bearing a cross-reactive idiotype. *J. Immunol.*, **114**, 1548–1553.

van Dalen, A., Seijen, H. G., and Gruber, M. (1967). Isolation and some properties of rabbit IgM. *Biochim. Biophys. Acta*, **147**, 421–426.

Davis, B. J. (1964). Disc electrophoresis: II. Method and application to human serum proteins. *Ann. N. Y. Acad. Sci.*, **121**, 404–427.

Deutsch, H. F. (1967). Preparation of immunoglobulin concentrates. In C. A. Williams and M. W. Chase (Eds) *Methods in Immunology and Immunochemistry* volume 1. Preparation of Antigens and Antibodies, pp. 315–321. Academic Press, New York and London.

Ey, P. L., Prowse, S. J., and Jenkin C. R. (1978). Isolation of pure IgG1, IgG2a and IgG2b immunoglobulins from mouse serum using protein A-Sepharose. *Immunochemistry*, **15**, 429–436.

Fahey, J. L. (1967). Chromatographic separation of immunoglobulins. In C. A. Williams and M. W. Chase (Eds) *Methods in Immunology and Immunochemistry* volume 1. *Preparation of Antigens and Antibodies*, pp. 321–332. Academic Press, New York and London.

Fahey, J. L., McCoy, P. F., and Goulian, M. (1958). Chromatography of serum proteins in normal and pathological sera: the distribution of protein-bound carbohydrate and cholesterol, siderophilin, thyroxin-binding protein, B_12-binding protein, alkaline and acid phosphatases, radioiodinated albumin and myeloma proteins. *J. Clin. Invest.*, **37**, 272–284.

Flodin, P. and Killander, J. (1962). Fractionation of human serum proteins by gel filtration. *Biochim. Biophys. Acta*, **63**, 403–410.

Forsgren, A. (1968). Protein A from *Staphylococcus aureus*. V. Reaction with guinea pig γ-globulins. *J. Immunol.*, **100**, 921–926.

Forsgren, A. and Sjoquist, J. (1966). Protein A from *S. aureus*. I. Pseudo-immune reaction with human γ-globulin. *J. Immunol.*, **97**, 822–827.

Fuchs, S. and Sela, M. (1978). Immunoadsorbents. In D. M. Weir (Ed.) *Handbook of Experimental Immunology* Volume 1, *Immunochemistry*, pp. 10.1–10.6. Blackwell, Oxford.

Goding, J. W. (1976). Conjugation of antibodies with fluorochromes: modifications to the standard methods. *J. Immunol. Methods*, **13**, 215–226.

Goding, J. W. (1978).Use of staphylococcal protein A as an immunological reagent. *J. Immunol. Methods*, **20**, 241–253.

Gordon, A. H. (1969). *Electrophoresis of Proteins in Polyacrylamide and Starch Gels*. North Holland Publishing Company, Amsterdam.

Goudswaard, J., van der Donk, J. A., Noordzij, A., van Dam, R. H., and Vaerman, J. P. (1978). Protein A reactivity of various mammalian immunoglubulins. *Scand. J. Immunol.*, **8**, 21–28.

Hannon, R., Haire, M., Wisdom, G. B., and Neill, D. W. (1975). The use of indirect immunofluorescence to evaluate the gel filtration method of fractionating human immunoglobulins. *J. Immunol. Methods*, **8**, 29–36.

Haustein, D. and Warr, G. W. (1976). Use and abuse of Sepharose-conjugated antibodies for the isolation of lymphocyte-surface immunoglobulins. *J. Immunol. Methods*, **12**, 323–336.

Heide, K. and Schwick, H. G. (1978). Salt fractionation of immunoglobulins. In D. M. Weir (Ed.) *Handbook of Experimental Immunology* volume 1. *Immunochemistry*, pp. 7.1–7.11. Blackwell, Oxford.

Hjelm, H. (1975). Isolation of IgG3 from normal human sera and from a patient with multiple myeloma by using Protein A-Sepharose 4B. *Scand. J. Immunol.*, **4**, 633–640.

Inman, J. K. (1975). Thymus-independent antigens: the preparation of covalent, hapten-ficoll conjugates. *J. Immunol.*, **114**, 704–709.

Inman J. K. and Dintzis, H. M. (1969). The derivatization of cross-linked polyacrylamide beads. Controlled introduction of functional groups for the preparation of special-purpose, biochemical adsorbents. *Biochemistry*, **8**, 4074–4082.

James K. (1973). Preparation of antilymphocytic antibodies. In D. M. Weir (Ed.) *Handbook of Experimental Immunology*, pp. 32.1. Blackwell, Oxford.

Jonsson, S. and Kronvall, G. (1974), The use of protein A-containing *Staphylococcus aureus* as a solid phase anti-IgG reagent in radioimmunoassays as exemplified in the quantitation of alpha-fetoprotein in normal human adult serum. *Eur. J. Immunol.*, **4**, 29–33.

Kessler, S. W. (1975). Rapid isolation of antigens from cells with a staphylococcal protein A-antibody adsorbent: parameters of the interaction of antibody-antigen complexes with Protein A. *J.Immunol.*, **115**, 1617–1624.

Kessler, S. W. (1976). Cell membrane antigen isolation with the staphylococcal protein A–antibody adsorbent. *J. Immunol.*, **117**, 1482–1490.

Klein, O. (1972). Immunoadsorption sur Sepharose 4B. Comparaison de differentes techniques d'elution d'anticorps anti-immunoglobulines. *Rev. Europ. Etudes Clin. Biol.*, **17**, 525–529.

Kronvall, G., Grey, H. M., and Williams, R. C. (1970a). Protein A reactivity with mouse immunoglobulins. Structural relationships between some mouse and human immunoglobulins. *J. Immunol.*, **105**, 1116–1123.

Kronvall, G., Seal, U. S., Finstad, J., and Williams, R. C. (1970b). Phylogenetic insight into evolution of mammalian Fc fragment of G globulin using staphylococcal protein A. *J,. Immunol.*, **104**, 140–147.

Kronvall, G. and Williams, R. C. (1969). Differences in anti-protein A activity among IgG subgrouips. *J. Immunol.*, **103**, 828–833.

Lachmann, P. J. and Hobart, M. J. (1978). Complement Technology. In D. M. Weir (Ed.) *Handbook of Experimental Immunology* volume 1. *Immunochemistry*, pp. 5A.1–5A1.23, Blackwell, Oxford.

Levy, H. B. and Sober, H. A. (1960). A simple chromatographic method for preparation of gamma globulin. *Proc. Soc. Exp. Biol. Med.*, **103**, 250–252.

Lowry, O. H., Rosebrough, N. J., Farr, A. L., and Randall, R. J. (1951). Protein measurement with the folin phenol reagent. *J. Biol. Chem.*, **193**, 265–275.

Maarten, J. D., Tol. V., Veenhoff, E., and Seijen, H. G. (1978). Rabbit IgM: its isolation in high yield by a convenient procedure using serum from trypanosome-infected animals. *J. Immunol. Methods*, **21**, 125–131.

Mackenzie, M. R., Gutman, G. A., and Warner, N. L. (1977). The binding of murine IgM to staphylococcal A protein. *Scand. J. Immunol.*, **7**, 367–370.

Marchalonis, J. J., Atwell, J. L., and Goding, J. W. (1978). 7S immunoglobulins of a monotreme, the Echidna, *Tachyglossus aculeatus:* two distinct isotypes which bind A protein of *Staphylococcus aureus. Immunology*, **34**, 97–103.

Marchalonis, J. J., Warr, G. W., Smith, P., Begg, G. S., and Morgan, F. J. (1979). Structural and antigenic studies of an idiotype-bearing murine antibody to the arsonate hapten. *Biochemistry*, **18**, 560–565.

Medgyesi, G. A., Fiist, G., Gergely, J., and Bazin, H. (1978). Classes and subclasses of rat immunoglobulins: interaction with the complement system and with staphylococcal protein A. *Immunochemistry*, **15**, 125–129.

Muller-Eberhard, H. J. and Osterland, C. K. (1968). Zone electrophoresis on powder blocks. In C. A. Williams and M. W. Chase (Eds) *Methods in Immunology and Immunochemistry*, volume 2. *Physical and Chemical Methods*, pp. 57–67. Academic Press, New York and London.

O'Carra, P., Barry, S., and Griffen, T. (1974a). Interfering and competing adsorption effects in bioaffinity chromatography. In W. B. Jakoby and M. Wilchek (Eds) *Methods in Enzymology* volume 34. *Affinity Techniques: Enzyme Purification:* Part B, pp. 108–126. Academic Press, New York and London.

O'Carra, P., Barry, S., and Griffin, T. (1974b). Spacer arms in affinity chromatography: use of hydrophilic arms to control or eliminate nonbiospecific adsorption effects. *FEBS Lett.*, **43**, 169–175.

O'Farrell, P. H. and O'Farrell, P. Z. (1977). Two dimensional polyacrylamide gel electrophoretic fractionation. *Method Cell Biol.*, **16**, 407–420.

Ornstein, L. (1964). Disc electrophoresis: I. Background and theory. *Ann. N. Y. Acad. Sci.*, **121**, 321–349.

Parikh, I. and Cuatrecasas, P. (1977). Affinity chromatography in immunology. In M. Z. Atassi (Ed.) *Immunochemistry of Proteins* volume 2, pp. 1–44, Plenum, New York and London.

Parikh, I., March, S., and Cuatrecasas, P. (1974). Topics in the methodology of substitution reactions with agarose. In W. B. Jakoby and M. Wilchek (Eds) *Methods in Enzymology* volume 34. *Affinity Techniques, Enzyme Purification:* Part B, pp. 77–102. Academic Press, New York and London.

Patrick, C. L. and Virella, G. (1978). Isolation of normal human IgG3. Identical molecular weight for normal and monoclonal gamma-3 chains. *Immunochemistry*, **15**, 137–139.

Peacock, A. C. and Dingman, C. W. (1968). Molecular weight estimation and separation of ribonucleic acid by electrophoresis in agarose–acrylamide composite gels. *Biochemistry*, **1**, 668–674.

Porath, J. (1960). Gel filtration of proteins, peptides and amino acids. *Biochim. Biophys. Acta*, **39**, 193–207.

Porath, J. and Flodin, P. (1959). Gel filtration: a method for desalting and group separation. *Nature (Lond)*, **183**, 1657–1959.

Potter, M., Rudikoff, S., Vrana, M., Rao, D. N., and Mushinski, E. B. (1977). Primary structural differences in myeloma proteins that bind the same haptens. *Cold Spring Harbor Symp. Quant. Biol.*, **41**, 661–666.

Saltvedt, E. and Harboe, M. (1976). Binding of IgA to protein-A-containing staphylococci—relationship to subclasses. *Scand. J. Immunol.*, **5**, 1103–1108.

Segrest, J. R., Jackson, R. L., Andrews, E. P., and Marchesi, V. T. (1971). Human erythrocyte membrane glycoprotein: a reevaluation of the molecular weight as determined by SDS-polyacrylamide gel electrophoresis. *Biochem. Biophys. Res. Commun.*, **44**, 390–395.

Smithies, O. (1955). Zone electrophoresis in starch gels. Group variations in the serum proteins of normal human adults. *Biochem. J.*, **61**, 629–641.

Sober, H. A. and Petersen, E. A. (1958). Protein chromatography on ion exchange cellulose. *Fed. Proc.*, **17**, 1116–1126.

Sober, H. A. and Petersen, E. A. (1959). Variable gradient device for chromatography. *Anal. Chem.*, **31**, 857–862.

Stanworth, D. R. and Turner, M. W. (1978). Immunochemical analysis of immunoglobulins and their sub-units. In D. M. Weir (Ed.) *Handbook of Experimental Immunology* volume 1. *Immunochemistry*, pp. 6.1–6.102. Blackwell, Oxford.

Svedberg, T. and Pederson, K. O. (1940). *The ultracentrifuge*. Oxford University Press.

Ternynck, T. and Avrameas, S. (1972). Polyacrylamide–protein immunoadsorbents prepared with glutaraldehyde. *FEBS Lett.*, **23**, 24–78.

Tiselius, A. (1937). Electrophoresis of serum globulin. II. Electrophoretic analysis of normal and immune sera. *Biochem. J.*, **31**, 1464–1477.

Tiselius, A. Porath, J., and Albertsson, P. A. (1963). Separation and fractionation of macromolecules and particles. *Science*, **141**, 13–20.

Tombs, M. P., Cooke, K. B., Burston, D., and Maclagan, N. F. (1961). The chromatography of normal serum proteins. *Biochem. J.*, **80**, 284–292.

Vaerman, J. P., Heremans, J. F., and Vaerman, C. (1963). Studies of the immune globulins of human serum. I. A method for the simultaneous isolation of the three immune globulins (γss, γ1M and γ1A) from individual small serum samples. *J. Immunol.*, **91**, 7–10.

Warr, G. W. and Hart, I. R. (1979). Binding of canine IgM and IgG to protein A of *Staphylococcus aureus*: a simple method for the isolation of canine immunoglobulins from serum and the lymphocyte surface. *Am. J. Vet. Res.*, **40**, 922–926.

Weber, K. and Osborn, M. (1969). The reliability of molecular weight determinations by dodecyl sulphate polyacrylamide gel electrophoresis. *J. Biol. Chem.*, **244**, 4406–4412.

Weston, P. D. and Avrameas, S. (1971). Proteins coupled to polyacrylamide beads using glutaraldehyde. *Biochem. Biophys. Res. Commun.*, **45**, 1574–1580.

Williams, C. A. and Chase, M. W. (Eds) (1968). *Methods in Immunology and Immunochemistry* volume 2. *Physical and Chemical Methods*. Academic Press, New York and London.

Williams, J. W. (1963). *Ultracentrifugal Analysis in Theory and Experiment*. Academic Press, New York and London.

Williamson, A. R. (1978). Isolelectric focusing of immunoglubulins. In D. M. Weir (Ed.) *Handbook of Experimental Immunology* volume 1. *Immunochemistry*, pp. 9,1–9,31, Blackwell, Oxford.

Antibody as a Tool
Edited by J. J. Marchalonis and G. W. Warr
©1982 John Wiley & Sons Ltd

Chapter 4

Principles of Antibody Reactions

IVAN OTTERNESS
*Department of Pharmacology, Pfizer Central Research,
Groton, CT 06340, USA*

and

FRED KARUSH
*Department of Microbiology, School of Medicine,
University of Pennsylvania, Philadelphia, PA 19104, USA*

I. INTRODUCTION

The purposeful application of antibody to the solution of biological and chemical problems provides the core of the discipline immunochemistry. The fundamental framework that allows us to understand the use of antibody is based upon two concepts: first, that antibody has binding sites for antigenic determinants, each site possessing both a high degree of selectivity for the specific determinant and a high affinity for it; and second, that once antibody has bound antigen, the system changes in a way which may be detected biologically, chemically or physically and which allows a measurement to be made of the extent of the binding. The elaboration of these two principles provides the key to understanding immunochemical reactions.

Before these principles are expanded, it is useful to establish a focus for our discussion by asking what kind of questions can be answered using immunochemical techniques. At the simplest level, since antibody reacts with antigen, that reaction provides a means for the *detection of antigen*. More refined measures of the interaction such as radioimmunoassay, precipitation assays, enzyme linked assays, competitive binding assays, and immunodiffusion or immunoelectrophoretic assays provide a means of *quantitating the antigen*. Immunodiffusion in gels and competitive binding assays can be used to obtain *structural information* regarding antigenic homologies and dissimilarities as well as conformational or aggregational changes. These

97

approaches focus attention on the antigen itself. The principal biological function of antibody is not to supply us with immunochemical tools to study antigens, but rather to provide several host defense systems against infection and, presumably, neoplasia. Thus it is important to characterize the nature of the antigen–antibody reaction to understand how antibody carries out its natural biologic function. In addition, to apply antibody optimally as an immunochemical tool, it is important to understand the basic reaction so that its potentialities can be fully utilized.

Four parameters are critical for the description of the antibody–antigen reaction. The *class of antibody*, although frequently not a variable in the reaction, is a prime determinant of whether many biological end points such as complement fixation or mast cell degranulation can be used to detect antibody–antigen complex formation. It also plays a role with respect to the ease of complex precipitation and the flexibility of the hinge region. The *structure of the antigen* plays an even more important role; whether antigenic sites are repeating or non-repeating, the number and spacing of the sites as well as their detailed structure each play a role in the induction of antibody formation and in the characteristics of the final antigen–antibody interaction. The *affinity constant* for the reaction is probably the single most important overall parameter of the reaction since it determines the sensitivity of detection of the antigen. The lower the affinity constant the greater the amount of antibody and/or antigen that is required for measurable reaction. Finally there is the question of the *specificity of the reaction*. Antibody directed precisely against the antigen in question leaves less chance of undesirable cross-reactions to extraneous or even related antigens. It is frequently this exquisite selectivity that makes antibody such a valuable research tool.

II. MONOVALENT LIGANDS

A. An Overview: Heterogeneity

We start our description of the antibody–antigen reaction by defining two types of heterogeneity. The first we will call 'epitope' heterogeneity. By this we mean antibody directed against different determinants on the same antigen. Thus antibodies made to myoglobin (Atassi, 1975), lysozyme (Atassi, 1978), and staphylococcal nuclease (Sachs *et al.*, 1972a,b) have been shown to be made up of subpopulations of antibody each directed against different amino acid clusters of the parent molecule. Epitope heterogeneity has also been demonstrated by genetic studies with lymphocyte antigens such as the H-2 complex and with the erythrocyte antigens, for example, the M, Rh, and ABO loci. It should be clear that an epitope is the antigenic determinant complementary to the antibody combining site. The concept of epitope heterogeneity is of particular importance in the understanding of cross-reactions of antibodies with whole antigens. There is a second type of heterogeneity, one that we will define as 'clonal' heterogeneity. It arises when different antibody populations are directed against the same determinant. The term clonal is used to emphasize the origins of the heterogeneity. Antibody arising from a single clone of lymphocytes will be homogeneous in affinity constant, variable region sequences, idiotype, and the epitope it is directed against. Although clonally heterogeneous antibody reacts with the same epitope determinants, it will be heterogeneous with respect to variable region sequence, idiotype, and affinity constant. For example, anti-phosphorylcholine antibody, although directed against the same chemical moiety, demonstrates heterogeneity by affinity constant measurement and by analysis of the amino acid sequence of the variable region. Thus clonal heterogeneity leads to the fine differences in specificity, affinity, and cross-reactivity demonstrated in different antibody subpopulations directed against the same epitope.

B. Homogeneous Antibody

The reaction of antibody with its homologous epitope or more generally any monovalent hapten or ligand is governed by the Law of Mass Action. Thus:

$$\text{Antibody} + \text{Ligand} = \text{Antibody}-\text{Ligand} \tag{1}$$

The concentrations of free and bound ligand may be measured in a number of ways briefly summarized in Table 1.

When antibody is homogeneous, that is composed completely of antibody molecules of a single amino acid sequence in their variable region, the binding is characterized by a single affinity constant. If we define R as the concentration of ligand bound to antibody, C as the concentration of free ligand in the reaction mixture, B as the concentration of free antibody sites, then it follows that

$$K = \frac{R}{B \cdot C} \tag{2}$$

where all concentrations are in moles/litre or its equivalent, millimoles/millilitre. This form is not very useful so it is customary to rearrange the equation into linear form after making the substitution $B = (N-R)$ where N is the total concentration of antibody sites in the reaction, then

$$R/C = NK - RK \tag{3}$$

If the concentration of antibody molecules, A, is accurately known, then:

$$N = nA \tag{3a}$$

S. M. Griffith
National Forage Seed Production Research Center
Oregon State University
3450 S.W. Campus Way
Corvallis, Oregon 97331-7102

Table 1. Methods for the determination of free and bound monovalent ligand
concentration

Method	Brief description	Reference
I. Measurements *in situ*		
a. Equilibrium dialysis	Dialysis is carried out across a membrane permeable to ligand, but not antibody. Total ligand concentration is measured on each side of the membrane. On the antibody side, one obtains the sum of the free and bound ligand concentration; on the other side, the concentration of free ligand. It is an absolute experimental method	Eisen and Karush (1949) Karush and Karush (1971)
b. Fluorescence quenching	Irradiation of antibody at 295 nm leads to fluorescence emission at 345 nm. Certain ligands such as dinitrophenol and azophenyl-arsonate quench, that is decrease, the fluorescent emission when bound to antibody. This method can be extended to non-fluorescent ligands with the use of 'reporter' groups. A useful method for relative binding values, but not for absolute values with heterogeneous antibody populations since different antibody subpopulations may quench with different efficiency	Velich *et al.* (1960) Eisen and Siskind (1964) Gopalakrishnan and Karush (1975)
c. Fluorescence enhancement	Similar to fluorescence quenching except that the exciting light is re-emitted at a longer wavelength instead of being quenched. Thus an increase in fluorescence at the longer wavelength is measured after binding. Again different antibody populations enhance with different efficiencies so the method is not absolute	Parker *et al.* (1967)
d. Fluorescence depolarization	A fluorescent-labelled ligand depolarizes plane polarized light during the time period between its absorption and re-emission due to its rotary Brownian motion. Combination of ligand with antibody retards the ligand's rotary motion decreasing depolarization. The change in depolar-	Danliker *et al.* (1965)

Table 1. *Contd.* Methods for the determination of free and bound monovalent ligand concentration

Method	Brief description	Reference
	ization with increasing ligand allows a computation of free and bound ligand. It is an absolute method useful for fluorescent mono-valent ligands	
II. Separation methods		
	These methods rely on physical separation of the free and the antibody-bound ligand. In general they give relative equilibrium constants.	Kim *et al.* (1975)
	Before it can be accepted that they give absolute values, detailed comparisons with an absolute method must be carried out to demonstrate the separation technique does not disturb the equilibrium	Seppälä (1975)
a. Coupling of anti-body to an insoluble substrate	The insolubilized antibody can be sedimented without carrying down free ligand. Ligand will sediment only when bound to antibody	Wide (1969)
b. Selective precipitant for anti-body	Ammonium sulphate, ethanol, etc. may be used to precipitate antibody. Ligand is not precipitated unless it is bound to antibody	Strupp *et al.* (1969)
c. Selective adsorption of free ligand	Charcoal, for example, may be used to adsorb the free ligand. This allows the determination of the ligand bound to antibody	Herbert *et al.* (1965)

where n is simply the number of combining sites per molecule. Defining r as the concentration of bound ligand divided by the concentration of antibody

$$r = R/A \qquad (3b)$$

Substituting definitions (3a) and (3b) into equation (3), one obtains directly the Scatchard equation (Scatchard, 1949).

$$r/C = nK - rK \qquad (4)$$

The number of binding sites per molecule of antibody and the affinity constant can be directly determined by plotting data according to equation (4) and obtaining the so-called Scatchard plot.

Antibody as a Tool

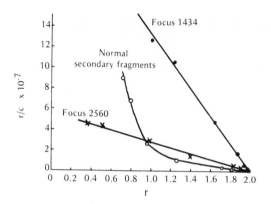

Figure 1. Ligand binding curves constructed from equilibrium dialysis data with homogeneous antibody from focus No. 1434 (O) and focus No. 2560 (X), and pooled antibody from four normal secondary fragments (O). *r* represents the moles of α,H-[³H]acetyl-DNP lysine bound per mole of antibody at the equilibrium free hapten concentration *C*. From Klinman (1969)

An example of a Scatchard plot of homogeneous antibody is shown in Figure 1 along with a companion plot of heterogeneous antibody. *K* is determined from the slope and *n* is determined from the *x* intercept. The problem of evaluating *K* for a heterogeneous population will be discussed later. It is important to note that homogeneous binding, that is antibody–ligand binding associated with a single affinity constant, is the exception rather than the rule. It appears to occur particularly with certain carbohydrate antigens, for example, pneumococcal vaccine (Pappenheimer *et al.*, 1968; Katz and Pappenheimer, 1969; Jaton *et al.*, 1970), streptococcal vaccine (Krause, 1970; Ghose and Karush, 1973), and digoxin (Smith *et al.*, 1970). Homogeneity has been found rather infrequently with antibodies elicited to typical determinants. The homogeneous binding to vasopressin (Wu and Rockey, 1969) and to aspirylaminocaproate (Hoffman and Campbell, 1969) are exceptional. By contrast, the use of special procedures to obtain antibody, e.g. monofocal antibody (Klinman, 1969; Klinman *et al.*, 1977), monoclonal hybridomas (see Chapter 9) or myelomas of defined specificity (Eisen *et al.*, 1967) routinely leads to homogeneous binding.

Conceptually it is convenient to rearrange equation (2) into the form of the Langmuir adsorption isotherm. Noting that

$$R = N\left(\frac{KC}{1 + KC}\right) \tag{5}$$

and defining the extent of reaction as

$$\alpha = R/N \tag{5a}$$

which is just the fraction of reacted antibody sites, then

$$\alpha = \frac{KC}{1 + KC} \tag{5b}$$

Thus the extent of the reaction for a monovalent ligand depends on the concentration of free ligand and on the affinity constant of the antibody. Also at $\alpha = 1/2$, $KC = 1$ or

$$K = 1/C \tag{5c}$$

Thus the concentration at which the binding sites are half saturated with ligand can be used as an exact estimate of K in the case of homogeneous antibody and as an estimate of the median K in the case of heterogeneous antibody.

C. Antibody, Restricted Heterogeneity

Since antibody is so infrequently homogeneous, it must be considered to be composed of a plurality of clonotypes (Kreth and Williamson, 1973) each of which is homogeneous. Thus it is appropriate to generalize equation (5) to:

$$R = N_1 \frac{K_1 C}{1 + K_1 C} + N_2 \frac{K_2 C}{1 + K_2 C} + \dots \tag{6}$$

or written in more compact form

$$R = \sum_{i=1}^{m} \frac{N_i K_i C}{1 + K_i C} \tag{7}$$

where now antibody is composed of a number of clonotypes, each of which is defined by two parameters, its concentration in solution (N_i) and its affinity constant (K_i). The use of this equation to describe ligand binding is exact but its application is only practical when there are a few dominant clonotypes, i.e. m the number of clonotypes is small, preferably no more than two or three. Under those circumstances, it may be considered that curve fitting will give a concrete representation of the true state of the system, particularly if N_i can be independently determined by analytical isoelectric focusing or the K_i of the dominant antibody population can be determined after preparative isoelectric focusing.

D. Heterogeneous Antibody

With heterogeneous antibody such as anti-DNP, it becomes an impossible task to determine the true set of N_i and K_i because of the large number of clonotypes in the antibody population (Kreth and Williamson, 1973). A general approach to this problem was formulated (Bowman and Aladjem,

1963), but the computational difficulties have left it unused to date. A simpler curve fitting approach based upon equation (7) was applied by Werblin *et al.* (1972), Mukkur *et al.* (1974), and Erwin and Aladjem (1976). The value of curve fitting must be conceived of as giving a rough approximation of the distribution function of affinity constants of subgroups of clonotypes. Thus Werblin *et al.* (1973) found that the binding function of antibody of a single rabbit immunized to DNP changed considerably with time (Figure 2a) and they empirically represented the non-uniform distribution by a set of evenly spaced K_i's (Figure 2b). Erwin and Aladjem (1976) developed a similar curve fitting function, but with several advantages. First, it estimates the amounts of antibody whose K_i is either too low or too high to be determined accurately in the concentration range of ligand used. Second, they determined the smallest number of subpopulations that would give a good representation of the data. In Figure 3a, a derived distribution is shown for the binding of p-[${}^{131}I$]phenylarsonate to its rabbit antibody with m, the number of assumed subpopulations, equal to 14. When they minimized the number of assumed subpopulations, three were found to give an equivalent fit (Figure 3b) as judged by the statistical test chi square, i.e. chi square was 13 for $m = 14$ and 12.5 for $m = 3$. The best Sips distribution (see below) had a chi square of 29, a much poorer fit.

In general, with pooled sera or whenever there is a large number of clonotypes, according to the Law of Large Numbers (Feller, 1966, 1968) the distribution function, here the distribution of affinities, will tend to be grouped about a central mean and have regular moments. As such the distribution could be reasonably approximated by a normal (Gaussian) distribution about a mean K denoted K_0. Karush and Sonnenberg (1949) assumed that the free energies (proportional to ln K) showed a dispersion defined by the normal distribution.

$$P(K) = \frac{1}{\sigma\sqrt{\pi}} e^{-(\ln K/K_0)^2/\sigma^2} \tag{8}$$

It can be shown, setting v for $\ln(K/K_0)/\sigma$, that:

$$r/n = 1 - 1/\pi \int_{-\infty}^{\infty} \frac{e^{-v^2}}{1 + K_0 C e^{v\sigma}} \, dv \tag{9}$$

This function proved to give a good representation of hapten binding data (Karush, 1956). Since the function must be integrated numerically, it is much more convenient to use another, unimodal distribution, the Sips function (Sips, 1948; Nisonoff and Pressman, 1958)

$$r = \frac{n(KC)^a}{1 + (KC)^a} \tag{10}$$

or

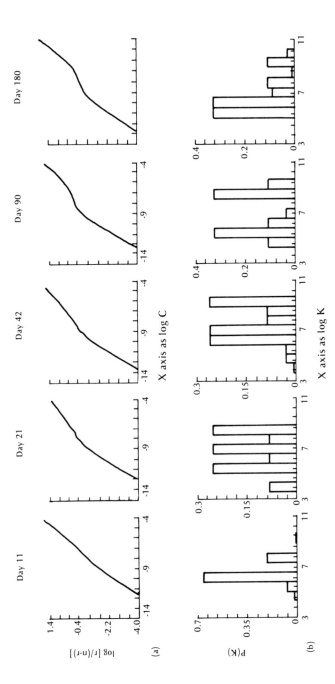

Figure 2. Change in the ligand binding characteristics of the antibody rabbit 1352-11 with time after immunization with DNP–bovine gamma globulin. Binding measured with DNP–lysine. (a) Binding data plotted according to equation (11). (b) Histograms for the computed distribution of binding constants according to the method of Werblin *et al.* (1973). The value $P(K)$ is the probability of an affinity constant of magnitude K. Data and computations from Werblin *et al.* (1973)

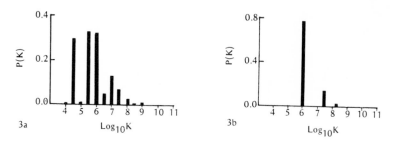

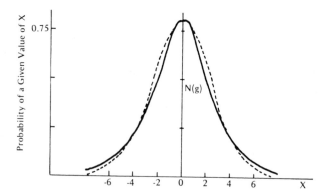

Figure 3. The computed distribution of affinity constants determined according to the method of Erwin and Aladjem is shown under two conditions: (a) where the number of subpopulations is assumed to be 14 and (b) where the number of subpopulations is minimized by a standard statistical procedure. From Erwin and Aladjem (1976)

$$\log [r/(n - r)] = a \log C + a \log K_0 \tag{11}$$

In the Sips plot, $\log [r/(n - r)]$ versus $\log C$ is graphed and the exponent a (the slope of the line) is a measure of the heterogeneity, $a = 1$ for a homogeneous system and $a < 1$ indicates heterogeneity with the more heterogeneous preparations being associated with a smaller a. A comparison of a Sips and a Gaussian distribution of affinity constants with similar dispersions from the mean is shown in Figure 4. Bruni *et al.* (1976) calculated the relationship of a to the dispersion σ about K_0

$$\sigma^2 = \pi^2(1 - a^2)/3a^3 \tag{12}$$

When the binding curve is smooth, i.e. there are no atypical inflection points, the Sips function is the most practical approach to the description of binding for heterogeneous antibody. Where this is not the case, the simplest analytical

Figure 4. A comparison of the Gaussian (--) and the Sips (--) distribution functions for similar mean and variance. The figure demonstrates the basic similarities of the two distributions

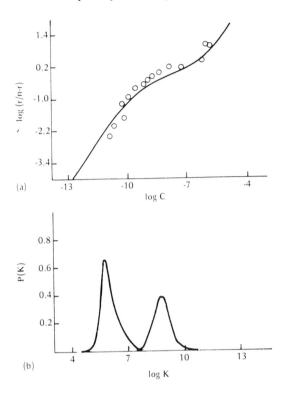

Figure 5. Hapten binding data with DNP-lysine and anti-DNP rabbit antibody taken 90 days after immunization with 0.5 mg DNP–bovine gamma globulin, (a) Data from Werblin *et al.* (1973) graphed according to equation (11). Calculated theoretical line and (b) bimodal distribution derived by the method of Bruni *et al.* (1976)

approach is to assume a bimodal distribution of affinity constants as described by Bruni *et al.* (1976).

With the limited range of experimental binding data available and the relatively large degree of error in the data, interpolation of the data to compute a tri- or polymodal distribution is not sound numerical analysis even though m in equation (7) may be shown by isoelectric focusing to be large. The representation of the data as a bimodal distribution appears reasonably verified experimentally (Bruni *et al.*, 1976). A plot of log $(r/n - r)$ against log C, equation (11), allows one to discriminate graphically whether the Sips function is a suitable description of the data. If the plot is linear, then the slope is simply the value a and the intercept I is just a log K, thus

$$K = 10^{I/a} \tag{13}$$

If the plot is not linear as in Figure 5a, the method of Bruni *et al.* (1976) can be used to derive a bimodal distribution (Figure 5b). Since m is in general large, it must be kept in mind that the use of a bimodal distribution is, like that of a unimodal distribution, a construct allowing an analytical representation of the data. In fact, if one could compute the distribution function of K, that is the probability of a given K or $P(K)$, one would not expect to find a continuous function but rather $P(K)$ would be made up of a series of delta functions, that is at certain values of K corresponding to the K_i of a particular clone, $P(K)$ would be finite; at all other values of K, $P(K)$ would be zero. A derived distribution of $P(K)$ is shown in Figure 3 computed according to the method of Erwin and Aladjem (1976). Note the difference between it and the computed continuous distributions for the Sips and normal distribution, Figure 4. The method of Erwin and Aladjem can readily represent continuous and discrete distributions too. Thus it is commensurate with the continuous distributions. To be consistent conceptually, it would be best to adopt the convention of reserving the delta function representation for experimental situations where a real association of particular K_i's with specific antibody subpopulations has been made, and to use continuous or bar graph functions whenever only an analytical representation of the data is made.

III. DISPLACEMENT ASSAYS

Much of the usefulness of antibody as an analytical tool results from its ability to elicit information about an antigenic determinant. In general, this type of information is obtained in a displacement assay. If it is structural information about the antigen that is desired, then an appropriate test ligand is used to probe the antibody binding site complementary to the antigen. It is assumed that the test ligand which displaces antibody from its homologous antigen at the lowest concentration is structurally most similar to the antigenic determinant. If it is simply the concentration of the antigenic determinant that is desired, then the degree of displacement of an appropriately labelled antigen by the unlabelled antigen allows one to determine its concentration. Standard curves are constructed empirically to calibrate the system thereby circumventing the problem of specifying the detailed workings of the system. In the exposition to follow we outline the general principles of displacement assays and leave the detailed description of radioimmunoassays and enzyme linked immunoassays to Chapter 6.

Let us first define our system using two equilibrium constants: the first, for free antigen, is defined by equation (2) and the second, for the test antigen or tracer (T), is defined by equation (14)

$$K_t = \frac{BT}{B \cdot T} \tag{14}$$

where now BT is the concentration of bound test antigen, T is the free concentration of test antigen and B is again the concentration of free antibody sites. Since the concentration of free antibody sites is

$$B = N - R - BT \qquad (15)$$

combining equations (2), (13), and (14), one obtains the relationship

$$R = \frac{NKC}{1 + K_t T + KC} \qquad (16)$$

Structural information can then be obtained in the following manner. The binding R is defined at some C with $T = 0$. Then for each test determinant T_i, R is determined as a function of concentration of added T_i at the same C. As an end point, either a plot of R versus the log of T_i or a convenient measure much as the concentration where T_i reduces R by 50%, i.e. the ID_{50}, can be used. The T_i with the lowest concentration at the 50% binding point is assumed to be the test determinant closest in structure to the antigen itself. Figure 6 shows an example of a structural similarity analysis for a dextran by determination of sugars detected by a human anti-dextran antibody.

Ideally when $K_t = K$, the test antigen should be identical to the antigen determinant. However, since K is often not known or not determined, it is assumed that when K_t is a maximum the test antigen is structurally similar to the antigen itself. It is further assumed that structural dissimilarities lower K_t in a transitive manner, i.e. when the ID_{50}'s are ordered such that $ID_{50} (1) < ID_{50} (2) < ID_{50} (3) ...$, then the structural 'likeness' to the native determinant will be ordered $T_1 > T_2 > T_3$. There are several potential objections to the use of this method which must be kept in mind: (1) one never knows if the 'minimum' ID_{50} is the 'best' structure or if there is a better structure one has not tested; (2) parts of the structure unrecognized by the antibody will play little, if any, role in the structural determination; (3) there is the theoretical possibility of heteroclitic antibody, that is antibody which binds better to a determinant different than the determinant to which it was elicited. Nevertheless, these objections detract but little from the power of the method for analysis of structural similarities with an antigen.

If one wishes rather to determine the concentration of the antigen, one uses the analogous equation:

$$BT = \frac{NK_t T}{1 + K_t T + KC} \qquad (17)$$

In this case we consider T as the tracer, that is an antigen that is labelled by radiochemical, enzymatic, or fluorescent techniques. Then the concentration of antigen in a solution can be determined by the displacement of the tracer from the antibody. Several things become immediately apparent: the

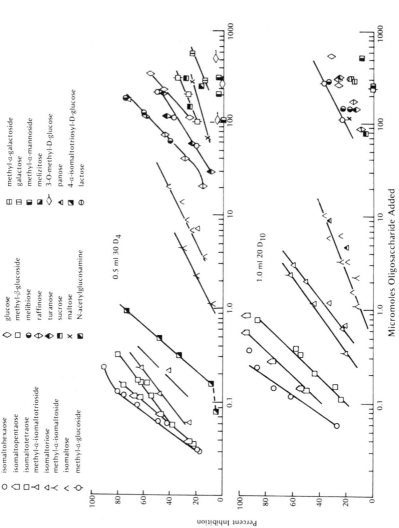

Figure 6. Inhibition by various sugars and sugar derivatives of precipitation of human anti-dextran by dextran. Conditions used: Top panel, 0.5 ml antiserum 30 D₄ containing 33 μg AbN; 10 μg clinical dextran N150 N; total volume 2.0 ml. Bottom panel, 1.0 ml antiserum 20 D₁₀ containing 31 μg AbN; 10 μg clinical dextran N150 N; total volume 2.5 ml. From Kabat (1957)

sensitive range of the displacement curve is in the range $0.1\ K_tT < KC < 10$ K_tT. Thus the choice of tracer and antibody concentration defines the measurement range. If tagging the antigen does not alter its binding, i.e. $K_t = K$, then the measurement range is simply $0.1 \cdot T < C < 10 \cdot T$ and the maximum sensitivity is at $T = C$.

A proviso must be entered. K_tT should ideally be much greater than 1. This gives maximum displacement in tracer binding as one goes from high to low antigen concentrations. As K_tT approaches or goes below 1 the sensitivity of the assay is lost because the amount of displacement is decreased. Finally as K_tT goes significantly below 1, there are two other complications which make the assay unreliable. First, the total amount of binding of tracer becomes very low and, although one can still displace what binding there is by increasing $KC > 1$, the low level of specific binding will leave the values of BT very sensitive to non-specific binding of tracer.

Second, the low value for K_tT suggests that BT may tend to dissociate during its separation from free T. Obviously then the sensitivity of the displacement assay may be estimated as $S = 0.1\ K^{-1}$ with $K_t = K$. Measurements at higher antigen concentrations do not represent a problem if antibody concentrations can be correspondingly increased.

Finally, the selectivity of the assay, that is the ability to discriminate between closely related antigens, may be examined using

$$BT = \frac{K_tT}{1 + K_tT + KC + K^*C^*} \tag{18}$$

where now C^* and K^* are respectively the free concentration and the affinity constant for the potentially competing antigen under test. For example, if one were measuring cGMP in the presence of cAMP, then K and C would be the affinity constant and free concentration of cGMP, K_t and T would be the affinity constant and free concentration of the labelled cGMP, here probably the iodinated succinyl cGMP, and K^* and C^* would represent the affinity constant and free concentration of cAMP. In the measurement of the potentially cross-reactive cyclic nucleotides cGMP and cAMP, concentrations of cAMP may be as much as 100-fold higher that cGMP, Steiner *et al.* (1972). Since typically $K_t \cong K$, only if $KC \gg K^*C^*$ will the system discriminate between the two antigens. If $C > C^*$, as in the measurement of cAMP in the presence of cGMP, the requirement for selectivity as measured in terms of K and K^* will be less severe. Conversely if $C^* \gg C$ in the measurement of cGMP in the presence of cAMP, then $K \gg K^*$ in order to have a valid measure of C in the presence of C^*. In terms of selectivity it means K/K^* should be $\geq 10^4$. This criterion appears to have been met, see for example, Frandsen and Krishna (1976).

IV. MULTIVALENT ANTIGEN

The combination of antibody with a monovalent ligand is best characterized as a simple association, governed by a single affinity constant. By contrast, the reaction of antibody with multivalent antigen leads to a plethora of secondary physical and biological *sequelae*. Among the more prominent effects as depicted in Figure 7 are precipitation, agglutination, complement fixation, cell surface receptor redistribution, and binding cooperativity. Since monovalent antibody (Fab) combined with multivalent antigen fails to exhibit these phenomena, the mechanistic requirement for their occurrence must be the presence of both multivalent antibody and multivalent antigen. Multivalence contributes a whole new dimension to antibody reactions and is obligatory for the occurrence of most of the important biological consequences of the antibody–antigen interaction.

A. Intrinsic Affinity

We begin our analysis of multivalent antibody–antigen interactions by first extending the definition of the reaction between a single monovalent ligand and its antibody. Amino acid sequence data and crystallographic structural determination have shown that the Fab regions of bivalent antibody are identical. This identity also implies equivalence of combining sites and affinity constants. The equivalence has been experimentally verified for monovalent ligand since the combining sites on IgG act independently (Nisonoff *et al.*, 1960; Skubitz *et al.*, 1977). Lack of cooperativity and independence of combining sites holds only for univalent ligands, it is lost when antibody binds to multivalent antigen. It is thus important to define as a point of reference the affinity constant of an independent antibody binding site with the equivalent, albeit hypothetical, monovalent ligand which corresponds to the homologous epitope of multivalent antigen. We call this the 'homologous intrinsic affinity constant' (HIAC), an extension of the 'intrinsic affinity constant' concept of Karush (1970). To make the definition more concrete, we will define HIAC explicitly for the situation depicted in Figure 8. We start by specifying the epitope concentration. In the case of a protein of non-repeating amino acid sequence such as lysozyme or albumin, the concentration of an epitope is identical to the concentration of the antigen since each epitope (antigenic determinant) occurs exactly once. The detailed delineation of an epitope can be followed in the work of Atassi (1978). By definition each epitope must be structurally distinct and have elicited its own unique set of antibodies. It is also obvious that in some situations, e.g. an anti-hapten antibody directed against a protein conjugated with the homologous hapten, there may be only a single type epitope—the hapten multiply substituted on the antigen surface. In that case the epitope

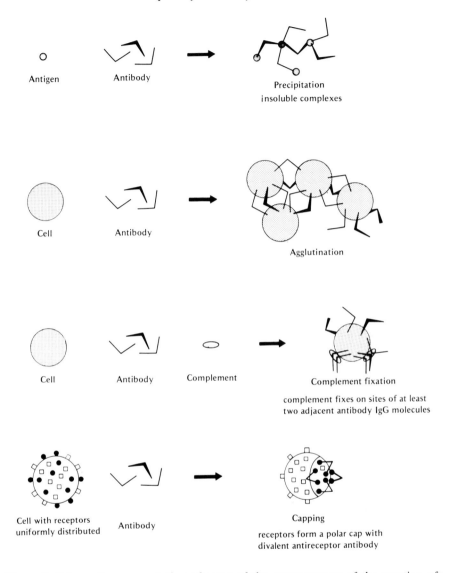

Figure 7. Schematic representation of some of the consequences of the reaction of multivalent antibody combining with multivalent antigen

concentration will be a multiple of the antigen concentration. With G as the total antigen concentration, G_j as the concentration of the jth epitope, N_j as the concentration of bivalent antibody against the jth epitope, it is a straightforward procedure to compute P_j, the probability that the epitope is free, that is unreacted, with its specific antibody.

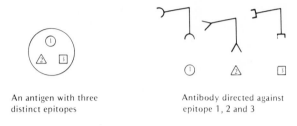

An antigen with three distinct epitopes

Antibody directed against epitope 1, 2 and 3

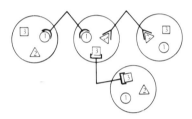

Antibody antigen reaction allows formation of aggregates, agglutinates and precipitates by cross-linking epitopes

Figure 8. Schematic representation of the interaction of a multivalent antibody with multivalent antigen that has non-repeating epitopes

$$P_j = \frac{\text{Free epitope concentration}}{G_j} \tag{19}$$

It then follows from the definition that the homologous intrinsic affinity constant is

$$K_t = \frac{(1 - P_j) \cdot G_j}{(2 \cdot N_j - (1 - P_j) \cdot G_j) \cdot P_j \cdot G_j} \tag{20}$$

It is important to define operationally the homologous intrinsic association constant K_j. Thus K_j may be experimentally estimated by the extent of reaction of the antibody with an equivalent monovalent ligand or of monovalent antibody with mono- or polyvalent ligand. For example, Pecht *et al.* (1971) measured an intrinsic association constant of antibodies directed against the loop peptide of lysozyme (amino acids 63–80), a large monovalent ligand. Hornick and Karush (1972) determined a monovalent affinity constant for DNP conjugated to the bacteriophage ϕX174 by two different methodologies. First, they used equilibrium dialysis to determine the affinity constant between the monovalent hapten DNP–lysine with divalent antibody. This is the 'intrinsic' affinity constant of Karush (1970). Second, they prepared monovalent antibody, both the 3.5S Fab fragment and the monovalent 7S hybrid against the ϕX174 DNP conjugate. This allows study of the antibody binding to the complete homologous epitope. They then determined the affinity constant using phage neutralization. The two experimental approaches for estimating the HIAC gave results that differed by a factor of 10, i.e. $3.3 \times 10^7 \, \text{M}^{-1}$ for the equilibrium dialysis method versus $3.3 \times 10^8 \, \text{M}^{-1}$ for neutralization by the 7S monovalent hybrid antibody. Presumably most of the difference arises because equilibrium dialysis measures the mean affinity constant whereas the neutralization technique selects for the high affinity fraction of the anti-DNP antibody. Use of homogeneous antibody would minimize differences between the two methods. Although the data demonstrate that the 'operational' definition of the homologous intrinsic affinity constant is not without ambiguities, the values, nonetheless, provide a bench mark against which one can examine effects of multivalency on affinity. Furthermore, the monovalent hybrid antibody technique would appear a particularly useful method for the general determination of HIAC since it would obviate the need to synthesize the monovalent homologous ligand required for use with bivalent antibody.

B. Functional Affinity, Definition with Monogamous Binding

When the association of multivalent antibody and antigen takes place, an affinity constant can be defined for the association of the kinetic units. Karush (1970) has suggested the term 'functional affinity' be used to characterize the interaction of antibody and antigen in those systems involving multivalent linkages. Thus in a formal way the functional affinity constant for antibody with n sites (B^n) and antigen with m sites (G^m) can be defined by the association of the two kinetic units:

$$B^n + G^m = B^n G^m \tag{21}$$

It should be clear that this is not to be equated with the intrinsic affinity constant

$$B^1 + G^1 = B^1 G^1 \tag{22}$$

Note that the association in equation (22) is accurately defined by the association of the two kinetic units. The association of equation (21) is effectively undefined (even though we have defined a K for the kinetic units) since we have not stipulated how many of the n B sites and the m G sites are combined. We only know how many B and G units are associated.

It is worth emphasizing that intrinsic affinity is normally examined in most studies of the structural relationship, complementarity, and kinetics of antibody interactions. By contrast, in most biological systems, it is the functional affinity that best describes the process since under those conditions it is the interaction of the kinetic units, the antibody and the bacteria, the antibody and virus or the antibody and cell that is of importance.

Hornick and Karush (1972) determined the functional affinity constant for the association of bivalent 7S anti-DNP antibody against dinitrophenylated ϕX174 (DNP-ϕX174). They demonstrated single hit kinetics, that is one antibody molecule would neutralize the DNP-ϕX174, and dissociation of that molecule would restore biological activity of the phage. The functional affinity constant for equation (21) can be written

$$K = \frac{G^m B^n}{[B^n - (G^m B^n)]G^m - (B^m B^n)]} \tag{23}$$

defining the probability of an unreacted neutralizing DNP site as P, then

$$P = 1 - \frac{G^m B^n}{G^m} \tag{24}$$

where G^m is the number of phage in the system since there is one neutralizing DNP site per phage (single kit kinetics) and $G^m B^n$ is the number G^m combined with antibody at the neutralization site. Thus

$$K = \frac{1 - P}{[B^n - G^m(1 - P)] \cdot P} \tag{25}$$

Now since for the DNP-ϕX174, $B^n \gg G^m$

$$K \cong \frac{1 - P}{B^n \cdot P} \tag{25a}$$

With 84% neutralization and an antibody concentration of $1.5 \times 10^{-11}\,\text{M}$, a functional affinity of $3.5 \times 10^{11}\,\text{M}^{-1}$ was obtained; an enhancement of 4 orders of magnitude over the nomologous intrinsic affinity constant. Since, in this case, there are multiple repeating epitopes (the DNP hapten on the surface of the ϕX174), the situation is probably best explained by multivalent monogamous binding as depicted in Figure 9. Thus, although only the single key site needs to be blocked with antibody to neutralize the phage, it is presumed that the monogamous binding of the second antibody site leads to the enhancement of functional affinity. A similar enhancement was obtained by Gopalakrishnan and Karush (1974) with a *p*-aminophenyl β-lactoside hapten conjugate of ϕX174. These experiments demonstate the great biological advantage of multivalency for antibody affinity since all bacterial and viral surfaces are composed of repeating antigenic determinants.

The functional affinity constant can, by analogy to the intrinsic affinity constant, be considered to be the ratio between the kinetic constants for the forward and the reverse reactions.

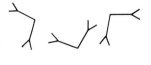

An antigen with
identical epitopes

Antibody directed
against the epitope

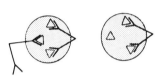

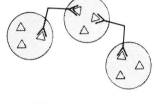

Monogamous binding

Bigamous binding

Figure 9. Schematic representation of antibody binding options when there are multiple identical epitopes on the antigen surface. In this case there is the possibility of both monogamous (binding of the antibody to only one antigen) and bigamous binding (binding which cross-links two or more antigen molecules through the antibody). The competition between bigamous and monogamous binding depends upon the flexibility of the antibody hinge region, and the spatial distribution and orientation of the epitopes on the antigenic surface

$$G^m + B^n \underset{k_f}{\overset{k_f}{\rightleftharpoons}} G^m B^n \tag{26}$$

$$K = k_f/k_r \tag{26a}$$

For a small monovalent ligand (Karush, 1978) k_f is generally in the range 4×10^5 to 2×10^8 $M^{-1} s^{-1}$. For the reverse reaction, the k_r's range from 3×10^{-5} to 900 s^{-1}. Since the K's vary from 10^4 to 10^{11} M^{-1} the dissociation reaction is the major determinant of the affinity constant. The data of Hornick and Karush (1972) show that the change from monovalent to multivalency has little effect on the rate constant of association, k_f, but greatly retards the rate of dissociation. Thus the primary effect of multivalency is to slow complex dissociation, a conclusion that accords well with theoretical expectations.

C. Affinity Constant, Protein Antigens

An affinity has also been frequently determined by workers using multivalent antigens such as albumin which lack repeating epitopes (Figure 8). Changes in affinity have been used principally as a probe of biological function, i.e. effects of immunodeficiency (Soothill and Steward, 1971; Alpers *et al.*, 1972), malaria (Steward and Voller, 1973), and adoptive transfer (Celada *et al.*, 1969). Hudson (1968) and Steward and Petty (1972) suggested calculation of affinity constants based upon ammonium sulphate precipitation of the anti-protein antibodies according to the method of Farr (1958). The measurement made in such a system allows the determination of the fraction of antigen combined with one or more antibodies. Thus the computed binding value measures neither the functional nor the intrinsic affinity constant. Since a free antigen molecule must have all of its epitopes uncombined with specific antibody, then where the total antigen concentration is G, the concentration of free antigen must be (Berzofsky *et al.*, 1976; Otterness, 1979)

$$\text{Free antigen} = \Pi P_j \cdot G \tag{27}$$

Where Π means the product $P_1 \cdot P_2 \cdot \ldots$ for all the epitopes. The fraction of antigen precipitated by ammonium sulphate, q, must be simply

$$q = 1 - \Pi P_j \tag{28}$$

Each P_j is different; it is determined by G_j, K_j, and N_j of equation (20), and no more can be done without drastic simplifying assumptions. Here we use two, first that the concentration of antibody against the jth epitope, N_j, is just the total antibody concentration N divided by the valence of the antigen, f, where valence is the maximum number of antibodies that can simultaneously combine with the antigen, a number that may be less that the number of epitopes because of overlapping combining sites or steric hindrance. Second, we make the assumption of Goldberg (1952) that all the P_j are equivalent, i.e. $P = P_j$. Then

$$P = (1 - q)^{1/f} \tag{29}$$

Determination of q then allows in principle the computation of K from equation (20) by substituting P from equation (29) where now the subscripts j can be dropped in equation (20). Hudson (1968) made the computation on several extensive sets of data using ammonium sulphate precipitation of a fluorescent-labelled albumin. He obtained the disconcerting result that the computed binding constant was a function of antigen concentration.

One can argue that it is necessary to go out to far antigen excess where on the average no large aggregates can be formed. Under those circumstances q is very small and

$$P \cong 1 - q/f \tag{30}$$

Thus an estimate of the intrinsic binding constant is just

$$K = \frac{qG}{(2N - qG) \cdot C} \tag{31}$$

where instead of the normal definition of the free antigen concentration $C =$

$G(1 - q)$ we find that $C = G(1 - q/f)$ and we have used 2 as the valence of the antibody and f as the valence of the antigen. Since this is just the binding constant as defined by Steward and Petty (1972) it suggests that in far antigen excess the calculated binding constant and the intrinsic affinity constants should coincide, a result that is merely another way of saying that antigen acts in far antigen excess as a monovalent ligand. Arend and Mannik (1974) used the Steward–Petty approach to compute association constants for HSA–anti–HSA and found the association constants again a function of antigen concentration.

There are several possibilities for this anomalous dependence of association constants upon concentration. The first is to postulate that as one goes to lower concentrations, one measures the effects of only the progressively higher affinity populations of antibody. This possibility appears excluded since the determined antibody concentration does not change with dilution. A more logical explanation of these results is that under most measurement conditions, it is the stoicheiometry of the reaction that is being measured since the concentrations generally used are not low enough to find measurable dissociation by the techniques used. This point of view appears validated by plotting the fraction of antigen bound versus the ratio of antigen to antibody (G/N) added to the reaction mixtures. One finds that the plot of fraction of antigen bound for each of the dilutions generally gives a single curve within experimental error. Thus the system has not normally been diluted sufficiently for measurable dissociation to take place and the K's measured are probably measures of stoicheiometry. By this criterion the K's for the HSA–anti–HSA system must be at least $10^{+9} M^{-1}$, that is of the same order of magnitude as for polypeptide hormones (Wu and Rockey, 1969; Berson and Yalow, 1959; Worobec *et al.*, 1972), rather than the low values commonly estimated by ammonium sulphate precipitation or ultracentrifugal analysis.

D. Cooperative Interactions

The binding of polyvalent antigen to antibody does not always lead to the same form of the Scatchard plot seen with monovalent ligand, that is linear when antibody was homogeneous and curved concave when antibody was heterogeneous (Figure 1). Scatchard plots presented by Paul *et al.* (1966), Matsukura *et al.* (1971), Weintraub *et al.* (1973), Bartels *et al.* (1972), Niederer (1974), and Celis *et al.* (1977) for multivalemt antigen show an initial convex region of the binding curve. Thus initially the r/c ratio increases with added antigen, and reaches a maximum beyond which the ratio falls in typical concave fashion (Figure 10). Although this phenomenon has been exploited in the development of a radioimmunoassay, Matsukura *et al.* (1971), there is no evidence supporting a particular mechanism for the effect except that

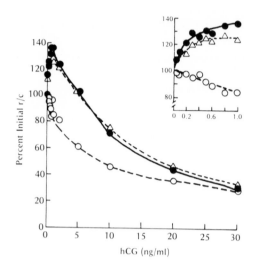

Figure 10. Radioimmunoassay standard curves using intact antibody (•–•), modified antibody (△---△), and univalent Fab (○---○). The enhanced tracer binding at small increments of hCG was observed with intact and modified antibody but not with Fab. Insert shows detailed binding data at low hCG concentration. From Weintraub *et al.* (1973)

antibody bivalency appears to be required. Weintraub *et al.* (1973) examined the binding of human chorionic gonadotropin (HCG) with anti-HCG. They used first the native antibody and the two papain cleavage products, the Fab_1 monovalent antibody and the modified antibody, apparently Fab_2. Both the native and the modified anti-HCG showed the convex Scatchard plot. By contrast, the Fab monovalent antibody gave a normal concave Scatchard plot suggesting that multivalency of antibody is critical for the phenomenon. Niederer (1974) verified in another system that the papain monovalent fragment failed to show the convex Scatchard plot. He suggested that this phenomenon is evidence for cooperative binding since if

$$B + G \overset{K_1}{\rightleftharpoons} BG \tag{32}$$

and

$$BG + G \overset{K_2}{\rightleftharpoons} BG_2 \tag{32a}$$

then if binding at the first site enhances the binding K of the second site, i.e. $K_2 > K_1$, a convex Scatchard plot is obtained. Bartels *et al.* (1972) assumed the equilibrium was

$$B + 2G \rightleftharpoons BG_2 \tag{33}$$

which is just equations (32) when $K_2 \gg K_1$. Obviously cooperative allosteric binding as formulated by Monod *et al.* (1965) would similarly provide an explanation. However, there is little supporting evidence for that point of view (Metzger, 1978) and the distance between the two binding sites is sufficiently great that it is difficult in practice to conceive that any of the above mechanisms would provide an explanation.

A simple explanation of the apparent cooperativity would be the existence of an energetic advantage to having adjacent antibody or antigen molecules, for example if the molecule (antigen or antibody) had an innate tendency for dimer or aggregate formation. This would result in an apparent enhancement of the affinity constant whenever the molecules could be in adjacent position where ε is the energy advantage of

$$K_{adj.} = Ke^{\varepsilon/RT} \tag{34}$$

adjacent compared to non-adjacent binding. The data of Celis *et al.* (1977) appear to focus attention on the antigen molecule. Since their antibody was covalently bound to agarose, cooperativity due to formation of more favourable energetic surface arrangements by antibody could not be expected to occur. The possibility of an energetic contribution by antigen dimerization was postulated by Metzger (1978), but lacks experimental documentation. It is clearly premature to attempt to define the causes of this apparent cooperativity.

E. Precipitin Reactions

The ability of multivalent antibody and antigen to precipitate formed the basis of the first quantitative assays of antibody and antigen interaction (Heidelberger and Kendall, 1929, 1935). Precipitation is routinely used as the first and frequently as the sole measure of antibody content. Precipitation in capillary tubes is rapid and may be used as a qualitative indication of antibody content.

The precipitation reaction of a typical protein antigen with bivalent antibody is shown in Figure 11. In the example, increasing amounts of egg albumin were added to a constant amount of rabbit anti-egg-albumin antibody and the precipitate allowed to form. The supernatant and precipitate were separated by centrifugation, the precipitate washed and then analysed according to Kabat and Mayers (1961). The analysis of the precipitate is most commonly carried out by determination of either the optical density of the dissolved precipitate or by nitrogen analysis of the precipitate. The results, typical for rabbit antibody, show that with increasing antigen the amount of precipitate increases steadily to a maximum and thereafter the amount of precipitate decreases with increasing antigen until effectively none is formed. When the supernatant from each precipitate is tested by adding a small amount of additional antibody or antigen to it, some

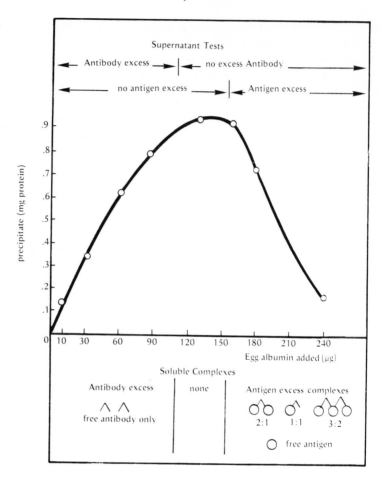

Figure 11. A precipitin curve showing the amount of precipitate formed between rabbit anti-egg-albumin antibody and egg albumin as a function of added egg albumin. At the top of the figure the results of supernatant analysis are shown. At the bottom of the figure are shown the soluble supernatant reactants computed. From Aladjem *et al.* (1966)

insight into the nature of the reaction is obtained (Heidelberger, 1939). At low antigen concentrations, that is before the point of maximal precipitation, additional precipitate is formed when excess antigen, but not when antibody, is added. That implies that after precipitation, antibody is left in the supernatant which is still available to precipitate additional antigen. Similarly, beyond the point of maximum precipitation, when excess antibody is added, but not when excess antigen is added, additional precipitate is formed. This implies an excess of antigen in the supernatant. Since in the region of maximal precipitation, addition of neither excess antibody nor excess antigen will cause formation of additional precipitate, this region of the precipitin curve is called the *equivalence zone*.

A number of theories have been proposed to describe the mechanism of the precipitation reaction (Heidelberger and Kendall, 1935; Teorell, 1946; DeLisi, 1974; Stensgaard, 1977; Goldberg, 1952; Amano *et al.*, 1963). Of particular note is the theory of Palmiter and Aladjem (1963) and Aladjem *et al.* (1965, 1966) which was formulated to provide a clear quantitative description of the reaction that could be readily tested experimentally. They used the simple device of computing the precipitate (*PT*) as the difference between the total antibody (*N*) and antigen (*G*) added into the reaction mixture less than in soluble complexes. Thus

$$PT = W_\mathrm{B}N + W_\mathrm{G}G - \underset{S}{\Sigma}(iW_\mathrm{G} + jW_\mathrm{B})m_{ij} \tag{35}$$

where m_{ij} is the molar concentration of a complex containing i antigen and j antibody molecules, and W_B and W_G are the conversion factors from moles/litre to weight of antibody and antigen, respectively, and S designates the sum over all soluble complexes. Aladjem chose to compute the concentrations of the complexes using the statistical mechanical approach pioneered by Stockmayer (1943) and Goldberg (1952). For refinement, the computational method of Amano *et al.* (1963) could be used for protein antigens with non-repeating epitopes. No satisfactory theory has been derived for computations in the case where monogamous binding takes place, but see Crothers and Metzger (1976) for a discussion of the problem. It should be further recognized that if cooperative effects (see Section IV.D) occur during precipitation, systematic deviations in computed complex distributions may be found. Aladjem *et al.* (1966) defined soluble complexes according to the earlier work of Singer (1957). Thus free, uncombined antibody and antigen were considered soluble, as well as the limiting complex for bivalent antibody, the {2 : 1} complex, that is two antigens bound with each antibody (o⌒o); also the {1 : 1} complex, one antibody, one antigen and the {3 : 2} complex, 3 antigens, 2 antibodies o⌒o⌒o were defined as soluble. The computed functional affinity constants were of the order of $10^9 \mathrm{M}^{-1}$ by chi square fit. Their computation suggests several important points of interpretation: (1) it is predicted that large complexes are formed only in the region of equivalence; (2) in the region of antibody or antigen excess it predicts that only small complexes are formed. Thus in antibody excess, most antigenic sites are combined with antibody, but few antibodies would have both sites bound to antigen, i.e. in the example typically a {1 : 3}⌒∞ or {2 : 5} ∞⌒∞ complex might be formed in antibody excess and {3 : 2}, {2 : 1}, {1 : 1}, and {4 : 3} complexes in antigen excess; and (3) that at least in some systems cross-linking does not appear to be required for precipitation.

These results also could be interpreted to suggest that in precipitating systems where a prozone exists (Figure 12), there is a requirement for

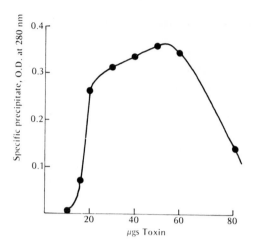

Figure 12. Quantitative precipitation of horse antitoxin antibody with the crystalline toxin MY. Note that with the horse antitoxin antibody, there is a failure of antibody and antigen to precipitate at high antibody/antigen ratio. The lack of precipitation in the antibody excess region is called a prozone. From Pappenheimer *et al.* (1972)

cross-linking before precipitation will take place (Palmiter and Aladjem, 1968). It also happens that some antibodies do not precipitate, for example, horse γG(T) antibody. Klinman and Karush (1967) demonstrated that the non-precipitating γG(T) antibody forms bivalent cross-links with antigen far less frequently than precipitating γGab antibody. That also seems to suggest that bivalent cross-linking is a critical part of the precipitation phenomena.

V. PRECIPITIN REACTIONS IN GELS

The antibody–antigen reactions described allow both sensitivity and selectivity of antigen detection via binding reactions, displacement reactions, and precipitin reactions. However, when more than a single antibody–antigen system is present, it is not easily recognized nor analysed using those reactions since measurement may consist, for example, of only the total amount of antibody and antigen precipitated. By contrast precipitin reactions in gels typically occur with the precipitate for each antigenic system being localized in spatially distinct areas. Thus these reactions are able to define the presence of multiple antigenic systems and delineate structural cross-reactivities between antigens. Precipitin reactions in gels, therefore, differ from those in liquid media by the wide variety of physical arrangements that are used to optimize the information obtained and by the differences in spatial display of the precipitating systems that result with each different arrangement. The topic has been extensively reviewed by Crowle (1973) and Williams and Chase (1971).

There are two general types of arrangements of gel and reactants that may be distinguished, simple and double diffusion. In simple diffusion the gel containing the antibody and the gel containing the antigen are juxtaposed, whereas in double diffusion the antibody and the antigen are separated by an intervening gel containing neither antibody or antigen. Precipitation usually occurs in the intervening gel. For more complex mixtures of antigens an electrophoretic step may be superimposed to obtain greater spatial resolution of the precipitating systems. Alternatively an electrophoretic step can be superimposed to speed the movement of the antigen into the antibody gel. In either case the procedure is called immunoelectrophoresis and again the physical arrangement of the reactants greatly affects the pattern of the precipitin lines obtained.

Precipitation in gels can also be used to determine antigen concentration. However, because the technique is normally limited to antigens that precipitate directly with antibody, excluding many low molecular weight as well as all univalent antigens, and because the sensitivity rarely gets down below 10 µg/ml, the technique has been principally of use for the quantification of serum proteins.

A. Simple Diffusion

There are a number of arrangements for simple diffusion that have been used to advantage. We will discuss only two: (1) simple diffusion in tubes (Oudin, 1946, 1948) because it is the system in which most of the principles of immunodiffusion were developed and tested; and (2) radial simple diffusion according to Mancini *et al.* (1965) because it is a principal method for determining serum concentrations of particular immunoglobulin classes.

Typically for simple diffusion in tubes, antibody in a dilute 0.2% melted agar solution is added to a height of around 4 cm in a 2 mm (inside diameter) tube. After the agar has solidified, 3 to 4 cm of an antigen solution are added to the tube. The tube is sealed and diffusion and immunoprecipitation are allowed to proceed at constant temperature. Precipitate begins to form in a few hours, but the best definition of the antigenic systems begins to take place after a few days with a convenient reading time being from day 4 to 7.

The analysis of immunodiffusion as with other diffusion processes begins with Fick's Law

$$\frac{\partial c}{\partial t} = D \frac{\partial^2 c}{\partial x^2} \tag{36}$$

and the definition of boundary conditions that will give a suitable solution. There are a number of fundamental assumptions. (1) Precipitation takes place in a zone where free antigen and antibody meet and combine to precipitate such that all the antibody and antigen are consumed in the precipitate, i.e. it is a complete sink, there is no free antigen below this region and no free antibody above it. (2) It is considered that the precipitation zone (or at least its leading edge) is of negligible thickness and thus it can be approximated by a moving plane. (3) The composition of the precipitate (at least at the leading edge) is constant. Thus if the ratio of antigen to antibody (G/B) is (R) then at the leading edge

$$G = R \cdot B \tag{37}$$

Although it is not critical for the development of a quantitative description of the immunodiffusion process, it is often assumed that the ratio R is not too different from the ratio G/B at the equivalence zone of the precipitin curve. The amount of precipitate (PT) formed is simply

$$PT = R \cdot B + B \tag{38}$$

Finally it is assumed that the precipitation zone acts as a sink only for the specific antibody and antigen, but allows unrelated antibody and antigen to pass through relatively unimpeded.

We indicate qualitatively the nature of the solution of diffusion equation (36) using the elementary theory of Becker *et al.* (1951). Those readers requiring a more quantitative result should consult Speirs and Augustin (1957). Becker *et al.* (1951) assumed that the initial antigen concentration (G_0) was high compared to the initial antibody concentration (B_0), thus the system can be treated as a one way diffusion of antigen into the antibody gel. The antigen concentration G at time t and a distance x into the antibody gel is then

$$G(x,t) = G_0(1 - 2/\pi^{1/2} \int_0^y e^{-y^2} \, dy) \tag{39}$$

where

$$y = x/(4Dt)^{1/2} \tag{40}$$

and the concentration of antigen at the leading front is defined by equation (37). When y is large, the integral in equation (39) can be expanded as

$$2/\pi^{1/2} \int_0^y e^{-y^2} \, dy \cong 1 - \frac{e^{-y^2}}{\pi^{1/2}} \left(\frac{1}{y} - \frac{1}{2y^3} + \frac{1 \cdot 3}{4y^5} - \ldots \right) \tag{41}$$

substituting equation (41) in equation (39) after neglecting terms of order $1/y^3$, then taking logarithms of each side

$$\ln(\pi^{1/2}G) = \ln G_0 + \ln y - y^2 \tag{42}$$

Again since y is large, we drop $\ln(y)$ as negligible compared to y^2, substituting G (equation 37) and converting to logarithms to the base 10, one finds

$$\log G_0 \cong \log (\pi^{1/2} R \cdot B_0) + x^2/t \cdot (9.2/D)^{-1} \qquad (43)$$

Thus at high G/B ratio, the logarithm of the initial antigen concentration is approximately proportional to the square of the distance migrated by the precipitation zone divided by the time. This equation can be used to determine diffusion coefficients with about a 10% error (Becker, 1971).

Using the expansion of the integral of equation (39) under conditions where y is small, after analogous substutions, one obtains

$$\log G_0 \cong \log (R \cdot B) + X/t^{1/2} \cdot 4.3(\pi D)^{1/2} \qquad (44)$$

When Oudin (1948) examined simple diffusion in tubes over a wide range of antigen concentrations, antibody held constant, he found the proportionality predicted by equation (44) to be more generally applicable. Thus $\log (G_0)$ is proportional to $x/t^{1/2}$. Further since x and $\log (G_0)$ are proportional at a fixed time, it provides a suitable method for the experimental determination of antigen concentration. Equation (44) predicts the correct proportionality. However, it applies principally in the region where antibody is significant; thus the diffusion of the antibody towards the antigen and the depletion of the antigen via the precipitation sink cannot be neglected (Speirs and Augustin, 1958) and this formulation is not quantatively exact.

In practice, convenience has led to the use of simple radial diffusion as the most common gel diffusion method of measuring concentrations of unknown antigens. The usual technique, that of Mancini *et al.* (1965) consists of a 3% agar gel containing a dilution of the antibody. Generally gels are poured only a millimetre or so in depth to conserve antibody and antigen and holes 2 mm in diameter are punched to receive antigen. The exact antibody dilution is chosen by running a standard series of antigen concentrations encompassing the desired measurement range of antigen for each antibody dilution and choosing the optimally discriminatory dilution. Immunodiffusion plates pre-made with various antibody specificities are available commercially. The advantage of simple radial diffusion is primarily in the great simplicity of sample preparation and handling, particularly with a large number of samples. Results are expressed as the diameter of the precipitin ring formed. Unlike simple diffusion in tubes where the supply of antigen may be large, in simple radial diffusion the supply of antigen is finite and, after a few days, its depletion results in the formation of a stable precipitin ring. It has been found empirically that the square of the terminal diameter (D^2) of the precipitate is directly proportional to the amount of antigen added to the centre well, that is volume (V) times antigen concentration, $(V \times G_0)$ and inversely proportional to the antibody concentration in the agar gel. Thus

$$D^2 = a + b \cdot V \cdot G_0/B_0 \qquad (45)$$

The convenience of running large numbers of samples makes it a simple task to include a standard curve with each set of measurements, an expedient that ensures the reliability of the procedure.

B. Double Diffusion

Double diffusion is the methodology generally applied to reveal multiple antigens in a preparation and to examine cross-reactivity, that is antigenic similarity. The procedure is quite simple. Usually a 0.5% agar gel is prepared with an appropriate pattern of wells. Typically, in Ouchterlony double diffusion, circular wells are used (Ouchterlony, 1958, 1962; Crowle, 1973), but rectangular (Elek, 1949; Zivković et al., 1976) and triangular wells (Jennings and Malone, 1954) may be used with good results. Wells are fitted with an appropriate dilution of antigen and antibody and allowed to diffuse towards each other at constant temperature. The time for good precipitin line development lengthens from overnight to 4 to 5 days as one goes from microscope slide size wells several millimetres apart to Petri dish size wells, a few centimetres apart. The amount of antigen and antibody required also increases and generally the clarity of spatial resolution improves.

Double diffusion may be used simply to enumerate the number of distinct antigens in the system. It is important to remember though that an antigen will only be detected when there is a precipitating antibody directed against it. Thus there is a requirement to utilize antisera to all the relevant antigens for a correct enumeration. This may require the use of a mixture of antisera or immunization with appropriate crude or concentrated mixtures of antigens. Since the location of the precipitin line for each antigen–antibody system is determined by the equivalent zone ratio R (equation 37) and the antibody and antigen concentrations, it is a rare event to obtain completely indistinguishable (overlapping) precipitin lines with a few antigenic systems present. However, when an antigen is present in considerable excess, instead of a sharp precipitin line, a very broad diffuse band of precipitate forms which may interfere with the discrimination of the different antigenic systems.

This application of double diffusion finds its principal use in the determination of antisera specificity for such uses as immunoprecipitation reactions for antigenic purification or quantification. Although this technique may be used for the enumeration of components in a mixture, it is less than ideal for that purpose. Polyacrylamide gel electrophoresis, for example, is a much simpler and a more generally applicable technique since the detection of a particular component in the mixture does not depend on the immunogenicity of the component nor on the presence of the specific antibody for its detection.

If it is necessary not only to enumerate but to identify the antigens present several techniques may be applied. (1) Specific staining for lipids, carbohydrates, and nucleic acids may be used. (2) Radiolabelled antigens, i.e.

radioautography (Thorbecke *et al.*, 1971) or antigen tagged with dye may be used to co-migrate with an untagged antigen. (3) Since the position of the precipitin line at a constant antibody concentration will shift towards the antibody well in excess antigen, the antibody can be absorbed with test antigen thereby moving the precipitin line of the antigen identical to the test antigen towards the antibody well or eliminating it all together. Alternatively the test antigen can be added to the antigen well. Again the precipitin line identical to the test antigen will be shifted towards the antibody well. (4) An adjacent well may be set up to examine the antigen mixture for cross-reactions with known antigens—see below. (5) Where the antigen to be identified is an enzyme, there may be a specific colour reaction that will identify it, see Uriel (1971) for a comprehensive listing. (6) If the choice is between a few well characterized antigens, the shape of the precipitin line may allow discrimination since the shape depends on the diffusion coefficients of the antigen and antibody. As a general rule, if antigen has a greater diffusion coefficient than antibody, the precipitin line will show curvature towards the antibody well, the higher the diffusion coefficient, the greater the curvature (Korngold and Leeuwen, 1957; Aladjem *et al.*, 1959). Conversely, if the diffusion coefficient is similar to that of antibody the precipitin line will be straight and, if the antigen has a lower diffusion coefficient, the line will be curved towards the antigen well. Since lower molecular weights generally have higher diffusion coefficients (except with highly asymmetric molecules), this also allows a rough ranking of antigens by size.

Double diffusion may also be used to examine cross-reactivity or antigenic similarity. Typically a well pattern is cut in agar such as is shown in Figure 13. Four patterns of cross-reactivity are recognized. The most common reaction is the 'Reaction of Independence'. It indicates that the antiserum does not recognize any epitopes that are common to both antigens. The 'Reaction of Identity' indicates that as far as the antiserum can discriminate, both antigens are identical, that is all the recognized epitopes are identical. Although strongly suggestive, it does not guarantee that the antigens are identical since in the absence of an appropriate specificity in the antiserum, existing epitope differences can go unrecognized.

The 'Cross-Reaction, Single Dissimilarity' indicates that the antiserum recognizes common epitopes between the two antigens, but that one antigen (G_1 in Figure 13) has at least one additional epitope which is absent in antigen G_2. The absence of these epitopes in antigen G_2 allows the formation of a spur, i.e. the antibody which does not react with G_2 diffuses through the precipitin line and reacts with G_1 to form the spur. Since much of the antibody against G_1 is consumed in the cross-reacting precipitin line, the spur is formed only with the left over non-cross-reacting antibody. Thus it is commonly noted that the spur forms a less dense precipitate than the primary line against the same antigen (here G_1). This type of pattern is commonly found where a

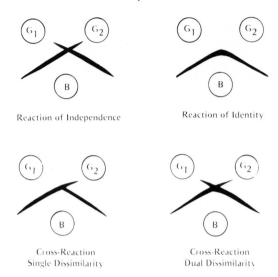

Figure 13. Illustration of the four basic precipitin patterns formed in double diffusion tests of antigenic similarity. In each case the well, labelled B, contains antibody, and the well, labelled G_1 and G_2, contains two different antigens. See the text for the interpretation of the reactions

molecule has been enzymatically cleaved or separated into subunits and the cleavage products or subunits are compared to the parent molecule. The former are deficient in epitopes posessed by the latter.

The 'Cross-Reaction, Dual Dissimilarity' pattern indicates a common epitope between both antigens but that each antigen has at least one epitope that is not in common with the other antigen. Thus the two precipitin lines coalesce but in addition they each also form a spur with antibody to the unique epitope. Again for the reasons mentioned above the spur will be less dense than the primary precipitin line, a fact which helps to distinguish this reaction from the reaction of independence. This type of reaction is commonly observed when comparing different products of an enzymatic cleavage.

The analysis of antigen similarity is the most unique application of immunodiffusion. It is used as the starting place for the determination of relationships between cell surface antigens and has been used extensively to examine systematic relationships in biology. In both cases, however, sequence analysis provides the absolute measure of similarity.

C. Immunoelectrophoresis

The superposition of an electric field on the process of immunodiffusion allows for much greater spatial resolution of the antibody–antigen precipitin lines (Grabar and Williams, 1953, 1955). This is particularly of value where one is looking for qualitative changes in the antigen distribution when there are numerous antigens present. For example, with whole sera there are simply too many antigens present to draw any meaningful conclusions from double diffusion analysis. Immunoelectrophoresis first separates each antigen according to its electophoretic mobility. Then a trough parallel to the direction of electrophoresis is filled with antibody, and precipitation is allowed to occur by immunodiffusion. The ability now to identify antigens by their electrophoretic mobility in addition to their precipitation pattern permits greatly improved observations of qualitative changes in the antigenic mixture.

Further improvements have been made in the technique which permit quantitation through use of two-dimensional (crossed) immunoelectrophoresis (Laurell, 1965; Clarke and Freeman, 1968). In two-dimensional electrophoresis, after the first electrophoretic separation of the antigen in the agar gel, a second agar gel now containing antibody is juxtaposed with the original agar slab. The separated antigen is now electrophoresed (the direction is perpendicular to the original direction of electrophoresis) into the antibody gel forming distinct peaks of precipitate. The areas of the peaks can be quantitatively related to the amount of antigen. Although this represents a definite quantitative improvement over standard immunoelectrophoresis, its principal use is determination of changes in serum components under pathological conditions, see for example Clarke and Freeman (1970).

VI. PERSPECTIVE

Recent developments in the preparation of homogeneous antibody based on the hybridoma technology (Melchers *et al.*, 1978) will, undoubtedly, provide homogeneous and biochemically defined immunological reagents for the assay of a wide variety of antigens. The ambiguities and limitations of serology will be eliminated as such reagents replace traditional antisera. As a consequence the treatment of the interaction of antigen with homogeneous antibody developed in this chapter will acquire increased applicability and relevance for both biological and analytical purposes. Immunochemistry will become an even more powerful tool for the detection, assay, and structural analysis of the wide variety of molecules encountered in living systems.

REFERENCES

Aladjem, F., Jaross, R. W., Paldino, R. L., and Lackner, J. A. (1959). The antigen–antibody reaction III. Theoretical considerations concerning the formation, location, and curvature of the antigen–antibody precipitation zone in agar diffusion plates and a method. *J. Immunol.*, **88**, 221–231.
Aladjem, F. and Palmiter, M. T. (1965). The antigen–antibody reaction V. A

quantitative theory of antigen–antibody reaction which allows for heterogenicity of antibodies. *J. Theoret. Biol.*, **8**, 8–21.

Aladjem, F., Palmiter, M. T., and Chang, Fu-Wu (1966). On the mechanism of the quantitative precipitin reaction. *Immunochemistry*, **3**, 419–424.

Alpers, J. H., Steward, M. W., and Soothill, J. F. (1972). Differences in immune elimination in inbred mice. The role of low affinity antibody. *Clin. Exp. Immunol.*, **12**, 121–132.

Amano, T., Syozi, I., Tokunaga, T., and Sato, S. (1963). A new statistical mechanical theory on the antigen–antibody reaction. *Biken J.*, **5**, 259–296.

Arend, W. P. and Mannik, M. (1974). Determination of soluble immune-complex molar composition and antibody association constants by ammonium sulfate precipitin analysis. *J. Immunol.*, **112**, 451–461.

Atassi, M. Z. (1975). Antigenic structure of myoglobin: The complete immunochemical anatomy of a protein and conclusions relating to antigenic structures of proteins. *Immunochemistry*, **12**, 423–438.

Atassi, M. Z. (1978). Precise determination of the entire antigenic structure of lysozyme: Molecular features of protein antigenic structures and potential of 'surface-simulation' syntheses—a powerful new concept for protein binding sites. *Immunochemistry*, **15**, 909–936.

Bartels, H. J., Hesch, R. D., and Hüfner, M. (1972). Das Phänomen ansteigen-der B/F-Kurven bei radioimmunochemischen bestimmungsmethoden. *Z. Klin. Chem. Klin. Biochem.*, **10**, 351–354.

Becker, E. L. (1971). Determination of diffusion coefficients of antigens by simple diffusion in tubes. In C. A. Williams and M. W. Chase (Eds.) *Methods in Immunology and Immunochemistry III*, pp. 174–180. Academic Press, New York.

Becker, E. L., Munoz, J., Lapresle, C., and Lebeau, L. (1951). Antigen–antibody reactions in agar. II. Elementary theory and determination of diffusion coefficients of antigen. *J. Immunol.*, **67**, 501–511.

Berson, S. A. and Yalow, R. S. (1959). Quantitative aspects of the reaction between insulin and insulin-binding antibody. *J. Clin. Invest.*, **38**, 1996–2016.

Berzofsky, A., Curd, J. G., and Schechter, A. N. (1976). Probability analysis of the interaction of antibodies with multideterminant antigens in radioimmunoassay: application to the amino terminus of the chain of hemoglobin S. *Biochemistry*, **15**, 2113–2121.

Bowman, J. D. and Aladjem, F. (1963). A method for the determination of heterogeneity of antibodies. *J. Theoret. Biol.*, **4**, 242–253.

Bruni, C., Germani, A., Koch, G., and Strom, R. (1976). Derivation of antibody distribution from experimental binding data. *J. Theoret. Biol.*, **61**, 143–170.

Celada, G., Schmidt, D., and Strom, R. (1969). Determination of activity of anti-albumin antibodies in the mouse. Influence of the number of cells transferred on the quality of the secondary adoptive response. *Immunology*, **17**, 189–198.

Celis, E., Ridaura, R., and Larralde, C. (1977). Effects of the extent of DNP substitution on the apparent affinity constant and cooperation between sites in the reactions of dinitrophenylated human serum albumin with anti-DNP and anti-HSA antibodies coupled to agarose. *Immumochemistry*, **14**, 553–559.

Clarke, H. G. M and Freeman, T. (1968). Quantitative immunoelectrophoresis of human serum proteins. *Clin. Sci.*, **35**, 403–413.

Clarke, H. G. M., Freeman, T., and Pryse-Phillips, W. E. M. (1970). Serum protein changes in Still's disease, rheumatoid arthritis and gout. *Brit. J. Exp. Path.*, **51**, 441–447.

Crothers, D. M. and Metzger, H. (1972). The influence of polyvalency on the binding properties of antibodies. *Immunochemistry*, **9**, 341–357.

Crowle, A. J. (1973). *Immunodiffusion*, 2nd edn. Academic Press, New York.

Dandliker, W. S., Halbert, S. P., Florin, M. C., Alonso, R., and Schapiro, H. C. (1965). The study of penicillin antibodies by fluorescence polarizations and immunodiffusion. *J. Exp. Med.*, **122**, 1029–1048.

DeLisi, C. (1974). A theory of precipitation and agglutination reactions in immunological systems. *J. Theoret. Biol.*, **45**, 555–575.

Eisen, H. N. and Karush, F. (1949). The interaction of purified antibody with homologous hapten. Antibody valence and binding constants. *J. Amer. Chem. Soc.*, **71**, 363–364.

Eisen, H. N., Little, J. R., Osterland, C. K., and Simms, E. S. (1967). A myeloma protein with antibody activity. *Symp. Quant. Biol.*, **32**, 75–81.

Eisen, H. N. and Siskind, G. W. (1964). Variations in affinities of antibody during the immune response. *Biochemistry*, **3**, 966–1008.

Elek, S. D. (1949). The serological analysis of mixed flocculating systems by means of diffusion gradients. *Brit. J. Exp. Path.*, **30**, 484–500.

Erwin, P. M. and Aladjem, F. (1976). The heterogeneity of antibodies with respect to equilibrium constants. Calculations by a new method using delta functions and analysis of the results. *Immunochemistry*, **13**, 873–883.

Farr, R. S. (1958). A quantitative immunochemical measure of the primary interaction between I*BSA and antibody. *J. Infect. Dis.*, **103**, 239–262.

Feller, W. (1966). *An Introduction to Probability Theory and Its Application*, volume II, p. 253. John Wiley, New York.

Feller, W. (1968). *An Introduction to Probability Theory and Its Application*, volume I, 3rd edn, p. 244. John Wiley, New York.

Frandsen, E. K. and Krishna, G. (1976). A simple ultrasensitive method for the assay of cyclic AMP and cyclic GMP in tissues. *Life Sciences*, **18**, 529–542.

Ghose, A. C. and Karush, F. (1973). Fractions of anti-lactose antibody and their temporal variation. *Biochem.*, **12**, 2437–2443.

Goldberg, R. J. (1952). A theory of antibody–antigen reactions. I. Theory for reactions of multivalent antigen with bivalent and univalent antibody. *J. Amer. Chem. Soc.*, **74**, 5715–5725.

Gopalakrishnan, P. V. and Karush, F. (1974). Antibody affinity. VIII. Multivalent interaction of anti-lactoside antibody. *J. Immunol.*, **113**, 769–778.

Gopalakrishnan, P. V. and Karush, F. (1975). Antibody affinity. VIII. Measurement of anti-lactose antibody by fluorescence quenching with a DNP-containing ligand. *J. Immunol.*, **114**, 1359–1362.

Grabar, P. and Williams, C. A. (1953). Méthode permettant l'étude conjuguée des propriétés électrophorétiques et immunochimiques d'un mélange de protéines. Application au sérum sanguin. *Biochim. Biophys. Acta*, **10**, 193–194.

Grabar, P. and Williams, C. A. (1959). Méthode immuno-électrophorétique d'analyse de mélanges de substances antigéniques. *Biochim. Biophys. Acta*, **17**, 67–74.

Heidelberger, M. (1939). Quantitative absolute methods in the study of antigen–antibody reactions. *Bact. Rev.*, **3**, 49–95.

Heidelberger, M. and Kendall, F. E. (1929). A quantitative study of the precipitin reaction between Type III pneumococcus polysaccharide and purified homologous antibody. *J. Exp. Med.*, **50**, 809–823.

Heidelberger, M. and Kendall, F. E. (1935). The precipitin reaction between Type III pneumococcus polysaccharide and homologous antibody. III. A quantitative study and a theory of the reaction mechanism. *J. Exp. Med.*, **61**, 563–591.

Herbert, V., Lau, K. S., Gottleib, C. W., and Bleicher, S. J. (1965). Coated charcoal immunoassay of insulin. *J. Clin. Endocrinol. Metab.*, **25**, 1375–1384.

Hoffman, D. R. and Campbell, D. H. (1969). Model systems for the study of drug hypersensitivity. I. The specificity of the rabbit anti-aspiryl system. *J. Immunol.*, **103**, 655–661.

Hornick, C. L. and Karush, F. (1972). Antibody affinity. III. The role of multivalence. *Immunochemistry*, **9**, 325—340.

Hudson, B. W. (1968). An investigation of the effect of antigen concentration on protein antigen–antiprotein association constant. *Immunochemistry*, **5**, 87–105.

Jaton, J. C., Waterfield, M. D., Margolies, M. N., and Haber, E. (1970). Isolation and characterization of structurally homogeneous antibodies from anti-pneumococcal sera. *Proc. Natl. Acad. Sci., USA*, **66**, 959–974.

Jennings, R. K. and Malone, F. (1954). Rapid double diffusion precipitin analysis. *J. Immunol.*, **72**, 411–418.

Jennings, R. K. and Malone, F. (1957). Objective double diffusion precipitin analysis. *J. Path. Bact.*, **74**, 81–92.

Kabat, E. A. (1957). Size and heterogeneity of the combining sites on an antibody molecule. *J. Cell. Comp. Physiol.*, **50**, suppl. 1, 79–102.

Kabat, E. A. and Mayer, M. M. (1961). *Experimental Immunochemistry*, 2nd edn, pp. 67–78. Charles Thomas, Springfield, Illinois.

Karush, F. (1956). The interaction of purified antibody with optically isomeric haptens. *J. Amer. Chem. Soc.*, **78**, 5519–5526.

Karush, F. (1970). Affinity and the immune response, *N.Y. Acad. Sci.*, **169**, 56–64.

Karush, F. (1978). The affinity of antibody: range, variability, and the role of multivalence. In G. Litman and R. A. Good (Eds.) *Immunoglobulins*, pp. 85–116. Plenum Publishing Corporation, New York.

Karush, F. and Karush, S. S. (1971). Equilibrium dialysis. In C. A. Williams and M. W. Chase (Eds.) *Methods in Immunology and Immunochemistry* volume IV, pp. 383–393. Academic Press, New York.

Karush, F. and Sonnenberg, M. (1949). Interaction of homologous alkyl sulfates with bovine serum albumin. *J. Amer. Chem. Soc.*, **71**, 1369–1376.

Katz, M. and Pappenheimer, A. M., Jr. (1969). Quantitative studies of the specificity of anti-pneumococcal antibodies Types III and VIII. IV. Binding of labeled hexasaccharides derived from S3 by anti-S3-antibodies and their Fab fragments. *J. Immunol.*, **103**, 491–495.

Kim, Y. T., Kalver, S., and Siskind, G. (1975). A comparison of the Farr technique with equilibrium dialysis for measurement of antibody concentration and affinity. *J. Immunol. Meth.*, **6**, 347–354.

Klinman, N. R. (1969). Antibody with homogeneous antigen binding produced by splenic foci in organ culture. *Immunochemistry*, **6**, 757–759.

Klinman, N. R. and Karush, F. (1967). Equine anti-hapten antibody. V. The precipitability of bivalent antibody. *Immunochemistry*, **4**, 387–405.

Klinman, N. R., Segal, G. P., Gerhard, W., Braciale, T., and Levy, R. (1977). Obtaining homogeneous antibody of desired specificity from fragment cultures. In E. Haber and R. M. Krause (Eds.) *Antibodies in Human Diagnosis and Therapy*, pp. 225–236. Raven Press, New York.

Korngold, L. and van Leeuwen, G. (1957). The effect of the antigens molecular weight on the curvature of the precipitin line in the Ouchterlony technique. *J. Immunol.*, **78**, 172–177.

Krause, R. M. (1970). Factors controlling the occurrence of antibodies with uniform properties. *Fed. Proc.*, **29**, 59–65.

Kreth, H. W. and Williamson, A. W. (1973). The extent of diversity of anti-hapten antibodies in inbred mice; anti-NIP (4-hydroxy-5-iodo-3-nitro-phenacetyl) anti-bodies in CBA/H mice. *Eur. J. Immunol.*, **3**, 141–147.

Laurell, C.-B. (1965). Antigen–antibody crossed electrophoresis. *Anal. Biochem.*, **10**, 358–361.

Mancini, G., Carbonara, A. O., and Heremans, J. F. (1965). Immunochemical quantitation of antigens by single radial immunodiffusion. *Immunochemistry*, **2**, 235–254.

Matsukura, S., West, C. D., Ichikawa, Y., Jubiz, W., Harada, G., and Tyler, F. H. (1971). A new phenomenon of usefulness in the radioimmunoassay of plasma adrenocorticotropic hormone. *J. Lab. Clin. Med.*, **77**, 490–500.

Melchers, F., Potter, M., and Wosner, N. (Eds.) (1978). Lymphocyte hybridomas. In *Current Topics in Microbiology and Immunology* volume 81. Springer-Verlag, New York.

Metzger, H. (1978). The effect of antigen on antibodies: recent studies. *Contemp. Top. Mol. Immunol.*, **7**, 119–152.

Monod, J., Wyman, J., and Changeux, J. -P. (1965). On the nature of allosteric transitions: A plausible model. *J. Mol. Biol.*, **12**, 88–118.

Mukkur, T. K. S., Szewezuk, M. R., and Schmidt, D. E., Jr. (1974). Determination of total affinity constant for heterogeneous hapten–antibody interactions. *Immunochemistry*, **11**, 9–13.

Niederer, W. (1974). The interpretation of paradoxical radioimmunoassay standard curves. *J. Immunol. Methods*, **5**, 77–82.

Nisonoff, A. and Pressman, D. (1958). Heterogeneity and average combining constants of antibodies from individual rabbits. *J. Immunol.*, **80**, 417–428.

Nisonoff, A., Wissler, F. C., and Woernly, D. L. (1960). Properties of univalent fragments of rabbit antibody isolated by specific absorption. *Arch. Biochem. Biophys.*, **88**, 241–249.

Otterness, I. G. (1979). Derivation of the Steward–Petty approximation. *Molecular Immunol.*, **16**, 171–172.

Ouchterlony, O. (1958). Diffusion-in-gel methods for immunological analysis. *Prog. Allergy*, **5**, 1–30.

Ouchterlony, O. (1962). Diffusion-in-gel methods for immunological analysis. II. *Prog. Allergy*, **6**, 30-154.

Oudin, J. (1946). Méthode d'analyse immunochimique par précipitation specifique en milieu gélifié. *Compt. rendu Acad. Sci.*, **222**, 115–116.

Oudin, J. (1949). La diffusion d'un antigène dans uns colonne de gel contenant les anticorps précipitants homologues. Etude quantitative des trois principales variables. *Compt. rendu Acad. Sci.*, **228**, 1890–1892.

Oudin, J. (1952). Specific precipitation in gels and its application to immunochemical analysis. In A. C. Corcoran (Ed.) *Methods in Medical Research* volume 5, pp. 355–378. Year Book Publishers, Chicago, Illinois.

Palmiter, M. T. and Aladjem, F. (1963). The antigen–antibody reactions. IV. A quantitative theory of antigen–antibody reactions. *J. Theoret. Biol.*, **5**, 211–235.

Palmiter, M. T. and Aladjem, F. (1968). On the composition of insoluble antigen–antibody complexes. *J. Theoret. Biol.*, **18**, 34–52.

Pappenheimer, A. M., Jr., Reed, W. P., and Brown, R. (1968). Quantitative studies of the specificity of anti-pneumococcal polysaccharide antibodies, Types III and VIII. III. Binding of a labeled oligosaccharide antibodies derived from S8 by anti-S8 antibodies. *J. Immunol.*, **100**, 1237–1244.

Pappenheimer, A. M., Jr., Uchida, T., and Harper, A. A. (1972). An immunological study of the diphtheria toxin molecule. *Immunochemistry*, **9**, 891–906.

Parker, C. W., Yoo, T. J., Johnson, M. C., and Godt, S. M. (1967). Fluorescent probes for the study of the antibody–hapten reaction. I. Binding of 5-dimethylaminonaphthalene-1-sulfonamido groups by homologous rabbit antibody. *Biochemistry*, **6**, 3408–3416.

Paul, W. E., Siskind, G. W., and Benacerraf, B. (1966). Studies on the effect of the carrier molecule on antihapten antibody synthesis. II. Carrier specificity of anti-2,4-dinitrophenyl-poly-l-lysine antibodies. *J. Exp. Med.*, **123**, 689–705.

Pecht, I., Maron, E., Arnon, R., and Sela, M. (1971). Specific excitation energy transfer from antibodies to dansyl-labeled antigen. Studies with the 'loop' peptide. *Eur. J. Biochem.*, **19**, 368–371.

Sachs, D. H., Schechter, A. N., Eastlake, A., and Anfinsen, C. B. (1972a). Inactivation of staphylococcal nuclease by the binding of antibodies to a distinct antigenic determinant. *Biochemistry*, **11**, 4268–4273.

Sachs, D. H., Schechter, A. N., Eastlake, A., and Anfinsen, C. B. (1972b). Antibodies to a distinct antigenic determinant. *J. Immunol.*, **109**, 1300–1310.

Scatchard, G. (1949). The attraction of proteins for small molecules and ions. *Ann. N.Y. Acad. Sci.*, **51**, 660–672.

Seppälä I. J. T. (1975). Disturbance of hapten–antibody equilibria by ammonium sulfate solutions. A source of error in antibody affinity determinations. *J. Immunol. Meth.*, **9**, 135–140.

Singer, S. J. (1957). Physical-chemical studies on the nature of antigen–antibody reactions. *J. Cell. Comp. Physiol.*, **50**, Suppl. 1, 51–78.

Sips, R. (1948). On the structure of a catalyst surface. *J. Chem. Physics*, **16**, 490–495.

Skubitz, K. M., O'Hara, D. S., and Smith, T. W. (1977). Antibody–hapten reaction kinetics: A comparison of hapten interactions with IgG and Fab preparations. *J. Immunol.*, **118**, 1971–1976.

Smith, T. W., Butler, V. P., Jr., and Haber, E. (1970). Characterization of antibodies of high affinity and specificity for the digitalis glycoside digoxin. *Biochemistry*, **9**, 331–337.

Soothill, J. F. and Steward, M. W. (1971). The immunopathological significance of the heterogeneity of antibody affinity. *Clin. Exp. Immunol.*, **9**, 193–199.

Speirs, J. A. and Augustin, R. (1958). Antigen–antibody reactions in gel. Single diffusion: theoretical considerations. *Trans. Faraday Soc.*, **54**, 287–295.

Steensgaard, J., Johansen, H. K. W., and Møller, N. P. (1975). Computer stimulation of immunochemical interactions. *Immunology*, **29**, 571–579.

Steiner, A. L., Pagliara, A. S., Chase, L. R., and Kipnis, D. M. (1972). Radioimmunoassay for cyclic nucleotides. II. Adenosine 3',5'-monophosphate and guanosine 3',5'-monophosphate in mammalian tissues and body fluids. *J. Biol. Chem.*, **247**, 1114–1120.

Steward, M. W. and Petty, R. E. (1972). The use of ammonium sulfate globulin precipitation for the determination of affinity of anti-protein antibodies in mouse serum. *Immunology*, **22**, 747–756.

Steward, M. W. and Voller, A. (1973). The effect of malaria on the relative affinity of mouse antiprotein antibody. *Brit. J. Exp. Path.*, **54**, 198–202.

Stockmayer, W. H. (1943). Theory of molecular size and distribution and gel formation in branched-chain polymers. *J. Chem. Physics*, **11**, 45–55.

Stupp, Y., Yoshida, T., and Paul, W. E. (1969). Determination of antibody–hapten equilibrium constants by an ammonium sulfate technique. *J. Immunol.*, **103**, 625–627.

Teorell, T. (1946). Quantitative aspects of antigen–antibody reactions I. A theory and its corollaries. *J. Hyg. Comb.*, **44**, 227–236.

Thanavala, Y. M. and Hay, F. C. (1978). Modifications of the Farr assay using ethanol–ammonium acetate precipitation and its application to the measurement of affinity of anti-HGG produced in several species. *J. Immunol. Methods*, **23**, 51–58.

Thorbecke, G. J., Hochwald, G. M., and Williams, C. A. (1971). Autoradiography of antigen–antibody reactions in gels. In C. A. Williams and M. W. Chase (Eds.) *Methods in Immunology and Immunochemistry* volume 3, pp. 343–357. Academic Press, New York.

Uriel, J. (1971). Color reactions for the identification of antigen–antibody precipitates in gels. In C. A. Williams and M. W. Chase (Eds.) *Methods in Immunology and Immunochemistry* volume 3, pp. 294–321. Academic Press, New York.

Velick, S. F., Parker, C. W., and Eisen, H. N. (1960). Excitation energy transfer and the quantitative study of the antibody hapten reaction. *Proc. Natl. Acad. Sci., USA,* **46**, 1470–1482.

Weintraub, B. D., Rosen, S. W., McCammon, J. A., and Perlman, R. L. (1973). Apparent cooperativity in radioimmunoassay of human chorionic gonadotropin. *Endocrinology,* **92**, 1250–1255.

Werblin, T. P. and Siskind, G. W. (1972). Distribution of antibody affinities: Technique of measurement. *Immunochemistry,* **9**, 987–1011.

Werblin, T. P., Young, T. K., Quagliata, F., and Siskind, G. W. (1973). Studies on the control of antibody synthesis. III. Changes in heterogeneity of antibody affinity during the course of the immune response. *Immunology,* **24**, 477–492.

Wide, L. (1969). Radioimmunoassays employing immunoabsorbants. *Acta Endocrinol.,* **S142**, 207–221.

Williams, C. A. and Chase, M. W. (1971). *Methods in Immunology and Immunochemistry,* volume 3. *Reactions of Antibody With Soluble Antigens.* Academic Press, New York.

Worobec, R. B., Wallace, J. H., and Huggins, C. G. (1972). Angiotension–antibody interactions. II. Thermodynamic and activation parameters. *Immunochemistry,* **9**, 239–251.

Wu, W.-H. and Rockey, J. H. (1969). Antivasopressin antibody, characterization of high-affinity antibody with limited association constant heterogeneity. *Biochemistry,* **8**, 2719–2728.

Zivković, T., Pokrić, B., and Pucar, Z. (1976). Determination of precipitating titers and diffusion coefficients by double diffusion in gels. *Anal. Chem.,* **48**, 1405–1412.

Antibody as a Tool
Edited by J. J. Marchalonis and G. W. Warr
© 1982 John Wiley & Sons Ltd

Chapter 5

Methods of Immune Diffusion, Immunoelectrophoresis, Precipitation, and Agglutination

AN-CHUAN WANG

*Department of Basic and Clinical Immunology and
Microbiology, Medical University of South Carolina,
Charleston, South Carolina 29403, USA*

I. INTRODUCTION

This chapter deals with several basic immunological techniques commonly used for detecting and measuring antigen–antibody reactions. Two types of reactions are discussed, the precipitation and agglutination reactions. The manifestation of humoral immune reactions depends primarily on the properties of the participating antigen and antibody molecules. If the antigen is soluble and has multiple antigenic determinants, the antigen molecules would likely be locked into a lattice by antibody molecules. The result would be the formation of a precipitate. On the other hand, aggregate formation in the presence of cellular antigens (e.g. bacteria or vertebrate blood cells) is referred to as agglutination.

The text begins with a brief description of one of the simple precipitation methods, the RING test. This is followed by in-depth descriptions of widely used immune diffusion techniques: the Ouchterlony method (Ouchterlony, 1958) for qualitative identification and the Mancini method (Mancini *et al.*, 1965) for quantitative measurement of precipitation reactions following diffusion of the antigen or both antigen and antiserum on a semi-solid agar medium. Two kinds of immunoelectrophoretic techniques are also discussed in detail; the simple immunoelectrophoresis on agar/agarose gel and the rocket immunoelectrophoresis on agarose gels. Among the agglutination reactions the passive haemagglutination reaction is a major one described at length herein. However, the direct haemagglutination reactions for the A, B, O, blood groups antigens and an example for bacterial agglutination reaction are also described in detail. Several excellent methodological books have been published (Kabat and Mayer, 1967; William and Chase, 1971, 1977; Garvey *et al.*, 1977; Weir, 1978). Readers are urged to refer to them for further information.

II. SIMPLE PRECIPITATION (THE RING TEST)

When the combination of antibody and antigen in solution results in visible aggregation, it is called a precipitation reaction. This reaction was recognized as early as 1897 by Krause, and was described in detail by Oudin (1946). The detection of soluble antigens or precipitating antibodies is usually accomplished by a ring test which is performed by layering the antigen solution carefully over a portion of an antiserum in a narrow test tube in such a manner that a sharp liquid interface is formed. Appearance of a turbid ring constitutes a positive test. This occurs as a result of diffusion of antigen and antibody towards each other until their respective concentrations are at a ratio optimal for precipitation. The ring test can be used for antigen or antibody identification as well as quantitative analysis. A general laboratory procedure for detecting antigen or antibody is as follows:

1. Laboratory Protocol for the Ring Test

(i)   Prepare borate-buffered saline (pH 8.5). In a 1 litre volumetric flask add 600 ml distilled water, 6.2 g boric acid, 9.5 g borax (sodium tetraborate, $Na_2B_2O_7 \cdot 10H_2O$), and 4.4 g NaCl. Mix to dissolve, add more water to the 1 litre mark

(ii) Mark five test tubes (6 mm × 50 mm) I to V respectively. Pipette 0.2 ml of the antiserum (e.g. rabbit) into tubes I and V, 0.2 ml of normal rabbit serum into tubes III and IV, and equal volumes of the antigen solution (approximately 0.5 mg/ml in borate-buffered saline) into tube II.

(iii) Overlay tubes, I, II, and IV with 0.2 ml of borate-buffered saline, III and V with the antigen solution. To prevent mixing at the interface, the top solution should be added very carefully and gently.

(iv) Wait a few minutes, then observe the tubes against a dark (black) background for turbidity-ring formation. Tubes I to IV contain negative controls, a ring in tube V but none of the other tubes is a positive reaction. A typical precipitation ring is shown in Figure 1.

Quantitative precipitation tests can also be used as a tool for establishing the equivalance zone for antigen–antibody reaction (Dean and Webb, 1926). This is important since excess of either antigen or antibody may prevent or decrease visible precipitate from forming even though there has been an antigen–antibody reaction. A procedure for determining the equivalence zone is exemplified as follows:

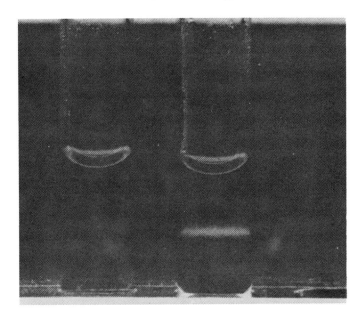

Figure 1. Simple precipitation between antigen and antibody in test tubes. The appearance of a precipitation ring in the right tube indicates a positive test. The tube on the left serves as a negative control

(i)   Label seven 6 mm × 50 mm tubes I to VII and place them in consecutive order in a tube rack. Add two drops of borate-buffered saline in tube VII with a Pasteur pipette.

(ii) Add four drops of the antigen solution (in serial twofold dilution, starting at 1 mg/ml for tube I to 0.03 mg/ml in tube VI) in each of the first six tubes respectively.

(iii) Add four drops of the antiserum to each tube, mix the tube contents immediately by flicking the tubes with a finger.

(iv) Observe the tubes carefully. The tubes will show varying degrees or turbidity almost immediately on being shaken. The tube first showing flocculation corresponds to the equivalence zone.

(v)   If tube I shows flocculation first, repeat steps (i)to (iv) with increased amount of antigen. If tube VI shows flocculation first, repeat steps (i) to (iv) with decreased amount of antigen.

The use of the ring test is no longer very advantageous because it consumes larger amounts of antiserum and antigens, is less sensitive, less descriminative, and not readily reproducible. It has generally been replaced by immune diffusion and immunoelectrophoretic methodology employing semi-solid agar and/or agarose gels.

III. IMMUNE DIFFUSION

Immune diffusion tests involve precipitation reactions between antigens and antibodies in a semi-solid rather than a liquid medium. In 1905, a physicist Bechhold first oberved immuno precipitates established in a gel. However, this observation was described purely from a physicist's point of view, thus it was ignored by immunologists at that time. The first detailed description of immune diffusion tests in tubes was made by Oudin (1946). This was followed a few years later by the establishment of the classical double diffusion technique of Ouchterlony (1958).

The diffusion of antigen and antibody in a gel medium has the advantage over diffusion in a liquid medium in that disturbances induced by currents are avoided. The gel forms a mesh-like structure stabilizing the liquid and preventing convective currents. Therefore, precipitation techniques in gels are easy to perform and have good reproducibility. A dilute (0.3–1.5%) agar gel is generally used as the semi-solid medium for immune diffusion reactions. The average pore diameter of such gels is larger than 30 nm, and thus allows free diffusion of most soluble glycoproteins. A dilute agar gel is translucent, the precipitate is clearly visible in it, and thus identification can easily be made.

Two types of gel diffusion methods have been used by immunologists. In the simple diffusion method, a concentration gradient is established for only one of the reactants. Antigen or antibody is incorporated into the gel at a comparatively low concentration. The other reactant, at a much higher concentration, is allowed to diffuse into the gels from an external source. In the double diffusion method, concentration gradients are established for both the antigen and the antiserum. Both reactants diffuse from separate external sources into a virgin gel. Both the simple and the double diffusion methods can be further characterized by the dimensions employed (i.e. one-, two-, three-dimensional methods).

A typical simple, one-dimensional immune diffusion system can be set up as follows:

A warm, agar-mixed antibody solution is poured into a test tube. After formation of the gel, a solution of the corresponding antigen (at a concentration higher than the antibody) is poured on top of the gel column, and the gel is incubated at room temperature. As the antigen diffuses into the gel column, antigen-antibody aggregates will be formed just below the interface between the solution and the gel. A precipitation band will be visible provided that the antibody concentration is above the threshold for precipitate formation. At the site of the precipitation the reactants are present at equivalent concentrations. As the diffusion continues, more and more antigen will come into the gel, and the excess antigen will gradually dissolve the initial precipitate. However, new precipitating aggregates will be formed in the adjacent part further down in the gel column. The continuation of this process of precipitation, dissolving, and reprecipitation creates the image of a slow migrating precipitate band with a sharp leading edge and an extended tail. The distance from the interface to the leading edge of the precipitate is proportional to the square root of the time of diffusion. An increase in the initial concentration of the external reactant increases the rate of migration of the precipitate while an increase in the concentration of the internal reactant has a retarding effect. If equivalent concentrations of the external and internal reactants are employed the precipitate is formed at the interface and remains stationary.

A. The Ouchterlony Method

The two-dimensional immune diffusion is best exemplified by the Ouchterlony technique (Ouchterlony and and Nilsson, 1978) which has been widely used for qualitative analysis of antigen–antibody reactions. A typical laboratory procedure for this method is outlined below:

1. Laboratory Protocol for the Ouchterlony Method

(i)   Coat large microscope slides (89 mm × 100 mm) with a thin film of hot 0.5% aqueous solution of noble agar (DIFCO laboratory), cool and dry the slides. For the preparation of these, cut a piece of filter paper the width of the slide and pre-warm the slides. Add a few drops of melted agar to one end of each slide. Spread the agar immediately by pulling it across the slide with the filter paper.

(ii)   Prepare phosphate-buffered saline (pH 7.2). Add 1.4 g of NaH_2PO_4, 8.8 g NaCl, and 900 ml of distilled water into a 1 litre volumetric flask, shake to dissolve the solid particles, adjust the pH to 7.2 with 4 M NaOH, then add more distilled water up to the 1 litre mark.

(iii)   Make 1.5% noble agar medium with the above buffer, warm to dissolve the agar and store the medium in 15 ml aliquots in large test tubes (12.7 mm × 150 mm) in a refrigerator.

(iv)   For each experiment, solubilize one tube of agar medium by heating in a boiling water bath for 10 minutes.

(v)   Place one precoated slide on a level surface, distribute approximately 14 ml of the hot medium evenly on the slide with a pipette, cool the agar at room temperature for 30 minutes.

(vi)   Cut wells into the agar using a patterned cutter (commercially available, e.g. LKB Instruments, Inc), remove agar from the wells using a Pasteur pipette attached to a vacuum line or a dropper bulb. An example of well pattern and antigen–precipitation is shown in Figure 2.

(vii)   Using 50 μl disposable micropipettes (Corning micro-sampling pipettes), fill the well with the antigen and antiserum solutions according to your experimental design.

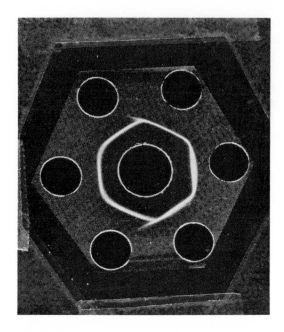

Figure 2. Precipitation between antigen and antibody in an agar gel. The centre well contains an anti-IgG antiseum. The three wells on the right contain IgG. The three wells on the left contain the Fc fragment of IgG. The spurs indicate that the anti-IgG antiserum contains antibodies to antigenic determinants not only at the Fc (common determinants) fragment but also to those at the Fab fragment of the IgG molecule

(viii)   Place the slide in a moist chamber and allow it to stand at room temperature for 1 to 2 days.

  (ix)   After formation of the precipitation lines, remove the unreacted proteins by soaking the slide in phosphate-buffered saline for 1 day.

   (x)   Take a picture at this time for a permanent record (optional).

  (xi)   Wrap the slide with a piece of filter paper. Allow the agar to dry overnight.

  (xii)   If the lines are not sufficiently clear, stain the dried slide with a stain of your choice (e.g. Coomassie Brilliant Blue: 0.1% dye in 10% acetic acid, 45% ethanol, and 45% H_2O) for 10 minutes.

 (xiii)   Remove the excess stain by soaking the slide in a de-stain solution (e.g. 10% acetic acid, 25% ethanol, and 65% H_2O).

 (xiv)   Dry the de-stained slide, take a picture (optional) and keep it in your file.

B. The Mancini Method

The gel immune diffusion techniques were modified by Mancini for quantitative determination of antigens (Mancini *et al.*, 1965). A diluted monospecific

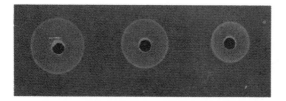

Figure 3. Precipitation haloes on a Mancini plate. The gel contains an anti-IgG antiserum diluted 1 : 160. The wells are filled with, from the left to right, 8 μg, 4 μg, and 2 μg of IgG respectively

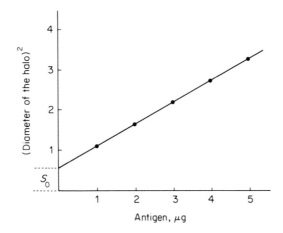

Figure 4. The calibration curve of an antigen by radial immunodiffusion

antiserum, against an antigen being studied in a mixture, is incorporated into a thin layer of agar gel. The sample that contains the corresponding antigen is then put into a well cut in the agar gel. As the antigens diffuse out from the well, only the specific antigen will react with the particular antibody in the agar. The reaction forms a halo of precipitation around the well, and after the halo has reached its maximal size, the area of the halo is directly related to the concentration of the antigen (see Figures 3 and 4). Subsequently, this single radial diffusion technique was modified by Vaerman *et al.*, (1969), in which antigen was incorporated into the gel and antibody was the diffusion reagent. This modified method has been referred to as the reversed method.

When purified antigen is available, a calibration curve can be made based on known concentrations of the antigen tested under identical conditions. A plot of the antigen concentration versus the area of precipitation should result in a straight line. Due to the presence of the well, the intercept is not at zero; the value of the intercept is related to the size of the well and the volume of the antigen. In laboratory practice, the square of the diameter instead of the area of the halo is generally plotted using the following equation:

$$S = So + K(Q_{Ag})$$

In this equation, S is the square of the diameter (in millimetres) of the halo; So is the intercept on the ordinate; K is the slope of the line; Q_{Ag} represents the concentration of the antigen.

In order to achieve accurate measurements, the thickness of the gel should be kept uniform across the plate and should be the same from one plate to another. The slope of the line is independent of the well size but varies inversely with the antibody concentration. As a result, the area of the precipitation halo also varies inversely with the concentration of the antibody. The rule of thumb is to use diluted antiserum for better sensitivity and conservation of reagents. However, there is a limit to which the antiserum can be diluted. This is because as the area of precipitation increases with dilution of the antiserum the halo also becomes fainter, and eventually becomes invisible. By finding out the optimal antiserum concentration, the Mancini method can be sensitive enough for measuring 20 ng of many protein antigens.

If the antiserum contains antibodies to more than one of the antigens in a mixture being studied, miltiple haloes may be observed. When a purified antigen and a sample containing a mixture of antigens are placed in nearby wells on the same gel, boundaries of the two haloes may fuse if the 'purified antigen' is also present in the mixture. On the other hand, boundaries of haloes due to non-identical antigens will cross each other in a two-way overlap. Haloes of cross-reacting but non-identical antigens may show one-way overlap or spur boundary.

1. Laboratory Protocol for the Mancini Technique

   (i)   Prepare pH 8.6, 0.5 M barbital buffer (for 1 litre use 10.3 g sodium diethylbarbiturate, 70 ml of 0.1 M HCl, 0.5 g sodium azide).
   (ii) Precoat slides (51 × 51 mm) with 0.5% agar in water (see above for detail).
   (iii) Prepare 2% agar in the barbital buffer and keep it melted in a 50 °C water bath.
   (iv) Make 1.5 ml each of 1 : 80, and 1:40, 1:160 dilutions of the antiserum with the barbital buffer in three test tubes (9 mm × 100 mm), and keep the antiserum dilutions warm in a 50 °C water bath.
   (v)   Add 1.5 ml of the melted agar into each of the three test tubes containing the respective antiserum dilutions. Mix the two solutions carefully to avoid air bubbles.
   (vi) Place three precoated slides on a perfectly level surface. Distribute 2.5 ml of the agar–serum mixtures evenly over the surface of the slides. Let the agar gels sit at room temperature for 20 minutes.

(vii) Cut wells in the agar gel, remove the agar from the wells and put a fixed amount (e.g. 2 μl) of properly diluted (usually in serial twofold dilutions) antigen and standard solutions into each well.

(viii) Incubate the slides in a moist chamber for 5 to 6 days until the reaction is complete (i.,e. the size of the halo no longher enlarges).

(ix) At the end of the incubation period, measure the diameter (millimetres) of the halo, and check the square of the diameter against a calibration plot made previously to find out the amount of the specific antigen being placed in each well. Figure 4 illustrates a typical calibration plot; at the end of the reaction, the slope assumes a straight line.

(x) If the precipitation haloes are too large or too small, the antiserum dilution should be adjusted accordingly.

IV IMMUNOELECTROPHORESIS

The immune diffusion technique is the method of choice when relatively simple antigen–antibody systems are studied, but this method has limited resolving power when mixtures of antigen–antibody systems are being investigated. The resolving power for analysing humoral immune reactions was greatly increased when Grabar and Williams (1953) combined the Ouchterlony double diffusion method with electrophoretic separation of antigens on the same gel, and the resultant technique has been designated immunoelectrophoresis. This initial methodology has since been modified for higher sensitivity and economy of reagents (Scheidegger, 1955). The technique has been widely used for detecting and identifying individual components in a multicomponent system; for determining the purity of a supposedly single component system; for evaluating the efficiency of a fractionation procedure for the isolation of a given material; and for recognizing abnormal proteins associated with many pathological conditions. The procedure is schematically illutrated in Figure 5. The sample to be examined for the presence of antigens is first separated into its component molecules by electrophoresis in an agar/agarose gel. After the electrophoretic step antiserum is introduced into troughs cut into the gel parallel to the path of electrophoretic migration and on both sides of the antigens. The reactants are then allowed to diffuse against each other, and precipitation arcs will form when antigens and antibodies meet at appropriate concentrations.

The gel is prepared in the same way as for regular immune diffusion plates. Buffers between pH 6 and 9 can be used and barbital or borate buffers are generally recommended. Theoretically, when an alkaline buffer is used, most proteins will be negatively charged and move through the gel to the anode. However, in practice, some proteins (e.g. IgG) actually migrate toward the cathode when agar is used as the semi-solid medium. This is due to the effect of

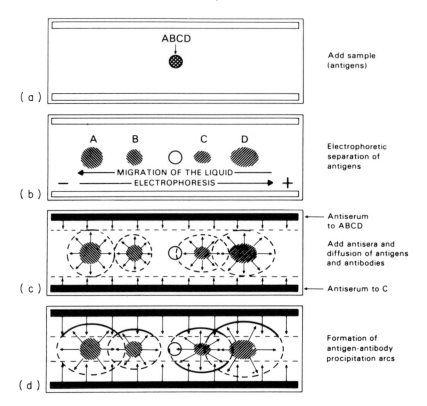

Figure 5. A schematic representation of immunoelectrophoresis, A, B, C, and D represent four non-cross-reactive antigens

electro-osmosis. Since the agar molecules are negatively charged and immobilized in the gel, the liquid in the gel assumes a positive charge and migrates towards the cathode. This net flow of liquid tends to carry all molecules towards the cathode and thus affects the electrophoretic mobility of all molecules. For this reason many people use agarose or a mixture of agarose and agar to avoid or reduce electro-osmosis effect.

Many elements can influence the efficiency of immunoelectrophoresis. These include the size of the well of origin, the distance between the well of origin and the trough, the concentrations of the antigen and antibodies, the purity of the agar and/or agarose, the pH and ionic strength of the buffer, the strength of the electric field and many others. The best conditions for a given unknown antigen–antibody system have to be determined empirically. However, the technique is flexible enough and many established procedures can be used satisfactorily for routine analysis in most of the situations. The following is a description of the protocol used in our laboratory to serve as an example.

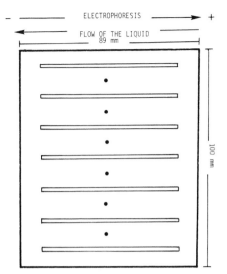

Figure 6. Pattern of an immunoelectrophoresis plate showing the locations where the troughs are to be cut

1. Laboratory Protocol for Immunoelectrophoresis

(i)   Prepare pH 8.6 barbital buffer: in a 2 litre volumetric flask, add 10.28 g sodium barbital, 1.84 g barbituric acid, 9.6 g boric acid, and 1.78 g of sodium hydroxide, dissolve them with distilled water to the 2 litre mark.

(ii) Prepare 1% agar/agarose medium: for 100 ml, boil 0.5 g of noble agar (Difco) and 0.5 g agarose (type 2, Sigma) in 100 ml barbital buffer. Divide the medium into 15 ml aliquots and store them in large test tubes (12.7 mm × 150 mm) in a refrigerator.

(iii) For each experiment, melt one tube of the medium in a boiling water bath for 10 minutes.

(iv) Place one precoated slide (see above for coating) on a perfectly level surface and distribute approximately 14 ml of the medium on the slide evenly with a pipette. Let the medium cool and solidify at room temperature for 30 minutes.

(v)   Cut wells with a patterned cutter which is commercially available and the one we use is illustrated in Figure 6. Fill the wells with antigens to be separated by electrophoresis.

(vi) Put the slide in a moist chamber between two buffer vessels. Connect the gel to the buffer via filter-paper wicks which are pre-soaked in the buffer. One side of the wet paper wicks covers approximately 5 mm of the gel and the other side hangs into the buffer.

(vii) Connect the buffer vessels with a power supply and applying a potential drop of 6 volts(V)/cm in the gel for approximately 45 minutes. Most of the serum proteins are fractionated under the above conditions. For separation of antigens in a special mixture, the length of time, voltage, and amperage should be adjusted empirically for best resolution.

(viii)   After completion of the electrophoretic separation, cut troughs on the gel using a patterned cutter (see Figure 6). Remove the gel from the trough with a disposable pipette to a mild vacuum line. Fill the troughs with specific antisera using a disposable pipette.

 (ix)   Put the plate on a level surface in a moist chamber and leave it at room temperature for 25 to 48 hours.

  (x)   After the precipitation arcs have developed, remove unreacted proteins by soaking the plate in normal saline overnight. Take a picture at this time (optional). The precipitation arcs formed between normal human serum and an antiserum against normal human serum are shown in Figure 7.

 (xi)   Dry the gel. If the precipitation arcs are not clear enough, stain (and de-stain) the gel as described earlier (see protocol for Ouchterlony method, see above).

(xii)   Take a picture for permanent record (optional).

V. ROCKET IMMUNOELECTROPHORESIS (RIEP)

The regular immunoelectrophoresis technique was modified by Laurell (1966) for quantitative analysis. The modified method is generally called rocket immunoelectrophoresis (RIEP). The reason for this is that at the end of the antigen-antibody reaction, rocket-shaped precipitation peaks are formed. The height of the precipitation peak is roughly proportional to the concentration of the antigen, and thus permits quantitative estimation of the antigen. Two major versions of this technique are commonly employed, namely the one-dimensional and two-dimensional methods.

A. One-dimensional RIEP

In this method a series of wells are cut along one side of an agarose gel that contains specific antibodies. The text material and dilutions of a standard antigen, at concentrations much higher than that of the antibodies used for calibration, are placed into the wells. Both the antigen and antibody migrate in the elctric field, and antigen-antibody complexes form and precipitate. Antigens are in excess at the leading boudary of the antigen migration. As the excess antigen migrates into the area of precipitation, the antigen–antibody complexes dissolve and re-form again further along the path of antigen migration. Along the outside edges of the migration path, the concentrations of antigen and antibody are at equilibrium, and thus the precipitation persists. As the electrophoresis progresses, all antigens at the moving front eventually will

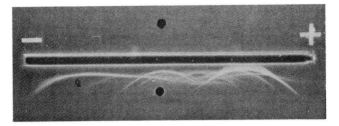

Figure 7. Precipitation arcs between antigens and antibodies after immunoelectrophoresis. The trough is filled with an antiserum directed towards normal human
serum. The lower well is filled with normal human serum, and the upper well is empty

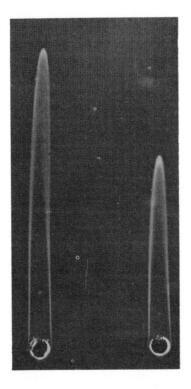

Figure 8. Rocket formation after one-dimensional rocket-immunoelectrophoresis.
The gel contains a diluted antiserum (1 : 160) towards IgG. The wells contain, from left
to right, 4 µg and 2 µg of IgG respectively

be complexed with antibody and the curves of the precipitation lines converge
to form a rocket-like shape. After this point is reached, the lines of
precipitation remain stationary regardless of the continuation of the electrophoresis. Examples of such rockets are shown in Figure 8. The area of

rocket is directly proportional to the antigen concentration, and indirectly related to the antibody concentration in the gel. The height of the rocket can be used as a rough estimate of the antigen concentration if electrophoresis is started immediately after the antigen application into the wells. The concentration of an antigen in an unknown sample can be determined by reference to standards of an identical antigen of known concentration run parallel to the sample on the same gel. A curve plotting concentration versus height of the standards can be constructed to facilitate estimation of the test antigen's concentration. Optimal concentrations of antigen and antibody must be determined empirically for each system. Highest sensitivity for antigen detection is when minimal antibody concentration is employed, and the hieght of the rocket increases inversely with antibody concentration. In actual practice the rocket heights between 10 and 50 mm give the best reproducible results for measurement. Also in actual practice, caution should be used to assure uniform gel thickness and sample volume. Furthermore, the total time for loading the samples into a given gel should be kept under 5 minutes, otherwise diffusion of the sample will cause shortening of the rockets. A typical laboratory protocol for one-dimensional RIEP using a LKB model 2117 multiphor apparatus is as follows:

   (i)   Prepare pH 8.8 RIEP running buffer. In a large jar, dissolve 65 g of sodium barbital, 10.34 barbital, 281 g glycine, and 226 g of Tris (hydroxymethyl)aminomethane with distilled water. Add more distilled water to a total volume of 10 litres.

   (ii)   Make 2% agarose with the above buffer.

  (iii) Melt 14 ml of the agarose in a 56 °C water bath.

  (iv) Make an appropriate dilution (e.g. 1 : 160; the exact dilution should be determined empirically for each system) of the antiserum with the RIEP running buffer, and warm the diluted antiserum in a 56 °C water bath.

   (v)   Mix 14 ml of the warm diluted antiserum with 14 ml of the warm 2% agarose thoroughly and gently to avoid air bubble formation.

  (vi) Distribute the mixture evenly on a 125 mm × 125 mm glass plate. Let the agarose solidify in a cold room (or a refrigerator).

 (vii) Cut wells with a patterned cutter parallel to the edges of, and approximately 30 mm from, the side where the cathode will be connected.

(viii) Fill the wells with the sample to be tested and various dilutions of the standard antigen.

  (ix) Fill the buffer trays, connect the gel to the buffer via wet wicks. Hook up the circulating water cooling system.

   (x)   Connect the electrodes to a power supply. Run the electrophoresis under constant voltage at 250 V (20 V/cm) for approximately 5 hours (or until the front edge of the rockets ceases to advance).

(xi)   At the end of the electrophoresis, turn off the power, and wash the agarose gel in normal (0.9% w/v) saline overnight. Take a picture at this time (optional).

(xii)   Dry the agarose gel by placing a piece of the filter paper over it (avoid trapping air bubbles when you put the paper on, and leave it at room temperature overnight.

(xiii) Rewmove the dried filter paper from the dried gel. Wet slightly with water if the filter paper adheres to the gel.

(xiv)   If the precipitation rockets are not clear enough, stain with Coomassie Brilliant Blue for 10 minutes, then de-stain with a de-stain solution (see above).

(xv)   Measure the heights of rockets to estimate antigen concentrations. Take a picture for permanent record (optional).

B. Two-dimensional RIEP

The one-dimensional RIEP can be used to measure the concentration of a given antigen in a mixtuyre of antigens if monospecific antiserum towards that antigen is available. It can also be used to measure the concentrations of a purified antigen with a polyspecific antiserum. But this technique has its limitations when neither a purified antigen nor a monospecific antiserum towards the antigen is available. The cross (or two-dimensional)-rocket immunoelectrophoresis is required for identifying or measuring the concentrations of multiple antigens in a mixed sample. In the early days, the cross-immunoelectrophoresis was mainly used for analysis of plasma proteins, but recently its application has been extended to encompass a variety of other protein systems (e.g. the complement components).

Two major steps are involved in this procedure. The first is a regular agarose gel electrophoresis. This step allows the separation of antigens in a given sample. Afterwards a large section of the unused gel (i.e without antigens) is cut off and in its place warm fresh agarose is added that contains a diluted antiserum. After solidification of the newly added agarose, electrophoresis is carried out again at a 90° angle to the previous direction. This second electrophoresis step allows the formation of multiple precipitation rockets corresponding to separated individual antigens complexed with the antibodies directed towards them. Figure 9 shows the precipitation rockets formed by native and converted C3 components after cross-RIEP. An exemplifying laboratory procedure, using a LKB model 2117 multiphor apparatus, is described below.

1. Laboratory Protocol for the Cross-Immunoelectrophoresis

(i)   Prepare a pH 8.8. running buffer (the same as that for one-dimensional RIEP, see above).

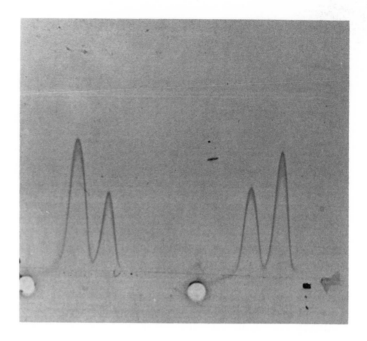

Figure 9. Rocket formation after cross-rocket immunoelectrophoresis. The gel contains a diluted antiserum (1 : 400) towards C3 (the third component of human complement system. The wells are filled with incubated samples (60 minutes at 37 ° C). The left well—normal human serum (1 : 4.3 dilution), right well—normal human serum (1 : 4.3 dilution) plus aggregated immunoglobulins (0.4 mg/ml). Courtesy of Dr R Boackle

(ii) Make 1% agarose with the above buffer and melt 60 ml of it in a 56 °C water bath.

(iii) Distrbute the warm agarose evenly on a 260 mm × 125 mm glass plate. Let the agarose solidify in a cold room (or refrigerator).

(iv) Cut a row of wells separated from one another by equal distance (e.g. 60 mm) with a patterned cutter. These wells are parallel to and 30 mm from the edge of the long side (260 mm) where the cathode will be connected for the second electrophoretic step (see Figure 10).

(v) Fill the wells with the antigen solutions.

(vi) Fill the buffer trays, connect the gel to the buffer via wet wicks and hook up the circulating water cooling system.

(vii) Connect the electrodes to a power supply, and run the electrophoresis parallel to the long side of the gel at 500 V (19 V/cm) for 80 minutes.

(viii) Cut two-thirds of the gel out, parallel to, and away from the antigens.

(ix) Make an appropriate dilution for the antiserum with the RIEP running buffer, and warm the diluted antiserum in a 56 °C water bath.

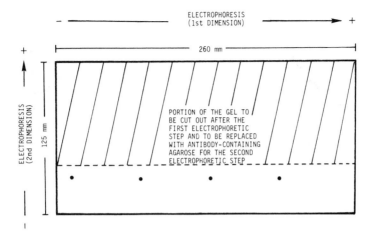

Figure 10. Pattern of cross-rocket immunoelectrophoresis plate showing the locations where the wells are to be cut. Shaded area indicates where the gel is to be cut away after the first electrophoretic step

(x)　Mix 20 ml of the diluted antiserum with 20 ml of the warm 2% agarose thoroughly.

(xi)　Distribute the warm mixture evenly in the space previously occupied by the removed agarose. Let the gel solidify in a cold room or refrigerator for 15 minutes.

(xii)　Repeat the electrophoresis process at a 90° angle from the direction of the previous electrophoretic step at 250 V for 5 hours.

(xiii)　After the termination of the elctrophoresis, measure the heights of the rockets and estimate the concentrations of various antigens. Take a picture (optional).

(xiv)　Dry the gel as described earlier (see above).

(xv)　If the precipitation rockets are not sufficiently clear, stain the gel with Coomassie Brilliant Blue and de-stain with a de-stain solution as described earlier (see Chapters 2 and 3).

(xvi)　Take a picture for permanent record (optional).

VI AGGLUTINATION REACTIONS

The agglutination of a particulate antigen by its specific antiserum has been a simple and effective way for analysing the antigen and/or antibody (Coombs and Fiset, 1954). Red blood cells and bacteria are commonly involved in the agglutination reactions. In this section, three types of agglutination methods will be described. These are direct haemagglutination, passive haemagglutination and bacterial agglutination methods.

A. Direct Haemagglutination

This has been the classic method for the detection of genetic alleles of red blood cell antigens (Race and Sanger, 1975). In 1900 Landsteiner studied the agglutination reactions between blood samples from different individuals and discovered A, B, AB, AND O blood types. The method has since then been widely used for the analysis of many other blood cell antigens including the Rh grouping. To serve as an example for the direct haemmagggglutination technique, a simple procedure for ABO blood grouping is outlined below.

One drop of blood is put in each of two circles on a glass microscope slide. A drop of anti-A serum is added to one of the circles and a drop of anti-B serum is added to the other circle. The drops in each circle are mixed throughly with clean applicator sticks and spread out to fill the circles. The slide is rotated with a circular rolling motion and observed for agglutination. Appropriate controls with blood cells of known A, B, O, and AB blood groups in reaction to anti-A and anti-B should be included. Another control containing a drop of normal human serum of the AB blood group and a drop of the red blood cells from the person being tested should give no agglutination. The pattern of agglutination should be as shown in Table 1. Table 1. Pattern of agglutination of red blood cells

Erythrocyte	Anti-A serum	Anti-B serum	Serum of an AB person
O	–	–	–
A	+	–	–
B	–	+	–
AB	+	+	-

B. Passive Haemagglutination

Passive haemagglutination, also called indirect haemagglutination, was developed approximately 40 years ago. The technique involves the adsorption of foreign antigens on to red blood cells and use of the agglutination of the coated cells as a means to observe the antigen–antibody reactions. Figure 11 illustrates the principle of passive haemagglutination and haemagglutination inhibition. The sensitivity of the passive haemmagglutination is usually quite good in comparison with any other conventional serological method. With some antigens, particularly bacterial polysaccharides, erythrocytes may be effectively coated by merely exposing them to the antigen. With most protein antigens, however, special chemical treatment of the cells is often necessary to achieve better coating and higher agglutinability.

Several ways for coating cells have been commonly used including the tannic acid (Boyden, 1951), the bisdiazotized benzidine (Pressman *et al.*, 1942), the

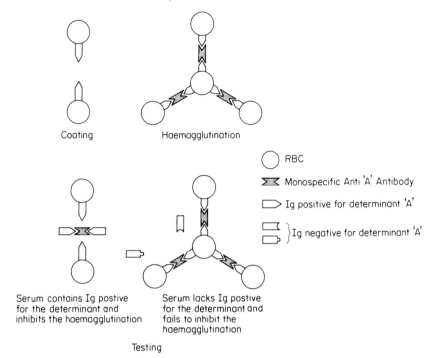

Coating   Haemagglutination

RBC

Monospecific Anti 'A' Antibody

Ig positive for determinant 'A'

} Ig negative for determinant 'A'

Serum contains Ig postive
for the determinant and
inhibits the haemagglutination

Serum lacks Ig postive
for the determinant and
fails to inhibit the
haemagglutination

Testing

Figure 11. A schematic representation of the principle for haemagglutination and haemagglutination inhibition. This figure was reproduced, with the permission of the Oxford University Press, from a book entitled *Basic Immunogenetics* by Fudenberg, Pink, Wang, and Douglas

carbodiimide (Johnson *et al.*, 1968), the difluorodinitrobenzene (Ling, 1961, and the chromic chloride, (Vyas *et al.*, 1968) methods. Passive haemagglutination tests have been commonly used for diagnosis of many microbial infections, because bacterial polysaccharides are spontaneously bound to erythrocytes. Such tests have been developed for the diagnosis of plague (e.g. *Vibrio fetus, Neisseria meningitis*, etc.). Passive haemagglutination techniques have also been widely used for analysis of protein antigens. The chromic chloride method has been successfully used for investigating the genetic markers of human immunoglobulins. A laboratory protocol, using cells coated by the chromic chloride method, is outlined below to serve as an example for passive haemagglutination methods.

1. Protocol for Passive Haemagglutination

(a) Coating of antigen to cells using chromic chloride

   (i)   Approximately 10 ml of freshly drawn type O, Rh+ red blood cells are

(ii)   washed five times with a phosphate-buffered saline (pH 7.3), using a 10-fold (in volume) of normal saline for each wash.

(ii)   Dissolve the antigen with normal saline; make the antigen concentrations at 5 mg/ml, 2.5 mg/ml, and 1 mg/ml respectively.

(iii)   Dilute the stock solution of 0.0375 M chromic chloride with normal saline; make 1 to 5, 1 to 10, 1 to 15, and 1 to 20 dilutions respectively.

(iv)   Mark each of 12 test tubes (7 mm × 50 mm) with the respective antigen and chromic chloride concentrations. To each tube add 0.1 ml of the antigen solution, 0.1 ml of the chromic chloride solution, and 0.05 ml of washed packed erythrocytes.

(v)   Agitate the tubes continuously for 5 minutes, and wash the cells in each tube four times, using 30-fold (in volume) normal saline for each wash.

(vi)   The coated cells are reconstituted as a 0.1% suspension in normal saline that contains 0.1% gelatine.

(b) Titration of the antiserum

(i)   Absorb the antiserum appropriately to make it monospecific to the antigen being coated on the erythrocytes.

(ii)   Heat the antiserum at 56 °C for 30 minutes to deactivate the complement system.

(iii)   Absorb the antiserum with washed and uncoated type O, Rh+ erythrocytes.

(iv)   To each of the first wells (left well in each row) in a microtitration plate (V-shaped, Dynatech, Inc.) add two drops of antiserum. To the rest of the wells, add one drop of normal saline containing 0.1% gelatine.

(v)   Make serial twofold dilutions of the antiserum using a microtitre loop holder calibrated for one drop.

(vi)   Add one drop of the 0.1% suspension of the coated cells to each well.

(vii)   Set up two negative controls: cell control (coated cells plus normal saline); antiserum control (uncoated cells plus antiserum).

(viii)   Mix the reagents gently with a fine jet of air.

(ix)   Cover the plate with a wide transparent adhesive plastic wrap and leave the plate at room temperature for 2 hours.

(x)   Centrifuge the plate at room temperature for 1 minute at 1500 r.p.m. using a special head for an IEC centrifuge.

(xi)   Keep the plate inclined at a 60° angle on an illuminated white platform for 15 minutes.

(xii)   Observe the wells for agglutination. There is a smooth run-down of the red blood cells when agglutination is absent; in contrast, agglutinated cells either remain as a button at the bottom of the well or come down in the vertex as a button. The highest dilution of antiserum capable of agglutinating the coated cells is taken as the haemagglutination titre of the antiserum.

(c) Haemagglutination inhibition

   (i)   Make an antiserum dilution equal to 4 agglutination units with normal saline containing 0.1% gelatine. An agglutination unit of an antiserum is that dilution equal to the titre of the antiserum.

  (ii)   To each of the first wells in a microtitration plate add two drops of the test sample (the inhibitor) and to each of the remaining wells add one drop of the normal saline containing 1% gelatine.

 (iii)   Make twofold serial dilutions of the inhibitor using a microtitre holder.

 (iv)   Add one drop of the 0.1% suspension of the coated cells and one drop of the diluted antiserum to each well.

  (v)   Set up appropriate controls: cell control (coated cell plus normal saline); agglutinator control (coated cells plus diluted antiserum).

 (vi)   Mix the reagents gently with a fine jet of air.

(vii)   Cover the plate with a wide transparent adhesive plastic wrap and leave the plate at room temperative for 2 hours.

(viii)   Spin the microtitration plate at 1500 r.p.m. for 1 minute in an IEC centrifuge.

 (ix)   Keep the plate inclined at a 60° angle on an illuminated white platform for 15 minutes.

  (x)   Observe the wells for haemagglutination; agglutination formation means no inhibition whereas absence of agglutination indicates inhibition.

C. Bacterial Agglutination

Bacteria can be agglutinated by specific antiserum directed towards them (Edwards and Ewing, 1972). Bacterial agglutination tests are employed both for identification of antibodies using known bacterial antigens and for identification of bacterial antigens using antisera of known specificity. The reactions are largely between the antigens making up the cell surface, capsule, flagella of the bacteria and the antibodies against them. Bacterial agglutination is very useful as a diagnostic tool (Boackle, *et al.*, 1982) for detection of bacterial infection (e.g. salmonellosis, brucellosis, leptospirosis, etc.). However one must be cautious in interpreting the data. Many normal individuals have antibodies against a variety of pathogenic micro-organisms due to previous active immunization through vaccination, infections, or exposure to other cross-reacting micro-organisms. Therefore, a rising titre of the respective antibody in the serum must be clearly demonstrated before a positive diagnosis can be made.

    Bacterial agglutination can be observed either by a test-tube or a slide method. For a successful test, it is essential to have pure bacterial strains maintained in culture. Non-viable bacterial suspensions are generally preferable to viable suspensions. It is often necessary to kill the bacteria to avoid autolysis of bacterial cells and danger of infection by the pathogens. A simple procedure for detection of anti-bacterial antibodies is outlined below:

(i) Number 10 test tubes (9 mm × 100 mm) I to X.

(ii) Pipette 1.8 ml of saline in tube number I and 1.0 ml of saline in each of the other tubes.

(iii) Add 0.2 ml of the antiserum into tube number I. Mix thoroughly by pulling the liquid up and down in the pipette; do this carefully to avoid air bubbles.

(iv) Make twofold dilutions of the antiserum. Transfer 1 ml of the mixture from tube I to tube II. Mix throughly as described above. Then using the same pipette transfer 1 ml from tube II to tube III, and mix the contents in tube III; repeat the procedure until tube IX. Discard 1 ml from tube IX after mixing. Tube X serves as the antigen control.

(v) Pipette 1 ml of the bacterial suspension (0.1% in phosphate-buffered saline) into each of the 10 tubes.

(vi) Shake and mix the contents of the tubes thoroughly.

(vii) Place the tubes in a 37 ° C water bath overnight.

(viii) Observe agglutination by flicking the bottom of each tube with a finger to resuspend the bacteria that have settled to the bottom. The antigen control tube (X) should have a uniform turbidity, whereas aggregates are formed in the tubes where agglutination occurred. The highest dilution of the antiserum capable of causing agglutination is defined as the titre of the antiserum.

REFERENCES

Boackle, R. J., Virella, G., Wang, A. C., Fudenberg, H. H. (1982). Immunodiagnosis: antibodies in body fluid. In A. J. Nahmias and R. J. O'Reilly (Eds) *Immunology of Human Infections, Part II*. pp. 515–543 Plenum Publ., New York.

Boyden, S. V. (1951). The absorption of proteins on erythrocytes treated with tannic acid, and subsequent hemagglutination with antiprotein sera *J. Exp. Med.*, **93**, 107–120.

Coombs, R. R. A. and Fiset, M. L. (1954). Detection of complete and incomplete antibodies to egg albumin by means of a sheep red cell-egg albumin antigen unit. *Brit. J. Exp. Pathl.*, **35**, 472–477.

Dean, H. R. and Webb, R. (1926). The influence of optimal proportions of antigen and antibody in the serum precipitation reaction. *J. Path. Bact.*, **29**, 473–492.

Edwards, P. R. and Ewing, W. H. (1972). *Identifiction of Enterobacteriaceae*, 3rd edn. Burgess Publ. Minneapolis.

Garvey, J. S., Cremer, N. E., and Sussdorf, D. H. (1977). *Methods in Immunology*, 3rd edn. W. A. Benjamin Inc., Publ. London.

Grabar, P. Williams, C. A. (1953) Methode permentent l'etude conjuguue des proprietes electrophoretiques et immunoclinique d'm melange de proteins. Applica-tion au serum sanguin. *Biochem. Biophy. Act.*, **10**, 193–194.

Johnson, H. M., Smith, B. G., and Hall, H. E. (1968). Carbodiimide hemagglutination.

A study of some of the variables of the conflicting reaction. *Int. Arch. Allergy*,**33**, 511–520.

Kabat, E. A. and Mayer, M. M. (1967). *Experimental Immunochemistry*, 3rd edn. Charles C. Thomas Publ. Springfield, Ill. USA.

Laurell, C. B. (1966). Quantitative estimation of proteins by electrophoresis in agarose gel containing antibodies. *Anal Biochem*, **15**, 45–52.

Ling, N. R. (1961). The coupling of protein antigens to erythrocytes with difluorodinit-robenzene. *Immunology*, **4**, 49–54.

Mancini, G., Carbonara, A. O. and Heremans, J. F. (1966). Immunological quantitation of antigens by single radial immunodiffuision. *Immunochemistry*, **2**, 235–254.

Ouchterlony, O. (1958). Diffusion-in-gel methods for immunological analysis. *Progess in Allergy*, **5**, 1–78.

Ouchterlony, O. and Nilsson, L. A. (1978). Immunodiffusion and immunoelectrophoresis. In D. M. Weir (Ed.) *Handbook of Experimental Immunology*, Volume 1. *Immunochemistry*, 3rd edn., pp. 19.1–19,44. Blackwell Scientific Publ., Oxford.

Oudin, J. (1946). Methode d'analyse immunochemique par precipitation en milieu gelifie. *C. R. Acad. Science*, **222**, 115–116.

Pressman, D., Campbell, D. H., and Pauling, L. (1942). The agglutination of intact azoerythrocytes by antisera homologous to the attached group. *J. Immunol.*, **44**, 101–105.

Race, R. R. and Sanger, R., (1975). *Blood Groups in Man*, 6th edn. Blackwell Publ., Oxford.

Scheidegger, J. J. (1955). Une micro-methode l'immunoelectrophorese. *Int. Arch. Allergy*,**7**, 103–110.

Vaerman, J. P., Labacq, A. M., Scolari, L., and Heremans, J. F. (1969). Further studies on single radial immunodiffusion. II. the reversed system: Diffusion of antibodies in antigen-containing gels. *Immunochemistry***6**, 297–293.

Vyas, G. N., Fudenberg, H. H., Pretty, H. M., and Gold, E. R. (1968). A new rapid method for genetic typing of human immunoglobulins. *J. Immunol.*, **100**, 274–279.

Weir, D. M. (Ed.) (1978). *Handbook of Experimental Immunology*, volume 1. *Immunochemistry*, 3rd edn. Blackwell Scientific Publ., Oxford.

William, C. A. and Chase, M. W. (Eds) (1971). *Methods in Immunology and Immunochemistry*,, volume 3. Academic Press, London.

William, C. A. and Chase, M. W. (Eds) (1977). *Methods in Immunology and Immunochemistry*, volume 4. Academic Press, London.

Antibody as a Tool
Edited By J. J. Marchalonis and G. W. Warr
© 1982 John Wiley & Sons Ltd.

Chapter 6

Principles of Radioimmunoassays and Related Techniques

LEONARD BENADE
Microbiological Associates,
Bethesda, MD 20816, USA

and

JAMES N. IHLE
Cancer Biology Program, NCI Frederick Cancer Research Center,
P.O. Box 8, Frederick, Maryland 21701, USA

I. INTRODUCTION

The advent of the radioimmunonassay (RIA) in the 1960s precipitated a phenomenal surge of interest in immunochemical methodlogy. First described by Berson and Yalow in 1960, the assay was initially developed to measure levels of insulin in the blood (Berson and Yalow, 1959; Yalow and Berson, 1959; Yalow, 1959). Because of the remarkable sensitivity and specificity afforded by the technique, it has been adopted for the detection and quantification of minute levels of innumerable substances (Hunter, 1967; Skelley *et al.*, 1973; Yalow, 1978; Colt *et al.*, 1971; Raud and Odell, 1969). It has also been widely employed to compare homology between macromolecules and has proved an invaluable tool for the detection of subtle differences in closely related antigens of which viral proteins are prime examples (Barbacid *et al.*, 1978; Benade *et al.*, 1978; DeCleve *et al.*, 1976; Ihle *et al.*, 1976; Stephenson *et al.*, 1975; Strand and August, 1975; Teramoto and Schlom, 1978; Scolnick *et al.*, 1972). Moreover, the rapidity and ease with which many samples can be processed has virtually revolutionized clinical serology.

The RIA is based on the principle that the amount of a labelled antigen (tracer) bound by a fixed level of antibody is inversely proportional to the amount of unlabelled antigen present. In other words, the unlabelled antigen competes with the labelled antigen for antibody binding. Thus, a 'dose–response' curve for serial dilutions of samples containing unknown levels of a particular antigen can be compared to a standard curve derived from dilutions of a known quantity of the purified antigen. The key to the sensitivity, specificity, and precision of the assay is the antibody. The RIA is one of many related techniques known collectively as ligand-binding assays (other examples of ligand-binding assays, e.g. enzyme immunoassay and immunoradiometric assay will also be considered in this chapter). The sensitivity of these assays is determined by the specificity of the binding reagent and its affinity for the ligand. The extreme specificity and high affinity of antibodies for antigenic determinants ideally suits them for this role.

The extent of antigen binding obtained with antibodies is a function of both their affinity (strength of binding to antigenic determinants) and capacity (the number of available binding sites). Considering the following equilibrium conditions in an immunoassay (Potts *et al.*, 1967),

$$Ag + Ab \underset{k_2}{\overset{k_1}{\rightleftharpoons}} Ag \cdot Ab$$

the affinity is described by K_a (the quilibrium or affinity constant):

$$\frac{(Ag \cdot Ab)}{(Ag)(Ab)} = k_1/k_2 = k_a$$

Since an antiserum consists of a heterogeneous population of antibodies with varying specificities and affinities, the observed K_a really represents an average of many values.

The principle of the radioimmunoassay is remarkably simple. If the amount of antibody (binding capacity) is limited to the amount of labelled antigen (in excess), then unlabelled antigen present in the reaction mixture will compete for the available binding sites. Thus, in an assay which consists of a series of serial dilutions of a sample containing the unlabelled antigen, the amount of bound labelled antigen will be seen to vary inversely with the concentration of unlabelled antigen. It remains then simply to separate and determine the relative amounts of bound and free labelled antigen. A comparison of the 'dose–response' curve thus generated with a standard curve established with serial dilutions of a known quantity of unlabelled antigen allows a precise determination of the amount of unlabelled antigen present in the original sample. Moreover, comparison of the patterns of inhibition of binding can provide important information concerning the immunological relatedness of various antigens.

The development of a radioimmunoassay for a particular antigen involves several aspects, all of which will contribute to the precision, sensitivity, specificity, and reproducibility of the assay. These include the purification of the antigen to homogeneity under conditions which do not alter its immunological properties relevant to the samples to be tested. Next, a specific antiserum must be chosen which ideally will have higher titres of high avidity antibodies which at the same time are immunologically specific. For the assay, procedures must be developed to radiolabel the antigen to high specifity without significantly altering its immunological properties. Optimal reaction conditons must next be established to provide precision and sensitivity for the assay. Lastly, the data must be analysed both with regard to the quantitative and qualitative patterns of inhibition of binding. In this chapter, the latter aspects specifically associated with performing radioimmunoassays will be discussed. Theoretical aspects of RIAs will be discussed as necessary to develop a practical appliction. For more extensive discussions of the theory behind RIAs there are several excellent reviews to which the reader is referred (Hunter, 1967; Skelley *et al.*, 1973).

II. RADIOLABELLING OF ANTIGENS

The sensitivity of radioimmunassays is highly dependent on the specific activity (Ci/mmol) to which the antigen can be radiolabelled. Although a variety of approaches using both *in vivo* and *in vitro* labelling are currently available, a few are particularly well suited for the requirements necessary for radioimmunoassays. The most widely used method involves iodination of the antigen with either ^{125}I or ^{131}I using chloramine-T as the catalyst. Chloramine-T is the sodium salt of the *N*-monochloro derivative of *p*-toluene sulphonamide which in aqueous solutions is a mild oxidizing reagent. The mechanism by which chloramine-T causes iodination of proteins is not known, but probably involves formation of cationic iodine. Iodination can be accomplished in aqueous solutions under mild conditions of pH and ionic strength and, in most cases, results in little if any denaturation of the antigen. Iodinations can not be done, however, in solutions containing reducing agents such as mercaptoethanol, dithiotreitol, etc. The predominant product of the reaction is mono- and di-iodotyrosine, although iodine may also react with sulphydryl groups, histidines, or with tryptophan. Under the general conditions used, specific activities of a 100 μCi/μg protein can routinely be obtained. This value, however, is quite variable and is dependent on the number of tyrosines available and their accessibility for iodination. The choice between ^{125}I or ^{131}I is primarily one of convenience, although the specific activity of ^{131}I is generally higher than ^{125}I, and the half-life (8 days) is considerably less than that for ^{125}I (60 days). Therefore, for routine assays which are done over periods of time, ^{125}I is the most useful isotope. Both ^{125}I and ^{131}I readily concentrate in the thyroid gland and are toxic. Therefore, extreme care should be taken while performing iodinations. Iodinations should only be done in a well ventilated fume hood equipped with activated charcoal filters. In addition, lab coats, safety glasses, and gloves should be used during the reaction and fractionation steps.

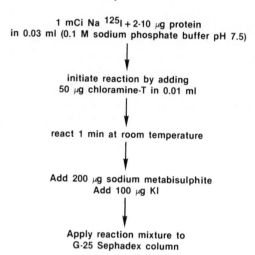

Figure 1. Reaction sequence for a typical protein iodination using chloramine-T. The concentrations of chloramine-T can be varied to modify the extent of iodination. In some cases, tyrosine (200 μg) can be substituted for sodium metabisulphate to terminate the reaction. When carrier protein is required, it should be added after the addition of KI.

A typical reaction sequence is shown in Figure 1. For iodination, the reaction is started by adding chloramine-T to a mixture of antigen and isotope. Iodination is generally complete within 1 minute at room temperature and the reaction is stopped by either adding sodium metabisulphate to reduce excess chloramine-T or by adding excess tyrosine. Since sodium metabisulphite can often cause protein denaturation, adding tyrosine is often preferred. All that remains to be done is to separate the labelled antigen from any free label. This can be most conveniently done by using Sephadex G-25 columns. Generally, low concentrations of KI are added to facilitate exchange of any non-covalently bound labelled iodine. Alternatively, or in addition, the sample can be dialysed to remove free iodine. Since iodinations are down with very low concentrations of proteins, it is sometimes necessary to add 'carrier' proteins such as BSA after the iodination to minimize denaturation due to dilution during the fractionation.

In some cases chloramine-T iodination has not proved usable due to either denaturation of the antigen by oxidation, alteration of immunological properties by modification of tyrosines, or lack of tyrosine residues; for such cases alternative approaches are available. A particularly useful reagent has been developed by Bolton and Hunter (1973) which is currently commercially available. This reagent, di-iodo[125] 3-*p*-hydroxyphenyl propionic acid *N*-hydroxysuccinimide ester, under appropriate conditions, conjugates with the amino group of lysine or the *N*-terminus of the antigen, thereby introducing the label. It is available supplied in dry benzene since in the presence of water it rapidly hydrolyses. For iodinations, the benzene must first be evaporated off and the antigen introduced to the dry reagent. Reactions generally take from 1–24 hours and products are separated from the reactant by gel chromatography. Another approach less commonly used involves lactoperoxidase iodination of proteins (Marchalonis, 1969). For this approach there are commercially available kits in which lactoperoxidase and glucose oxidase are supplied immobilized on an acrylic resin. To iodinate a protein, the sample is added with sodium iodide and buffer to the reaction mixture and the reaction is started by adding D-glucose. The glucose oxidase continuously produces hydrogen peroxide which in turn is used by lactoperoxidase to oxidase the radioiodide. The reaction products are first separated from the resin by centrifugation and then from unreacted iodide by gel chromatography. In general, this approach is milder than reactions with chloramine-T, but the specific activities attained are considerably less.

Another new reagent available for iodinations is 1,3,4,6-tetrachloro-3α,6α-diphenylglycoluril (Markwell and Fox, 1978) which is sold commercially as IODO-GEN. As with chloramine-T, the predominant reaction products are substituted tyrosines. The reagent is first dissolved in an organic solvent and placed in an appropriate reaction vessel. The solvent is subsequently evaporated away leaving the reaction vessel coated with the reagent—this is necessary since the reagent is not soluble in aqueous solutions—and the radioiodine added. Reactions generally require 10–15 minutes at room temperature. The iodinated antigen is subsequently separated free from radioiodine as above. This reagent is as effective as chloramine-T, but in many cases is without the adverse effects on antigen immunological reactivity.

III. ANTISERA: REQUIREMENTS FOR RIA

One of the most important considerations in developing a RIA is the antiserum. Properties such as avidity, titre, and specificity will directly affect the assay. Ideally, an antiserum should be titred with high avidity antibodies which minimally cross-react with related antigens. Since the production of antisera is discussed elsewhere, only the properties affecting the RIA will be considered here. The important characteristics of an antiserum can be assessed from the titration curves against labelled antigen. To determine the titre of the antserum, serial dilutions of the antiserum are incubated with a constant amount of labelled antigen in the absence of unlabelled antigen (Berson and Yalow, 1964; Raud and Odell, 1969). All other parameters such as reaction volume, temperature, pH, incubation time, and method of separation should be identical to those that will be used in the RIA. The titration is plotted as per cent bound versus the log of the antiserum dilution

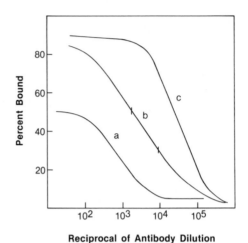

Reciprocal of Antibody Dilution

Figure 2. Representative titration curves. Illustrated are typical titration curves obtained when the per cent bound is plotted versus the reciprocal of the antibody dilution. Curve a illustrates lack of complete precipitation of the labelled antigen. Curve b illustrates data obtained from a high titred, low avidity antiserum. Curve c illustrates the data obtained from a high titred, high avidity antiserum. See text for details.

(Raud and Odell, 1969). The titre of the antiserum is arbitrarily defined as the dilution of the antiserum which precipitates 50% of the labelled antigen. The steepness of the plot of precipitation between complete reaction and no binding is related to the avidity of the antibody. Thus, an antiserum with a very sharp loss in binding has high avidity, whereas an antiserum giving a very protracted curve of binding has low avidity. For RIAs antisera with higher avidity will generally give the most sensitivity and specifity.

Some general characteristics of titration curves are illustrated in Figure 2. The most important characteristic of the titration curve is to assess the percentage of the labelled antigen precipitated at high concentrations of antisera. Ideally, 95–100% of the labelled antigen should be precipitated, however, in practice this is not always obtained. Failure to see maximum precipitation can be due to a variety of factors including impure antigens used for iodination or the presence of free label. Both of these factors can be detected by polyacrylamide gel electrophoresis of the iodinated antigens. More importantly, however, lack of complete precipitation can occur as a consequence of partial protein denaturation during the iodination procedure. Similarly the maximum precipitation of a particular antigen preparation may decrease with storage implicating again denaturation of the protein. When such effects are observed, altering the iodination conditions or storage buffers may alleviate the problem.

The effect of different avidities of antibody is also illustrated in Figure 2. In the example, antiserum b has high titres of low-avidity antibodies since binding activity occurs at high dilutions of the antiserum, but the range of incomplete binding is quite broad. Conversely, antiserum c has high titres of high avidity antibodies because binding activity occurs at high dilutions of antiserum and the range of incomplete binding is quite narrow. Antisera which produce the sharpest slopes of binding provide the most sensitive RIAs. As noted above, the avidity of an antiserum for the native antigen may be different from that for the iodinated antigen. This effect can be assessed by comparing the titration curves using only the iodinated antigen versus titration curves using 10% iodinated antigen and 90% native antigen, in both cases the absolute antigen concentration being the same. If the titration curves are identical, the avidity for the iodinated antigen is comparable to that for the native antigen. If the curve for the iodinated antigen alone is displaced to the right, it is likely that the avidity for the iodinated antigen is less that that for the the native antigen. In this case, the sensitivity of the RIA will be proportionally less.

The titre of the antiserum and the sensitivity of the RIA are dependent on the specific activity of the labelled antigen. A high specific activity affords greater sensitivity. The effect of increasing the specific activity of the tracer is to increase the titre of a given antiserum and to decrease the amount of unlabelled antigen required for competition, thus increasing the sensitivity.

Titre is a function of both the affinity constant (K_a) and the concentration of free antibody binding sites (Ab). The antibodies in an antiserum represent a heterogeneous array of binding sites and affinities, but the concentration of antigen giving 50% saturation of an appropriate antiserum dilution closely approximates the average association constant (Odell *et al.*, 1971):

$$K_a = \frac{(Ag \cdot Ab)}{(Ag)(Ab)}$$

When Ab is at 50% saturation,

$$\frac{(Ag \cdot Ab)}{(Ab)} \quad 1/1$$

and therefore,

$$K_a = 1/(Ag) = 1/\text{moles/litre}) = L/M$$

Antibodies generally show K_a values ranging from 10^9 to 10^{11} L/M. Although the K_a's for certain antibodies may be lower, such antibodies may not be suitable for use in RIAs. In other words, K_a is the volume in litres necessary to dilute 1 mol of the antibodies to a point where 50% of a minimal amount of labelled antigen will be bound.

The sensitivity of the assay is also a function of the avidity. The quantity of antigen bound at 50% saturation defines the sensitivity of the system and this value is related to K_a by the equation

$$K_\mathrm{a} = \frac{1}{(\mathrm{Ag})}$$

at 50% saturation. This then defines the smallest quantity of antigen detectable (sensitivity) at optimal conditions for a given antiserum.

The affinity constant may be obtained from an arithmetic plot of bound/free label (B/F) on the ordinate versus bound label on the abscissa (Scatchard analysis) (Scatchard, 1949). This yields a straight line for the theoretically ideal assay involving only one species of binding sites. The negative slope of the line gives the K_a in L/M. Practically speaking, such a straight line is never observed because of the heterogeneity of antibodies present in an antiserum. Instead, the Scatchard plot shows a curvature where the steepest slope is indicative of the antibody binding site with the greatest avidity. As the slope increases so does the theoretical limit of detection (sensitivity). The intercept defines the binding capacity or maximum number of binding sites. These features of the Scatchard analysis make it ideal for selecting the best bleedings during the course of an immunization by comparing the quality, concentration, and average avidity of the antibodies.

Two parameters which must be considered in selecting the dilution of antiserum to use are assay sensitivity and precision (Berson, 1970). Sensitivity is defined by the smallest quantity of the antigen detectable in the assay. Precision represents the ability to measure between any two points on the assay curve. Precision is enhanced when the antiserum dilution detects differences in antigen levels by significant displacement of label within the range of interest, whereas sensitivity is enhanced at lower displacement. However, as maximum sensitivity is approached, interference by cross-reactive substances and non-specific binding of labelled antigen can increase to an impractical level (Travis, 1979). Thus, assay conditions are optimal when set such that maximum binding (B_o) of labelled Ag in the absence of unlabelled Ag approaches 50% or a B/F ratio of 1. As per cent B_o increases so does precision, but sensitivity decreases and vice versa. The best compromise is simply to work in a range of B_o = 30–50% (Raud and Odell, 1969).

As stated above, the precision of the assay tells us with what confidence we can measure between two points on the response curve. This, of course, depends on the variation obtained in repeated determinations of antigen concentration in the same sample. Precision is expressed as the coefficient of variation (CV) which is the standard deviation (SD) observed for multiple determinations divided by their mean:

$$CV = SD/ \times \chi\ 100$$

where SD

$$\Sigma_\chi^2 \frac{- n(\Sigma_\chi/n)^2}{n - 1}$$

Precision depends on the slope of the assay curve (i.e. the relative displacement of labelled antigen between points on the curve). In other words, the extent of variation at a given titre decreases (increasing precision) with increasing displacement between bound and free tracer at the concentration of antigen around which the variation is determined.

A critical aspect of any radioimmunoassay is its specificity, defined as freedom from interference by any substances other than the one being analysed. Because antibodies are directed towards a relatively small portion of a protein molecule and because antisera are a heterogeneous mixture of antibodies recognizing a variety of determinants, a given antiserum may bind other substances to varying degrees. Substances that are different but are cross-reactive may compete partially but with an altered slope of the binding curve. This results from binding with a decreased affinity. Closely related but non-identical substances may yield a competition curve whose slope is identical over a wide range but does not reach completion. This would indicate that the cross-reactive substance shares most but not all of the antigenic determinants of the initial antigen.

Other factors in RIAs may alter the avidity or extent of binding of antibodies for specific antigens non-specifically. These potential sources of interference include ionic strength, pH, and detergent concentration. Optimal conditions can be most conveniently established by comparing standard titration curves obtained under various conditions. As noted above, the optimal conditions will yield a titration curve having the higher titre and the sharpest slope. Yet another source of interference derives from non-specific binding of the tracer (e.g. to the walls of the reaction vessel). This 'background' is determined by averaging the c.p.m. bound in multiple negative control tubes in the absence of sample and substituting a homologous normal serum for the antiserum in question.

IV. SETTING UP THE ASSAY

The radioimmunoassay is generally carried out in small glass or plastic tubes containing final reaction volumes varying from 200–500 μl. We have found that disposable borosilicate glass tubes (10mm × 75mm) are convenient and have used these almost exclusively. Occasionally, with certain antigens which show a high degree of non-specific adherence to glass, it is necessary to use either plastic or siliconized glass tubes. Low molarity phosphate-, Tris-, or borate-buffered saline solutions are most commonly employed as diluents. Though the majority of assays are carried out at pH 7.0–7.2, optimal results are not necessarily guaranteed in this range. The sensitivity of the cAMP RIA described by Steiner *et al.*, (1972) was significantly enhanced with increased ionic strength to 0.05 M and a lower pH (5.5–6.2). Fischer *et al.* (1974) reported that the specificity of an immunoassay for human parathyroid hormone was several fold greater at pH 5.0 than at pH 8.6, apparently because of conformational alterations in the antigens. Thus, while the majority of RIAs may well be optimally run at neutrality, it is prudent to study the effects of pH, buffers, and ionic strength for each individual assay in order to maximize sensitivity, specificity, and reproducibility.

Serial dilutions of each sample are made in tubes containing the RIA buffer (when practical, samples should be tested in duplicate or triplicate). The dilution factors used depend upon the assay and the precision required. For the viral antigens we have studied twofold or threefold dilutions will give sufficient points within the range of concentrations giving partial competition to define the competition curve. This will vary with assays, however, primarily as a function of the antibody and should be determined for each assay. A series of 'standard' tubes containing dilutions of a known amount of the unlabelled antigen should be run with each assay if an accurate estimation of the amount of antigen in the unknown samples is to be made. Particular attention should be given to positive and negative controls for the assay. These controls are known positive and negative samples of the same nature (e.g. cell-free extract, disrupted virions, etc.) as the unknown samples to be tested. Finally, two sets of replicate tubes are necessary to determine the maximum binding and the background. The number of counts that will be bound at the dilution of antibody used in the assay is known from the titration curve, however, because of possible inter-assay variation, several tubes should be set up with all assay reagents in the absence of sample. The background level of non-specific binding to serum proteins and vessel walls can be estimated from replicate tubes containing all the reagents but substituting an equivalent dilution of homologous non-immune serum for the antiserum.

The next step is the addition of the primary antibody. The antiserum is prepared so that its dilution in the final reaction volume will equal the predetermined titre (generally a dilution at which 50% of the tracer is bound in the absence of unlabelled antigen). At very high dilutions of antibody it may be desirable to perform dilutions in RIA buffer supplemented with 0.1–1% bovine serum albumin, ovalbumin, or homologous normal serum.

The antibody is generally allowed to react with the sample for 30–60 minutes prior to the addition of the tracer to allow any unlabelled antigen present to bind first. This is not critical in some cases since the binding reactions are rapidly reversible and attainment of equilibrium after addition of the labelled antigen is quickly re-established. However, in cases in which dissociation occurs slowly, the incubation with unlabelled antigen first can significantly increase the sensitivity of the assay. The number of c.p.m. of labelled antigen commonly added ranges from 10^4 to 10^5 for ^{125}I-labelled antigens. This will, of course, be dependent on the quality and specific activity of each preparation of tracer. As would be expected from the above discussions, the sensitivity of the assay increases with lower concentrations of antigens but the precision will generally decrease.

Suitable incubation times vary from minutes to days, but 1–3 hours is usually convenient and adequate for most assays. The incubation temperature is initially (15 to 60 minutes) at 37 °C to accelerate attainment of equilibrium and subsequently at 4 °C. The avidity of antibody binding at equilibrium is optimal at approximately 4 °C and decreases with increasing temperature (Karush, 1956).

Next it is necessary to separate the bound from the free tracer in one of several ways. The two most popular methods are the use of a precipitating second antibody or formalin-fixed suspensions of the protein-A-containing bacterium *Staphylococcus aureus*. The second antibody or antiglobulin (a heterologous antiserum prepared against the homologous immunoglobulin) should be titred to determine the amount necessary to precipitate the optimal amount of the first antibody. If necessary, a small titration can be performed along with the initial assay. Increasing amounts of the antiglobulin reagent are added to a series of tubes containing all the assay reagents. A visual examination is usually sufficient to determine the first tube at which the maximum flocculent precipitate is formed. The amount of antiglobulin added to that tube is then added to each of the assay tubes which are then incubated at 37 °C. As before, a 1–3 hour period should suffice. At the end of this period, flocculent precipitates should be visible in all the tubes. It then remains to add 0.5–1 ml of RIA buffer to dilute the free label, spin down the precipitate containing the bound label, aspirate the supernatant, and determine the radioactivity remaining in the tube. If necessary, the precipitate may be washed to reduce further the background.

The double antibody technique has some limitations that must be considered. First, it must be recognized that anti-immunoglobulin sera are quite complex and vary considerably in their charcteristics of general binding activity and reactivity with specific classes of immunoglobulins. In general, such antisera will have low reactivities against IgM antibodies and in certain antisera, particularly early bleedings in which IgM antibodies may predominate, the lack of precipitation of IgM will interfere with the assay. In essence, IgM will compete for IgG binding. Secondly, the equivalence point for precipitation may be quite sharp with many antiglobulin sera, so that in the assays the ratios of immunoglobulin sera must be very precise. This aspect will vary considerably with different preparations of antiglobulin and must be examined for each preparation. Lastly, the commercial preparations of antiglobulin are quite expensive considering the amounts typically used in the assay. When a large number of routine assays is expected, it is advisable and relatively simple to prepare the antiglobulin sera.

The relatively recent discovery of the immunoglobulin-binding properties of 'protein-A', which are present in the surface of some strains of *S. aureus.*, has led to a convenient simplification of the last step of the radioimmunoassay (Goding, 1978; Premkumar-Reddy *et al.*, 1977; Wong and Harris, 1979). The binding of protein-A to immunoglobulins, preferentially to the IgG fraction, is rapid and takes only 5–10 minutes at room temperature. No titration is necessary; the protein-A is added in vast excess in the form of a suspension of the bacteria (fixed in formalin and washed in the RIA buffer). There is no prozone effect as seen when antiglobulin is in excess. The pellets obtained with these bacteria when the suspensions are diluted and centrifuged are good and firm. Another advantage is that only very low levels of carrier immunoglobulin are necessary. The drawback to the use of protein-A as a second reagent is that it does not bind all immunoglobulin subclasses equally well. Rabbit immmunoglobulins are bound especially well, but goat and mouse immunoglobulins are bound poorly in comparison. Moreover, the binding of protein-A is primarily to all or some of the IgG subclasses of immunoglobulins depending on the species of origin (Goding, 1978) and is mediated by the Fc fragment of the IgG molecule.

A variety of additional approaches have been used to separate bound versus free antigen, although these techniques are more specialized for a particular type of antigen. In general, any technique (electrophoresis, chromatography, gel diffusion, etc.) can be used to separate bound versus free antigen. Irrespective of the technique, however, two general considerations must be met. First, since antigen–antibody reactions are reversible, the separation should be achieved rapidly to minimize dissociation of complexes. Second, the separation system itself should not disrupt antigen–antibody complexes. Any technique which fulfils these criteria can be used for RIA systems.

V. PRESENTATION AND INTERPRETATION OF DATA

Radioimmunoassay data are displayed by plotting B/F (ratio of bound to free tracer), per cent bound (of total tracer), per cent B/B_o, B/T (ratio of bound to total c.p.m.), or any other partition index between bound and free tracer (all of which are inversely proportional to concentration of Ag) on the ordinate versus Ag on the abscissa (Bliss, 1970; Ekins and Newman, 1970; Midgley *et al.*, 1969; Rodbard *et al.*, 1969; Rodbard and Catt, 1972). If B/F is plotted against the arithmetic dose of sample, a curvilinear function is obtained (Figure 3B). If, however, per cent bound on the ordinate is plotted versus the log dose of sample, a sigmoidal curve results (Figure 3A). Another possibility is to plot logit B versus the log dose of sample which then yields a straight line (Figure 3C). For convenience, the sigmoidal semilog plot or the arithmetic plot are usually used.

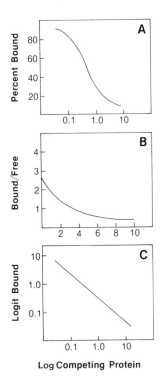

Figure 3. Representative plots of radioimmunoassay data. See text for details.

The original data of Berson and Yalow used B/F as a partition index (Berson and Yalow, 1959;Yalow and Berson, 1959; Yalow and Berson, 1960). The use of B/F as a response parameter is derived strictly from a treatment of the system according to mass action equations. Considering, however, that the resulting curves are neither linear nor log linear and the scatter of determinations differs markedly at different points along the curve (Midgley *et al.*, 1969), the per cent bound plotted agaiınst log (Ag) generally gives a straight line in the steep central portion of the sigmoidal curve and appears to be the method of choice for presentation of RIA data.

Typical per cent bound versus log (Ag) plots of RIA data are shown in Figure 4 and will be used to illustrate aspects of interpreting RIA data. The primary use of RIA techniques is to quantitate the amount of a particular antigen in an unknown sample. In this case, the inhibition curve of the unknown is compared with a standard inhibition curve obtained with known concentrations of antigen (compare lines a and b). For this calculation, any point in the linear portion of the inhibition curve can be used. In general, the steeper the linear portion of the curve is for a particular assay, the more

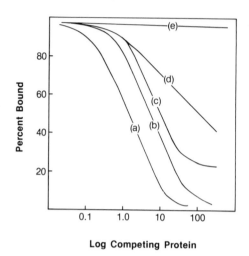

Figure 4. Representative plots of radioimmunoassay data illustrating the effects of cross-reactive antigens. See text for details.

precise the assay will be. For reasons considered below, quantitative determinations are only justified if the pattern of competition, i.e. the slope and extent of competition, are identical to the standard inhibition curve.

The sensitivity of an RIA for quantitating an antigen in an extract depends upon a variety of factors discussed above which will vary with each assay. In our experience with a variety of viral proteins, the range of variation has been anywhere from 50 ng to 0.1 ng of native antigen giving a 20% inhibition of competition in a typical assay. In quantitative assays, the typical upper limit of cell extract protein that can be assayed is about 1 mg. Above this level the assay is prone to non-specific interference which precludes making accurate determinations. Therefore, the typical lower limits of detection of an antigen have ranged from 0.1 ng to 50 ng of competing antigen per milligram of extract or sample. Most RIA assays for proteins should fall within this range under appropriate conditions of a high specific antigen and a high avidity antiserum.

Typical patterns of cross-reactivity in inhibition assays are also illustrated in Figure 4. Cross-reactivity of related antigens in RIA can give rise to two types of alterations of the patterns of inhibition relative to the standard inhibition curve. The most generally observed effect is a reduced slope of competition. This results from the ability of a cross-reactive antigen to bind antibody, but with much less avidity than the primary antigen. Consequently, the antigen concentrations required to compete are higher and inhibition occurs over a broader range of antigen concentrations. A second effect is to alter the extent of the competition curve (line c). In this case, inhibition comparable to the standard may occur over a region of the inhibition curve but complete inhibition is not obtained. In this case, the cross-reactive antigen has antigenic determinants in common with the test antigen and thus can compete effectively for the antibodies recognizing such determinants, but it lacks some determinants. Thus in the competition mixture, one class of antibodies is competed out while one class remains available to bind antigen. The 'plateau' observed then represents the equilibrium situation for the second class of antibodies relative to the labelled antigen concentration. Since this equilibrium is determined by the avidity and concentration of this class of antibodies, the degree of lack of competition (i.e. per cent bound when the cross-reactive antigen is in excess) bears little relationship to the extent of antigenic relatedness and will vary with individual antisera and the concentrations of antibody used in the assay.

A number of potential artefacts exist with competition assays that must be considered. For example, one common artefact occurs when the test extract contains proteases that can degrade the labelled antigen. Such extracts yield competition curves which may bear remarkable similarity to the competition with standards. This effect can be controlled by adding protease inhibitors such as PMSF (phenylmethylsulphonyl fluoride) or by monitoring the status of the labelled antigen after incubation (e.g. by SDS–polyacrylamide gel electrophoresis). Similarly, an extract may contain factors which bind the labelled antigen and in effect compete for antibody binding of the antigen. Conversely, lack of inhibition can be due to degradation of the antibody. This can be detected by adding known concentrations of antigen to the extract and running an inhibition assay.

VI. A PRACTICAL EXAMPLE OF RIA

Although RIA techniques will be quite individualized as defined by the characteristics of a particular antigen and the requirements of the investigator, the range of potentials of an RIA can be best illustrated by an example situation. This example comes from our work in characterizing the expression and relatedness of retroviruses (C-type viruses) in mice. In general, the approaches should be applicable to any protein RIA. Retroviruses contain seven structural proteins including p15, p12, p30, p10, coded for by the *gag* gene region; reverse transcriptase, coded for by the *pol* gene; and gp71, and p15E, coded for by the *env* region. The proteins p15, p12, p30, p10, and gp71 can be purified relatively easily by conventional techniques and can be iodinated to high specific activity without significant denaturation by the chloramine-T techniques given above. An RIA can be easily established for each protein using either monospecific antisera prepared against the purified proteins or antisera prepared against disrupted purified virus. Note that in the latter case, the existence of antibodies against other viral proteins does not interfere with the assay as long as the iodinated antigens are homogeneous. In either case, the appropriate antiserum is titrated against the iodinated antigen using the double antibody technique described above to separate free from bound antigen. The titrations are done in a buffer containing 0.01 M Tris buffer, pH 7.5, 0.1 M NaCl, and 0.01% Triton X-100. The latter was included in the titrations since in the competitions, viruses disrupted with Triton X-100 were used. In the titrations for p10, a buffer consisting of 0.01 M Tris, 0.2 M NaCl, 0.1% bovine serum albumin, and 0.1% Triton in siliconized glass tubes was used since p10 has the property of binding to glass under the normal buffer conditions and thus giving unacceptable background levels. In all the titrations the antisera were successively diluted by two-fold into 10 tubes. The titrations were started at a 1 : 50 dilution of the antiserum (0.004 ml of immune serum in 0.2 ml) and carrier normal serum (0.002 ml) was added to the second tube and 0.004 ml to the remaining tubes to give equivalent serum concentrations to all tubes. After dilution and addition of carrier, the labelled antigen was added and the reactions incubated at 37 °C for 2 hours and overnight at 4 °C. The complexes were subsequently precipitated by the addition of 0.1 ml of antiglobulin. This amount of antiglobulin was predetermined by examining the precipitates obtained with 0.004 ml of normal serum in 0.2ml of RIA buffer and various amounts of antiglobulin. The amount of antiglobulin giving the optimal visual precipitation was chosen. After incubation for 1 hour at 37 °C and 3 hours at 4 °C, the samples were then diluted with 1.0 ml of buffer and the precipitates were collected by centrifugation and washed twice with the titration buffer (1.0 ml). The serum dilution giving 50% of maximum precipitation of each antigen was subsequently used in the competition assays.

For the RIA, either antigen or disrupted virus was serially two-fold diluted in 0.2 ml of the appropriate buffer for 10 tubes. The starting concentrations of proteins were known from previous experience; however, in some cases, serially dilutions of 3-, 5- or even 10-fold may be used to determine the appropriate range of concentrations. In this case, two-fold dilutions were used to give the maximum number of points in the partial competition region such that the shape of the competition curve could be accurately defined. To the diluted samples, 0.05 ml of buffer containing antisera to give the final desired dilution and normal serum to give a final concentration of 0.004 ml per tube was added. After incubation at 37 °C for 1 hour, 0.01 ml of iodinated antigen in the RIA buffer was added and the samples were incubated at 37 °C for 2 hours and overnight at 4 °C. To precipitate the complexes, the appropriate amount of antiglobulin (0.1 ml) was added and the complexes washed as above. Control samples included tubes with only normal serum (background controls) or immune sera plus normal serum (positive controls).

The experimental approach was designed to determine the origin of an unusual virus (HIX) initially detected as a variant of the parental (MoLV) by changes in its host range characteristics. To characterize the virus, it was examined in RIAs for the MoLV proteins p15, p12, p30, p10, and gp71 and the ability of HIX virus to compete in the RIAs was compared with several prototype murine C-type viruses. The results obtained are shown in Figure 5 and readily demonstrate several characteristics of murine C-type viruses as well as the properties of the HIX virus. In this example, the results have been plotted as the per cent precipitation observed relative to the control rather than the per cent bound. In the RIAs for p30 and p10, all the prototype viruses as well as the HIX virus compete completely and with identical slopes of competitions. This suggests that these proteins are very homologous among the viruses examined and that the relative concentrations of the proteins in the virus preparations are comparable. The homology of these viral proteins has also been demonstrated by comparison of amino acid sequences. In contrast, the RIAs for p15, p12, and gp71 show quite specific patterns of competition in that among the prototype viruses only the MoLV will compete completely for the MoLV proteins. Thus, these proteins are 'type-specific' and readily distinguishable among viruses and can be used to type an unknown virus. Note that among the other prototype viruses some compete but with distinctly altered slopes and extents of competition due to the presence of related proteins. With regard to the HIX virus, the data demonstrate that the virus contains a p12 and p15 which are homologous to the MoLV protein since the extent and slope of competition are identical to that given by the prototype MoLV proteins. However, the HIX virus is not completely identical to the MoLV since in the RIA for gp71 HIX does not compete identically to MoLV. Based on these results, it was suggested that the HIX virus was derived from the MoLV parental virus and that either by mutation or a recombinational event, the gp71 was altered which, in turn would be responsible for its altered host range characteristics. Indeed, in subsequent studies employing tryptic peptide mapping, it was confirmed that the HIX virus arose by recombination within the gp71 gene region and, thus had a gp71 composed of regions derived from both parental MoLV and a second, BALB : virus-2, type of virus. Nevertheless, this type of experimental example demonstrates the usefulness of a RIA both to quantitate the amounts of antigens present and to examine the relatedness of antigenic determinants.

VII. RELATED ASSAYS

A. Enzyme Immunoassays (EIA)

Several recently developed and increasingly popular modifications of the radioimmunoassay utilize an enzyme instead of the radioactive label (Engrall, 1977; Teramoto and Schlom, 1978). The enzyme may be linked to the antigen, the primary antibody, or the antiglobulin. One thus avoids the risks and difficulties associated with the use of isotopes such as ^{125}I and [131]I. The assays are often highly sensitive and the enzyme 'label' can be quantitated without expensive or sophisticated counters using a simple colorimetric device. In addition to the advantages of practicality and economy, the reagents have a long shelf-life. However, a potential problem always exists for steric hindrance of the enzyme when linked to a large molecule or during formation of the antigen–antibody complexes. Other complications are those which are common to all enzyme assays, such as pH, the temperature effects, and interface or inhibition by other substances in the reaction. Two important observations led to the development of the EIAA: (1) antigens or antibodies can be attached to an enzyme without a significant reduction in either the enzymatic or immunological activity; and (2) antigen/antibody can be adsorbed on to an inert carrier or solid surface (such as the plastic well of a microtitre plate) without loss of activity or specificity.

In a homogeneous enzyme immunoassay one has the advantage of not having to separate bound label from free. Both phases are present together when the activity is determined. Depending on the system or the enzyme chosen, the activity of the enzyme may be either inhibited or converted from an inactive to an active form when it is bound to antibody. In other words, the enzyme label would be free to catalyze its substrate only when unbound in the former case or when bound in the latter case. In a typical EIA, the antigen–enzyme complex and the unlabelled antigen compete for a limited number of antibody binding sites. The specific substrate for the enzyme is then added and the change in enzyme activity (a function of the bound enzyme) may be determined by a colorimeter or spectrophotometer.

An alternative form of EIA is the enzyme-linked immunosorbent assay (ELISA) (Engrall, 1977). For this assay the immunoreactants are immobilized on a solid phase and either the antigen, primary antibody, or antiglobulin is coupled with enzyme. The basic steps are as follows:(1) antigen/antibody is adsorbed to the solid phase (i.e. plastic surface); (2) antibody or antigen is allowed to react with the immobilized agent; (3) enzyme coupled antiglobulin is then added to bind the antigen/antibody complex; and (4) the substrate for the enzyme is added and the reaction results in a colour change such that the amount of antigen/antibody complex is directly proportional to the change in optical density.

B. Solid-phase Radioimmunoassays

The so-called solid-phase radioimmunoassays (Colombatti and Hilgers, 1979; Premkumar-Reddy *et al.*, 1977; Rosenthal, *et al.*, 1973; Wiktor *et al.*, 1972) were originally developed to eliminate the centrifugation step normally used to concentrate the bound phase or antigen–antibody complex so that the free labelled antigen in solution can be aspirated. The antigen or antibody is

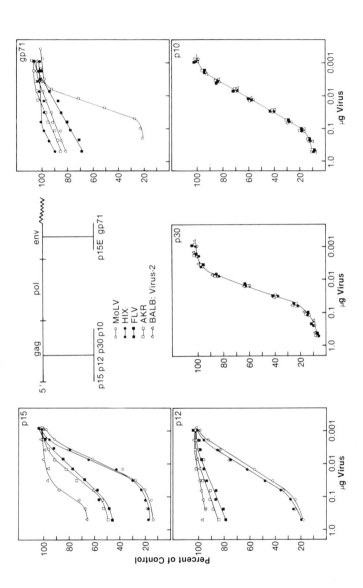

Figure 5. Characterization of a recombinant C-type virus by radioimmunoassay. Radioimmunoassays for the MoLV structural proteins p15, p12, p30, p10, and gp71 were developed as described in the text. In the centre is illustrated the genomic structure of C-type viruses and the locations within the genome of the various proteins. The prototype viruses include Moloney leukaemia virus (MoLV), Friend leukaemia virus (FLV), an AKR leukaemia virus and a murine xenotropic virus, BALB:virus-2. These viruses represent the major classes of serologically distinguishable murine C-type viruses.

complexed to a solid phase such as disk, glass beads, test tube walls, or the plastic wells of microtitre plates. Rather recently, solid phase assays using microtitre plates have been widely employed for screening the monoclonal antibodies produced by hybridoma cell cultures (Nowinski *et al.*, 1979). In this case, antigens are adsorbed to the surface of polyvinyl microtitre wells by incubation overnight in buffer at 37 °C. The solution containing the antigen may be evaporated to dryness by incubating the plate without a cover in an unhumidified incubator. This, however, is not necessary, overnight incubation in a sealed plate is sufficient. Serial dilutions of antibody are added after the bound antigen has been preincubated with bovine serum albumin (BSA) to reduce non-specific binding. The amount of antibody bound to the complexed antigen is determined by measuring the extent to which it either inhibits the specific binding of an ^{125}I-labelled antibody to the antigen (indirect technique) or increases the binding of ^{125}I-labelled antiglobulin or protein-A (direct technique: Rosenthal *et al.*, 1973). One hour incubations at room temperature are carried out for the primary antibody and the labelled second antibody or antiglobulin. Incubations with labelled protein-A may be considerably shortened.

C. Automated RIAs

There are several commercially available automated immunoassay systems available. Assays such as the EIA which do not require a physical separation of bound versus free are readily adaptable to such a system. However, it is the requirement for flexibility in the separation of the immunoassay procedure that has hindered the development and practicality of automation. Many of the systems now available are intended for use with the reagents and protocols supplied by the manufacturer and are not easily adapted to other assays.

Recently, a solid-state radioimmunoassay system was described for the automated analysis of samples in microtitre plates (Kennel and Tennant, 1979). An antiglobulin bound to Sepharose beads is used to bind antigen–antibody complexes. The beads are then separated from the free antigen by an automated cell harvester (Otto Hiller Co., Madison, Wisconsin) designed for use with the microtitre system. The assay was developed to test for virus-positive cells and allowed the authors to analyse up to 1000 clones a day in a sensitive and reproducible manner.

D. Immunoradiometric Assay

The immunoradiometric assay was originally developed by Miles and Hales (1968, 1969). This technique utilizes a labelled antibody rather than an antigen tracer. An excess of the labelled antibodies are incubated with the sample containing antigen. All antibodies not bound to antigen are then removed by an immunadsorbent consisting of antigen coupled to a solid phase. The remaining radioactivity is, therefore, a measure of the antigen present in the sample.

Labelling the antibody is a convenient means to circumvent occasional problems encountered with radioiodination of antigens. Such problems may arise with polypeptide antigens lacking tyropsine residues or with haptens.

A variation of the above procedure is the 'two-site assay' (Woodhead *et al.*, 1974). This involves the coupling of unlabelled antibody to an insoluble matrix which is then used to bind the antigen in the sample.

Most antigens have more than one immunoreactive determinant and, consequently, the amount of antigen adhering to the immunoadsorbent can be determined following incubation with labelled antibody.

A criticism of the immunoradiometric assay is that it requires much larger amounts of specific antisera than conventional RIAs. An alternative is to label an antiglobulin (or protein-A) and react this with the specific antibody prior to its use in the assay (Woodhead *et al.*, 1974).

Although the primary reason for the development of the immunoradiometric assay was to increase the sensitivity obtainable with a given antiserum, such an advantage over the conventional RIA has not been demonstrated. This could be due to minor reductions in avidity during the course of labelling and isolating the antibody.

VIII. CONCLUSIONS

The usefulness of RIA techniques is now fully established. Assays have been developed for a remarkable range of biological agents including steroids, polypeptide hormones, and complex proteins. Theoretically, if a purified antigen is available and an antiserum can be obtained, the essential elements exist to develop a RIA. The major uses of a RIA are to quantitate levels of an antigen and to assess qualitatively the relationship among similar antigens. The values of quantitative determinations are many. First, the techniques are relatively rapid and simple, thus, allowing a number of samples to be examined in a relatively short period of time. This aspect has considerably simplified quantitation of a variety of substances which previously could only be measured by more tedious biological assays. Quantitation has also been made possible for proteins, such as viral or cellular structural proteins, for which there are no biological or enzymatic assays and for which the only previous quantitative assays available were relatively insensitive complement fixation assays. Quantitation of specific enzymes has also been simplified, particularly in cases in which purifications were required prior to quantitation due to interfering factors in crude extracts or existence of interfering enzyme activities. It should be noted, however, that in general, a RIA assay is less sensitive for quantitating an enzyme than using enzyme activity. Neverthe-less, the use of RIAs has considerably expanded the ability to quantitate biologically relevant materials.

The added advantage and additional feature is the ability to discriminate among very closely related molecules. It is this aspect of the assay that utilizes the capabilities of antibodies to their fullest. Thus, RIAs can tell us not only how much of an antigen is present, but also whether it is precisely identical to the standard antigen with reference to the antibody being used. Thus, complete and equivalent competition can give us confidence that what we are attempting to quantitate is, in fact, what is being measured. Conversely, the ability of RIAs to discriminate among closely related proteins can be used to assess relatedness. Thus, 'typing' of viruses can be accomplished very rapidly and with minimal amounts of even impure preparations. Even more remarkably, the degree of specificity can be somewhat controlled by the characteristics of the antiserum. Thus, there is sensitivity, precision, and remarkable flexibility that can be developed into a RIA when utilized to its fullest capabilities.

REFERENCES

Aubert, M. L. (1970). Critical study of the radioimmunological assay for the dosage of the polypeptide hormones in plasma. *J. Nucl. Biol. Med.*, **14**, 85–104.

Barbacid, M., Robbins, K. C., Hino, S., and Aaronson, S. A. (1978). Genetic recombination between mouse type-C RNA viruses: a mechanism for endogenous amplification in animal cells. *Proc. Natl. Acad. Sci. USA*, **75**, 923–927.

Benade, L. E., Ihle, J. N., and DeCleve, A. (1978). Serological characterization of B-tropic viruses of C57BL mice: possible origin by recombination of endogenous N-tropic and xenotropic viruses. *Proc. Natl. Acad. Sci. USA*, **75**, 4553–4557.

Berson, S. A. and Yalow, R. S. (1959). Recent studies on insulin-binding antibodies. *Ann. N.Y.Acad. Sci.*, **82**, 338–344.

Berson, S. A. and Yalow, R. S. (1964). Immunoassay of protein hormones. *In* G. Princus, K. V. Thimann, and E. B. Astwood (Eds) *The Hormones*, p. 557. Academic Press, New York.

Berson, S. A. and Yalow, R. S. (1966). Iodoinsulin used to determine specific activity of iodine-131. *Science*, **152**, 205–206.

Bliss, C. I. (1970). Dose–response curves for immunassays. *In* J. W. McArthur and T. Colton (Eds) *Statistics in Endocrinology,* MIT Press, p. 431, Cambridge, Mass.

Boiocchi, M. and Nowinski, R. C. (1978). Polymorphism in the major core protein (p30) of murine leukemia viruses as identified by mouse antisera. *Virology,* **64**, 530–535.

Bolton, A. E. and Hunter, W. M. (1973). The labeling of proteins to high specific radioactivity by conjugation to an ^{125}I-containing acetylating agent. Application to the radioimmunassay. *J. Biochem.*, **133**, 529–539.

Colombatti, A. and Hilgers, J. (1979). A radioimmunoassay for virus antibody using binding of ^{125}I-labeled protein A. *J. Gen. Virol.*, **43**, 395–401.

Colt, E.W.D., Miles, L. E. M., Becker, K. L., and Shah, N. J. (1971). A sensitive new assay for calcitonin employing labeled antibody. *J. Clin. Endocrinol. Metab.*, **32**, 285–289.

Dalrymple, J. M., Teramoto, A. Y., Cardiff, R. D., and Russell, P. K. (1972). Radioimmune precipitation of group A arboviruses. *J. Immunol.*, **109**, 426–433.

DeCleve, A., Lieberman, M., Ihle, J. N., and Kaplan, H. S. (1976). Biological and serological characterization of radiation leukemia virus. *Proc, Natl. Acad. Sci. USA*, **73**, 4675–4679.

Ekins, R., and Newman B. (1970). Theoretical aspects of saturation analysis. *Acta Endocrinol.*, **64**, Suppl. 147, 11–30.

Engrall, E. (1977). Quantitative enzyme immunoassay (ELISA) in microbiology. *Medical Biology*, **55**, 193–200.

Erlich, H. A., Cohen, S. N., and McDevitt, H. O. (1978). A sensitive radioimmunassay for detecting products translated from cloned DNA fragments. *Cell*, **13**, 681–689.

Fischer, J. A. Binswanger, U., and Dietrich, F. M. (1974). Human parathyroid hormone. Immunological characterization of antibodies against a glandular extract and the synthetic amino-terminal fragments 1–12 and 1–34 and their use in the determinant of immunoreactive hormone in human sera. *J. Clin Invest.*, **54**, 1382–1394.

Gerloff, R. K.., Hoyer, B. H., and McClaren, L. C. (1962). Precipitation of radiolabeled poliovirus with specific antibody and antiglobulins. *J. Immunol.*, **89**, 559–570.

Goding, J. W. (1978). Use of *Staphylococcal* protein A as an immunological reagent. *J. Immunol. Methods*, **20**, 241–253.

Greenwood, F. C. Hunter, W.M. and Glover, J. W. (1963). The preparation of ^{125}I-labeled human growth hormone to high specific radioactivity. *Biochem, J.*, **89**, 114–123.

Heineman, W. R. Aderson, C., and Halsell, H.B. (1979). Immunoassay by differential pulse polography. *Science*, **204**, 865–866.

Hunter W. M. (1967). The radioimmunoassay, *In* D. M. Weir (Ed.) *Handbook of Experimental Immunology* pp. 14.1–14.40, F. A. Davis Co., Philadelphia, Pennsylvania.

Ihle, J. N. Denny, T., and Bolognesi, D. P. (1976). Purification and serological characterization of the major envelope glyocproptein from AKR murine leukemia virus and its reactivity with autogenous immune sera from mice. *J. Virol.*, **17**, 727–736.

Ihle, J. N., Yurconic, M., Jr., and Hanna, M. G., Jr. (1973). Autogenous immunity to endogenous RNA tumor virus: radioimmune precipitation assay of mouse serum antibody levels. *J. Exp. Med.*, **138**, 194–208.

Karush, F., (1965). The interaction of purified anti-beta lactoside antibody with haptens. *J. Amer. Chem. Soc.*, **79**, 3380–3384.

Kennel, S. J. and Tennant, R. W. (1979). Assay of mouse-cell clones for retrovirus p30 protein by use of an automated solid-state radioimmunassay. *Virology*, **97**, 464–467.

Marchalonis J. J. (1969). An enzymic method for the trace indication of immunoglobulins and other proteins. *Biochem. J.* **113**, 299–305.

Markwell, M. A. and Fox, C. F. (1978). Surface-specific iodination of membrane proteins of viruses and eucaryotic cells using 1,3,4,6-tetrachloro-3α, 6α-diphenylglycoluril. *Biochemistry*, **17**, 4807–4817.

Midgley, A. R. Jr., Niswender, G. D., and Regar, R. W. (1969). Principles for the assessment of the reliability of radioimmunoassay methods (precision accuracy, sensitivity, specificity). *Acta Endocrinol.*, **63**, Suppl. 142, 163–180.

Miles, L. E. M. and Hales, C. M. (1968). Labeled antibodies and immunological assay systems. *Nature*, **219**, 186–189.

Miles, L. E. M. and Hales, C. N. (1969). The use of labeled antibodies in the assay of polypeptide hormones. *J. Nucl. Biol. Med.*, **13**, 10.

Miyachi, Y. and Crambach, A. (1972). Structural integrity of gonadotropins after enzymatic iodination. *Biochem. Biophys. Res, Comm.*, **46**, 1213.

Nowinski, R. C. and Kachler, S. L. (1974). Antibody to leukemia virus widespread occurrence in inbred mice. *Science*, **185**, 869–871.

Nowinski, R. C., Lostrum, M. E., Tom, M., Stone, M. R., and Burnette, W. N., (1979). The isolation of hybrid cell lines producing monoclonal antibodies against murine leukemia viruses: Identification of six antigenic determinants on the p15(E) and gp70 envelope proteins. *Virology*, **93**, 111–126.

Odell, W. D., Abraham., G. A., Showsky, W. R., Hescox, M. A., and Fisher, D. A. (1971). Production of antisera for radioimmunoassays. In W.D. Odell and W. H. Daughaday (Eds) *Principles of Competitive Protein Binding Assays*, pp. 57–88. J. B.. Lippincot Co., Philadelphia, Pennsylvania.

Potts, J. T., Jr., Sherwood, L. M., O'Riordan, J. L. H., and Aurbach, G. D. (1967). Radioimmunoassay of polypeptide hormones. *Advan. Intern. Med.*, **13f1**, 183–240.

Premkumar-Reddy, E., Devare, S. G., Vasuder, R., and Sarma, P. S. (1970). Simplified radioimmunoassy for viral antigens: use of *Staphylococcus aureus* as an adsorbent for antigen–antibody complexes. *J. Nat, Cancer Inst.*, **58**, 1859–1861.

Raud, H. R. and Odell, W. D. (1969). The radioimmunoassay of human thyrotropin. *British J. Hosp. Med.*,2, 1366–0000.

Rodbard, D., Bridson, W.,and Rayford, P. L. (1969). Rapid calculation of radioimmunoassay results. *J. Lab. Clin. Med.*, **74**, 770–781.

Rodbard, D., and Catt, K. J. (1972). Mathematical theory of radiological assays: the kinetics of separation of bound from free. *J. Steroid Biochem.*, **3**, 255–273.

Rodbard, D., and Lewald, J. E. (1970). Computer analysis of radioligand assay and radioimmunoassay data. *Acta Endocrinol.*, **64**, Suppl. 147, 79–92.

Rosenthal, J. D., Hayoshi, K., and Notkins, A. L. (1973). Comparison of direct and indirect solid-phase microradioimmunoassays for the detection of viral antigens and antiviral antibody. *Appl. Microbiol.*, **25**, 567–573.

Scatchard, G. (1949). The attraction of proteins for small molecules and ions. *Ann. N.Y. Acad. Sci.*, **51**, 660–000.

Scolnick, E. M., Parks, W. R., and Livingston, D. M. (1972). Radioimmunoassay of mammalian type-C viral proteins. I. Species specific reactions of murine and feline viruses. *J. Immunol.*, **109**, 570–577.

Simpson, J. S. A., Campbell, A. K., Ryan, M. E. T., and Woodhead, J. S. (1979). As stable chemiluminescent-labeled antibody for immunological assays. *Nature*, **279**, 646–647.

Skelley, D. S., Brown, L. P., and Beschn, P. K. (1973). Radioimmunoassay. *Clinical Chem.*, **19**, 146–188.

Steiner, A. L., Porter, C. W., and Kipnis, D. S. (1972). Radioimmunoassay for cyclic nucleotides. *J. Biol. Chem*, **247**, 1106–1124.

Stephenson, J. R., Reynolds, R. K., Ronick, S. R., and Aaronson, S. A. (1975). Distribution of three classes of endogenous type-C RNA viruses among inbred strains of mice. *Virology*, **67**, 404–414.

Strand, M. and August, J. T. (1975). Structural proteins of mammalian oncogenic RNA viruses : multiple antigenic determinants of the major internal protein and envelope glycoprotein. *J. Virol.*, **13**, 171–180.

Teramoto, Y. A. and Schlom, J. (1978). Radioimmunoassays that demonstrate type-specific and group specific antigen reactivities for the major internal structural protein of murine mammary tumor viruses. *Cancer Res.*, **38**, 1990–-1995.

Travis J. C. (1979). *Fundamental of RIA and Other Ligand Assays*, p. 168. Radioassay Publishers, Asnaheim, California.

Wiktar, T. J., Koprowski, H., and Dixon, F. J. (1972). Radioimmunoassay procedure for rabies-binding antibodies. *J. Immunol.*, **109**, 464–470.

Woodhead, J. W., Addison, G. M., and Hales, C. N. (1974). The immunoradiometric assay and related techniques. *Br. Med. Bull.*, **30**, 44–49.

Wong, B. L. and Harris, P. K. W.(1979). Use of protein A as a radioimmunoassay tool. *The Ligand Quarterly*, **2**, 40–41.

Yalow, R. S. (1978). Radioimmunoassay: a probe for the fine structure of biologic systems. *Science*, **200**, 1236–1245.

Yalow, R. S. and Berson, S. A. (1959a). Assay of plasma insulin in human subjects by immunological methods. *Nature*, **184**, 1648–1649.

Yalow, R. S. and Berson, S. A. (1959b). Immunoassay of endogenous plasma insulin in man. *J. Clin. Invest.*, **39**, 1157–1175.

Yalow, R. S. and Berson, S. A. (1970). Radioimmunoassays. In J. W. McArthur and T. Colton (Eds) *Statistics in Endocrinology* p. 378. MIT Press, Cambridge, Massachusetts.

Antibody as a Tool
Edited by J. J. Marchalonis and G. W. Warr
© 1982, John Wiley & Sons Ltd.

Chapter 7

Immunofluorescence Analysis

DOMINICK DELUCA

*Department of Biochemistry, The Medical University of South Carolina,
Charleston, South Carolina 29425, USA*

I. INTRODUCTION

Immunofluorescence technology provides a very important connection between biochemical or immunological approaches and cytological methods in the study of many varied biological problems. Cellular products which can be isolated and characterized by the biochemist can also be localized on or in cells using immunofluorescence techniques. The method, first outlined by Albert M. Coons in 1941 and further refined in 1942 and in 1950, has been used extensively over the past two decades in a myriad of applications covering nearly the entire biomedical spectrum. Although the technique is somewhat less sensitive than other cytological methods (e.g. immunoautoradiography) it does have the very real advantage of being capable of detecting components on living cells. Rapid progress has recently been made in instrumentation, such that fluorescence techniques can now be applied to give one of the most sensitive and specific methods available for the purification of living cells. Cells sorted in this way for characteristic surface markers can then be used to study their functions in various biological systems.

Immunofluorescence analysis is blessed with the advantages of immunochemical methodology such as exquisite specificity and sensitivity. It is also fraught with many of the same problems as any immunological method; potential non-specific artefacts and lack of pure native fluorescent reagents (e.g. antibodies) with which to work. Therefore, all experiments using the technique require strict controls for non-specific staining, and the use of the purest fluorescent tracer reagents available. The purpose of this chapter is to provide the reader with a general outline of the methodology involved in immunofluorescence, and its limitations. Much more detailed information can be obtained from any one of several excellent monographs on the subject, or from other publications cited in the References. A few practical procedures which might be commonly useful in the biomedical laboratory are given in the Appendix.

II. PREPARATION OF FLUORESCENT-LABELLED ANTIBODIES AND ANTIGENS

A. Purification of Antibodies and Antigens

The production of specific antisera and the purification of specific antibodies through the use of immunoadsorbents has been thoroughly described in Chapters 2 and 3. Every effort should be made to document the specificity of the antiserum to be used as a fluorescent tracer. Since even the most carefully prepared and absorbed sera can still be contaminated with unwanted antibodies, the best material to use would be monoclonally derived antibodies from plasma cell hybridomas (Chapter 9). For routine work, particularly using the direct immunofluorescence method, conjugates of specific antisera can be purchased from commercial suppliers. These antisera are usually prepared by accepted procedures and will give good results. However, adequate control experiments documenting the specificity of these reagents should be performed by the investigator for his own application.

As with antibody tracers, antigens used for fluorescent tracing should be as pure as possible, and be relatively stable molecules so that they will not easily denature under the conditions used for fluorochrome conjugation.

B. Fluorescent Dyes

Although many substances will fluoresce when excited by light of the appropriate wavelength, only a limited number of dyes exhibit the characteristics required of a useful immunofluorescent tracer. One of the most important of these characteristics is a stable high quantum yield (or efficiency of converting quanta of exciting light into quanta of fluorescent light). Another important consideration is that the wavelengths of exciting and emitted light must be appropriate for the illumination and filtration systems in the instrument used, as well as being in high contrast with any background autofluorescence emitted by the specimen. Finally, the fluorochrome must be in a form which can be chemically bound to antibodies or antigens without denaturing them.

Four fluorescent dyes have been used by most investigators; fluorescein, shown as isocyanate (FIC) and isothiocyanate (FITC) in Figure 1, 1-dimethylamino-naphthalene-5-sulphonyl chloride (DANSC), tetramethylrhodamine isothiocyanate (TRITC), and tetraethylrhodamine sulphonyl chloride (lissamine rhodamine B-200) (Figure 1). DANSC and tetraethylrhodamine have not been widely used as compared with their counterparts with similar spectral

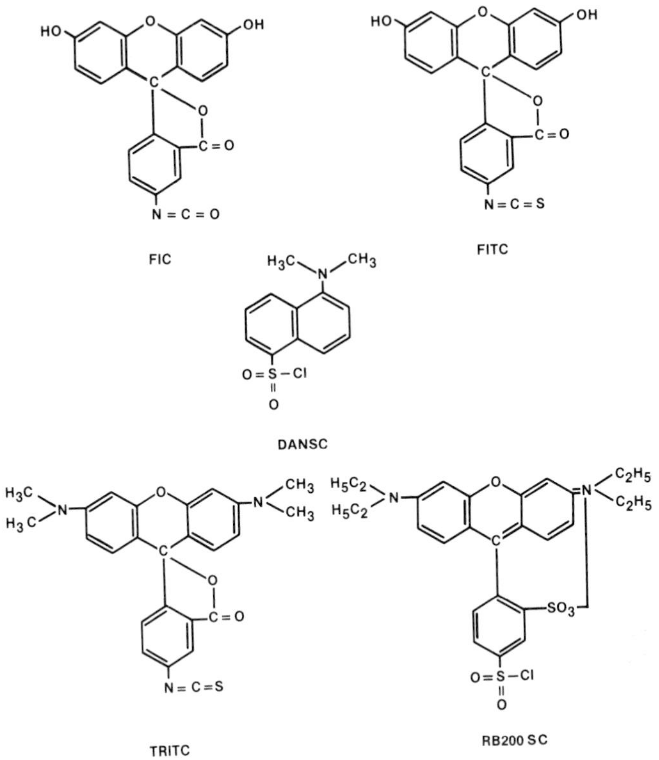

Figure 1. Structural formulae for some commonly used fluorochromes. FIC = fluorescein isocyanate, FITC = fluorescein isothiocyanate, DANSC = dimethyl-amino-naphthalene-5-sulphonyl chloride, TRITC = tetramethylrhodamine isothiocyanate. RB200SC = lissamine rhodamine B200 sulphonyl chloride. FIC and FITC give an apple-green fluorescence. DANSC gives a yellowish fluorescence emission. TRITC and RB200SC give a reddish orange fluorescence. Note the basic similarity in structure between these fluorochromes and the relatively small structural changes which can result in a large spectral shift in fluorescence emission (e.g. between FITC and TRITC)

characteristics, FITC and TRITC, either because of low quantum efficiency compared with the other fluorochromes, or the lack of pure, commercially available, supplies of the dye in a form suitable for easy conjugation to proteins.

Recently, a new rhodamine derivative, called XRITC, has been made available. This fluorochrome, which can be purchased from Research Organics, Cleveland, Ohio, USA, is sometimes used as a substitute for TRITC when single cells are to be assayed by flow cytofluorometry. The absorption spectrum of XRITC is more compatible with the emission of some lasers used in this technology (see the section on flow cytofluorometry).

In the past, commercially available preparations of FITC and TRITC were often contaminated with degradation products and other compounds which resulted in poor protein labelling. In recent years Baltimore Biological Laboratories (BBL) have produced crystalline preparations of chromatographically pure FITC and TRITC which usually give good results, However, some batches of these fluorochromes can still be contaminated, (e.g. Branddtzaeg, 1973) and the presence of impurities combined with the relatively short shelf-life of these reagents can result in poor protein labelling. The purity of a given preparation of FITC can be checked by thin layer chromatography using precoated silica gel plates (Kawamura, 1977) and a chloroform–methanol (85 : 15, v/v) solvent system. FITC can be purified from badly contaminated commercial preparations by silicic acid column chromatography (Kawamura, 1977) or it can be extracted directly from scrapings of FITC spots on silica thin layer plates. Fluorochromes should always be stored in a dry atmosphere, and they should not be unnecessarily exposed to light.

C. Conjugation of Fluorochromes to Proteins

The reactive group of FITC and TRITC, the isothiocyanate, reacts primarily with epsilon amino groups of lysine residues at alkaline pH, and with the amino terminus of polypeptides. The sulphonyl chlorides of DANSC and tetraethylrhodamine also react at alkaline pH with primary amino groups. Many commercial preparations of fluorochromes, particularly TRITC, are quite insoluble in aqueous solutions. Acetone can be used to dissolve the fluorochrome, but dimethylsulphoxide (DMSO) is less harmful to the protein (Bergquist and Nilsson, 1974). Thus, protein solutions of 10–15 mg/ml in carbonate–bicarbonate buffer pH 9.5 (see Appendix), are mixed with FITC at a ratio of 20 µg/mg of protein. For TRITC, the ratio is usually about 10 µg/mg protein. The reaction is usually performed at room temperature in the dark and a plateau level of labelling is attained after about 1–2 hours (The and Feldkamp, 1970). If the protein being labelled is especially subject to denaturation, labelling can be performed at 4 °C, but the reaction will proceed at a slower pace and may require 18–24 hours to go to completion. Some workers advocate the dialysis method of fluorescent labelling (Clarke and Shepard, 1963) in which a solution of the protein to be labelled is placed in dialysis tubing, and allowed to dialyse overnight in the cold versus an alkaline buffered solution containing the fluorochrome. Since the protein is exposed to rather dilute concentrations of both fluorochrome and the organic solvent required to solubilize the fluorochrome, protein denaturation is said to be reduced, and the number of fluorochrome molecules bound per protein molecule is considered to be more uniform among all the protein molecules in the solution (but see discussion by Goding, 1976).

D. Separation of Fluorochromated Conjugates from Unreacted Fluorochromes

Unreacted dye can be removed from conjugates by dialysis, but a much faster and simpler method is molecular sieving by the low exclusion limit Sephadex® or Bio-Gel® media for column chromatography (see Chapter 3). The columns can be quite small; a 3.5 cm × 1 cm 'Quik Sep' column of Sephadex G-25 marketed by Isolabs, Akron, Ohio can handle 0.5 ml of conjugate containing up to 10 mg of labelled protein. Conjugates labelled with rhodamine derivatives tend to be more difficult to separate from the unreacted dye, and longer columns may have to be used. Of course, large amounts of conjugate will also require longer columns, and many methods call for columns of 10–30 cm in length. A good rule of thumb is to allow 2 cm per millilitre of FITC-labelled protein solution and about 8 cm of column per millilitre of TRITC-labelled protein solution (assuming the inner diameter of the column is 1.5 cm). The coloured conjugates can easily be seen moving down the column, and can be collected directly. The conjugates will be diluted about twofold. Unreacted dye should be left very near the top of the column, and should be visible as a brightly coloured band.

Another important advantage of gel filtration is that it allows for an easy and rapid change of buffers and pH due to the fact that the components of the original buffer will migrate with the unbound fluorochrome, and the conjugated protein will migrate into the buffer with which the column had been equilibrated. For example, a Sephadex or Biogel column can be pre-equilibrated with 0.01 M phosphate buffer, pH 8, such that the conjugate will be eluted in the correct buffer for charge fractionation (see below).

E. Fractionation of Fluorochromated Proteins on the Basis of Charge

When an ε-amino group is bound to a fluorochrome, the positive charge usually associated with that group at neutral pH is lost. If the fluorochrome involved also carries a net negative charge, as does fluorescein, the end result is a net change in charge for that site (i.e. substitution of a negative charge for a positive one). Heavily conjugated protein molecules will have a large difference in net charge from their native state, and because of this additional negative charge, they often produce non-specific staining by binding to positively charged components on the specimen. On the other hand, protein molecules which are underconjugated or unconjugated will lack sensitivity in the fluorescence assay and will even compete for specific binding sites with more ideally labelled molecules. Every conjugate consists of a mixture of these overcoupled, undercoupled, and ideally coupled molecules, the ratios of which may influence the results obtained.

To separate the molecules of fluorochromated proteins on the basis of their net charge, DEAE column chromatography is employed (e.g. Riggs *et al.*, 1960). The conjugate is run into a 2.0 cm × 11.5 cm column of DEAE–cellulose or DEAE–Sephadex at low ionic strength, and the progressively higher

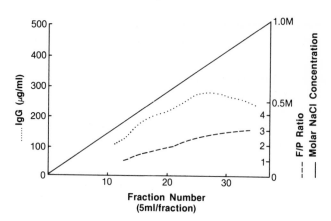

Figure 2. DEAE column chromatography elution profile for FITC-labelled IgG (from Goding, 1976) showing total protein and fluorochrome load as a function of the fraction number and the salt concentration of the eluting buffer. Reproduced by permission of Elsevier/North-Holland Biomedical Press

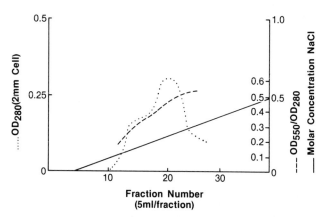

Figure 3. DEAE column chromatography elution profile for TRITC-labelled IgG (from Goding, 1976) showing total protein and fluorochrome load as a function of the fraction number and the salt concentration of the eluting buffer. Note the greater charge heterogeneity of the FITC-conjugated protein relative to the less disperse elution profile of protein conjugated with the hydrophobic, uncharged TRITC molecule. Reproduced by permission of Elsevier/North-Holland Biomedical Press

negatively charged molecules are eluted from the column with a continuous, increasing gradient of sodium chloride (see Appendix). The initial peak of protein eluted from the column will be unlabelled (Figures 2 and 3) and the following fractions will have progressively more fluorochrome bound per molecule of protein (i.e. a higher F/P ratio as measured below).

III. MEASUREMENT OF THE DEGREE OF FLUOROCHROME SUBSTITUTION OF PROTEINS AND CHARACTERIZATION OF FLUORESCENT CONJUGATES

DEAE column chromatography will separate the protein molecules of the fluorescent conjugate on the basis of the extra negative charges added to the protein by the fluorochrome. The amount of protein and fluorochrome in a given fraction of conjugate can be determined spectrophotometrically or through the use of micro-Kjeldahl, Folin, or biuret methods but it must be kept in mind that fluorochrome, protein, or coloured protein products from protein assays may have overlapping absorbance curves. One of the easiest methods to measure the amount of protein and fluorochrome is to measure the absorbance of the conjugate at 280 nm for protein and at the absorption maximum for bound fluorochrome, and apply correction values for the absorbance of fluorochrome at 280 nm. The following formulae for determining the concentration of protein in FITC conjugates, and their F/P ratio (fluorochromes per protein molecule) are from Nairn, 1969

$$\text{Concentration of protein} = \frac{OD_{280} - (0.36 \times OD_{496})}{\text{Extinction coefficient } (OD_{280}) \text{ of proteins}}$$

where 0.36 is the ratio of OD_{280}/OD_{496} for bound FITC (Jobbagy and Kiraly, 1966; Wood *et al.*, 1965).

$$\text{F/P ratio} = \frac{OD_{496} \times \text{MW factor}}{1.9 \times \text{protein concentration}}$$

MW factor = molecular weight of protein $\times 10^{-5}$.

The above formulae can be used to determine the approximate values for molar concentrations of protein, and F/P ratios. The determination of absolute values, particularly for the molar concentration of fluorochrome bound in conjugates, is complicated by the fact that the absorption maxima (Schiller *et al.*, 1953) and extinction coefficients for fluorochromas change after conjugation to protein. Thus, the extraction coefficient of unbound FITC was found to be 0.219 (for a 1 µg/ml solution) but that of FITC bound to protein was only 0.176–0.190 (McKinney *et al.*, 1964). A similar 15–20% drop in extinction for bound versus unbound FITC was reported by Wood *et al.* (1965) and Jobbagy and Kiraly (1966). Brighton and Johnson (1971), using [14C]FITC as an independent label, found that the number of FITC molecules bound per molecule of protein was 1.13-fold higher when determined by radioactivity than by absorption methods using the extinction coefficient of unconjugated FITC. Jobbagy and Jobbagy (1973) also found a similar discrepancy (a factor of 1.10) using absorption methods. On the basis of such measurements, extinction coefficients for bound fluorochromes can be determined, but since the apparent extinction coefficient of bound FITC changes with increasing conjugation (Johnson and Brighton, 1971; see also Nairn, 1976, p. 41) an absolutely accurate extinction for bound fluorochrome is not available.

A further complication in the determination of absolute F/P ratios is introduced by the fact that impurities in commercial FITC preparations, which have different absorbance, colour, and fluorescence characteristics than that of the pure dye, bind equally well to proteins (Frommhagen and Spendlove, 1962). The presence of these contaminants makes the choice of a suitable FITC standard very difficult indeed. Thus, if the absolute value of FITC bound to a protein is an important consideration, then only purified FITC can be used for the conjugation, and for the standard. The measurement of absorbance maxima for each fluorochrome (e.g. about 490 nm and 552 nm for unbound FITC and TRITC respectively and 496 nm and 555 nm for bound FITC and TRITC) can be confirmed by the investigator. Since, for FITC, the extinction coefficient of the bound dye is about 75% that of the free dye, the concentration of bound FITC can be calculated from the formula below from Goldman, 1968 (p. 123):

$$\frac{\text{Concentration free FITC standard} \times \text{OD}_{496} \text{ of the conjugate}}{\text{OD}_{490} \text{ of the FITC standard} \times 0.75}$$

The foregoing considerations probably also apply to the other fluorescent dyes, especially with regard to their unavailability as pure substances. Conjugates of immunoglobulin and crystalline tetramethylrhodamine isothiocynate isomer R (TRITC) and amorphous TRITC were compared in separate studies by Amante *et al.* (1972) and Bergquist and Nilsson (1974). It was found by Amante *et al.* that unknown amounts of non-reactive, low molecular weight contaminants in commercial preparation of amorphous TRITC made an accurate determination of the amount of utilizable fluorochrome very difficult. They also found that although the fluorochrome to protein ratio was kept constant at 30 µg amorphous TRITC/mg of protein (in this case immunoglobulin), the recovery of more optimally labelled conjugates after DEAE fractionation (as defined by their ability to specifically stain rabbit plasma cells) was improved if the protein concentration during conjugation was reduced from 10 mg/ml to 4 mg/ml. The authors surmised that at higher protein concentrations the protein molecules were either too close together to allow uniform reaction with fluorochrome or that reaction with low molecular weight contaminants in the amorphous TRITC preparation formed a very acidic protein conjugate which could not be eluted from DEAE cellulose. Amante *et al.* also found low recovery of optimal immunoglobulin conjugates made with commercial crystalline TRITC preparations. However, recovery could not be improved by lowering the protein concentration, and the authors considered the fact that crystalline TRITC, unlike amorphous TRITC, was insoluble in aqueous solution and had to be solubilized in acetone before addition to the protein to be an important factor in the loss of protein. The use of dimethylsulphoxide (DMSO) to dissolve fluorochromes results in less protein denaturation (Bergquist and Nilsson, 1974). According to Amante *et al.*, conjugates made with crystalline TRITC are quite homogeneous with respect to charge and DEAE chromatography is not required. Amorphous TRITC conjugates, however, are more charge heterogeneous, and DEAE chromatography must be performed to separate undercoupled and overcoup led molecules from the conjugate.

Spectrophotometric analysis of crystalline and amorphous TRITC conjugates showed that a red spectral shift occurs when amorphous TRITC is conjugated to protein, but no spectral shift occurs when crystalline TRITC is conjugated to immunoglobulin (Amante *et al.*, 1972, Bergquist and Nilsson, 1974). The determination of TRITC/protein ratio is, therefore, more straightforward for conjugates made with crystallline TRITC than with amorphous TRITC, especially since the latter shows two absorbance peaks (at about 515 nm and 550 nm). Crystalline TRITC conjugates give a single absorption band at 555 nm.

For conjugates made with crystalline TRITC, then, the following formula for TRITC/protein (IgG) ratio have been given by Amante *et al.* (1972)

$$\underline{M} \text{ TRITC}/\underline{M} \text{ IgG} = \frac{OD_{555} \text{ nm} \times 6.6}{\text{Protein concentration (mg/ml)}}$$

where 6.6 is the ratio of the coefficient of OD_{555} nm absorbance of 1 $\underline{M}$ TRITC (0.041) and the factor to convert protein concentration of IgG into $\underline{M}$(0.00625). This formula can be used for other proteins by simply substituting the proper conversion factor to obtain the micromolar concentration of the particular protein for the one used for IgG in the formula.

Unfortunately, the more easily characterized conjugates made with crystalline TRITC are the least fluorescent (Bergquist and Nilsson, 1974), although acceptable conjugates made with crystalline TRITC can be obtained. The balance, then, between what would be considered overcoupling, and ideal coupling is empirical, and depends on the needs of the investigator and the experimental system used. For instance, tissue sections with large surface areas containing numerous cells, some in different tissues, are more likely to stain non-specifically with a given conjugate than a suspension of cells. This point is illustrated by the fact that some rhodamine-labelled proteins, which are commonly used as counterstains for fluorescein-labelled antibodies in tissue sections because they bind non-specifically to much of the tissue in the section, give perfectly acceptable results if they are used as a probe for antigen receptors on the surface of lymphocytes in suspension.

It should also be noted that the higher the fluorochrome load, the lower the quantum yield of fluorescence per fluorochrome as compared with unbound fluorochrome (as shown by Sokol *et al.*, 1962 for FITC). For example, the fluorescence from a conjugate with an F/P ratio of 2 can be as high as 70% of the emission of free FITC molecules, but this value drops to 10% at an F/P ratio of 24. The molecular weight of the protein to be labelled should also be taken into account. Large molecules can bind a larger amount of fluorochrome, without suffering denaturation or too large a change in charge density, than can small molecules.

Finally, since, according to Nairn (1976) the antigenicity of proteins is not usually affected by conjugation with fluorochromes, as is antibody activity, the use to which the conjugate will be put is also a determining factor. For instance, antibody protein conjugates of lower F/P ratios should be suitable for antibody binding work, while higher F/P ratios for proteins to be used as antigens might be more satisfactory (and could be expected to give increased sensitivity). As a general rule of thumb, F/P ratios of about $1/10^5$ molecular weight (that is about 1–2 for IgG or IgA, 5–10 for IgM, and as high as 30 for a large protein antigen such as keyhole limpet haemocyanin) should give good results.

A. Absorption of Fluorescent Protein Conjugates with Tissue Powders

If the antibodies used to make a given fluorescent conjugate are sufficiently pure, and have not been denatured during the conjugation process, the specificity of the reaction of these fluorescent antibodies should be good enough for most applications. However, in some fluorescent antibody techniques, particularly those involving the staining of small amounts of antigens in tissue sections, the removal of small amounts of denatured antibodies or antibodies which cross-react with the tissue is in order. Absorption of conjugates with acetone or fluorocarbon preparations of tissue powders from the organ to be examined, or from another organ of an animal of the same species, is a popular means of removing unwanted background fluorescence from tissue sections. Many workers advocate the use of mouse liver powder, which is commercially available, for absorptions of fluorescent conjugates. Kawamura (1977) provides several procedures for the preparation and use of tissue powders.

B. Storage and Stability of Fluorescent Protein Conjugates

In our laboratory, fluorescent conjugates of antigens and antisera are routinely stored at 4 °C in the presence of 10^{-2} M sodium azide. It must be noted, however, that living cells cannot be exposed to conjugates containing azide at physiological temperature. The fluorochrome and azide must be applied at 0 °C and washed from the cells before they are warmed up. Under these conditions, our conjugates are still usable after some 3 months, although their fluorescence intensity may decrease somewhat. Other methods of storage, such as freezing small aliquots at -20 °C or -70 °C can also be used successfully, but cycles of freezing and thawing should be avoided. Kawamura (1977) reports that frozen or lyophilized antisera lose some activity after 1–2 years due to denaturation, whereas Nairn (1976) finds little change in the degree of conjugation, solubility, or immunological activity of conjugates stored at -70 °C for 2 years.

C. Fluorescence Characteristics of Fluorochromes and their Conjugates

Put very simply, if a molecule is irradiated with a photon of electromagnetic radiation of the appropriate wavelength and energy, the electrons circling the atoms of the molecules become redistributed from the 'ground state' into higher energy orbitals. Such molecules are said to be in an 'excited state'. Most substances in the excited state very rapidly lose the extra energy they have absorbed through intermolecular collisions, but a few compounds have a structure and a sufficiently stable excited state (about 10^{-8} s) such that their electrons will revert directly to a lower energy orbital distribution, and an emission of a photon of electromagnetic energy lower than that of the original (or exciting) photon will occur. Each such fluorochrome has a characteristic absorption and emission spectrum (Figure 4D and H).

This process, formally termed fluorescence if the excited state is 10^{-8} s, and phosphorescence if the reversion from the excited state to the ground state takes place over a longer period of time after the exciting radiation is removed, is not completely efficient. The degree of efficiency of energy conversion, or quantum yield, is defined as the ratio of emitted photons to absorbed photons and is dependent on the structure of the fluorochrome. In the range of the electromagnetic spectrum used in immunofluorescence, the most quantum efficient molecule is fluorescein. Rhodamine derivatives are about one-third as efficient as fluorescein (Pringsheim, 1949), and rhodamine conjugates are not as bright as fluorescein conjugates when these are excited by UV or blue light (e.g. Lewis and Brooks, 1964). However, under optimal excitation conditions (i.e. excitation with green light) rhodamine compares much better with fluorescein (Faulk and Hijmans, 1972).

The brightness of fluorescent emission is also dependent on the intensity and wavelength of the exciting light, and environmental factors such as the viscosity, fluorochrome concentration, and pH of the solution. Most fluorochromes are best excited by light of wavelengths corresponding to the absorbance of the fluorochrome. Some emission of fluorescence accompanies

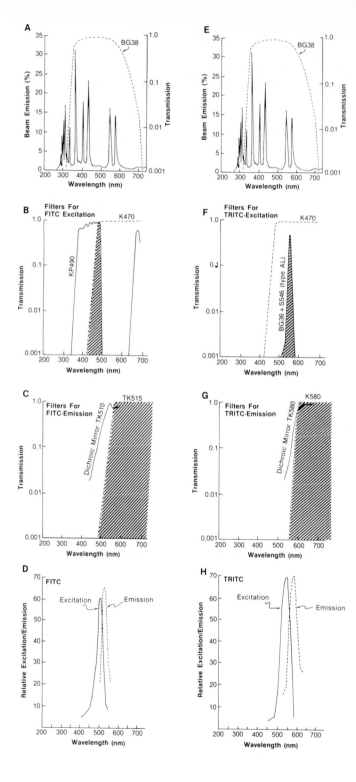

irradiation of fluorochromes with higher energy (shorter wavelength) light. However, most of the increased energy absorbed by the fluorochrome is dissipated by higher energy state transitions which do not result in fluorescence emission, and most of the final fluorescence emission is identical in wavelength to the emission given by radiation at the peak absorbance of the fluorochrome. The pH of the medium is a particularly important variable in fluorescence emission, and fortunately, the optimal pH for fluorescence emission by the most commonly used fluorochrome, fluorescein (pH 7–8), is compatible with that of most biological systems. The quantum efficiency of dilute solutions of fluorochrome is optimal, but as concentrations become higher, more and more energy is lost due to intermolecular collisions, and efficiency decreases (self-quenching). The addition of some other dyes, heavy metals, or other substances also quenches fluorescence emission. A more detailed and highly readable treatment of fluorescence theory is given by H. A. Ward and J. E. Fothergill in Nairn's *Fluorescent Protein Tracing* (1976).

The fluorescence characteristics of conjugates are very similar to those of the fluorochromes used to make them (but see discussion above concerning characterization of fluorescent conjugates). Absorption spectra are also similar except for a slight shift in fluorochrome absorption towards a longer wavelength, and the addition of absorption bands characteristic of the proteins to which the dye is bound. It should be remembered that high energy light can cause not only some decomposition of the fluorochrome (resulting in colour shifts), but may also result in breakdown of the chemical linkage of the dye to the protein (Nairn, 1976, p. 52). With these facts in mind, the wavelength of exciting light used for a given conjugate should be the lowest energy (longest wavelength) absorption peak of the fluorochrome component of the conjugate.

Figure 4. (A–D) Selective filtration of the emission of the 200 W high pressure mercury lamp (A) for the selective excitation of FITC (excitation and emission curves are shown in D). Much of the lamp's heat, long wavelength red radiation and short wave UV radiation are filtered out by a BG-38 filter (Figure 4A). Figure 4B shows the isolation of the optimal wavelengths of light for FITC excitation (cross-hatched) by the combination of a KP490 interference filter and K470 cut-off filter. Figure 4C shows how the dichroic mirror in this vertical fluorescence illumination system, TK510, and suppression filter, TK515, isolates the fluorescence emission of FITC (cross-hatched) Figure 4 (E–H) illustrates the selective filtration system used for TRITC, starting with the same BG-38 filtered emission from the 200 W high pressure mercury lamp (E) used for FITC excitation. The 546 nm 'spike' of the lamp's emission is isolated by the filters K470 and BG36 + S546 (type AL) as illustrated by the hatching shown in Figure 4F. Figure 4G illustrates the isolation of TRITC emission (hatched area) in a vertical illumination system using a TK580 dichroic mirror and a K580 suppression filter. The excitation and emission spectrum for TRITC are shown in Figure 4H for comparison. (Based on data presented by Koch, 1972)

IV. INSTRUMENTATION

The primary considerations in any detection system for immunofluorescence analysis are: (1) the selection of an appropriate light source which will excite only the fluorochrome used as a tracer and not stimulate any autofluorescence in the specimen; (2) the removal of this exciting light before it reaches the recording device of the system (the eye, photomultiplier tube, or photographic emulsion); while, (3) recording the light emitted by the fluorochrome. Given the overlapping excitation and emission curves for the commonly used fluorochromes (Figure 4D and H), this is no mean task. The following account provides some of the most commonly used approaches to this problem, as well as an introduction to some of the currently available technology for processing fluorescence-tagged specimens. More detailed information can be obtained from sources quoted in the text, as well as the manufacturers of the instruments described.

A. Light Sources in Fluorescence Methodology

Figure 5 presents a comparison of the spectral intensity distributions of some light sources commonly used in light microscopy. The most useful light sources are those that produce the greatest intensity of light in the absorbance region of the fluorochrome tracer without producing as much radiation in other regions of the spectrum. No light source, other than the appropriately chosen laser (see below), fits the ideal criterion, and lasers are not commonly used in routine microscopy due to their expense and the risk of injury due to accidental exposure of the eye to an unfiltered laser beam. The high pressure mercury arc lamps (100 or 200 watt (W)) are the light sources of choice for routine applications since the appropriate 'spikes' of light energy at about 496 nm and 546 nm (near the absorbance maxima for FITC and TRITC, respectively) are easily isolated by utilizing the appropriate narrow beam pass interference filters. The greater energy produced by these lamps at 546 nm relative to 496 nm is a happy coincidence, since TRITC conjugates are not nearly as quantum efficient as FITC- conjugates, these lamps will therefore excite both fluorochromes satisfactorily. Such is not the case with other light sources (such as the zenon lamps or halogen lamps) shown in Figure 5, and the near continuous emission of these lamps makes isolation of desired wavelengths more difficult.

The lamp of choice for all types of fluorescence microscopy is the 200 W high pressure mercury lamp. The 100 W lamp produces a more intense beam for a sensitive probe of cell surface fluorescence when used, for example, with a vertical fluorescence illuminator (see below). However, since the size of the arc of the 100 W lamp is much smaller than that of the 200 W lamp, it does not fill the entrance pupil of dark ground condensers and it is not generally suitable for transmitted light fluorescence. Both types of lamps are housed in similar

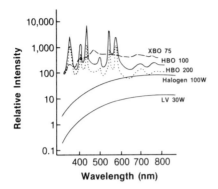

Figure 5. A comparison of the spectral emission intensities of some lamps commonly used for fluorescence work, compared with a low voltage lamp (LV30 W). XBO 75 = the high pressure 75 W zenon lamp. HBO 100 = the high pressure 100 W mercury lamp. HBO 200 = the high pressure 200 W mercury lamp. The 50 W high pressure mercury lamp (not shown) gives a similar spectral emission to the 100 W and 200 W models, but with lower intensity. The halogen 100 W lamp is a low emission lamp which has limited applications for fluorescence microscopy

lamp housings made by the major microscope manufacturers (see instruction manuals) with adjustment for positioning the lamp and focusing the lamp beam. Many lamp housings also have holders for various heat and primary light filters. High pressure mercury lamps are rated for 200 hours' use, assuming each firing of the lamp lasts for 2 hours. If the lamp is burned for a shorter length of time per firing, the lamp life will be shorter. In practice, lamp-life is quite variable, some lasting longer than 400 hours with others lasting only 50 hours. If a lamp burns out early, a claim can often be filed with the manufacturer. Read the literature enclosed with a new lamp carefully to determine the manufacturer's policy for claims. It is a very good idea to keep a record of the use of a lamp and replace it before the end of its rated life. This is done not only because the intensity of the lamp decreases with usage, but also because of the chance of explosion of the high pressure (70 atm) bulb upon burnout. A lamp explosion can cause expensive damage to the lamp housing and if anything flammable is near the housing, a fire can result.

When replacing a lamp, be sure not to touch the bulb as fingerprints can be permanently etched into the glass upon starting, which could affect the light output. Read instructions carefully, and pay close attention to the voltage and amperage ratings of a given lamp (designated as L_1 or L_2 on Osram lamps). Many lamp power supplies have an adjustable L_1 or L_2 circuit to match the lamp. When first starting the lamp, let it run for at least 2 hours so that the arc will 'burn-into' the electrodes, assuring flicker-free future operation. Modern high pressure lamps do not require a long warm-up period before maximum intensity is reached. After turning off the lamp, it should not be re-fired until it has cooled off (about 15 minutes). The lamp should also not be handled while it is hot since the glass envelope is fairly thin and is under a great deal of pressure until the mercury vapour has cooled off.

B. Selective Filtration of Fluorescence Excitation and Emission in Microscopy

High pressure lamps radiate a great deal of heat, and this is usually filtered out by a 2 mm KG-1 filter (from Leitz) inserted in the lamp housing. In our Leitz system, heat and unwanted red light is filtered from the lamp's emission with 1 or 2 BG-38 filters 4 mm in thickness (also from Leitz, Figure 4A and E). Also in the lamp housing is a K-470 cut-off filter (Figure 4B and F) which does not transmit any wavelengths of light below 470 nm (which will often excite tissue autofluorescence), while transmitting the wavelengths of light useful for FITC and TRITC excitation. These filters are exposed to intense heat, and should be removed from the beam when not in use.

For most practical fluorescence microscopy, where FITC and TRITC are used as tracers, the filter systems illustrated in Figure 4 are routinely used in our laboratory to select from the lamp's emission the best wavelength to excite the fluorochromes (Figure 4A and B for FITC and E and F for TRITC) and to detect their emission (Figure 4C for FITC and 4G for TRITC). These filter components are commonly sold as integrated systems by the major microscope manufacturers (e.g. Ernst Leitz GmbH Wetzlar and Carl Zeiss) who also provide a great deal of literature on fluorescence microscope systems. In the set up shown in the figure, a vertical fluorescence illuminator (illustrated in Figure 6, see below), is used, and one of the 'filters' in this system is actually a dichroic mirror which reflects the appropriate exciting wavelengths of light down through the microscope's objective lens, and transmits light emitted by the specimen (TK510 for FITC, in Figure 4C and TK580 for TRITC, in Figure 4G).

The filter systems illustrated in Figure 4 isolate the emission of the mercury lamp which best matches the absorption bands of fluorescein or tetramethylrhodamine while eliminating the ultraviolet wavelengths which are usually those causing the most excitation of tissue autofluorescence. However, in some applications, such as in the examination of tissue sections or for the use of other fluorescent tracers, other filtration systems which preserve tissue autofluorescence, are useful. For example, tissues which give blue autofluorescence upon exposure to UV light offer an excellent contrast for areas stained with FITC and also give the observer an opportunity to orient the specific staining in the tissue.

Finally, the mode of fluorescence excitation used, either transmitted up through the specimen with a darkfield condenser (see the section below on illumination) or down on to the specimen using a vertical illuminator, will dictate slight changes in the filtration system used. For instance, additional

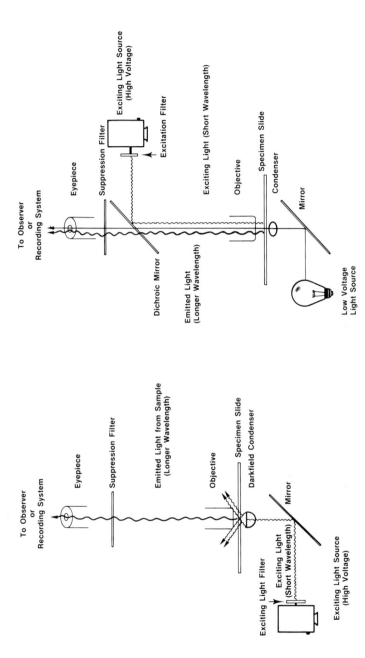

Figure 6. A schematic diagram giving a comparison between transmitted and vertical illumination systems for fluorescence. The vertical illumination system is shown with a low voltage transmission illumination system (e.g. phase contrast) which can be used concomitantly with the fluorescence system

secondary filters to remove exciting light which comes through the specimen in transmission excitation may have to be incorporated into the system to provide sufficient contrast with the background of the specimen. Table 1 presents some filter systems recommended by Leitz for various purposes (Koch, 1972). This publication 'Fluorescence microscopy; instruments, methods, applications' is available from Leitz dealers, and also contains more detailed information on modern filtration systems, as does Nairn (1976).

C. The Fluorescence Microscope

1. Illumination Systems

Two basic sorts of illumination systems are commonly used in fluorescence microscopy, transmission illumination and vertical illumination (Figure 6).

In transmission illumination, the exciting light is directed through the specimen by the use of a darkfield condenser which focuses the light so as to prevent direct light from entering the objective lens. The use of a darkfield condenser thus lessens the need for extensive secondary filtration. The condenser should have a large aperture to collect as much exciting light as possible from the lamp, and it should give good transmission of ultraviolet, as well as visible, light. Since light can be scattered and absorbed by microscope slides, these should be kept as thin as possible. The transmission of light through the gap between the condenser and the slide can be facilitated through the use of a drop of immersion oil placed to fill the gap between the condenser and the slide.

The vertical illumination system depends upon a dichroic mirror to reflect exciting illumination from the light source down through the objective lens of the microscope. Fluorescent light emitted by the specimen and collected by the objective lens is not reflected by the mirror, but passes through it, to be analysed by the detection system (the eye, a photomultiplier tube, or photographic emulsion). Because it is the objective lens which focuses the light on to the specimen, this lens must have a high numerical aperture (i.e. must efficiently collect light) and in addition must effectively transmit UV light as well as the other excitation and emission wavelengths used by the system. Immersion objectives are to be preferred, and the inconvenience of oil immersion objectives with wet mounted specimens can be circumvented through the use of water immersion objectives especially made for vertical fluorescence work.

In general, transmission illumination is the system of choice for low magnification work, because the intensity of the beam of exciting light on the specimen is not dependent upon the magnification of the objective lens. Thus the operator can easily control the intensity of the exciting light while rapidly

Table 1

Exciting radiation	Broad-band transmitted light	Broad-band vertical light	Selective excitation transmitted light	Selective excitation vertical light	Dichroic mirror (vertical light)/suppression filter (both vertical and transmitted light)	Additional suppression filters (optional)
Ultra-violet	1 mm UG1 2 mm UGl	2 mm UGl			TK400/K400	K430
Violet	3 mm BG3	(2 ×) 3 mm BG3		KP425 + 3 mm BG3	TK455/K460	K460
Blue	1.5 mm BG12 3 mm BG12 2 × 3 mm BG12	3 mm BG12	K480 + KP490	K480 + 2KP490 or KP500	TK510/K515	S525 (Type AL)
Green				K480 + KP560 + 2 mm BG36	TK580/K580	K610

scanning a specimen. Also, dry rather than oil immersion objectives can be more readily used with the transmission system, thus avoiding the difficulties presented when immersion oil begins to fluoresce after exposure to air and to intense irradiation with exciting light.

For higher magnification work ($\times$ 400–1000), the vertical illumination system: (1) gives a lower fluorescence background (although flare of exciting light within the lens may pose a problem); (2) gives a perfect focus of exciting light on to the specimen within the field of the lens; (3) avoids interference from the slide or thick specimens which can absorb or scatter exciting light when transmission illumination is used; and (4) is compatible with other forms of transmission illumination, such as phase contrast, which can be used simultaneously. For further comparisons between these illumination systems for various purposes see Kawamura, 1977 (p. 110).

2. Optics

As stated in the previous section, microscope objectives should have a high numerical aperture (light gathering ability) and a high transmittance for the wavelengths of light used in microscopy. The lenses themselves should not fluoresce when exposed to exciting light (especially UV light). Achromats are generally better in this regard than apochromats (Nairn, 1976, p. 88). The lowest magnification objective that can generally be used is $\times$ 10, and, at such low magnification, non-immersion lenses with lower numerical aperture can be used with transmission illumination. Dry objectives of $\times$ 63 (NA 0.80) are useful since immersion oil is often difficult to work with. However, for high magnification work involving weakly fluorescent specimens, $\times$ 63 oil immersion objective of NA 1.32 would be preferable to the dry objective since the final yield of fluorescent light varies with the square of the numerical aperture. Water immersion lenses (sold by Leitz) of $\times$ 25 (NA 0.60), $\times$ 50 (NA 1.0), and $\times$ 100 (NA 1.2) can be used for both vertical and transmission illumination, without the difficulties encountered with the use of oil immersion lenses. Finally, for use with the darkground condensers commonly used in transmission fluorescence microscopy, high power objective lenses with an adjustable iris diaphragm are useful to block out unwanted diffracted light. The rings of phase contrast objectives, however, cause a considerable light loss when employed with a darkground condenser as these should only be used with vertical illuminators.

As with the numerical aperture of objectives, the intensity of the final fluorescent image will vary inversely with the square of the magnification of the eyepieces. For example, the intensity of fluorescent light transmitted through a $\times$ 10 eyepiece is four times greater than the fluorescence intensity of light transmitted by a $\times$ 20 eyepiece. For this reason, the lowest magnification eyepiece possible should be used. I have found that $\times$ 6.3 to $\times$ 12.5 eyepieces give good results, depending on the application.

For more details on fluorescence optics see Kawamura (1977), Nairn, (1976), and Koch (1972).

3. Photomicrography of Fluorescent Specimens

The main problem to be overcome in fluorescence photomicrography is that of recording the weak fluorescent image on film before it fades or changes colour during intense irradiation. The use of high speed daylight film (e.g. Kodak Tri-X Pan ASA 400 for black and white or Kodak Ektachrome ASA 400 for colour) helps reduce the exposure time, especially if the films are push developed after exposure to even higher ASA ratings. The increased grain of films developed in this manner is not that important in most fluorescence applications because of the inherent granularity and high contrast of good fluorescent preparations. Colour transparencies using high speed daylight films are used routinely in our laboratory since the same photograph can be used for colour slides and for black and white publication prints. Polaraoid 107 black and white film offers a high ASA rating (3000) and other types of Polaroid film can be obtained with an ASA rating of 10,000. However, because of the large format of Polaroid film, the advantage of increased ASA rating is negated somewhat due to the loss of light intensity which occurs as the light rays diverge to expose a large piece of film.

Any camera which can be adapted for use with a microscope can be successfully used in photomicrogaphy of fluorescent material. However, since fluorochromes (FITC much more so than TRITC) fade with irradiation (the rate of fading being dependent on the fluorochrome and its environment), there is usually only one chance to photograph a particular field, and the precise exposure control provided by an automatic exposure meter is extremely useful. Also, photographs taken with such cameras are generally of better qualtiy and are more reproducible since the exposure meter automatically compensates for fluorescence fading. The major microscope manufacturers offer very sophisticated automatic cameras with spot metering capability which work very well, but are also quite expensive. If expense is a problem the operator can, with experience, estimate the exposure time with some degree of success. If one must guess at exposure times, however, it is best to use black and white films since these have a broader exposure latitude than colour film. It should also be pointed out that the photomultiplier tubes of some automatic exposure systems can have different sensitivities to different colours of light. For example, since the photomultiplier tube of the automatic camera is less sensitive to red light than to green light, exposures of TRITC-stained material (which also fades less quickly than FITC) will be too long unless the film speed is rated on the meter approximately fourfold higher than the speed at which the film will be developed.

No matter what sort of exposure control is used, the exposure should be made as short as possible to avoid colour shifts in the film due to reciprocity failure, as well as damage , fading, and fluorescent colour shifts in the specimen due to irradiation. Exposure times can be reduced not only by using faster film, but also by minimizing fading. This can be accomplished by using the proper selective excitation light for the fluorochrome involved, and avoiding higher energy exciting light which promotes rapid fading. Also, the mounting medium can strongly influence both the brightness and fading of the specimen. Dry mounted material fades twice as rapidly as material mounted in buffered (pH 7.1) glycerol (buffering at pH 8.6 is even better) and material mounted in xylol-miscible reagents (e.g. isobutylmethacrylate) fades comparatively slowly (Nairn, 1976, p. 106). Finally, it should be obvious that the effects of fading should also be minimized by irradiating the specimen for as short a time as possible before beginning the exposure, and by using FSA tubes which are capable of transmitting 100% of the light directly to the camera rather than diverting some light to the eyepieces during exposures. Most of the foregoing points are covered in more detail by Nairn (1976) and Koch (1975).

4. Fluorescence Microphotometry

For much fluorescence work, some comparison of image brightness between different preparations is required. Experienced observers can make subjective assessments of brightness particularly if the samples are coded such that the determination of fluorescence intensity can be made without prejudice. However, an objective and quantitative assessment of fluorescence brightness is very difficult to obtain visually.

Microphotometer devices, using voltage-stabilized current, can provide an objective value for fluoresence intensity. These instruments, available from the major microscope manufacturers, are usually mounted on the microscope much like a camera, with a beam splitter to divert the light into the photomultiplier tube. Also incorporated into the microscope set up for microphotometry is an iris diaphragm to limit the area of the specimen to be measured by the sytem and to eliminate as much background as possible. The voltage supply of both the photomultiplier and the lamp must be stabilized to prevent spurious readings.

Recently, sophisticated microphotometry systems have been introduced in which microprocessor-controlled automatic scanning of specimens can be used in concert with a computer operated 'graphic tables' microphotometer system to quantify fluorescence intensity of tissue sections in the form of contour maps (Ploem *et al.*, 1978). Automatic scanning methods can also be used for precise measurement of the fluorescence intensity of fluorescent Sepharose beads by microphotometer-equipped inverted fluorescence microscopes. Similarly, a direct fluorescent immunoassay using solid phase coupled antigen (or antibody) can be performed using a fluorometer to measure fluorescence intensity. This method has been used with several interesting fluorochromes (Wiedes, 1978), as well as FITC or TRITC.

Since the photomultiplier tube will register many colours of light, with varying efficiency, the exciting light should be as 'pure' as possible to prevent the stimulation of unwanted autofluorescence. Often, when such selective filtration is used, the sensitivity of the instrument is impaired. A further problem is that in some cases, sample preparation may influence the autofluorescence level. For example, aldehyde fixatives, which are sometimes used to preserve suspensions of fluorescent cells (e.g. Warr *et al.*, 1979), will produce enough autofluorescence in the cells when excited with broad band blue light to obscure specific fluorescence as measured by photometer. When selective FITC excitation (i.e. about 490 nm) is used, too little exciting light is left to stimulate measurable specific fluorescence with these instruments. Unfixed cells, however, have much less autofluorescence, and these can be successfully used with broad band blue light excitation and the photometer (e.g. Marchalonis *et al.*, 1978). Laser illumination, with its much more powerful monochromatic excitation avoids this difficulty and this light source has found wide appeal in automatic cytofluorometry (see below). Lasers have also been used in microscope-coupled photomultiplier systems (e.g. Bergquist, 1975). Accurate and reproducible photometer measurements require the use of appropriate fluorescence standards. Small capillary tubes filled with a standard fluorescent solution (Sernetz and Thaer, 1970) fluorescent conjugated beads (van Dalen *et al.*, 1973) or glass slides impregnated with a fluorescent mineral can be used for this purpose (Jogsma *et al.*, 1971).

5. Video Intensification Microscopy

Recently, silicon-intensifier target video cameras, 1000–10,000 times more sensitive than conventional TV cameras, have become available through security system suppliers. These cameras have certain advantages over the unadapted eye or conventional photographic film in the analysis and recording of fluorescent images. Aside from their extreme sensitivity (which can rival flow cytometry measurements in some applications), the use of a video tape recorder and a TV monitor allows for the recording of a fluorescent image almost
intantaneously, before any bleaching of the fluorescence or damage to the specimen occurs due to irradiation with high energy exciting light. Video recorders are available which can record and play back images at normal speed or 1/108 speed, thus allowing for time lapse photography of fluorescent material in living cells to be performed (Willingham and Pastan, 1978). Since the recorder can also take single frames of the image, any given frame can be 'frozen' on the TV monitor for photography using a Polaroid cathode ray tube camera. If negatives of the TV image are required, Polaroid positive/negative

film can be used for photography such that a working print and a negative can be made of the same exposure. We have found such a system particularly useful in determining the distribution of various fluorescent ligands on the surface of lymphoid cells.

D. Flow Cytofluorometry and the Fluorescence Activated Cell Sorter

One of the most important technological advances made in immunofluorescence analysis over the past decade has been the development of flow cytofluorometry. Using a powerful laser beam for the excitation of fluorochrome-labelled single cells passing through a laminar fluid flow chamber, these machines can easily analyse the fluorescence emission of thousands of cells in a fraction of the time required to do the same job manually with a microscope photometer system. These instruments can also automatically determine the size and viability of a given cell as well as its fluorescence emission for two different fluorochromes (e.g. FITC and TRITC) simultaneously. The data can then be analysed, usually through the use of a computer system, and any given parameter, or combination of parameters, can be used to separate physically the appropriate cell type from the rest of the population. The essentials of a flow cytofluorometer with sorting capability are as follows: (1) a laminar flow cell into which a stream of labelled cells is injected; (2) a laser light source to excite fluorescence of the cells in the stream formed by the flow system; (3) photomultiplier tube systems to measure the emitted fluorescence as well as to determine the degree of laser light scattered by each cell (the degree of light scatter is proportional to cell size and viability); (4) an electronic analysis system to correlate the data; (5) a mechanism for placing a given cell into a droplet which can be separated from other droplets on the basis of the fluorescence, size, and viability characteristics of the cell inside. A schematic diagram which illustrates the basic principles involved in flow cytofluorometry and fluorescence-activated cell sorting is shown in Figure 7. These principles will now be discussed in more detail below.

In the configuration illustrated in Figure 7 (the Becton Dickson FACS II), cells in medium are forced into a laminar flow of sheath water. Because of the laminar flow characteristics of the flow system, the fluids do not mix, and the cells flow nearly single file with the stream towards a nozzle which is vibrating at ultrasonic speed. As the cells flow out of the nozzle, before droplets actually form, they are illuminated with the beam from an argon ion laser tuned to emit the appropriate wavelength of light to excite the fluorochrome. Scattering of this exciting light is proportional to the size of the cell as well as its viability. The degree of low angle scatter is measured by a detector on the other side of the droplet stream. The degree of emitted fluorescence is measured, after appropriate filtration, by a photomultiplier tube placed at right angles to the cell stream.

To decrease electronic noise in the fluorescence channel, the circuit is not

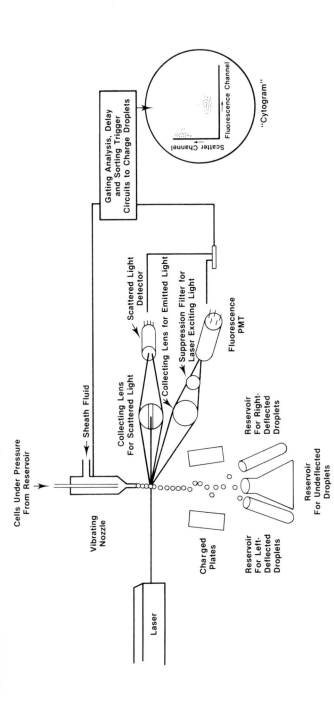

Figure 7. A schematic diagram illustrating the basic principles behind the operation of a fluorescence-activated cell sorter (FACS). The collection lens for the fluorescence photomultiplier tube is at a 90° angle to the laser beam illuminating the fluorescent cells before droplets are formed. The laser light is blocked out on the other side of the droplet stream, except for the narrow angle scatter light which is collected by the scattered light detector. Both fluorescence and light scatter signals are analysed and correlated by the electronic circuits of the machine (shown on an oscilloscope as a 'cytogram'). These correlated data are used to trigger the charged plates and other components to separate the desired cells from the rest of the population (see text).

activated unless the scatter channel determines that a cell is in the beam (this process is called 'scatter gating'). If the fluorescence is of the intensity selected by the operator and the cell meets other criteria such as size and viability, the droplet containing that cell is charged (either positively or negatively) as it is formed. In fact, the stream is actually charged long enough so that two charged droplets are formed for every positive cell to ensure that the cell is not missed. The sorted cells in the charged droplets are then deflected into the appropriate reservoirs, while the unselected cells in the uncharged droplets drop directly into another reservoir. In this manner, fluorescent cells can be sorted at the rate of about 5000 cells per second. (See Herzenberg *et al.* (1976) and Loken and Herzenberg (1975) for more details on the operation of the FACS).

Before the instrument can perform its sorting function, the various signals for fluorescence emission and light scattering must be analysed ('gated') and delayed so that the electronic pulses which charge the droplets occur at the time at which the droplet containing the selected cell is formed. This is accomplished by electronic circuits which also cancel signals from cells too close to one another in the stream to place in separate droplets (coincidence correction). Indeed, a great deal of work done with flow cytofluorometry does not require sorting, but involves extensive analysis of the acquired data through the use of additional computer software (e.g. Warner *et al.*, 1980). In this context, less expensive instruments (e.g. the cytofluorograf series made by Ortho Instruments), without sorting capability, can be used with simple data analysers to provide useful information on the distribution of fluorescence intensities among a population of stained cells (e.g. DeLuca *et al.*, 1979).

Most cytofluorometers include an oscilloscope which presents a scatter plot, or cytogram, of the information gathered by the system. As illustrated in the cytogram in Figure 8, each dot represents a cell analysed by the instrument which has been assigned a 'channel number' (or arbitrary unit of fluorescence) and a light scatter channel number (arbitrary size value). The position of each spot correlates the relative degree of fluorescence intensity (x axis) with the degree of light scatter (y axis) of the cell it represents. In the illustration shown in Figure 8, two populations of cells can be defined. One population, which consists of relatively large, weakly fluorescent cells, is shown on the cytogram as a collection of spots along the y axis. The other population, which is more strongly fluorescent, is smaller than the low fluorescence population and these cells are shown as a collection of spots along the x axis, reflecting their heterogeneity of fluorescence intensity. If a histogram of fluorescence intensity only were generated from the data shown in the cytogram of Figure 8, the graph shown below the cytogram would result. The fluorescence of the two populations in terms of arbitrary units is shown. The cytofluorograph analysis from which the figure was taken divides the entire range of fluorescence and light scatter detectable at the gain settings used into 100 channels. More advanced instruments give even better channel discrimination (i.e. 1000

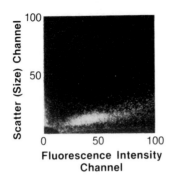

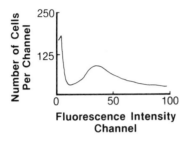

Figure 8. A sample cytogram from an Ortho Instruments Cytofluorograf model 4800 A with a 2100 distribution analyser. The cell suspension analysed consists of large non-fluorescent fish red blood cells (shown as a collection of spots along the *y* axis) and of smaller highly fluorescent lymphocytes from fish spleen stained with FITC anti-fish immunoglobulin (shown as the collection of spots running primarily along the *x* axis). A very small proportion of smaller fluorescent material (antigen–antibody aggregates, dead cells, and other debris) can be seen below the collection of living cells on the *x* axis.

A histogram of the fluorescence intensity versus number of cells for the cytogram is shown below for comparison

channels can be analysed by these instruments). For sorting, the operator can select (or 'gate') the machine to sort between any channels desired, based on both fluorescence and scatter signals. This ability is extremely useful and it allows the operator to reject dead cells and clumps from these analyses since dead cells give a lower scatter than live cells and clumps give a higher scatter than single cells. In some more sophisticated systems, two fluorescence signals (one for FITC and one for TRITC) obtained when the fluorochromes are excited by a laser tuned to emit light of a wavelength (514 nm) intermediate between the absorption peaks for the two fluorochromes, can be used so that cells can be analysed on the basis of their fluorescence intensity of FITC, TRITC, or both fluorochromes, as well as scatter (Loken *et al.*, 1977). Recently, krypton-ion lasers have been adapted for use in flow cytofluorometry. These have been used simultaneously with argon-ion lasers to excite FITC and TRITC (or the new 'XRITC' fluorochrome) in two colour fluorescence analysis. The use of two lasers, each of which is tuned to emit exciting light at the peak absorbance for each fluorochrome, provides a better resolution between the two different coloured products than would be obtained using a single laser emitting exciting light at a wavelength intermediate between the absorption peaks for each fluorochrome.

The argon laser's emission at 488 nm is used to excite FITC and the 530 nm emission of the krypton laser is used to excite TRITC. These wavelengths agree fairly well with the absorption spectrum of each fluorochrome (see Figure 4D for FITC and Figure 4H for TRITC). However, since the absorption and emission spectra for FITC and TRITC overlap somewhat, the resolution of components analysed by two-colour cytofluorometry can be enhanced further by using XRITC instead of TRITC. This fluorochrome's absorption spectrum (peak 570 nm, excited by the 568 nm line of the krypton laser) and emission spectrum (peak 600 nm) is shifted to the right of TRITC's, allowing for more efficient discrimination between FITC and XRITC when dual laser illumination is used.

Computer analysis is usually performed to express the data as a simple histogram of number of cells in a given channel of fluorescence intensity or of scatter (Figure 8), but more complicated systems utilizing data storage and retrieval can be used to create striking three-dimensional histograms for two-colour fluorochrome analysis (e.g. McGrath *et al.*, 1978).

Several manufacturers (e.g. Ortho Instruments, Westwood, Massachusetts, USA and Coulter Electronics, Hialeah, Florida, USA) have instruments on the market which differ somewhat in their operation from the FACS II. For example, some models have a coulter orifice incorporated into the flow cell such that cell volume can be determined by the increase in electrical resistance across the orifice as the cell passes through. Technological advances in this area have been very rapid, and the reader would be well advised to enquire into recent progress (and even future advances) before considering the purchase of a particular machine. It should be borne in mind that the operation of these instruments is usually best left in the hands of a qualified and experienced technician. Because of their high cost, and the attendant expenses involved in their operation, FACS are usually purchased as a department resource to assure that the machine receives usage adequate to justify its cost.

A final comment regarding the use of cell sorter technology involves an understanding of some of the limitations of these instruments. First, since the sorter can purify only about 5000 cells per second (3×10^5/minute or 3×10^6/hour) under the best of conditions, those experimenters who wish to use large numbers of purified cells in their work should consider using other bulk cell separation methods, if possible. In addition, cell sorters are generally incapable of providing an absolutely pure population of fluorescent cells if the frequency of such cells in the original unsorted population is low (e.g. 1%). In such cases, other less efficient bulk purification methods (e.g. binding to and release from ligand-coated plastic dishes) can be used first to purify partially the population before cell sorting is performed (e.g. Nossal *et al.*, 1978). Finally, flow cytometry is best performed in conjunction with fluorescence microscopy, since the human observer can most easily determine such characteristics of the preparation as the distribution of the fluorochrome in the cell (e.g. inside or outside the cell surface) as well as the cellular nature of the fluorescence staining (i.e. debris may mimic cellular staining in flow cytometry). The analysis of light scatter characteristics can usually be used to distinguish among these possibilities, as well as to determine cell viability and size. However, the proper interpretation of these data requires some experience, and it is recommended that the operator of the flow cytometer be well versed in general fluorescence methodology, including fluorescence microscopy, as well as some of the biological aspects of the cells being analysed.

For further information about the theory and practice of flow cyto fluorometry, including a description of the instruments currently available, the reader is referred to the book *Flow Cytometry and Sorting* by Melamed *et al.* (1979).

V. FLUORESCENCE METHODOLOGY

In this section I will attempt to acquaint the reader with the general principles of immunofluorescence assays. No attempt will be made to cover the myriad of techniques developed for particular analyses (see Nairn, 1976 or Kawamura, 1977). However, some basic methods used in our laboratory are outlined in the Appendix.

A. Direct and Indirect Immunofluorescence

Immunofluorescence analysis basically entails the use of a fluorescent-labelled tracer (usually an antigen or antibody) to localize other antigens or antibodies in tissues or on cells. For direct immunofluorescence, the fluorescent reagent alone is added to the specimen, the excess washed off, and the specimen examined (Figure 9). The indirect method, also illustrated in Figure 9, involves the use of a 'middle layer' of non-fluorescent antigen or antibody (although this, too, can be labelled) followed, after washing, with fluorescent-labelled reagent. This reagent is usually an antibody ((Fab)$_2$ fragments are best) directed against the 'middle layer', but other reagents can be used for this purpose. One of these is protein-A, which can be used to detect the binding of IgG subclasses (Ey *et al.*, 1978). Another form of indirect immunofluorescence is the use of an avidin conjugated 'middle layer' detected with fluorochrome conjugated biotin (Goding, 1980; Heggeness and Ash, 1977).

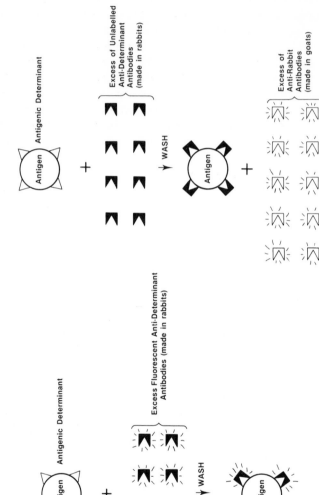

Figure 9. A schematic illustration of direct immunofluorescence (on the left) and indirect immunofluorscence (on the right). Note that the indirect method allows for the binding of more fluorescent antibody, and is, therefore, more sensitive than the direct method

As can be seen from the diagram, the indirect assay is more sensitive than the direct assay since the 'layering' of reagents increases the total number of determinants available to the fluorescent reagent, and the total number of fluorochromes bound to the specimen is increased. However, the indirect method is also more difficult to control, and the increase in background may be a poor trade-off for increased sensitivity.

For both methods adequate controls must be run. For example, in both direct and indirect systems, absorption of the test antiserum or prior incubation of the specimen with unlabelled antigen (if the tracer is an antigen) is essential to determine if the staining is specific or if it is due to some non-specific mechanism (e.g. overcoupling of the tracer with fluorochrome). This sort of control should also be supplemented by additional testing to ensure that binding of tracer is *not* inhibited by the addition of an *unrelated* protein. Indirect assays may require additional controls, in addition to the ones listed above. For example, the middle layer could be omitted to ensure that the fluorescent tracer in the final layer is specific for binding to the 'middle layer' only, and not to other components of the specimen. In addition, controls utilizing a 'middler layer' consisting of unrelated antibody (or 'normal serum') must be performed. Running the assay with various concentrations of reagents is a useful way to 'dilute out' potential non-specific staining. A final word on controls involves the need to include 'intrinsic' or totally unstained specimens as a means of assessing autofluorescence and other artefacts. This point is particularly important if the specimen is tested for the first time. It is amazing to see the frequency of non-specific artefacts which look 'real' until experience and control experiments determine their true nature.

It should be mentioned here that indirect assays can also be performed using enzyme (e.g. horseradish peroxidase)-conjugated reagents, instead of fluorochrome-labelled reagents. Ligand binding is detected through the use of a histochemical substrate for the enzyme which forms an insoluble, coloured precipitate upon cleavage by the enzyme (e.g. Avrameas *et al.*, 1978). These enzyme-conjugated reagents, now available through commercial suppliers, have an advantage over fluorescent conjugates in that, theoretically, the reaction can be run as long as necessary to detect whatever binding occurs. In addition, these methods can be easily adapted for use in the electron microscope (Kraehenbuhl *et al.*, 1978). Since the turnover number of some enzymes can be quite high, the potential sensitivity of these methods can be on the order of a few bound molecules. However, one must contend with additional controls in these systems, the most important of which is a determination of the intrinsic enzyme activity of the specimen. Some tissues have considerable amounts of the mammalian counterparts of the enzymes commonly used in immunoenzyme techniques, and these must be dealt with (either by irreversible inhibition before the addition of the immunoenzyme reagent, or by careful manipulation of the enzyme assay conditions) before interpretable results can be obtained. Finally, it must be remembered that the substrates used in immunoenzyme assays can often migrate from the exact binding site of the enzyme, before precipitation occurs, which can cause artefacts in ligand localization. These problems can be circumvented using controlled enzyme reaction conditions (DeLuca *et al.*, 1974).

B. Specimen Preparation

Many methods of specimen preparation have been developed to deal with the problems encountered in studying particular tissues (see Nairn, 1976 and Kawamura, 1977). For cell suspension work, unfixed cells, which have been gently teased into balanced salt solution supplemented with a source of protein (e.g. 5% foetal calf serum), are often used. Suspension of tissue culture monolayers can be made by gentle trypsinization of the monolayer (e.g. DeLuca *et al.*, 1979a), but one must keep in mind that the trypsin may remove some of the cell surface proteins. Suspensions should consist of viable cells, since dead cells will non-specifically take up fluorochrome-labelled tracer. Methods exist for the removal of dead cells from suspensions (e.g. Von Boehmer and Shortman, 1973, for lymphoid cells). After staining, cell suspensions should be examined immediately, but if the analysis method will tolerate some degree of autofluorescence, the cells can be fixed in 1% *p*araformaldehyde and stored for some time (weeks) before analysis (DeLuca *et al.*, 1979b).

If internal, rather than cell surface, structures are to be stained, cell suspensions can be smeared or spun down on to a slide using a cytocentrifuge (monolayers of tissue-cultured cells grown on glass coverslips can be used too) and fixed with methanol before staining to make internal structures accessible to fluorescent reagents (e.g. Raff *et al.*, 1976). It should be obvious that only antigens which are not denatured by such treatment can be examined in this manner, and that other unwanted fluorescence reactions may occur.

Solid tissues can be examined by a number of methods. One of the most common of these is frozen sections; the usual histological embedding methods (e.g. those using hot paraffin) have limited application since they denature many tissue antigens. Small pieces of tissue (2 mm × 4mm) on pieces of filter paper or aluminum foil placed in a small tube can be snap frozen in acetone and dry ice. Nairn (1976, p. 132) advocates the direct dipping of the tissue into liquid nitrogen and isopentane ($-160°C$) over the usual snap freezing procedure. For very small pieces of tissue, the filter paper can be placed on a microtome chuck which already has a small amount of frozen embedding medium (e.g. Tissue-Tek OCT compound from the Ames Company, Indiana, USA) on it. More embedding medium can be placed over the tissue, and the entire affair rapidly frozen. The entire block must then be sectioned until the tissue is found.

Microtomy is usually done in a special cabinet at $-20\,°C$ using a microtome suitable for use at low temperatures. Sections from less than 1 µm to 12 µm thick can be cut depending on the temperature (the colder the better) and the type of tissue. After cutting, sections are transferred to clean, cold slides, and the back of the slide touched with a fingertip to melt the section. Cutting thin sections requires skill and patience, and is probably best done, initially, under the supervision of experienced personnel.

Some tissues, such as lymph nodes and spleen, will leave monolayers (imprints) of cells after being touched to a slide. Such impressions have been used to give excellent results for cytological studies even though the retention of normal architecture of the tissue is poor.

Other methods for tissue sectioning and sample preparation are given by Nairn (1976) and Kawamura (1977).

C. Fixation

In addition to making intracellular structures accessible to fluorescent reagents, fixation also serves: (1) to prevent the loss of some cellular materials; and (2) to extract some substances which might interfere with antigen–antibody reactions (e.g. lipids). Clearly, the choice of fixative will depend on the stability of the antigen, the ability of the fixative to preserve the localization of the antigen (as well as the histology of the specimen), and the amount of tissue autofluorescence induced by the fixative. This latter consideration restricts the use of many of the best fixatives for the preservation of cell structure (e.g. glutaraldehyde). The most commonly used fixation technique involves the dipping of slides into 95–100% ethanol, at room temperature for a few seconds to a few minutes, followed by air drying. Many variations of this theme have been applied for various purposes (see Nairn's (1976) excellent section on the handling of specific tissues). In general, the lower the fixation temperature and the shorter the time of fixation, the less fixation will occur. Short fixation times tend to localize the antigens and reduce tisue autofluorescence; the author has found that dipping frozen sections in 100% acetone at room temperature for 1–2 s, followed by air drying, will give good results with foetal thymus tissue.

No fixation method is totally adequate for any given tissue. Problems with denaturation and non-specific artefacts induced by fixation abound. The individual experimenter must determine, through adequately controlled experimentation, which method of sample preparation is best for the tissue being studied.

D. Staining, Mounting and Observation of Specimens

Staining of cell suspensions for membrane immunofluorescence is usually done at 0 °C to prevent ingestion of the fluorescent ligand (capping and endocytosis) by the cell. It is wise to do the staining in medium containing an excess of some immunologically irrelevant proteins (e.g. 5% foetal calf serum), although there are instances where non-specific sticking of serum components to the tissue prevents specific ligand staining. After 30–60 minutes of incubation, the cells are washed extensively (three or four times) by centrifugation, resuspended in a small amount of medium, and a drop is placed on a microscope slide and overlaid carefully with a coverslip. Alternatively, the cells can be brought up in 1% paraformaldehyde in cacodylate buffer (0.1 M sodium cacodylate, pH 7.2) for storage (see Appendix). For routine work, we have found that a solution of 90% glycerine with phosphate-buffered saline at pH 7.3 mixed drop for drop on the slide with the fixed cell suspension and covered with a coverslip makes a good temporary mount (although a higher pH will enhance FITC fluorescence, it is not good for unfixed cells). It is possible, with fixed cells, to allow the cells to stand on the slide for a few hours in the cold, so that they adhere firmly to the slide before observing (and particularly photographing) them. Slides of fixed cells can be stored for at least a month by sealing the edges of the coverslip carefully with nail polish.

The general procedure for staining tissue sections is the same as that outlined above for cell suspensions. The section is flooded with the fluorescent tracer at the appropriate concentration, incubated in a moist chamber, and washed repeatedly by dipping the slide into a Coplin jar containing phosphate buffered saline. Consecutive sections on the same slide can be incubated with different reagents, but care must be taken to see that the reagents do not mix. Sections can be marked (e.g. with a diamond pencil) on the underside of the slide for easy location.

Under the microscope, FITC-stained preparations give a characteristic apple-green colour as opposed to the pale yellow-green or blue autofluorescence usually seen with tissues and cells. TRITC preparations give an orange-red fluorescence. It is recommended that narrow band, specific excitation for each fluorochrome be used (see the section on fluorescence microscopy), particularly in double immunofluorescence using both fluorochromes, to provide the best specific contrast of each fluorochrome to the background.

APPENDIX I

A. Preparation of Fluorescent Reagents

1. Antibodies

The purest available antibody preparation should be used. Material isolated from specific immunoadsorbents or hybridoma antibodies is ideal. The following procedure for fluorochrome conjugation of the total IgG fraction of whole rabbit serum is essentially the same as that reported by Goding (1976). The procedure for isolating IgG from serum using a column of protein-A covalently bound to Sepharose is described in the Appendix to Chapter 3. The IgG from 10 ml of rabbit serum (which should be about 50–60 mg in approximately 10 ml), is dialysed overnight at 4 °C against carbonate–bicarbonate buffer (17.3 $NaHCO_3$, 8.6 g Na_2CO_3 per litre of distilled H_2O, pH 9.3).

A concentration of protein for fluorochrome conjugation that is convenient and near optimal is 5 mg/ml. The dialysed IgG fraction is placed in a beaker with a small magnetic stirrer at room temperature. About 25 µg of FITC per milligram IgG or 10 µg of crystalline TRITC dissolved at a concentration of 1 mg/ml in diemethylsulphoxide is added dropwise with slow stirring. These fluorochromes can be obtained from Baltimore Biological Laboratories, Cockeysville, Maryland USA. The solution is left stirring for 2 hours at room temperature, with the beaker covered with aluminium foil to keep out light.

After coupling, the solution is passed over a 3 cm × 30 cm Biogel P-6 Column (Bio-Rad Laboratories, Richmond, California, USA) equilibrated with 0.01 M phosphate buffer at a flow rate of 1.5 ml/minute. The first coloured band off the column is collected for DEAE–Sephadex chromatography. Unbound fluorochrome should still be left near the top of the column by the time the conjugated protein is eluted. TRITC conjugates often have an additional band of intermediate mobility and undetermined nature which can contaminate the first protein band if the column is too short. If this contamination occurs, longer columns can be run, or the material can be rechromatographed.

A 20 ml plastic syringe filled with DEAE–Sephadex A50 (Pharmacia, Uppsala, Sweden) equilibrated with 0.01 M potassium phosphate, pH 8, is used for ion exchange chromatography. The column must be pre-equilibrated with 0.5–1 M phosphate buffer (pH 8) for 1–2 days, then re-equilibrated with 0.01 M phosphate (pH 8) for 1 day before use. The column should then be washed with several column volumes of 0.01 M potassium phosphate to ensure equilibration before adding the conjugate. After the conjugate has run into the column, wash with 0.01 M phosphate. The conjugated protein will bind to the column. The conjugate is then eluted using a linear gradient of 0 to 1 M NaCl in 0.01 M phosphate (pH 8). About 200 ml of salt gradient should suffice. Fractions of 5 ml should be collected (see Figures 2 and 3).

FITC conjugates are characterized by reading the OD_{280} and OD_{496} for each fraction, and the formula given in the section on the degree of fluorochrome substitution of proteins is used to determine the protein concentration and F/P ratio. Fractions of TRITC conjugates are characterized by the OD_{550}/OD_{280} ratio. An F/P ratio of 2–3 for FITC conjugates and an OD_{550}/OD_{280} ratio of about 0.5 for TRITC conjugates should give good results in immunofluorescence, and DEAE column fractions which give similar values can be pooled. However, before pooling, various fractions should be tested to determine which conjugation ratio is optimal for the investigator's own system. Many immunofluorescence procedures are best done using (Fab')$_2$ fragments rather than whole antibody in order to avoid binding by the portion of the molecule to receptors on many mammalian cells. The final conjugate, after overnight dialysis versus 0.2 M acetate buffer (37 ml of 0.2 M sodium acetate plus 63 ml of 0.2 M acetic acid, pH 4.5), is digested wih 10 mg pepsin per gram of IgG. The digestion is allowed to proceed for 12 hours at 37 °C and is followed by dialysis against PBS. The digest is then passed over protein-A Sephadex 4B as described in the Appendix to Chapter 3, to remove any residual Fc pieces or whole IgG.

Conjugates can then be stored frozen at −60 °C or kept in the refrigerator with sodium azide added at final concentration of 10^{-2} M.

2. Antigens

Conjugation of pure protein antigens with fluorochromes can be done by following the procedure outlined for IgG except that DEAE chromatography is usually omitted. However, if non-specific staining with antigen occurs, purification of the lower conjugated protein fractions by DEAE chromatography may eliminate this problem. Since many commercial preparations of antigens contain a large amount of ammonium sulphate, extensive dialysis of Sephadex chromatography must be done before conjugation.

B. Preparation of Tissues

1. Snap Freezing of Blocks of Tissue

Small pieces of fresh tissue placed on filter paper are put into small glass tubes. The tubes are then immersed into a slurry of dry ice and acetone until solidly frozen. Nairn (1976 p. 372) advocates the use of a slurry of isopentane and liquid nitrogen (−160 °C) in the following method. Isopentane (50 ml) is poured into an insulated vessel and liquid nitrogen is carefully poured with slow stirring with a glass rod (hand and eye protection should be used) until the isopentane begins to solidify. If the mixture begins to get too hard (white, with a toffee-like consistency) wait until it begins to thaw before use. Tissue (2 mm thick by 4–5 mm) on the tip of a triangle of aluminium foil is dipped directly into the slurry. After a few minutes, samples frozen by the isopentane method are transferred to tubes equilibrated at −20 °C, and then can be stored at −60 °C.

2. Dispersal of Single Cells

Cells can be dispersed from many organs by simply teasing the tissue into balanced salt solution using fine mouse-toothed forceps. A solution of

0.12–0.25% trypsin and 0.02% EDTA in phosphate buffered saline can be used to disperse cells from very small pieces of tissue which cannot be handled with forceps. The tissue can be placed on a small plastic dish containing a millilitre or so of trypsin–EDTA for 30 minutes at 37 °C. The cells can then be dispersed by gently pipetting the pieces of tissue up and down with a Pasteur pipette. This treatment does not perceptibly decrease the fluorescence binding of anti-immunoglobulin to the surface of immunoglobulin bearing B-lymphocytes in spleen (Mandel and Kennedy, 1978), but the possibility that the trypsin may remove surface antigens from any given tissue must be taken into account.

C. Immunofluorescence Staining

1. Double Membrane Immunofluorescence of Antigen and Immunoglobulin on Lymphoid Cells

The procedure for detecting cell surface immunoglobulins described here uses an indirect or 'sandwich' method, in which the specific first antibody is unconjugated, and is then detected by a fluorochrome-conjugated second antibody which can react with the first antibody. This method is more sensitive and easier to design controls for than the direct method, in which the first antibody is fluorochrome conjugated. The direct method can be carried out exactly as described below for the binding of the first antibody in the sandwich method.

The following procedure describes sequential binding of a TRITC-labelled protein antigen and a FITC-labelled anti-immunoglobulin reagent to lymphocytes, in a double labelling procedure. In practice, either procedure can be used independently of the other, exactly as described.

Conjugates stored for long periods of time may become aggregated, and aggregates can non-specifically bind to the specimen. Centrifuging the conjugate at $10,000 \times g$ for 30 minutes will remove the larger aggregates. The cells to be stained should be washed in a protein-containing balanced salt solution (e.g. Eisen's balanced salt solution plus 5–10% foetal calf serum) and brought up in a small volume of the same medium (e.g. 50–100 μl) containing about 10^7 cells. In the example presented here, TRITC-labelled antigen is used first, followed by an indirectly detected FITC anti-immunoglobulin reagent, to ensure that the binding of the antigen by cell surface immunoglobulin receptors is not inhibited by prior reaction of these receptors with the anti-immunoglobulin. Thus, 50–100 μg of TRITC antigen (in 50 μl of phosphate buffer plus 10^{-2} M NaN_3) is added to the cells (giving a final concentration of 0.5–1.0 mg/ml of antigen and 5×10^{-3} M NaN_3) and incubated for 1 hour at 0 °C. It is good practice to try several concentrations of antigen or antibody to ensure that the best staining versus background is achieved. The azide and low temperature help ensure that the cells do not endocytose the antigen. The cells are then washed twice with 5 ml of medium, and resuspended in 50–100 μl of medium, as before. If a very small number of cells are being stained, cell losses can be minimized by washing the cells twice with 1 ml of 100% FCS in small conical 'bullet tubes'. The first layer of chicken anti-mouse (Fab')$_2$ immunoglobulin fragment serum (0.1 mg/ml final concentration of globulin on a 1 : 10 dilution of serum) is then added to the cells and incubated as before. The first layer antibody can be raised in any appropriate species, for example rabbit, chicken, sheep, or goat. The rabbit reagent is the most commonly used. However, for mouse lymphoid cells, the chicken reagent can detect a wider range of surface immunoglobulins (i.e. for B and T cells). After another series of washes, the cells are finally incubated with a 1 : 10 dilution of (Fab')$_2$ fragments of goat anti-rabbit (or chicken, etc. as appropriate) immunoglobulin-labelled with FITC (reagents of this nature can be obtained ready made from Cappel Laboratories, Cochranville, Pennsylvania, USA). After a final washing with medium, the pellet of cells can be brought up in a small volume of medium for immediate examination, or the cells can be fixed in a solution of 1% *p*-formaldehyde in 0.1 M cocodylate buffer (pH 7.2) for storage.

The fixative is made by adding 2 g of *p*-formaldehyde powder (from Polysciences, Warrington, Pennsylvania, USA) to 100 ml of distilled water at 70 °C. After mixing, the solution is allowed to cool, and 1 M NaOH is added dropwise until the solution clears. Then, 100 ml of 0.2 M sodium cacodylate is added. The pH of the final solution should be about 7.2, and can be adjusted, if necessary, with 0.2 M HCl.

The microscopic appearance of antigen-binding lymphoid cells is that of a smooth or patched ring of fluorescence around the outer edge of the cell when observed with the edge in focus (Figure 10). Upon focusing up and down, patches of antigen over the entire cell surface will go in and out of focus. Cells should also be checked by phase microscopy (use of the vertical fluorescence-transmitted low voltage light combination is indicated here) to ensure the integrity and viability of the cell. Cells with obviously disrupted membranes (or 'blebs' of membrane) or which have a 'flat' appearance in phase contrast, are probably dead and are binding conjugate non-specifically. Such cells, in fact, are often autofluorescent, and they usually do not have reagent localized as a surface ring, but have very bright fluorescent material internal to the membrane. Some living cells may also take up fluorescent reagents non-specifically into their cytoplasm. The frequency of antigen-binding cells for a given antigen depends upon the amount of antigen added (DeLuca *et al.*, 1979) but a plateau frequency of binding cells should be approximately 0.1–1%, depending on the antigen and the type of lymphoid cells examined.

Antibody staining of cell membranes is essentially the same as that described above for antigen. It should be noted that in double immunofluorescence, the overlapping excitation and emission curves of FITC- and TRITC-labelled conjugates occasionally leads to some cross-excitation between

A

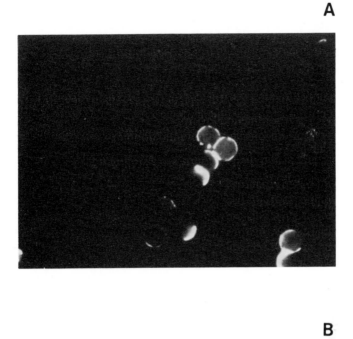

B

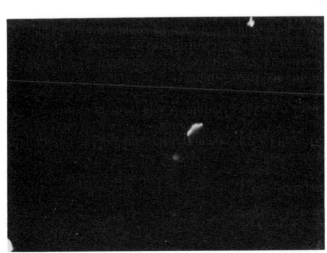

Figure 10. Double membrane immunofluorescence. Trout spleen cells stained with FITC–anti-trout immunoglobulin and TRITC–keyhole limpet haemocyanin (KLH) Figure 10A. Selective excitation for FITC shows many immunoglobulin-bearing cells. Figure 10B. Selective excitation for TRITC of the same cells shows one cell that strongly binds both reagents.

fluorochromes. For example, cells very brightly stained with TRITC-labelled conjugates may show some yellow fluorescence when the cells are excited for FITC fluorescence. This slight TRITC fluorescence under FITC excitation is not to be confused with the apple-green colour of FITC fluorescence, but it may be a problem in black and white photography of double labelled samples.

2. Immunofluorescence of Frozen Tissue Sections

Frozen tissue sections on slides are quickly dipped into a Coplin jar of 100% dry acetone for about 1 minute at room temerature. The slide is then washed several times in a Coplin jar containing phosphate buffer saline (PBS). The sections are marked on the opposite side of the slide with a diamond pencil for easy identification, and the area around the section side of the slide with a china pencil marker or melted paraffin wax. Various dilutions of antisera are then carefully placed dropwise on the sections with a Pasteur pipette or a wire loop.If sections on the same slide are being incubated with different reagents, make sure these stay within the marked areas. Incubation is at room temperature in a moist chamber (a large Petri dish with some damp paper towels inside will suffice) for 30 minutes. Washing is accomplished by repeated dipping in Coplin jars containing PBS. For indirect immunofluorescence, the second layer of fluorescent reagent is incubated on the section as above. After washing, the sections can be mounted and observed.

Since fixed material is used, cytoplasmic as well as membrane fluorescence can be observed. The specificity of the staining must be established with suitable controls.

D. Photomicrography

The following account describes the use of a fully automatic spot metering camera (e.g. on the Zeiss photomicroscope III) for double (FITC and TRITC) membrane immunofluorescence photomicrography. Consult the appropriate instruction manuals before using your camera. Kodak ektachrome 400 daylight colour transparency film is used. The ASA setting on the camera is 800 for FITC exposures (or transmitted light exposures) and 3200 for TRITC exposures. The camera should be set for spot metering and an area on the cell surface with a fluorescent spot which can be used to determine the exposure should be centred in the spot metering circle. It is important that the cell is not moving in the slightest degree, since the exposure may take as long as 3 minutes. I routinely use fixed cells mixed on a slide with 90% glycerine in PBS and left with a coverslip for several hours to ensure that the cells have adhered firmly to the slide before photography. Be very careful to focus precisely and to use a cable release to trip the shutter. Automatic exposure can be performed in the order TRITC, then FITC, then TRITC again (TRITC is less subject to fading than FITC) to make sure the cell has not moved during exposure. A transmitted light (e.g. phase contrast) photograph can then be taken. The distribution of fluorescent material for each fluorochrome can then be determined on the final photographs. Film should be professionally 'push-developed' at an ASA rating of 800.

REFERENCES

Amante, L., Ancona, A., and Forni, L. (1972). The conjugation of immunoglobulins with tetramethylrhodamineisothiocyanate. A comparison between the amorphous and crystalline fluorochrome. *J. Immunol. Methods*, **1**, 298–301.

Avrameas, S., Antoine, J-C., Kargenti, E., and Gonatas, N. K. (1978). The study of lymphocyte membranes using immunoenzymatic techniques. In W. Knapp, K. Holubar, and G. Wick (Eds) *Immunofluorescence and Related Staining Techniques*. Elsevier, North-Holland.

Beergquist, N. R. and Nilsson, P. (1974). The conjugation of immunogloublins with tetramethylrhodamine isothiocyanate by utilization of dimethysulfoxide (DMSO) as a solvent. *J. Immunol. Methods*, **5**, 189–198.

Bergquist, N. R. and Nilsson, P. (1975). Laser excitation of fluorescent copolymerized immunoglobulin beads. *Ann. N.Y. Acad. Sci.*, **254**, 157–162.

Brandtzaeg, P. (1973). Conjugates of immunoglobulin G with different fluorochromes. I. Characterization by anionic-exchange chromatography. *Scand. J. Immunol.*, **2**, 273.

Brighton, W. D. and Johnson, E. A. (1971). Conjugation parameters determined with ^{14}C-FITC. *Ann. N.Y. Acad Sci.*, **177**, 501–505.

Clark, H. F. and Shepard, C. C. (1963). A dialysis technique for preparing fluorescent antibody. *Virology*, **20**, 642–644.

Coons, A. H., Creech, H. J., and Jones, R. N. (1941). Immunological properties of an antibody containing a fluorescent group. *Proc. Soc. Exptl. Biol. Med.*, **47**, 200–202.

Coons, A. H., Creech, H. J., Jones, R. N., and Berliner, E. (1942). The demonstration of pneumococcal antigen in tissues by the use of fluorescent antibody. *J. Immunol.*, **45**, 159–170.

Coons, A. H. and Kaplan, M. H. (1950). Localization of antigen in tissue cells. II. Improvements in a method for the detection of antigen by means of fluorescent antibody. *J. Expt. Med.*, **91**, 1–13.

DeLuca, D., Kripke, M. L., and Marchalonis, J. J. (1979a). Induction and specificity of antisera from mice immunized with syngeneic UV-induced tumors. *J. Immunol.*, **123**, 2696–2703.

DeLuca, D., Warr, G. W., and Marchalonis, J. J. (1979b). The immunoglobulin-like T-cell receptor. II. Codistribution of Fab determinants and antigen on the surface of antigen binding lymphocytes of mouse thymus. *J. of Immunogenetics*, **6**, 359–372.

Ey, P. L., Prowse, S. J., and Jenkin, C. R. (1978). Isolation of pure IgG_1, IgG_{2a}, and IgG_{2b} immunoglobulins from mouse serum using protein A-sepharose. *Immunochemistry*, **15**, 429–436.

Faulk, W. P. and Hijmans, W. (1972). Recent developments in immunofluorescence. *Progr. Allergy*, **16**, 9–39.

Frommhagen, L. H. and Spendlove, R. S. (1962). The staining properties of human serum proteins conjugated with purified fluorescein isothiocyanate. *J. Immunol.*, **89**, 124–131.

Goding, J. W. (1980). Antibody production by hybriodmas. *J. Immunol. Methods*, **39**, 285–308.

Heggeness, M. H. and Ash, J. F. (1977). Use of avidin–biotin complex for the localization of actin and myosin with fluorescence microscopy. *J. Cell. Bio.*, **73**, 783–788.

Herzenberg, L. A., Sweet, R. G., and Herzenberg, L. A. (1976). Fluorescence-activated cell sorting. *Sci. Amer.*, **234**, 108–117.

Jobbagy, A. and Jobbagy, G. M. (1973). FTC-insulin conjugates. II. Chemical characterization of fluorescein thiocarbamized–insulin conjugates. *J. Immunol. Methods*, **3**, 399–410.

Jobbagy, A. and Kiraly, K. (1966). Chemical characterization of fluorescein isothiocyanate–protein conjugates. *Biochem. Biophys, Acta*, **124**, 166–175.

Jogsma, A. P. M., Hijmans, W., and Ploem, J. S. (1971). Quantitative immuno fluorescence standardization and calibration in microfluorometry. *Histochemie*, **25**, 329–343.

Johnson, E. A. and Brighton, W. D. (1971). The properties of some ^{14}C-fluorescein-–protein conjugates. *J. Immunol. Methods*, **1**, 91–99.

Kawamara, A. (1977). *Fluorescent Antibody Techniques and Their Applications*, 2nd edn. University of Tokyo Press, Tokyo and University Park Press, Baltimore, London and Tokyo.

Koch, K. (1972). *Fluorescence Microscopy: instruments, methods, applications.* Leitz GmbH, Wetzlar.

Koch, K. F. (1975). *Fluorescence Photomicrography. Sonderdruck aus Leitz Mitteilungen fur Wisenschaft u. Technik-Bd.* **6**, **4**, 149–156.

Lewis, V. J. and Brooks, J. B. (1964). Comparison of fluorochromes for the preparation of fluorescent-antibody reagents. *J. Bact.* **88**, 1520–152.

Loken, M. R. and Herzenberg, L. A. (1975). Analysis of cell populations with a fluorescence-activated cell sorter. *Ann. N.Y. Acad. Sci.*, **254**, 163–171.

Loken, M. R., Parks, D. R., and Herzenberg, L. A. (1977). Two color immuno fluorescence using a fluorescence-activated cell sorter. *J. Histochem. Cytochem.*, **25**, 899–907.

Mandel, T. E. and Kennedy, M. M. (1978). The differentiation of murine thymocytes *in vivo* and *in vitro*. *Immunology*, **35**, 317–331.

Marchalonis, J. J., Bucana, C., Hoyer, L., Warr, G., Hanna, M. G., Jr., and Szenberg, A. (1978). Visualization of a guinea pig T-lymphocyte surface component cross-reactive with immunoglobulin. *Science*, **199**, 433–435.

Melamed, M. R., Mullaney, P. F., and Mendelsohn, M. L. (1979). *Flow Cytometry and Sorting*. John Wiley and Sons, New York, Chichester, Brisbane, Toronto.

McGrath, M. S., Decleve, A., Lieberman, M., Kaplan, H. S., and Weissman, I. L. (1978). Specificity of cell surface virus receptors on radiation leukemia virus and radiation-induced thymic lymphomas. *J. Virol.*, **28**, 819–827.

McKinney, R. M., Spillane, J. T., and Pearce, G. W. (1964). Factors affecting the rate of reaction of fluorescein isothiocyanate with serum proteins. *J. Immunol.*, **93**, 232–242.

Nairn, R. C. (1969). *Fluorescent Protein Tracing*, 3rd edn. Churchill Livingston, Edinburgh, London, and New York.

Nairn, R. C. (1976). *Fluorescent Protein Tracing*, 4th edn. Churchill Livingstone, Edinburgh, London, and New York.

Nossal, G. J. V., Pike, B. L., and Battye, F. L. (1978). Sequential use of hapten-gelatin fractionation and fluorescence-activated cell sorting in the enrichment of hapten-specific B lymphocytes. *Eur. J. Immunol.*, **8**, 151–157.

Ploem, J. S., Tanke, H. J., Al, I., and Deelder, A. M. (1978). Recent developments in immunofluorescence microscopy and microfluorometry. In: Immunofluorescence and related staining techniques. W. Knapp, K Holubar, and G. Wick, eds. Elsevier/North Holland.

Pringsheim, P. (1949). *Fluorescence and Phosphorescence.* Wiley (Interscience), New York.

Raff, M., Megson, M., Owen, J. J. T., and Cooper, M. D. (1976). Early production of intracellular IgM by B-lymphocyte precursors in mouse. *Nature*, **259**, 254.

Riggs, J. L., Loh, P. C., and Eveland, W. C. (1960). A simple fractionation method for preparation of fluorescein-labeled gamma globulin. *Proc. Soc. Exptl. Bio. Med.*, **105**, 655–658.

Schiller, A. A., Schager, R. W., and Hess, E. L. (1953). Fluorescein-conjugated bovine albumin: physical and biological properties. *J. Gen. Physiol.*, **36**, 489–506.

Sernetz, M. and Thaer, A. (1970). A capillary fluorescence standard for microfluorometry. *J. Microsc.*, **91**, 43–52.

Sokol, F., Hulka, A., and Albrecht, P. (1962). Fluorescent antibody method. Conjugation of fluorescein-isothiocyanate with immune globulin. *Folia Microbiol. (Prague)*, **I**, 155–161.

The, T. H. and Feltkamp, T. E. W. (1970). Conjugation of fluorescein isothiocyanate to antibodies. I. Experiments on the conditions of conjugation. *Immunology*, **18**, 865–875.

Von Boehmer, H. and Shortman, K. (1973). The separation of different cell classes from lymphoid organs. IX. A simple and rapid method for removal of damaged cells from lymphoid cell suspensions. *J. Immunol. Methods*, **2**, 293.

Von Dalen, J. P. R., Knapp, W., and Ploem, J. S. (1973). Microfluorometry on antigen–antibody interaction in immunofluorescence using antigens covalently bound to agarose beads. *J. Immunol. Methods*, **2**, 383–392.

Warner, N. L., Dailey, M. J., Richey, J., and Spellman, C. (1980). Flow cytometery analysis of murine B cell lymphoma differentiation. *Immunological Reviews*, **48**, 197–243.

Warr, G. W., DeLuca, D., and Griffin, B. R. (1979). Membrane immunoglobulin is present on thymic and splenic lymphocytes of the trout, *Salmo Gairderi. J. of Immunol.*, **123**, 910–917.

Willingham, M. C. and Pastan, I. (1978). The visualization of fluorescent proteins in living cells by video intensification microscopy (VIM). *Cell*, **13**, 501–507.

Wood, B. T., Thompson, S. H., and Goldstein, G. (1965). Fluorescent antibody staining. III. Preparation of fluorescein-isothiocyanate-labeled antibodies. *J. Immunol.*, **95**, 225–229.

Antibody as a Tool
Edited by J. J. Marchalonis and G. W. Warr
© 1982 J. Wiley & Sons Ltd

Chapter 8

Principles of Immunoelectron Microscopy

LAWRENCE C. HOYER and CORAZON BUCANA
*Cancer Biology Program, NCI Frederick Cancer Research Center,
P. O. Box B, Frederick, Maryland 21701, USA*

I. INTRODUCTION

Immunoelectron microscopy (IEM) is a term that refers to any procedure involving the use of the electron microscope to visualize electron-dense markers applied through an antigen–antibody reaction. This technique developed very rapidly from procedures introduced by Coons (1961) and Singer (1959). Coons demonstrated the feasibility of visualizing antigen–antibody reaction(s) using the light microscope and a fluorescein-labelled antibody to localize the corresponding antigen in smears of cells or in tissue sections. Although this technique has been widely used and improved upon, there are limitations to its sensitivity and resolving capabilities. Consequently, the search for better sensitivity and greater resolution quickly led to the application of Singer's technique for conjugating globulins with an electron dense marker, ferritin, to produce a label of molecular dimensions which could be resolved by the transmission electron microscope. This method enabled the visualization of antigen–antibody reactions at the ultrastructural level through the use of ferritin-labelled antibodies. Since the first papers (Rifkind *et al.*, 1960; Smith *et al.*, 1960) using these techniques were published, numerous works have followed attesting to the sensitivity and wide application of the immunoferritin approach. Over the ensuing years, the immunoferritin technique has been improved upon, and other markers have been substituted for ferritin. Some of the more successful markers have been viruses (Hammerling *et al.*, 1969), latex beads (Molday, 1977), enzymes (Avrameas, 1970), haemocyanin (Karnovsky *et al.*, 1972), and assorted heavy metals such as uranium (Sternberger *et al.*, 1963) and gold (Faulk and Taylor, 1971; Horisberger and Rosset, 1977).

Some of these markers involve methods that are more indirect than others. For example, Nakane and Pierce (1966) reported a technique for conjugating enzymes with antibodies and rendering the enzyme electron dense by

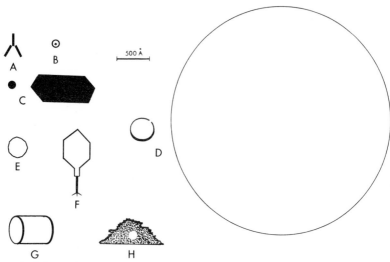

Figure 1. Schematic representation (drawn to relative scale) of various markers used for immunoelectron microscopy. A. Unconjugated antibody; B. Ferritin; C. Gold; D. Latex spheres; E. Small plant virus; F. Phage; G. Haemocyanin; H. Peroxidase

subsequent histochemical reactions. Also, the early techniques of linking peroxidase to specific antibodies (Nakane and Pierce, 1966; Avrameas and Uriel, 1966) have been modified to indirect methods in order to enhance amplification of the markers (Mason *et al.*, 1969; Sternberger and Cuculis, 1969) and improve sensitivity (Sternberger *et al.*, 1970).

Initially IEM techniques were developed for transmission electron microscopy (TEM); however, the visualization of markers with the transmission microscope is tedious and time consuming if one wishes to demonstrate the distribution of surface label rather than its mere presence. The development of scanning electron microscopy (SEM) has provided a means for easily viewing a large number of whole cells for the distribution of antigens and other cell surface moieties. At first, due to the lower resolution capabilities of SEM as compared to TEM, larger markers, such as viruses (Hammerling *et al.*, 1969; Aoki *et al.*, 1971), latex beads (Molday *et al.*, 1975) and haemocyanin (Revel, 1974) were used. But as the resolution of the SEM improved, smaller markers, such as ferritin (Marchalonis *et al.*, 1978) and gold (Horisberger *et al.*, 1975; Baigent and Muller, 1980), were used (Figure 1). Consequently, correlative SEM and TEM studies could now be conducted comparing new techniques and markers to the widely accepted immunoferritin method (Hoyer *et al.*, 1979), as well as using sequential SEM to TEM studies for more conclusive verification (Bucana *et al.*, 1976a,b). Immunoelectron microscopy must now be viewed at two distinct levels: With TEM it is possible to determine the intracellular and cell surface localization of antigens. However, the major limitation of TEM is the small area of the cell that can be examined. With SEM the distribution of

Table 1. Examples of applications of IEM

Specimen	Marker used	Reference
1. Cell fractions		
a. Endoplasmic reticulum Golgi lipoprotein	Ferritin	Matsuura and Tashiro, 1979
b. Myosin	Ferritin	Rikihisa and Mizuno, 1977a
c. Phagolysosomes	Ferritin	Rikihisa and Mizuno, 1977b
d. Viral antigen	Ferritin	Morgan *et al.*, 1961a
2. Prokaryotic cells		
a. Bacteria	Ferritin	Hsu *et al.*, 1963
		Rifkind *et al.*, 1964
b. Yeast	Gold	Horisberger and Rossett, 1977
c. Virus	Bacteriophage	Molday, 1977
3. Eukaryotic cells		
a. Thymocytes	SBMV	Stackpole *et al.*, 1971
b. Hepatocarcinoma	Ferritin	Bucana and Hanna, 1974
c. Erythrocytes	Gold	Horisberger and Rosset, 1977
d. Lymphocytes	Gold	Geoghegan *et al.*, 1978
	Latex beads	Molday, 1977
	Ferritin	de Petris and Raff, 1972
e. Spleen cells	HRPO	de Petris, 1978
4. Parasites		
a. *Trypanosoma*	Ferritin	Vickerman and Luckins, 1969
b. *Toxoplasma*	Ferritin	Matsubayashi *et al.*, 1966

cell surface labelling is demonstrated more quickly and a larger number of cells may be evaluated easily.

In this chapter, we present an overview of IEM as it is applied to the identification of cell surface labels and their distribution patterns. We hope to enable the reader to decide more easily a) when to use IEM, b) what markers and reagents to use, c) what basic procedures to follow, and d) how to interpret data gained from its use.

II. APPLICATIONS OF IEM

Immunoelectron microscopy techniques have been applied to a variety of systems in order to visualize the presence and/or distribution of antigens or antibodies. The techniques have been widely used in eukaryotic cells, prokaryotes, and parasites, as well as in the localization of antigens on isolated cell fractions (de Petris, 1978; Rifkind *et al.*, 1962). In most cases, IEM is preceded by immunofluorescence assays since the latter are faster and easier to do. Examples of the application of various IEM techniques for the visualization of antigens or antibodies are presented in Table 1.

III. WHEN TO USE IEM

Immunoelectron microscopy can provide information regarding the ultrastructural identification of antigenic sites as well as the topographical distribution of antigens. In addition, the sensitivity of IEM is greater than that of immunofluorescence and consequently may be a better technique to use when antigenic sites or other receptors are not numerous. IEM has been used successfully as a corroborative technique in conjunction with immunofluorescent studies. Frequently, electron microscopic studies are difficult to interpret without previous insight derived from other experimental procedures such as immunofluorescence observations at the light microscope level. The immunofluorescence technique can be a valuable time saver in determining the specificity of reagents and procedural techniques. Because IEM requires a great deal of time, it should be used as a technique only when the same information cannot be obtained by a simpler method (see Table 2).

IV. MARKERS USED FOR IEM

In selecting a marker for IEM, it is important to consider the resolution of the microscope, the availability of the marker, the ease with which the marker can be conjugated to the antibody without loss of reactivity, and the type of information to be obtained from the experiment. The resolution of the microscope is the primary limiting factor in the choice of an IEM marker. At the present time, the SEM has a lower resolution than the TEM. In general, field emission SEM can achieve 30 Å resolution; SEM with a LAB_6 gun can achieve 70 Å; and conventional SEM can achieve around 100 Å. TEM, however, will give 2–3 Å resolution. All markers can be used for TEM, but special consideration is required in the selection of a marker for SEM. At the SEM level, the quality and thickness of the metal coating used on biological specimens can obliterate small labels or alter the characteristic shape of large labels. It is also important to consider what type of information is desired from a particular experimental design, and to select a marker accordingly. To aid in this selection, some of the more commonly used markers (Figure 1) are discussed with their respective advantages and disadvantages in various applications.

A. Ferritin

Ferritin is one of the smaller (120 Å) and more widely used markers for TEM. The procedure for conjugating ferritin to antibodies has been reviewed in detail by Wagner (1973) and de Petris (1978) and is discussed in the section on conjugation of markers. It is sufficient to say that most antibodies may be easily conjugated to ferritin (Kishida *et al.*, 1975). Conjugated ferritin can be used for either direct or indirect labelling, and, since the ferritin is small, it reduces the possibility of steric hindrance and is an ideal label for thin section TEM (Figure 2). Its SEM (Figure 3) application is somewhat limited because of technical difficulties in resolving single particles or small patches of ferritin and the inability to confirm particles by X-ray or other techniques.

B. Gold

Colloidal gold < 100 Å to > 1000 Å (Revel, 1974; Hoyer *et al.*, 1979) has been used successfully at both TEM (Figure 4) and SEM (Figure 5) levels. It is electron dense and has the advantage that particles can be made to any desired size that can easily be identified by X-ray analysis. This is particularly useful for mapping surface moieties at the SEM level. However, the presence of larger particles of gold on the sample severely damages the knife when cutting thin sections. Also, there is some evidence that certain antibodies may not attach readily to the gold (Romano and Romano, 1977).

C. Latex Spheres

For versatility, the latex spheres (Figure 6) would be one of the more useful markers introduced in recent years. The spheres can be made in sizes ranging from 300 Å to 3400 Å with methacrylate derivatives containing hydroxyl and carboxyl functional groups (Molday, 1976; Molday, 1977). In addition to being visible with both TEM and SEM, they have been used as markers for immunofluorescence (Molday, 1977), autoradiography (Molday *et al.*, 1975), and as magnetic microspheres that can be used for cell separation by means of a magnetic field (Margel *et al.*, 1979). These spheres are prone to non-specific sticking. In addition, they are relatively large and may introduce steric hindrance. However, in situations where the antigens of interest are not numerous, the latex sphere can be a very useful marker. When large spheres (> 500 Å) are used, there is considerable loss of resolution with regard to surface distribution. This suggests that an alternative technique such as immuno-fluorescence should be considered.

D. Viruses

The spherical bacterial virus *Escherichia coli* f2 phage and the southern bean mosaic virus (SBMV) (Hammerling *et al.*, 1969; Matter *et al.*, 1972) have been exploited as surface markers at both the TEM and SEM level. The tobacco mosaic virus has been used primarily for SEM because of its large size and distinctive shape. The central nucleic acid core of these viruses can be stained densely with uranyl and lead acetate to render them readily visible with TEM.

Viruses are only suitable for surface labelling and are used frequently for replica techniques (Smith and Revel, 1972). They have been used primarily as

Table 2. Comparison of techniques used for visualization of antigen–antibody reactions

	Immunofluorescence	Immunoelectron microscopy TEM	SEM	Immunoenzyme
1. Label	Flourescein, rhodamine	Ferritin, virus, gold	Ferritin, virus, gold, latex, haemocyanin, other heavy metal	Peroxidase antiperoxidase, acid phosphatase
2. Equipment for visualization	Light microscope with UV light source	TEM microscope	SEM	TEM, SEM and/or bright field microscope
3. Types of samples examined	Frozen sections, single cells, tissue culture cells, bacteria, parasites	Tissues, single cells, tissue culture cells, bacteria, parasites, viruses, subcellular fractions	Same as TEM	Tissues, single cell
4. Specificity	Dependent on quality of reagents			
5. Quantification	Cytophotometer or use the cytofluorograph or cell sorter	Very tedious; serial sectioning and X-ray analysis required	Very tedious and may require other techniques for verification of label	
6. Advantages	Simple; fast; allows screening of large numbers of cells, conjugation of	High resolution of labelled components	High resolution 3-dimensional analysis. Large number of cells	Permanent slides can be made; LM requires inexpensive equipment; mol. wt. of labelled

| 7. Disadvantages | reagents and purification of conjugate is simple; labelled reagents available commercially; double labelling is easy | Very demanding technique; bias in cell sampling | Very demanding techniques conjugation with large particles may give misleading results because of steric results; other methods needed to verify label, e.g. X-ray technique | may be screened | ab fe-ab. and should be ideal for intracellular localization of ag |
| | Preparations fade, sensitivity limited by optical resolution | | | | LM sensitivity limited by optical resolution; acid Pase gives variable results; indirect labelling with peroxidase is preferred |

8. Sources of error   Non-specific reagents and insufficient controls

9. Controls   1. Inhibition test should be successful
   2. Negative labelling with non-homologous ab
   3. Negative labelling when the homologous-labelled ab is absorbed with specific ag
   4. In indirect and complement methods, there should be no fluorescence when 1st antibody is replaced with PBS, or normal serum, or non-homolous ab
   5. The more controls, the better

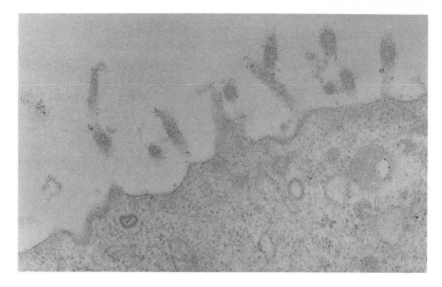

Figure 2. TEM micrograph of line 10 cell directly labelled with rabbit anti-line 10 conjugated ferritin. Note the plasma membrane labelling with electron dense marker.

indirect labels, because for direct labelling, large quantities of high concentrations of viruses are needed for efficient conjugation of viruses to antibodies (de Petris, 1978). The hybrid antibody technique makes it possible to attach the viruses to the antigen (Hammerling *et al.*, 1968), but this method has severe limitations due to the necessity of producing a hybrid antibody to the particular antigen of interest. The need for indirect labelling and the large size of the virus considerably reduce the resolution for the localization of a membrane molecule.

E. Haemocyanin

Haemocyanin is very similar to viruses in its use as a marker. It cannot be used for intracellular labelling, but because of its large size (linear dimension approximately 300 Å) and distinctive shape (cylindrical) it is very useful for SEM (Figure 7) and replica studies. Furthermore, the resolution for the localization of membrane molecules is approximately the same as that of viruses. Haemocyanin may be conjugated with antibodies by the same procedures used for ferritin conjugation (Karnovsky *et al.*, 1972) or may be used unconjugated in an indirect technique (Smith and Revel, 1972).

The most commonly used haemocyanin is extracted from the haemolymph of either the marine whelk *Busycon canaliculatum* or the giant keyhole limpet *Megatura crenulata* (Karnovsky *et al.*, 1972; Wofsky *et al.*, 1974). Although

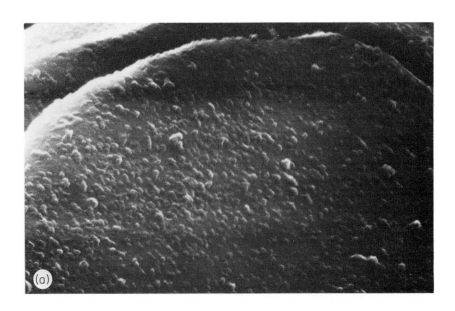

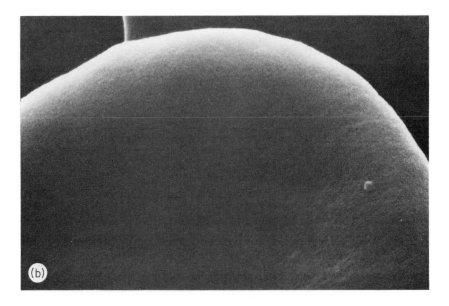

Figure 3. SEM micrograph of (a) Human red blood cell directly labelled with rabbit anti-human B-conjugated ferritin; (b) Human red blood cell negative control

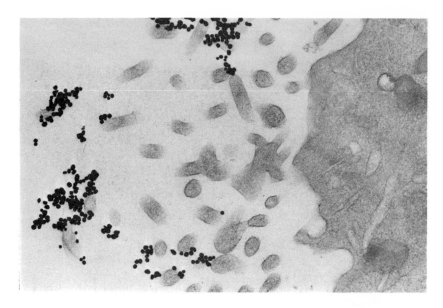

Figure 4. TEM micrograph of line 10 cell directly labelled with rabbit anti-line 10
conjugated gold

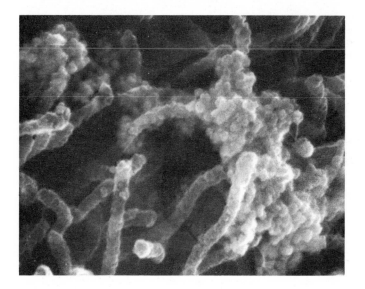

Figure 5. SEM of line 10 cell incubated sequentially with Guinea pig (Ig) anti-BCG,
ferritin goat anti-guinea-pig Ig, rabbit (Ig) anti-line 10 and gold protein-A. Individual
large gold particles. 500 Å (arrow G) and the smaller ferritin molecules (arrow F) are
sometimes seen in the labelled area of the cell

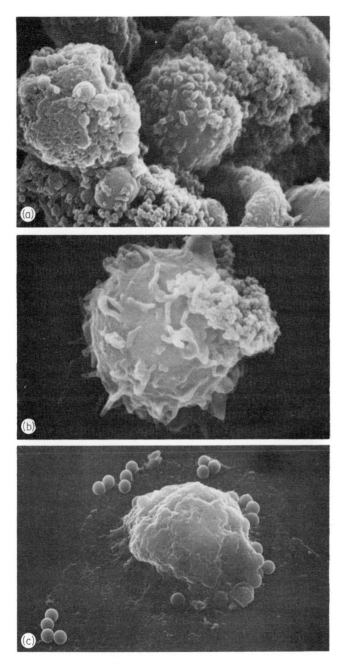

Figure 6 (a) SEM micrograph of a section of guinea pig spleen with B cells labelled with latex beads. (b) Guinea pig B cell labelled with latex beads. (c) Guinea pig macrophage phagocyting latex beads

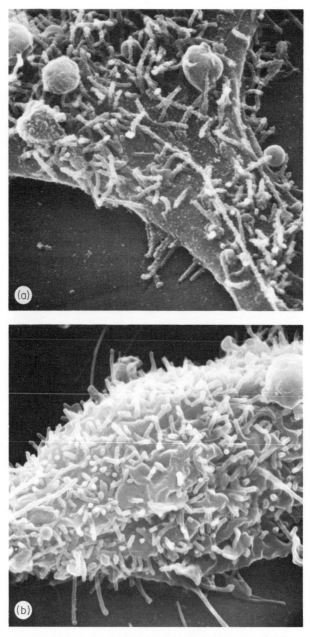

Figure 7. C11D mouse L cell fibroblast labelled for teratoma-defined antigen rabbit anti-mouse-teratoma antiserum followed by haemocyanin coupled to goat-anti-rabbit IgG; (b) Control C11D cell with non-immune rabbit serum substituted for the rabbit anti-mouse-teratoma antiserum. Photograph courtesy of Dr Bruce Wetzel

commercially lyophilized haemocyanins are available, they are often unsuitable as IEM markers since the polymeric molecules are fragmented.

F. Peroxidase

Horseradish peroxidase (HRPO) is one of the more widely used enzymes that may be attached to an antibody and acted upon by a suitable enzyme substrate yielding a large number of visible product molecules per antibody molecule. This label may be used to detect membrane antigens or receptors by directly conjugating them to an antibody or other protein (Nakane and Pierce, 1966; Avrameas, 1970). After the antibody–enzyme complex has reacted witht the membrane antigen, the cell is incubated with a suitable substrate that produces a local insoluble precipitate. This precipitate becomes electron dense after post-fixation with osmium tetroxide. The amorphous precipitate is not sutiable for surface replicas or SEM, but is probably one of the most sensitive markers available for TEM. It is important, however, to be extremely conscious of the parameters of the enzymatic reaction, for if the reaction is very strong, there may be diffusion of the stain over the cell surface and to adjacent cells. This phenomenon can result in false positive results. Thus, it is important to have controlled conditions to distinguish between non-specific staining and the more intense specific staining. This method is useful when a large number of cells need to be scanned, or when general characteristics of surface antigen distribution are desired.

G. Unconjugated Antibodies and Lectins

Unconjugated antibodies and lectins are only practical as surface markers, since they lack sufficient contrast to be used as intracellular labels. Cells labelled with this type of marker must be carefully prepared and sectioned. Where the marker is perpendicular to the cell membrane in a thin section, it can be readily identified by its size and shape provided that it is a minimum size, and the specimen has been stained properly. To achieve the needed contrast, the specimen is stained *en bloc* with 0.5% uranyl acetate before dehydration and embedding. Thin sections are re-stained with uranyl acetate and lead citrate. Even with this staining, individual molecules are not always distinguishable; however, clusters or patches of the molecules can be detected easily when compared to the appropriate controls. Unconjugated antibodies and lectins are good markers in certain experimental situations in which very accurate correlations are desired between ultrastructure and distribution of the marker. This approach also eliminates artefacts from conjugating the antibody or lectin to a marker. It is evident that these labels would not be useful for SEM studies because of their small size (they have a 'Y'-shaped structure with arms that are 40 Å in diameter and 70 to 85 Å in length) (Sarma *et al.*, 1971).

V. CONJUGATION OF MARKERS

When conjugating antibodies to markers, it is imperative that careful consideration be given to the reagents and coupling agents used. In general, the reagents used should be as pure as possible because the impurities in the reagents may affect the pattern of labelling and result in artefacts (Taylor *et al.*, 1971; de Petris and Raff, 1972; de Petris, 1978). Conjugation results may also vary with the source of IgG, species of IgG. or the concentration of the antisera. Consequently, it is advisable to consult the literature for procedural variations that are similar to your experimental design. It is accepted that bifunctional coupling agents can covalently conjugate antibodies to protein markers such as ferritin or HRPO. Of the coupling agents that have been successfully used, three have gained wide acceptance. These agents are glutaraldehyde (Avrameas, 1969), used in the one-step procedure, and isocyanate reagents, toluene-2, 4-diisocyanate and *m*-xylylene diisocyanate (Singer and Schick, 1961), that are usually used for the two- or three-step methods. For procedural details refer to Appendix I.C.

The one-step method simply involves mixing the antibody, ferritin, and the coupling agent, glutaraldehyde, together in appropriate proportions. This procedure will yield conjugates of suitable quality for most applications. In addition, because of its hydrophylic nature, glutaraldehyde has less effect than other coupling agents on the solubility of the proteins to which it binds. However, it is impossible to prevent the formation of some antibody dimers and marker dimers, or large mixed aggregation, as well as, alteration or inactivation of some antibody molecules. The two-step procedure reduces or eliminates these problems and has the advantage that the unreacted antibody can be recovered and used again. Glutaraldehyde can be used for the two-step approach (Otto *et al.*, 1973; Kishida *et al.*, 1975) but is not recommended because its two functional sites have identical reactivity that may result in ferritin–ferritin aggregates. Diisocyanates (Singer, 1959; Singer and Schick, 1961) largely avoid this problem because the second reaction site has a much slower reaction rate. This reaction rate, however, can be accelerated by elevating the temperature, thereby facilitating the coupling of the antibody to this site. A slight disadvantage of diisocyanates is that they must be stored very carefully because they tend to polymerize and precipitate upon contact with air. If a precipitate has formed in toluene-2, 4-diisocyanate during storage, it must be removed by centrifugation before using whereas precipitates in *m*-xylylene diisocyanate can be removed by distillation (Andres *et al*, 1973).

Kishida *et al.* (1975) introduced a three-step method for ferritin–immunoglobulin conjugates using water-soluble carbodiimide as a coupling reagent. The advantage of this procedure is that intra- and intermolecular reactions of ferritin are blocked by succinylation. This method is of particular value in producing monovalent antibody or Fab conjugates that can be especially useful for redistribution studies.

Antibodies can be conjugated to HRPO in a manner similar to that used for ferritin, (Avrameas, 1969; Avrameas and Teruynck, 1971; Nakane and Kavaoi, 1974) (see Appendix I. C). Both the one- and two-step methods yield about 2% bound HRPO to antibody, but the one-step procedure produces a larger proportion of large aggregates. The three-step method can result in up to 70% of the HRPO being coupled to IgG, but the conjugate contains few monomers and consists mainly of polymers (Boorsma and Streefkerk, 1976).

Antibodies can also be conjugated with haemocyanin (Karnovsky *et al.*, 1972) and latex-spheres (Molday *et al.*, 1975) by a one-step glutaraldehyde procedure (Karnovsky *et al.*, 1972) for use in direct labelling experiments. The difficulty that arises with haemocyanin is that it has a great propensity for forming aggregates; consequently, it is necessary to use a much lower antibody concentration than that used for conjugating IgG with ferritin (see Appendix I.C).

Antibodies can be attached to colloidal gold particles by an electrostatic charge rather than the covalent bonding previously discussed for other markers. We, as well as others (Romano and Romano, 1977; Goodman *et al.*, 1980), have found that the pH of the gold solution to be labelled needs to be elevated above the pI of the protein in order to create a sufficient charge differential for the protein to stick to the gold. We also believe that highly purified antibodies or, better yet, monoclonal antibodies (Hoyer *et al.*, 1980) can be attached more easily to the gold, and will yield a more satisfactory marker. The details for preparing colloidal gold and for labelling antibodies with it are given in the Appendix.

VI. MEMBRANE LABELLING TECHNIQUES

A. Direct IEM

The direct methods of IEM are one-step procedures in which the labelled antibody is applied directly to the cell (Figure 8A-C). As mentioned earlier, the label can be an unconjugated or a conjugated antibody. In either case, carefully washed cells are exposed to the marker, washed thoroughly after labelling, and prepared for electron microscopic viewing. Generally, the labelled antibody is directed against a single antigen, group of antigens or haptens (Wofsy, 1974).

The direct methods are good approaches when high resolution is desired for the localization of surface antigens. Since these methods involve a single incubation, there is less probability of non-specific labelling, and they may provide quantitative data in that the number of bound marker molecules is directly proportional to the number of surface antigen molecules. Also studies

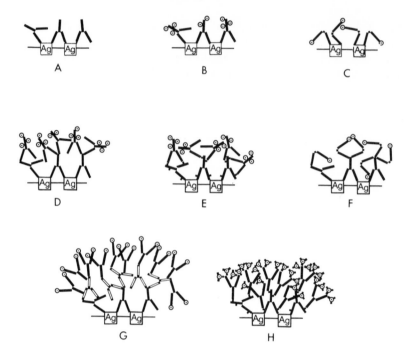

Figure 8. Schematic represenation of direct and indirect labelling. A. Direct antibody
B. Direct antibody conjugated with marker; C. Direct hybrid antibody conjugate with
marker; D. Indirect antibody conjugated with marker; E. Indirect hapten antibody
conjugated with marker; F. Indirect hybrid antibody conjugated with marker; G.
Mixed antibody bridge; H. Hapten bridge

of the redistribution of surface molecules as a function of cross-linking are
more easily interpreted when a single layer of antibodies is used.

The limitations to direct labelling are (a) conjugation of marker molecules to
a specific antibody is often inefficient and (b) the direct conjugation of
antibodies requires large quantities of marker and high-titre antisera.

B. Indirect IEM

Indirect methods of IEM use one or more unlabelled antibodies followed by
the labelled anti-immunoglobulin (Figure 8D, E). In a simple two-layer
approach, the unlabelled antibody binds directly to the antigen; this reaction
site is visualized by the binding of a labelled antibody specific to the first
immunoglobulin. The unlabelled antibody is often referred to as a bridge.
Currently there are many variations of indirect methods, each of which has
advantages and disadvantages that should be carefully considered before a
particular approach is selected.

Some of the variations of the indirect bridge methods are as follows: the first is the hybrid antibody approach in which an antibody is directed against a surface antigen. Then a hybrid antibody is applied, followed by the marker (Hammerling *et al.*, 1968). The hybrid antibody has two binding sites, one directed against the antibody and the other directed against the marker (Figure 8F).

The second variation is the mixed antibody bridge method which consists of three or four steps depending on whether the marker is used in a conjugated or unconjugated form. The first antibody is directed against the surface antigen. Additional antibodies are directed against the initial antibody and then the marker is applied (Figure 8G). This serves to amplify the response and is particularly useful when there are restricted or few antigenic sites and when a specific antibody is in short supply and does not allow direct conjugation with the marker. The mixed antibodies are possible sources of non-specific labelling, so consequently it is important to wash the cells extensively after each incubation, test different dilutions of each antibody, and run proper controls. Therefore, this technique must be used with care.

The third variation is the hapten bridge method which uses an intermediate bridging antibody directed against a hapten that was chemically attached to the first antibody and to the marker (Figure 8H). The marker molecule, when applied, reacts with the remaining free binding sites of the intermediate anti-hapten antibody. However, as with all indirect methods, there is substantial reduction in resolution, and the potential for non-specific labelling is greatly increased. The additional manipulations of the cells could result in artefacts and cellular changes, as well as loss of label.

VII. SAMPLE PREPARATION FOR CELL LABELLING

A. Adherent Cells

Adherent cells, whether they are tissue culture cells or cells taken directly from the animal, can be attached to cover glasses cleaned with alcohol and then dried. The cover glasses can be either glass or plastic, but, when immunof-luorescence techniques are used for preliminary evaluation of reagents, plastic coverslips should be avoided because of their fluorescent properties. Freshly plated cells should be given sufficient time to adhere firmly, or if trypsin or mechanical dissociation is required to free the cells before plating, it may be necessary to wait 12 hours or more before labelling to permit the cells to regenerate a normal cell surface. Most enzymatic dissociations remove many surface antigens and may expose subsurface antigens which may react to the antibody being used. Once the cells have returned to normal, they must be washed with buffer or serum-free media to remove excess serum and cell debris that could produce superfluous labelling. Non-adherent cells can also be attached to cover glasses by using polylysine-coated coverslips (Mazia *et al.*,

1975), but it is advisable to label the cells before attachment to prevent non-specific sticking of labelled antibody to the cover glass.

Cover glasses containing the sample are inverted over a drop of the test antibody in a moist chamber (such as the one available from Bellco, 930-22222 Vineland, New Jersey). Washing is achieved by rinsing with buffer from a wash bottle or by transferring cover glasses from one well of buffer to another in a six-well Linbro plate (Costar #3506, Cambridge, Massachusetts). After incubation the cover glasses are transferred to a six-well Linbro plate, fixed with glutaraldehyde and processed for TEM according to a published procedure (Bucana *et al.*, 1976).

An alternative procedure that is routinely used in our laboratory is to use 13 mm cover glasses. Cover glasses containing the sample are placed in six-well Linbro plates; 0.1–0.2 ml of test serum is placed on top of the cover glass to form a convex drop and incubated for 30 minutes with the plate cover on. Washing is achieved by flooding the cover glass with several changes of buffer. This is done several times without allowing the sample to dry between incubations. The cover glass is lifted periodically from the bottom of the dish to prevent trapping of reagents that may have seeped under during incubation. This procedure is followed during all subsequent washing steps. Subsequent incubations are carried out in the same well using enough reagent to cover the samples. After the last wash, samples are fixed and processed for TEM or SEM.

B. Suspension Cells

Suspension cells should be washed and resuspended as single cells. Cells can be washed by repeated centrifugation and resuspension in buffer. After incubation with conjugated antibody, the cells can be washed by the preceding procedure or by layering the cells and excess conjugate antibody over a 2–4 cm layer of a high-density medium such as albumin or sucrose and centrifuging the cells through the dense layer. The conjugate antibody will remain on top and is removed with the supernatant. The cell pellet is resuspended and washed several times with buffer to remove the high-density medium. Prolonged and violent washing may remove monovalent antibodies or ligands or low-affinity antibodies and in extreme cases it may be necessary to fix the cells before washing. In some cases, it may be advisable to incubate the cells in bovine serum albumin before incubation with the antibody. This is believed to prevent non-specific sticking.

Cells labelled in suspension are usually processed in a small volume (0.1–0.5 ml) at relatively high cell concentration (10^6–10^7 cells/ml) to avoid dilution or waste of the conjugate. Generally, conjugates containing 20–50 µg/ml of active conjugated antibody are sufficient to label 10^7 cells/ml. Ferritin–IgG conjugates made from whole IgG fraction may contain ferritin concentrations of 5–15 mg/ml. It is advisable to refer to the literature to find appropriate concentrations to use for specific cell types and experimental conditions.

Generally, unfixed cells are used for labelling, but there may be redistribution of the antigens (Frye and Edidin, 1970) or pinocytosis (Taylor *et al.*, 1971) of the antibody or marker on unfixed cells incubated at 37 °C. This can be overcome by incubating unfixed cells at 4 °C, but the binding is substantially slower and incubation times of 30–60 minutes are required rather than 5–10 minute incubation time at room temperature or 37 °C. Another alternative is the mild fixation of the cells before incubation or, if indirect techniques are being used, a mild fixation after the first incubation at 4 °C is recommended.

When the cells are pre-fixed with glutaraldehyde or formaldehyde to immobilize surface components, it is advisable to wash the cells thoroughly with buffer three or four times to assure removal of residual reactive aldehyde groups. These groups may also be inactivated by washing with isotonic 0.05 M ammonium chloride (Nicolson, 1971). The pre-fixed cells are incubated with the conjugated antibody for 30–60 minutes at room temperature, washed with buffer, and post-fixed with glutaraldehyde and 1–2% osmium.

When using indirect methods, it is advisable in some situations to fix the cells after one or more of the incubations have been completed. The cells are basically treated as if they were being pre-fixed. It has been reported that fixation frequently alters the antigenic properties of membrane molecules (Gatti *et al.*, 1974), whereas fixation with 4% formaldehyde for up to 1 hour or 2% glutaraldehyde for 2 hours does not completely destroy the antigenic determinants of a cell-bound antibody (de Petris, 1978; Biberfeld *et al.*, 1974). This fixation prevents pinocytosis, capping, or shedding of the antibody before the label can be added.

The cells can be labelled in any physiological buffer solution or serum-free culture medium provided it does not contain substances that are capable of interfering with binding. Thus, it is advisable to avoid the use of complex mixtures such as serum, and to be certain that the cells have been washed free of these substances and cell debris before labelling. In order to ensure that tissue cells remain in good condition, small amounts (0.1–0.2% up to 1–2%) of bovine serum albumin may be added. Although the albumin binds weakly and reversibly to cell membranes (Blaisie *et al.*, 1969) it does not interfere with specific labelling at low concentrations and may reduce non-specific binding of the label (de Petris and Raff, 1972).

C. Intracellular Labelling

Intracellular location of antigens requires the alteration of the plasma membrane in order to make the cells permeable to the conjugates. A number of techniques have been employed. For example, free cells are fixed for 5 minutes in 5% formalin in phosphate buffer, frozen, and cut 10 μm thick in a cryostat. The thawed sections are exposed to the conjugate, washed with cold buffer, fixed in glutaraldehyde and osmium vapours, dehydrated,and embedded for thin sectioning (Morgan *et al.*, 1961a). Tissue culture cells may be rendered permeable by simply freezing and thawing (Morgan *et al.*, 1961b). Other methods have been reported in which digitonin solution (Dales *et al.*, 1965), or gentle homogenization of the cells was used (Pierce *et al.*, 1964; Matsuura and Tashiro, 1979). More recently, Willingham and Yamada (1979) have developed a primary fixation method using a mixture of water-soluble carbodiimide that preserves the ultrastructural morphology of cells, yet produces a permeable membrane that allows the labelled antibody to label intracellular structures.

D. Solid Tissue Labelling

In solid tissue, it is usually necessary to dissociate the tissue to some extent before attempting to label extracellular sites (Andres *et al.*, 1962a, b). This can be accomplished by a short fixation of small tissue blocks in phosphate-buffered formalin, followed by mincing or teasing the blocks into tiny fragments before placing them in the conjugated solution. Alternatively, after fixation the tissue blocks can be quickly frozen, 10–50 μm sections cut in a cryostat, and the sections reacted with the conjugate (Rifkind *et al.*, 1964).

VIII. REAGENTS

A. Buffers and Fixatives

Basically, the purposes of buffers and fixatives are the same for both TEM and SEM. One purpose is to preserve cell structure with as little alteration from the living state as possible. Another purpose is to assure that this preservation is adequate to prevent disruption of the cells during dehydration, embedding, sectioning, staining, critical point drying and exposure to the electron beam. Ideally, a good fixative should preserve every facet of the cell integrity, but unfortunately the ideal fixative has not been found. Thus, it is important to select a buffer and a fixative that will preserve the features of primary interest with as little disruption as possible to the remainder of the cell.

Some of the more common buffers and fixatives are given in the Appendix, however, it would be impossible to list all the variations and applications of buffers and fixatives in this chapter. There are some basic considerations such as pH, osmolarity, temperature, etc. which affect the quality and type of fixation used for IEM work. Furthermore, changes in the buffer system may result in changes in osmolarity; consequently, some of the published data concerning different buffers should be considered cautiously (Hayat, 1970).

B. pH

In general, the best preservative technique for most animal tissue is to keep the pH of the fixative between 7.2 and 7.4. A pH in this range is close to the pH of the tissue and will help to prevent radical changes in the tissue pH resulting from death and fixation. Changes in pH will also affect the rate of penetration of the fixative into the cell, as well as the activity of many proteins and enzymes.

C. Osmolarity

In relatively compact tissue, small changes in osmolarity do not appear to have any noticeable effect. IEM work, however, is often done on dissociated tissue or single cell suspensions which are sensitive to osmotic changes. There are numerous reports that indicate changes in morphology with very small changes in osmolarity (Luft, 1956). The addition of appropriate electrolytes can lessen the amount of extraction of cellular materials. In order to maintain an isosmotic balance between the cell's content, the buffer, and fixative, a non-electrolyte such as sucrose, can be added.

D. Temperature

In IEM work, in which the investigator is interested in the distribution of a surface antigen, the cells are pre-fixed at room temperature, 37 °C, or the labelling procedure is conducted at 4 °C. Fixation is usually done at the same temperature as the incubation temperature to prevent any movement of cell surface antigens. The effects of temperature on the rate of fixation should also be considered. In general, higher temperatures increase the rate of penetration and fixation of cell constituents, as well as the rate of autolytic changes, whereas lower temperatures do the opposite. Thus, fixatives that penetrate and fix rapidly (i,e, acrolein) do not need to be carried out at high temperatures or for long durations of fixation. On the other hand, fixatives that penetrate and fix more slowly (i.e osmium tetroxide) require longer fixation times. Such fixatives are best applied at lower temperatures to minimize cellular extraction. Fixatives that penetrate slowly, but fix rapidly, such as glutaraldehyde, can be used at higher temperatures with reduced fixation time or at lower temperatures with increased fixation time. Formalin, which penetrates rapidly and fixes slowly, is best used for short pre-fixations to stabilize the cell membrane, provided one of the other fixatives is used as a post-fixative to preserve the fine structure of the cell. The most important thing to remember is to avoid long fixations at high temperatures if at all possible.

E. Antisera and Ligands

Many of the antibodies used as reagents for IEM studies today are commercially available and are almost exclusively molecules of the gamma-G globulin class (IgG). Some cells bear receptors for the corboxy terminal of Fc portion of the IgG molecule. To avoid the possibility of artefactual binding of IgG to cells by this region it is advisable to remove or destroy the Fc region. This is usually achieved enzymatically. Under appropriate conditions digestion with papain produces from one IgG molecule two Fab fragments each with one binding site. Pepsin digestion produces an $(Fab')_2$ fragment with two binding sites. The specificity of an antibody or its Fab fragments is primarily determined by the amino acid sequence of the segments of the heavy and light polypeptide chains that form its antigen-combining site. These sequences vary in different immunoglobulin molecules, and an individual antiserum will contain the products of a number of 'clones', each with a different amino acid composition at the combining site. Margolies *et al.* (1975) have pointed out that these clones are able to bind with comparable or different affinity to the same hapten or to the same antigenic determinant of a macromolecular antigen. In general, the antibodies used for cell surface labelling are directed against antigen molecules or parts of molecules accessible on the outer surface of the membrane.

The details of antigen and antibody preparation and conjugation are discussed in Chapter 3.

IX. MEANINGFUL INTERPRETATION OF DATA

As with all experimental work, controls are an integral part of the experimental design, and proper controls are of the utmost importance for IEM work. Throughout this chapter, we have alluded to potential hazards and procedural errors that could produce erratic and erroneous results. Simple procedural errors such as cell preparation, pH, temperature, etc. produce artefacts that can negate the results of the most meticulously designed experiment, and for that reason they will be emphasized once again.

A. Cell Preparation and Handling

As far as possible, the cells used for IEM studies should come from a common source. If, for example, several animals are needed to obtain a sufficient quantity of cells, it is advisable to pool the cells at the outset to be certain all the cells will receive equal treatment. After careful washing, the cells should be checked for viability and normal morphology. Dead or dying cells tend to be sticky and may show non-specific labelling. It is important that all samples receive the same number of washes and that they be prepared consistently. The latter is very important for SEM preparations where improper drying or coating can leave residual materials on one set of samples and not on another. These residual materials when viewed in the SEM can be mistaken for a label or can obliterate the label.

It is advisable to use the same buffer system throughout to avoid formation of precipitates that can result from mixing two different buffers or osmolarity changes. It is recommended that fixatives and stains, as well as any water that may be used should be filtered. These precautions are extremely important in preparing samples where the marker is a precipitated stain reaction or the marker is to be evaluated by SEM. Improperly washed cells (use serum-free buffers or media) will frequently produce non-specific labelling. In the case of suspension cells, it is important to thoroughly resuspend the cells with each washing to avoid trapping or blocking of the marker. In this regard, plated cells are easier to work with because there is no difficulty with clumping.

B. Experimental Controls

Many problems encountered in the interpretation of IEM results can be eliminated by using a well-characterized system and procedure in the experimental design. The two major sources of errors of non-specific labelling are: (1) non-specific absorption of one or more of the immunoreagents; and (2) the binding of anti-membrane antibodies directed against unidentified membrane components other than the antigens under study. Immune sera may contain natural antibodies that presumably resulted from previous natural immunizations. These natural antibodies can react with cell surface antigens producing false positive results. In most situations, natural antibodies are present in very low titre, and their influence is usually negligible because of the unavoidable dilution which accompanies preparation of the conjugate. Natural antibodies can also be eliminated by using specific antibodies purified by immunoprecipitation or immunoabsorption techniques.

Non-specific absorption of irrelevant conjugate is primarily the result of denatured or aggregated complexes. With careful preparation of the conjugate these complexes can be removed by centrifugation and column separation techniques. Carefully selected controls run in parallel with experimental samples are necessary for meaningful evaluation of labelling. Controls are somewhat simplified for direct labelling methods. First, incubation of the cell sample with a conjugated normal IgG or conjugated antiserum not directed at the antigen of interest should give negative results. Second, inhibition of specific labelling can be demonstrated either by incubating the cells with a saturating amount of unconjugated antibody before incubation with conjugated antibody or by blocking the antigen-binding sites of the antibody with a specific hapten if available. Third, absorption of the conjugate with a specific purified antigen should prevent cell labelling. Fourth, incubation of known non-reactive cells with the conjugate should give negative results. Cell samples that contain more than one type of cell population, i.e. lymphoid cells, or whole blood, have a built in control because of the presence of non-reactive cells. Specific hapten blocking, removal of specific active conjugate, and negative cells are all suitable controls for detecting the presence of irrelevant antibodies or ligands in the reagents.

Controls for indirect methods are even more important and become more involved with each added step in the process. The causes for non-specific binding with the indirect methods are basically the same as those for direct methods of labelling. In addition, washing between successive incubations is very important to minimize trapping of the antibodies and label. To control for non-specific labelling with the indirect methods, aliquots of the cell sample should be used with each aliquot having only one of the specific reagents omitted. If possible, substitution of an equivalent amount of a non-reactive reagent such as normal serum for the one omitted should be made.

C. Verification Procedures for Markers

Verification of the marker is very important for IEM studies using the SEM. With thin section TEM, this is not a problem assuming all the proper controls have been run to eliminate the possibility of non-specific binding. However, this is not always sufficient in the case of SEM studies, for here precipitates or small blebs might be mistaken for label.

In addition to the standard controls already discussed, it is important to have a marker that has a distinctive size and shape, and if possible, that has enough mass to be detected by X-ray diffraction. With X-ray diffraction, the potential for surface mapping and quantitative measurements can be possible on large numbers of cells. Where these requirements are difficult to meet, sequential studies can be very useful (Bucana *et al.*, 1976), but such studies should be undertaken only when the information desired cannot be obtained by simpler methods.

ACKNOWLEDGEMENT

This research was sponsored by the National Cancer Institute under contract No.NO1-CO-75380 with Litton Bionetics Inc.

APPENDIX I

The solutions and procedures that follow are, for the most part, ones we have used in our laboratory for the preparation of tissue, cell suspensions, and cells grown on cover glasses and plastic culture dishes. Although these procedures work well for the tissue and cells in our studies, they may not be effective for all tissues or cells. Procedures we have not actually used are referenced. In these cases, it is advisable to refer to the literature regarding the particular tissue or cells of interest.

A. Buffers

1. 2.0 M Cacodylate
   Sodium cacodylate ~3 H$_2$O   214g
   Distilled water   up to 500 ml
       adjust pH to 7.3 with HCl
2. 0.2 S-collidine
   S-collidine (2,4,6-trimethyl pyridine)   13.135 ml
   1N HCl   40.00 ml
   Distilled water   up to 500 ml
3. 0.06 M S-collidine
   0.2 M S-collidine   300 ml
   Distilled water   up to 990 ml
4. 0.01 M Phosphate buffered saline (Frederick Cancer Research Center)
   Na$_2$HPO$_4$ (MW 141.96)   1.20g
   NaH$_2$PO$_4$ (MW 137.99)   0.22g
   NaCl   8.50g
   Distilled water   1000 ml
       adjust pH to 7.5
5. PBS(Dulbecco)
   NaCl   8.0g
   KCl   0.2g
   Na$_2$HPO$_4$ 1.15g
   KH$_2$PO$_4$ 0.2g
   Distilled water   up to 1000 ml
       adjust pH to 7.3 with NaOH.

B. Fixatives

1. 3% Glutaraldehyde/2% paraformaldehyde in 0.1 M cacodylate
   70% Glut   0.43 ml
   2 M Cacodylate   0.50 ml
   20% Paraformaldehyde   1.0 ml
   Distilled water   8.07 ml
       adjust pH to 7.3 with 1 N HCl
   10% Glut   10.0 ml
   2 M Cacodylate   1.65 ml
   20% Paraformaldehyde   3.30 ml
   Distilled water   18.05 ml
       adjust pH to 7.3 with 1 N HCl
2. 2% OsO$_4$
   OsO$_4$ 2 ml
   0.2 M Cacodylate   2 ml

3. 20% Paraformaldehyde
   | Paraformaldehyde | 20.0 g |
   | Distilled water | 100 ml |

   Heat while stirring to 60 °C, to dissolve powder then add a few drops of 40% NaOH until solution clears.
4. Stock 25% glutaraldehyde in Tyrode's solution
   | 70% Glutaraldehyde | 10.0 ml |
   | Tyrode's solution | 18.0 ml |
5. Working solution of 2.3% glutaraldehyde in s-collidine
   | Stock 25% glut/Tyrode; s solution | 9.2ml |
   | 0.06 M s-collidine | up to 100 ml |
   adjust pH to 7.3 or 300 mol.

C. Conjugation of Markers

1. Ferritin (Davis, 1974)

   a. One-step IgG
   Mix 15 mg/ml IgG, 45 mg/ml ferritin, and 0.025% glutaraldehyde.
   Let stand at 4 °C for 30–60 minutes.
   Terminate by adding lysine–HCl in PBS in a ratio of 25 mg/ml of conjugate.
   Let stand at 4 °C for overnight.
   b. Separation of conjugate (de Petris and Raff, 1972)
   Remove aggregates and centrifuge at low speed.
   Add cold ammonium sulphate to supernatant to achieve 15% final saturation and let stand for 30–60 minutes at 4 °C. Centrifuge to remove precipitate.
   Dialyse against PBS overnight.
   Centrifuge 3.5 ml conjugate 150,000 g at 4 °C through discontinuous sucrose in PBS for 3 hours (de Petris and Raff, 1972).
   The following gradients are used:

   0.5 ml of 0.4 M sucrose
   2.5 ml of 0.5 M sucrose
   2.5 ml of 1.0 M sucrose
   1.0 ml of 1.5 M sucrose
   2.0 ml of 2.0 M sucrose

   Sucrose layers and their contents are as follows:

   0.4 M, 0.5M unconjugated immunoglobulin
   1.0 M, 1.5 M conjugated ferritin

   Remove conjugated ferritin and dialyse overnight against PBS.

Concentrate with 40% cold saturated ammonium sulphate.

Resuspend in small volume of PBS and dialyse exhaustively against PBS.

Sterilize by filtration through a 0.22 μm Millipore filter.

Store at 4 °C.

c. One-step Fab fragments (de Petris and Raff, 1973)

Mix 2 mg Fab, 25 mg ferritin in 1 ml with 0.05–0.075% glutaraldehyde at 4 °C for 4–6 hours.

Follow separation procedure for one-step IgG.

d. Two-step (Singer and Schick, 1961; Rifkind *et al.*, 1964)

    (i) Toluene-2, 4-diisocyanate (TC)

    Ferritin (20–25 mg/ml) dissolved in 0.05 M PBS, pH 7.5, 4 °C.

    Stirring add 0.020–0.025 ml of TC (0.1 ml/100 mg of ferritin).

    Continue stirring for 25 minutes.

    Then centrifuge at 1500 g for 30 minutes to remove TC (pellet).

    Supernatant is stored at 4 °C for 1 hour to complete reaction.

    Add 1 part IgG to 4 parts ferritin by weight.

    Add 0.3 M borate buffer, pH 9.5, to give final molarity of 0. 1M.

    Warm to 37 °C and stir 1 hour.

    Add lysine or NH_4Cl to stop reaction.

    See separation under one-step procedure.

    (ii) *Meta*-xylylene-diisocyanate (XC)

    Ferritin (20–25 mg/ml) dissolved in 0.05 M PBS, pH 7.5, 4 °C and 1 part borate buffer 0.3 M, pH 9.5

    Add XC, stir 45 minutes at 4 °C.

    Add lysine or NH_4Cl to stop reaction.

    See purification of ferritin.

e. Three-step (Kishida *et al.*, 1975)

Ferritin (100 mg/ml) in 6 ml of H_2O saturated with sodium succinate at room temperature.

Cool to 4 °C.

Add 0.53 g of succinic anhydride and keep for 1 hour at 4 °C.

Raise temperature to 22 °C for 1 hour.

Run on 6% agarose column.

Elute at 4 °C with 0.1 sodium phosphate buffer, pH 7.0.

Concentrate ferritin peak at 4 °C to 30 mg/ml in an Amicon ultrafiltration cell (Amicon Corp, Lexington, Massachusetts).

Add 15 mg cold succinylated ferritin in 0.5 ml of 0.01 PBS.

Add 37 mg carbodiimide [1-ethyl-3-(3-dimethylaminopropyl)] carbodiimide hydrochlorides (EDCI) and 23.4 mg of *N*-hydroxysuccinimide.

Let stand for 3 hours and filter through Sephadex G-200 column (0. 9 cm × 80 cm and equilibrate with 0.01 M phosphate buffer.

Immediately mix IgG or Fab with concentrated fraction of ferritin peak.

For IgG or Fab activated ferritin with 4.4 mg IgG (vol. 2/3ml) for 28 hours at 4 °C.

For Fab use 10 mg activated ferritin in 5.6 ml with 3.4 mg Fab in 1.7 ml of 0.1 M sodium phosphate buffer, pH 7.3, for 24 hours at room temperature.

Stop by adding glycine (400 mg).

Separate by filtration through 6% agarose gel column (use 0.9 cm × 60 cm for IgG and 2.5 cm × 90 cm for Fab).

2. Horseradish Peroxidase

a. One-step glutaraldehyde (Avrameas, 1969)

Mix 5 mg antibody, 12 mg HRPO in 1 ml of 0.1 M phosphate buffer, pH 6.8, with 0.05 ml 1% glutaraldehyde.

Let stand at room temperature for 2 hours.

Dialyse against PBS.

Centrifuge 60,000 g for 30 minutes.

Store supernatant at 4 °C.

b. Two-step (Avrameas and Ternynck, 1971)

(i) Glutaraldehyde

HRPO 15 mg in 2 ml 0.1 M phosphate buffer, pH 6.8, containing 1.25% glutaraldehyde.

Let stand at room temperature for 18 hours.

Separate by filtration through Sephadex G-25 column (60 cm × 0.9 cm) and equilibrate with 0.15 M NaCl.

Concentrate to 1 ml by ultrafiltration.

Add 1 ml 0.15 M NaCl containing 5 mg purified antibody or 2.5 mg purified Fab fragments.

Add 0.1 ml of 1 M carbonate–bicarbonate buffer, pH 9.5.

Let stand for 24 hours at 4 °C.

Stop by adding 0.1 ml of 0.2 M lysine (2 hours).

Dialyse exhaustively against buffered saline.

Separate conjugate from free antibody or Fab fragments through Sephadex G-200 column (100 × 2 cm).

Precipitate with 50% saturated ammonium sulphate.

Dialyse against buffered saline.

Centrifuge at 20,000 g, for 20 minutes.

Store at 4 °C.

(ii) Benzoquinone (BQ) (Termynck and Avrameas, 1976)

Add 6 mg BQ in 0.2 ml ethanol to 3mg IgG or Fab in 0.7 ml of 0.15 M NaCl and 0.1 ml of 1 M phosphate buffer, pH 6.

Filter through Sephadex G-25 column (0.9 × 4 cm), equilibrate in 0.15 M NaCl.

Add to first fraction 0.12 ml 1% HRPO solution.

(4 molar excess for optimal yield) and enough 1 M carbonate–bicarbonate buffer.

Adjust to pH 9 with final concentration of 0.1 M (total vol. of mixture not to exceed 3 ml) and let stand for 15 hours at room temperature.

To stop reaction add 0.1 M lysine for 4 hours or longer and dialyse against PBS at 4 °C.

c. Three-step periodate (Nakane and Kawaoi, 1974)

HRPO (5 mg) dissolved in 1 ml 0.3 M sodium bicarbonate, pH 8.1.Add 0.1 ml 1% fluorodinitrobenzyene in absolute ethanol.

Mix gently for 1 hour at room temperature.

Add 1 ml 0.04–0.08 M $NaIO_4$ in distilled H_2O and stir for 1 hour at room temperature.

To stop reaction add 1 ml 0.16 M ethylene glycol in distilled H_2O. Let stand for 1 hour at room temperature.

Dialyse against three 1 litre changes of 0.01 M sodium carbonate buffer, pH 9.5 at 4 °C.

Add 5 mg of IgG in 1 ml of buffer to 3 ml activated HRPO solution.

Mix for 2–3 hours at room temperature.

Add 5 mg of sodium borohydride to stabilize. Let stand for 3 hours at 4 °C.

Dialyse against PBS at 4 °C.

Centrifuge to remove precipitate.

Separate through Sephadex G-100 or G-200 column (85 × 1.5 cm).

Equilibrate with PBS.

Conjugate in first peak at 280 nm.

Pool and store at 20 °C with 10 mg/ml bovine serum albumin.

3. Haemocyanin (Karnovsky *et al.*, 1972)

264 mg haemocyanin and 28 mg IgG dissolved in 50 ml of 0.1 M phosphate buffer, pH 6.8.

Stir at 20 °C.

Add 1 ml 50% glutaraldehyde to give final concentration of 0.1%.

Stir for 2 hours.

Dialyse against PBS, pH 7.0, overnight at 4 °C.

Centrifuge 2000 g to remove precipitate.

Sterilize using a 0.45 μm Millipore filter.

4. Latex spheres (Molday *et al.*, 1975)

5. Preparations of gold particles

Heat 10 ml distilled H_2O under reflux.

Add 10 μl of 10% (wt/vol) gold chloride.

Add desired amount of 1% sodium citrate (controls size of gold particles).

Reflux 30 minutes.

Cool in ice.

Adjust pH to PK_I of protein being used with 0.2 M potassium carbonate solution.

Centrifuge 500 g for 20 minutes.

6. Labelling of antibodies with gold
Add 1 mg/ml protein to colloidal gold.
Suspend in 1 : 10 ratio.
Agitate 2 minutes.
Add 20% NaCl to produce final concentration of 1% NaCl.
Add polyethylene glycol solution (MW 20,000) to a final concentration
of 1%.
Centrifuge at 500 g for 10 minutes (remove aggregates and unbound
gold).
Centrifuge supernatant at 20,000 g for 1 hour.
Resuspend pellet in 0.1 м phosphate buffer, pH 7.3, with 4%
polyvinylpyrrolidone (MW 10,000) containing 0.2 mg/ml polyethylene
glycol.
Centrifuge 500 g for 10 minutes to remove aggregates before using.
Store at 4 °C.

D. Cell Preparation and Incubation for IEM

Wash cells with PBS or serum-free media three times.

Direct
Incubate cells with conjugated antibody at 4 °C for 30 minutes.
Wash cells with PBS or serum-free media at 4 °C three times.
Fix (follow standard fixation schedule) for 1 hour.

Indirect
Incubate cells with first antibody at 4 °C for 30 minutes.
Wash cells with PBS or serum-free media at 4 °C three times.
Incubate cells with second conjugated antibody at 4 °C for 30 minutes.
Wash cells three times with PBS or serum-free media at 4 °C.
Fix [follow standard (fixation) schedule] for 1 hour.

Note: Cells may be pre-fixed with 1% glutaraldehyde for 5 minutes or 1%
formalin for 10 minutes. If immunofluorescence is to be used, the cells should
be pre-fixed or post-fixed with formalin.
   If cells are for sequential studies for LM to TEM, it is essential that after the
LM work is completed the cells are fixed with glutaraldehyde and OsO_4.

E. Fixation Schedule for TEM

3% glutaraldehyde/2% paraformaldehyde/0.1 м cacodylate at pH 7.3	60 minutes
0.1 м Cacodylate rinse, three times,	10 minutes each

1% OsO$_4$/0.1 M cacodylate	60 minutes
Distilled water rinse, two times,	2 minutes each
1% Aqueous UAc (filtered)	45–60 minutes
Distilled water rinse	2 minutes
35% ETOH	5–10 minutes
50% ETOH	5–10 minutes
70% ETOH	5–10 minutes
80% ETOH	5–10 minutes
90% ETOH	5–10 minutes
95% ETOH	5–10 minutes
100% ETOH, three times,	5–10 minutes each
50% Spurr's	15 minutes
75% Spurr's	30 minutes
100% Spurr's	60 minutes
100% Spurr's	2 hours
100% Spurr's	Embed

Note: Fixations and dehydration should be done at room temperature unless otherwise specified.

F. O-T-O Fixation Schedule for TEM

3% Glutaraldehyde/2% paraformaldehyde/0.1M cacodylate at pH 7.3	60 minutes
0.1 M Cacodylate rinse, three times	5–10 minutes each
1% OsO$_4$/0.1 M in cacodylate	60 minutes
0.1 M cacodylate, rinse, five times,	5 minutes each
Thiocarbohydrazide-saturated (filtered)	10 minutes
Distilled water rinse, five times,	5 minutes each
2% OsO$_4$ or OsO$_4$ vapours	10 minutes
Distilled water rinse, two times,	2 minutes
1% Aqueous UAc (filtered)	30–60 minutes
Distilled water rinse	2 minutes
35% ETOH	5–10 minutes

May follow standard schedule or use Spurr's low viscosity medium applicable for SEM to TEM and monolayer cultures on coverslips.

50% ETOH	5–10 minutes
70% ETOH	5–10 minutes
80% ETOH	5–10 minutes
90% ETOH	5–10 minutes

95% ETOH	5–10 minutes
100% ETOH, three times,	5–10 minutes each
50% Resin	15 minutes
75% Resin	30 minutes
100% Resin	60 minutes
100% Resin	2 hours
100% Resin	Embed

G. Standard Fixation Schedule for SEM

3% Glutaraldehyde/2% paraformaldehyde/0.1M cacodylate at pH 7.3

	60 minutes
0.1 M Cacodylate rinse, three times,	5–10 minutes each
1% OsO_4/0.1 M cacodylate	60 minutes
Distilled water rinse, two times	2 minutes each
1% Aqueous UAc (filtered) (optional stain)	45–60 minutes
Distilled water rinse	2 minutes
35% ETOH	5–10 minutes
50% ETOH	5–10 minutes
70% ETOH	5–10 minutes
80% ETOH	5–10 minutes
90% ETOH	5–10 minutes
95% ETOH	5–10 minutes
100% ETOH, three times,	5–10 minutes each
50% Freon 13 and ETOH	5–10 minutes
70% Freon 13 and ETOH	5–10 minutes
80% Freon 13 and ETOH	5–10 minutes
90% Freon 13 and ETOH	5–10 minutes
100% Freon 13, three times,	5–10 minutes

Critical point dry with Freon 113.

Note: If CO_2 is used for critical point drying, then amyl acetate is used in place of Freon 13. If large pieces of tissues are to be critical point dried, increase the time for each step to permit adequate time for complete exchange.

H. Rapid Embedding

1. Rapid embedding of monolayers and suspensions
   Dehydration and infiltration:

| 20% ETOH–80% water | 30 seconds |

60% ETOH–40% Epon 812	5 minutes
30% ETOH–70% Epon 812	5 minutes
100% Epon 812	5 minutes

Embedding medium:

Epon	50 ml
DDSA	25 ml
NMA	25 ml three times for 10 minutes each
DMP-30	4 ml
dibutyl phthalate	1 ml

Polymerization:

55 °C for 3 days

2. Rapid embedding using Spurr's low viscosity medium

Dehydration and infiltration:

70% Acetone, two times,	3 minutes total
100% Acetone, three times,	5 minutes total
100% Acetone, 100% Spurr's,	10 minutes
100% Spurr's two times,	5 minutes total

Embedding:

100% Spurr's in *Beem* capsule

Polymerization: 95 °C for 60 minutes.

I. Resins

1. Spurr's

	Hard	Standard
Noneyl succinic anhydride (NSA)	26.0 g	26.0 g
4-Vinylcyclohexene dioxide (ERL-4206)	10.0 g	10.0 g
DER 736	4.0 g	6.0 g
Dimethylaminoethanol	0.4 g	0.4 g

Infiltrate with Spurr's:

50% Spurr's in ethanol 10–12 hours in uncovered vials or dishes

100% Spurr's (fresh mixture) 1 hour

100% Spurr's (fresh mixture) 1 hour

Embed in fresh mixture of Spurr's

50% Spurr's	10–15 minutes
75% Spurr's	30 minutes
100% Spurr's	1 hour
100% Spurr's	2 hours

Embed SEM to TEM

50% Spurr's	10 min at 70 °C
75% Spurr's	10 min at 70 °C
100% Spurr's	10 min at 70 °C

100% Spurr's	1 hour at room temperature
100% Spurr's	10 minutes at 70 °C
Embed	

Polymerization: 70 °C for 12–16 hours

2. Luft

Araldite	27.0 ml
DDSA	23.0 ml
DMP-30	0.75 to 1.0 ml

Keep at 4 ° C for a few weeks without catalyst
Polymerization:

Room temperature to 35 °C	overnight to 24 hours
Room temperature to 48 °C	12 to 24 hours
Room temperature to 60 °C	12 hours

Can be placed directly in 60 °C oven.

3. Quetol 651 (Ted Pella Inc.,Box 510, Tustin, California 92680)
Preparation of resin mixture:

Quetol	16.5 ml	33.0 ml
NSA	33.50	67.0 ml
DMP-30	0.875 ml	1.75ml

Infiltration and embedding procedures:

50% Quetol (in 100% ETOH)	20 minutes
75% Quetol	30 minutes
100% Quetol	1 hour
100% Quetol	2 hours
100% Quetol	Embed

Procedure: 1. Polymerize at 60 °C for 24 hours. NO AIR.
2. Close covers of *Beem* capsules.
3. Place Saran wrap over flat embedding moulds.
4. Place samples on rotator, if possible.

J. Poly-1-lysine

Poly-1-lysine (Sigman #P-1886) stored in freezer.

0.1 g	poly-1-lysine
100 ml	PBS

Store in dark bottle in refrigerator.
Procedure:

Place poly-1-lysine on cover glass and let stand for 30 minutes at 4°C.

Rinse with PBS and place cell suspension on cover glass. Allow 30 minutes for cells to settle and attach (4 °C).

Rinse with PBS and fix (follow standard fixation schedule).

REFERENCES

Andres, G. A., Hsu, K. G., and Seegal, B. C. (1973). Immunological techniques for the identification of antigens or antibodies by electron microscopy. In D. M. Weir (Ed.) *Handbook of Experimental Immunology*, volume 2, 2nd edn. Blackwell Scientific Publications, Oxford.

Andres, G. A., Morgan, C., Hsu, K. C..Rifkind, R. A., and Seegal, B. C. (1962a). Electron microscopic studies of experimental nephritis with ferritin-conjugated antibody. The basement membranes and cisternae of visceral epithelial cells in nephtritic rat glomeruli. *J. Exp. Med.*, **115**, 929.

Andres, G. A., Morgan C., Hsu, K. C., Rifkind R. A., and Seegal, B. C. (1962b). Use of ferritin-conjugated antibody to identify nephrotoxic sera in renal tissue by electron microscopy. *Nature*, **194**, 590.

Aoki, T., Wood, H. A., Old, L. J., Boyse, E. A., DeHarven, E., Lardia, M. P., and Stackpole, C. W. (1971). *Virology*, **45**, 858–862.

Avrameas, S. (1969). Coupling of enzymes to proteins with glutaraldehyde. Use of the conjugates for the detection of antigens and antibodies. *Immunochemistry*, **6**, 43–52.

Avrameas, S. (1970). Immunoenzyme techniques: enzymes are markers for the localization of antigens and antibodies. *Int. Rev. Cytol.*, **27**, 349–385.

Avrameas, S. and Ternynck, T. (1971). Peroxidase-labelled antibody and Fab conjugates with enhanced intracellular penetration. *Immunochemistry*, **8**, 1175–1179.

Avrameas, S. and Uriel, J. (1966). Methode de marquage d'antigens et d'anticorps avec des enzymes et son application en immunodiffusion. *Comptes Rendus de l'Academie des Sciences (Paris)* (D), **262**, 2543–2545.

Baigent, C. L. and Muller, G. (1980). A colloidal gold prepared with ultrasonics. *Experientia*, **36**, 472.

Biberfeld, P., Biberfeld, G., Molnar, Z., and Fagraeus, A. (1974;. Fixation of cell-bound antibody in the membrane immunofluorescence test. *J. Immunol. Methods*, **4**, 135–148.

Blaisie, J. K., Worthington, C. R., and Dewey, M. M. (1969). Molecular localization of frog retinal receptor photopigment by electron microscopy and low-angle X-ray diffraction. *J. Mol. Biol.*, **39**, 407–416.

Boorsma, D. M. and Streefkerk, J.G. (1976) Peroxidase conjugate chromatography. Isolation of conjugates prepared with glutaraldehyde or periodate using polyacrylami-de-agarose gel. *J. Histochem. Cytochem.*, **24**, 481–486.

Bucana, C. and Hanna, M. G., Jr. (1974). Immunoelectron-microscopic analysis of surface antigens common to *Mycobacterium bovis* (BCG) and tumor cells. *J. Nat. Cancer Inst.*, **53**, 1313–1323.

Bucana, C., Hobbs, B., Hoyer, L. C., and Hanna, M.G., Jr. (1976a). A technique for sequential examination of *in vitro* macrophage–tumor interactions using LM, SEM and TEM. *34th Ann. Proc. Electron Microscopy Soc. Amer.*, pp. 350–351.

Bucana, C., Hoyer, L. C., Hobbs, B., Breesman, S., McDaniel, M., and Hanna, M. G., Jr. (1976b). Morphological evidence for the translocation of lysosomal organelles from cytotoxic macrophages into the cytoplasm of tumor target cells. *Cancer Res.*, **36**, 4444–4458.

Coons, A. H. (1961). The beginnings of immunofluorescence. *J. Immunol.*, **87**, 499.

Dales, S., Gomatos, P. J., and Hsu, K. C. (1965). The uptake and development of reovirus in strain L cells followed with labeled viral ribonucleic acid and ferritin-antibody conjugates. *Virology.*, **25**, 193.

Davis, W. C. (1974) Use of antibodies for localization of components on membranes. In S. Fleischer and L. Packer (Eds) *Methods in Enzymology*, volume 32. *Biomembranes*, Part B, pp. 60–70, Academic Press, New York.

de Petris, S. (1978). In E. D. Korn (Ed.) *Methods in Membrane Biology*, Volume 9, pp. 1–201, Plenum Press, New York.

de Petris, S. and Raff, M. C. (1972). Distribution of immunoglobulin on the surface of mouse lymphoid cells as determined by immunoferritin electromicroscopy. Antibody-induced, temperature-dependent redistribution and its implications for membrane structure. *Eur, J. Immunol.*, **3**, 523–535.

de Petris, S. and Raff, M. C. (1973). Normal distribution, patching, and capping of lymphocyte surface immunoglobulin studied by electron microscopy, *Nature New Biol.*, **241**, 257–259.

Faulk, P. W. and Taylor, M. G. (1971). An immunocolloid method for the electron microscope. *Immunochemistry*, **8**, 1081.

Frye, L. D. and Edidin, M. (1970). The rapid intermixing of cell surface antigens after formation of mouse-human heterokaryons. *J. Cell Sci.*, **7**, 319–335.

Gatti, R. A., Ostborne, A., and Fagraeus, A. (1974). Selective impairment of cell antigenicity by fixation. *J. Immunol.*, **113.**, 1361–1368.

Geoghegan, W. D., Scillian, J. J., and Ackerwan, G. A. (1978). The detection of human B lymphocytes by both light and electronmicroscopy utilizing colloidal gold labeled anti-immunoglobulin. *Immunolog. Comm.*, **7**, 1–12.

Goodman, S. L., Hodges, G. M., Trejdosiewicz, L. K., Livingston, D. C. (1980). Colloidal gold probes—A further evaluation. *SEM*, **3**, 619.

Hammerling, U., Aoki, T., deHarven, E., Boyse, E. A., and Old, L. J. (1968). Use of hybrid antibody with anti-γG and anti-ferritin specificities in locating cell surface antigens by electromicroscopy. *J. Exp. Med.*, **128**, 1461–1473.

Hammerling, U., Aoki, T., Wood, H. A., Old L. J., Boyse, E. A., and de Harven, E. (1969). New visual marker of antibody for electromicroscopy. *Nature*, **223**, 1158–1159.

Hayat, M. A. (1970). *Principles and Techniques of Eectron Microscopy*, volume 1, pp. 5–105.

Horisberger, M. and Rosset, J. (1977a). Gold granular, A useful marker for SEM. In R. P. Becker and O. Johari (Eds) *Scanning Electron Microscopy*, II, pp. 75–82, Chicago Press, Chicago.

Horisberger, M. and Rosset, J. (1977). Colloidal gold, A useful marker for transmission and scanning electron microscopy. *J. Histochem Cytochem.*, **25**, 295–305.

Horisberger, M., Rossett, J., and Bauer, J. H. (1975). Colloidal gold granules as markers for cell surface receptors in the scanning electron microscope. *Experientia*, **31**, 1147.

Hoyer, L. C., Lee, J. C., and Bucana, C. (1979). Scanning immunoelectron microscopy for the identification and mapping of two or more antigens on cell surfaces. In R. P. Becker and O. Johari (Eds) *Scanning Electron Microscopy*, SEM III, pp. 629–636. Chicago Press, Chicago.

Hoyer, L. C., Lee, J. C., Bucana, C., Plentovich, D. (1980). Monoclonal antibodies specific for the guinea pig line 10 (L10) hepatocarcinoma. *Assoc. for Cancer Res.* **21**, 871.

Hsu, K. C., Rifkind, R. A., and Zabriskie, J. B. (1963). Fluorescent, electronmicroscopic, and immunoelectrophoretic studies of labeled antibodies. *Science*, **142**, 1471–1473.

Karnovsky, M. J., Unanue, E. R., and Leventhal, M. (1972). Ligand-induced movement of lymphocyte membrane macromolecules. II. Mapping of surface moieties. *J. Exp. Med.*, **136**, 907–930.

Kishida, Y., Olsen B. R., Berg, R. A., and Darwin, J. P. (1975). Two improved methods for preparing ferritin-protein conjugates for electronmicroscopy. *J. Cell Biol.*, **64**, 331–339.

Luft, J. H. (1956) Permanganate—a new fixative for electron microscopy. *J. Biophys. Biochem. Cytol.*, **2**, 799.

Marchalonis, J. J., Bucana, C., Hoyer, L., Warr, G. W., and Hanna, M. G., Jr. (1978). Visualization of a guinea pig T-lymphocyte surface component cross-reactive with immunoglobulin. *Science*, **199**, 433–435.

Margel, S. Zisblatt, S., and Rembaum A. (1979). Polyglutaraldehyde: A new reagent for coupling proteins to microspheres and for labeling cell-surface receptors. II. Simplified method by means of nonmagnetic and magnetic polyglutaraldehyde microspheres. *J. Immunol. Methods*, **28**, 341–353.

Margolies, M. N., Cannon, E., III, Strasberg, A. D., and Haber, E. (1975). Diversity of light chain variable region sequences among rabbit antibodies elicited by the same antigen. *Proc. Nat. Acad. Sci. USA*, **72**, 2180–2184.

Mason, T. E., Phifer, R. F., Spicer, S.S., Swallow, R. A., and Dreckin, R. B. (1969). An immunoglobulin–enzyme bridge method for localizing tissue antigens. *J. Histochem. Cytochem.*, **17**, 563–569.

Matsukayashi, H., Stahl, W., and Skao, S. (1966). Immunoelectron microscopy in experimental toxoplasmosin. *Proc. 1st Int. Conf. Parasitol.*, **1**, 159.

Matsuura, S. and Tashiro, Y. (1979). Immunoelectronmicroscopic studies of endoplasmic reticulum–golgi relationships in the intracellular transport process of lipoprotein particles in rat hepatocytes. *J. Cell Sci.*, **39**, 273–290.

Matter, A., Lisowska-Bernstein, B., Ryser, J. E., Lameline, J. P., and Vassalli, P. (1972). Mouse thymus-independent and thymus-derived lymphoid cells. II. Ultrastructural studies. *J. Exp. Med.*, **66**, 198–200.

Mazia, D., Schatten, G., and Sale, W. (1975). Adhesion of cells to surface coated with poly-lysine. *J. Cell Biol.*, **66**, 198–200.

Molday, R. S. (1976). Immunolatex spheres as cell surface markers for scanning electron microscopy. In M. A. Hayat (Ed.) *Principles and Techniques of Scanning Electron Microscopy*, volume 5, pp. 53–77. Van Nostrand Reinhold, New York.

Molday, R. S. (1977). Cell surface labeling technique for SEM. In R. B. Becker and O. Johari (Eds) *Scanning Eectron Microscopy* II, pp. 59–74, Chicago Press, Chicago.

Molday, R. S. (1977). Cell surface labeling technique for SEM. In *Scanning Electron Microscopy*, II, pp. 59–74, Chicago Press, Chicago.

Molday, R. S., Dreyer, W. J., Rembaum, A., and Yen, S. P. S. (1975). New immunolatex spheres: visual markers of antigens on lymphocytes for scanning electron microscopy. *J. Cell Biol.*, **63**, 75–88.

Morgan, C., Hsu, K. C., Rafkind, R. A., Knox, A. W., Rose, H. M. (1961b). The application of ferritin-conjugated antibody to electron microscopic studies of influenza virus in infected Cells. II. The interior of the cell. *J. Exp. Med.*, **114**, 833.

Morgan C., Rifkind, R. A., Hsu, K. C., Holden, M., Seegal, B. C. and Rose, H. M. (1961a). Electron microscopic localization of intracellular viral antigen by the use of ferritin-conjugated antibody. *Virology*, **14**, 292.

Nakane, P. K. and Kawaoi, A. (1974. Peroxidase-labeled antibody. A new method of conjugation. *J. Histochem. Cytochem.*, **22** 1084–1091.

Nakane, P. K. and Pierce G. B. Jr. (1966). Enzyme-labeled antibodies: preparation and application for the localization of antigen. *J. Histochem. Cytochem.*, **14**, 929–931.

Nicolson, G. L. (1971). Difference in topology of normal and tumour cell membranes shown by different surface distributions of ferritin-conjugates concanavalin A. *Nature New Biol.*, **233**, 244–246.

Otto, H., Takamiya, H., And Vogt, A. (1973). A two-stage method for cross-linking antibody globulin to ferritin by glutaraldehyde. Comparison between one-stage and two-stage method. *J. Immunol. Methods*, **3**, 137–146.

Pierce, G. B., Jr., Sir Ram, J. and Midgley, A. R., Jr. (1964). The use of labeled antibodies in ultrastructural studies. *Int. Rev. Expt. Path.*, **3**, 1.

Revel, J. P. (1974). Scanning electron microscope studies of cell surface morphology and labeling, *in situ* and *in vivo*. In R. P. Baker and O. Johari (Eds) *Scanning Electron Microscopy*, Part III, *Proceedings of Workshop on Advances in Biomedical Applications on the SEM*, pp. 541–548. Chicago, Illinois.

Rifkind, R. A., Hsu, K. C., and Morgan, C. (1964). Immunochemical staining for electron microscopy. *J. Histochem. Cytochem.* **12**, 131.

Rifkind, R. A., Hsu, K. C., Morgan, C. Seegal, B. C., Knox, A. W., and Rose, H. M. (1960). Use of ferritin-conjugated antibody to localize antigen by electron microscopy. *Nature (London)*, **187**, 1094.

Rifkind, R. A., Ossermann, E. F., Hsu, K. C., and Morgan, C. (1962). The intracellular distribution of gamma globulin in a mouse plasma cell tumor (X5563) as revealed by fluorescence and electron microscopy. *J. Exp. Med.*, **116**, 423–432.

Rikihisa, Y. and Mizuno, D. (1977a). Demonstration of myosin on the cytoplasmic side of plasma membranes of guinea pig polymorphonuclear leukocytes with immunoferritin. *Experimental Cell Research*, **110**, 87–92

Rikihisa, Y. and Mizuno, D. (1977b). Binding of markers on either side of plasma membranes to the cytoplasmic side of paraffin oil-loaded phagolysosomes. *Experimental Cell Research*, **110**, 93–101.

Romano, E. L. and Romano, M. (1977). Staphylococcal protein A bound to colloidal gold: a useful reagent to label antigen–antibody sites in electron microscopy. *Immunochemistry*, **14**, 711–715.

Sarma, V. R. Silverston, E. W. Davies, D. R., and Terry, W. D. (1971). The three dimensional structure at 6 Å resoltuion of a human γGl immunoglobulin molecule. *J. Biol. Chem.*, **246**, 3753–3759.

Singer, S. J. (1959) Preparation of an electron antibody conjugate. *Nature (Lond.)*, **183**, 1523.

Singer, S. J. and Schick, A. F. (1961). The properties of specific stains for electron microscopy prepared by conjugation of antibody molecules with ferritin. *J. Biochem. Biophys. Cytol.*, **9**, 519–537.

Smith, C. W., Metyger, J. F., Zacks, S. I., and Kase, A. (1960). Immune electron microscopy. *Proc. Soc. Exp. Biol. Med.*, **104**, 336.

Smith, S. B., and Revel, J. P. (1972). Mapping of concanavalin A binding sites on the surface of several cell types. *Develop. Biol.*, **27**, 434–441.

Stackpole, C. W., Aoki, T., and Boyse, E. A. (1971). Cell surface antigens: serial sectioning of single cells as an approach to typographical analysis. *Science*, **172**, 472–474.

Sternberger, L. A. and Cuculis, J. J. (1969). Method for enzymatic intensification of the immunocytochemical reaction without use of labeled antibodes (abstract), *J. Histochem. Cytochem*, **17**, 190.

Sternberger, L. A., Donati, E. J., and Wilson, C. E. (1963). Electron microscopic study on specific protection of isolated *Bordetella bronchiseptica* antibody during exhaustive labeling with uranium. *J. Histochem. Cytochem.*, **11**, 48.

Sternberger, L. A., Hardy, P. H., Jr. Cuculis, J. J., and Meyer, H. G. (1970). The unlabeled antibody method of immunohistochemistry. *J. Histochem. Cytochem.*, **18**, 315–333.

Taylor, R. B.., Duffus, W. P. H., Raff, M. C., and de Petris, S. (1971). Redistribution and pinocytosis of lymphocyte surface immunoglobulin molecules induced by anti-immunoglobulin antibody. *Nature New Biol.*, **233**, 225–229.

Vickerman, K. and Luckins, A. G. (1969). Localization of variable antigens in the surface coat of *Trypanosoma brucci* using ferritin-conjugated antibody. *Nature*, **224**, 1125–1126.

Wagner, M. (1973). Methods of labeling antibodies for electron microscopic localization of antigens. In J. B. G. Kwapinski and E. D. Day (Eds) *Research in Immunochemistry and Immunobiology*, volume 3, pp. 186–247, University Park Press, Baltimore.

Willingham M. C. and Yamada, S. S. (1979). Development of a new fixative for electron microscopic immuno-cytochemical localization of intracellular antigens in cultured cells. *J. Histochem. Soc.*, **27**, 947–960.

Wofsy, L. (1974). Probing lymphocyte membrane organization. In E.E. Sercarz, A. R. Williamson, and C. F. Fox (Eds) *The Immune System: Genes, Receptors, Signals*, pp. 259–269. Academic Press, New York.

Wofsy, L., Baker, P. C., Thompson, K., Goodman, J., Kimura, J., and Herry, C. (1974). Hapten-sandwich labeling. I. A general procedure for simultaneous labeling of multiple cell surface antigens for fluorescence and electron microscopy. *J. Exp. Med.*, **140**, 523–537.

Antibody as a Tool
Edited by J. J. Marchalonis and G. W. Warr
© 1982 John Wiley & Sons Ltd.

Chapter 9

Production of Monoclonal Antibodies by Cell Fusion

JAMES W. GODING
Walter and Eliza Hall Institute, Post Office,
Royal Melbourne Hospital, Parkville, Victoria 3050, Australia

1. INTRODUCTION

Antibodies may be used as versatile instruments for the analysis and purification of molecules contained within complex mixtures. Until recently, however, their usefulness has been restricted by limitations in the specificity of conventional antisera.

The specificity of the immune response is determined by many factors. These include:

(i) Genetic differences between the species of origin of the antigen and the species of the recipient.

(ii) Differences in responses between individuals within a species, governed by both genetic and poorly understood non-genetic factors.

(iii) Purity of the antigen. It is often impossible to purify the antigen sufficiently. Even seeningly minor amounts of impurities may result in significant amounts of unwanted antibodies.

(iv) Cross-reactions between structurally similar molecules., For example, most of the antibodies in antisera against the dinitrophenyl hapten will react with trinitrophenyl, although a minor subpopulation of antibodies might distinguish between the two.

All of these problems may be overcome by the use of cell fusion to generate continuous lines of antibody-secreting cells (hybridomas), a technique which was pioneered by Köhler and Milstein (1976). This technique essentially 'immortalizes' individual antibody-secreting cells from immunized animals, and allows the generation of unlimited quantities of homogeneous monospecific antibody against almost any antigen. The antigen used in the initial immunization need not be pure. All that is required is that the antigen be

273

capable of eliciting antibody, and that a detection system is available to allow screening for the clone secreting the desired antibody.

A typical fusion proceeds as follows. Mice are injected with antigen, and their spleens removed a few days after the last injection. A suspension of splenic lymphocytes is fused with myeloma tumour cells by addition of polyethylene glycol (PEG) or Sendai virus, and drugs are used to ensure that only hybrids between the tumour cells and the normal cells grow. After 10–20 days' growth, culture supernatants are tested for the presence of the desired antibody, and the relevant clones are isolated by limiting dilution. These clones may then be expanded to mass cultures and injected into mice, where they will form tumours secreting milligram amounts of antibody into the serum.

Hybridomas have now been made against a very wide range of antigens, including serum proteins, cell surface receptors, haptens, hormones, viruses, tumour antigens, histocompatibility antigens, enzymes, embryonic cells, and neurons. For an overview of the possibilities, see Melchers *et al.* (1978), Möller (1979), and Kennett *et al.* (1980).

The extreme specificity of monoclonal antibodies means that in general, one clonal product will identify one target molecule. Thus, monoclonal antibodies raise the exciting possibility of identifying and purifying a host of *previously unknown* molecules. It is likely that this will become the area in which they will have their biggest revolutionary impact. Hybridomas will be very important in neurobiology and embryology, where the processes of cell–cell recognition and morphogenesis must depend on as yet undefined cell surface macromolecules.

Hybridoma antibodies will also be invaluable in the classification of cells. More precise identification of the cell of origin of tumours by monoclonal antibodies may aid diagnosis and treatment of cancer. The possibility of 'arming' tumour-specific antibodies with drugs or toxins is being explored in many laboratories.

The production of 'hybridoma' antibodies has revolutionized serology. However, it should be emphasized that the production of monoclonal antibody-secreting cell lines involves considerable expenditure of time, effort, and money. It should not be undertaken without due appreciation of the need for commitment to meticulous care. In many cases, conventional approaches to antibody production will yield adequate results with far less effort. But for situations where extreme specificity is crucial, or where large quantities of homogeneous antibody are required, the results are well worth the effort.

This chapter is a personal view of the subject based upon the author's experience. The methods, approaches, and philosophies do not cover the literature exhaustively.

II. THEORETICAL PRINCIPLES

A. The Clonal Selection Theory

It is now well established that the immune system responds to antigen by selection, activation, and expansion of individual rare clones of lymphocytes which are pre-committed to a particular antigen (see Burnet, 1959). The mechanism of antibody diversification is still not well understood, although it is now clear that the number of germ line genes for antibody molecules is quite large (Weigert *et al.*, 1978). Each mature antibody-forming cell produces a single, homogeneous antibody, with very few exceptions. Thus, the diversity of the total serum antibody response to a given antigen is a result of the sum of the products of hundreds or thousands of individual clones.

In the normal immuneresponse, the antibody-forming cell is probably an 'end-stage' cell incapable of further differentiation. It is thought that antibody-secreting cells have a life of only a few days. However, an antibody-forming cell may undergo malignant transformation, resulting in the disease of multiple myeloma, in which large quantities of homogeneous immunoglobulin are present in the serum. In most cases of myeloma, antibody activity cannot be demonstrated, although extensive screening has shown antibody activity for a minority of myeloma proteins (Potter, 1977).

B. Cell Fusion

In certain situations, cells may fuse to generate multinucleate or hybrid products. Examples include the fusion of sperm and egg, and the generation of myotubules and osteoclasts (Ringertz and Savage, 1976). In general, though, spontaneous cell fusion is rare. However, almost any two cells may be made to fuse by the use of certain agents, notably Sendai virus and polyethylene glycol (PEG). The mechanism of fusion is poorly understood (Knutton and Pasternak, 1979).

Following fusion, multinucleated cells called *heterokaryons* are formed. If these cells undergo division, the nuclei fuse, and the daughter cells possess single nuclei containing chromosomes from each parental cell. The daughter cells are known as *hybrids*. While some hybrids are stable, there is a general tendency for the loss of chromosomes. In some instances, chromosomes from one parent are preferentially lost (Ringertz and Savage, 1976).

In 1975, Köhler and Milstein showed that fusion between normal antibody-secreting cells and myeloma cells could be achieved using Sendai virus. The resulting cells continued to secrete immunoglobulin from both, and retained the malignant properties of the myeloma parent. Thus, any single antibody-secreting clone could be immortalized. It rapidly became clear that, due to the clonal nature of the immune response, this technique could result in production of absolutely specific antibodies, even if the antigen was not pure. All that was needed was a way to select the desired clone.

C. HAT Selection

Fusion is a relatively rare event, even when PEG or Sendai virus is used. Thus, if tumour cells are fused with normal cells, the culture will be rapidly overgrown by unfused tumour cells. What is needed is a way to ensure that only hybrids will grow. By far the most popular strategy is that devised by Littlefield (1964). Its rationale is as follows.

The main biosynthetic pathways for purines and pyrimidines can be blocked by the folic acid antagonist aminopterin. However, the cell can still synthesize DNA via the so-called 'salvage' pathways, in which preformed nucleotides are recycled. These pathways depend on the enzymes thymidine kinase (TK) and hypoxanthine phosphoribosyl transferase (HPRT). Thus, if the cell is provided with thymidine and hypoxanthine, DNA synthesis can occur, *provided that the enzymes TK and HPRT are present.*

If one or other enzyme is absent, DNA synthesis ceases. The cell can, however, be 'rescued' by fusion with another cell which supplies the missing enzyme. Thus, if spleen cells (which possess TK and HPRT, but die in culture) are fused with myeloma cells lacking TK and HPRT, only the hybrid cells will grow in medium containing hypoxanthine, aminopterin, and thymidine (HAT medium).

Mutant myeloma cells lacking TK or HPRT are produced by use of toxic drugs. For example, thioguanine is incorporated into DNA via HPRT, resulting in cell death. Only HPRT$^-$ cells will survive thioguanine selection. Production of HPRT$^-$ cells is relatively easy, since the enzyme is coded for by a gene on the X chromosome. Cells possess only one active X chromosome (lyonization), and thus only a single mutation is needed to result in total loss of the enzyme. TK mutants are much more difficult to select, because two simultaneous rare events are required. It should be noted that not all thioguanine-resistant cells are HAT sensitive.

III. PRACTICAL ASPECTS

A. Immunization Protocol

Many different immunization protocols have been proposed. While no hard and fast rules exist, it does seem to be general experience that long immunization schedules with multiple doses of antigen are not necessary, and may indeed be counter-productive. Good results have been obtained after a single priming dose, or at the most one or two boosts. Adjuvants may help in some instances.

One factor does seem to be important. In general, experience indicates that the time between the last immunization and the time of fusion should be short. Three days seems to be optimal.

Most investigators have used the mouse as the recipient, although more recently several groups have reported success with rats (e.g. Ledbetter and Herzenberg, 1979).

B. Choice of Myeleoma Cell

Not all myeloma cell lines are suitable for fusion. Even certain sublines of known good lines have given poor results. The two lines which have given the best results are derived from MOPC-21 or MPC-11, which are murine tumours of BALB/c strain origin. These lines have been adapted to tissue cultures for many years. They secrete IgG1 and IgG2b respectively (see Melchers *et al.*, 1978 for details).

When myeloma cells are fused with normal antibody-forming cells, both the myeloma protein and the spleen cell protein will continue to be produced. Hybrids will secrete molecules containing all possible combinations of light and heavy chains. Most of these mixed molecules will be inactive.

Sevaral variants of MOPC-21 now exist, in which partial or total loss of synthesis of the myeloma protein has occurred. These include P3-Ns-1-Ag4-1 (abbreviated NS-1), which has lost heavy chain synthesis but still produces light chains, and X62-Ag8.653 (Kearny *et al.*, 1979) which synthesizes neither chain. A third line, Sp2/0-Ag14 (Shulman *et al.*, 1978) is itself a hybrid cell line which synthesizes neither chain.

Recently, a rat myeloma cell line has been described which has been shown to be useful for fusion (Galfrè *et al.*, 1979). This line is particularly attractive because of the much larger amounts of antibody obtainable from rats compared to mice.

In general, best results have been achieved when the phylogenetic distance between the normal spleen and the myeloma tumour has been small. Thus, mouse–mouse hybrids have been successful, as have rat–mouse. Rabbit––mouse hybridizations have been disappointing.

C. Assay Procedure

It cannot be stressed too strongly that the assay procedure is crucial to success. Unless the assay for antibody is quick, reliable, and inexpensive, success is unlikely. The more cultures that can be screened in a given time, the greater the chance of finding those with the desired properties. Speed is important because during the early phases of a hybridization, decisions regarding expansion and cloning must be made within a few days. If cells are allowed to overgrow, the resulting selective pressure will often result in overgrowth by non-producing cells.

The assay in use in the author's laboratory consists of a solid phase radioimmunoassay, performed in flexible 96-well polyvinyl chloride plates (Section IV.C). The plates are coated with protein, which is passively adsorbed to the plastic. Excess protein is removed and any remaining 'sticky' sites are saturated by washing with phosphate-buffered saline containing 1% bovine serum albumin. Wells are then filled with culture fluid. Following incubation, plates are washed again, and ^{125}I-labelled staphylococcal protein-A (which binds IgG; Goding, 1978) is added. Following a further wash, the wells are cut off and counted in a gamma counter. Further details are given in Section V.

The assay can be modified in many ways. For example, the use of isotope may be avoided by use of enzyme-linked immunosorbent assay (ELISA) (Kearney *et al.*, 1979). An elegant adaptation of the radioimmumoassay for cellular antigens has been described by Stocker and Heusser (1979). This modification avoids the need for multiple centrifugations.

D. Cloning Procedure

Once the culture wells containing the desired antibodies have been located, it is essential to clone the antibody-producing cells. This step is important because non-producing cells usually grow more rapidly than producing cells, and will eventually overgrow the culture. Cloning also makes it more probable that the final antibody will be homogeneous and monospecific. Since the hybrids are often unstable, it is important to reclone the cells periodically. Recloning may be essential to 'rescue' a failing culture.

In general, lymphoid cells in tissue culture do not grow well at very low densities. Most cloning procedures therefore use a population of inert 'feeder' cells (usually thymocytes) which support growth but do not themselves proliferate. The use of feeder cells allows cloning from individual cells with reasonable efficiency (20–70% is typical).

Probably the most popular method of cloning involves culturing small numbers (1–10) of hybrid cells in 96 well plates, each well containing 10^6 thymocytes. The strain of mouse providing the thymocytes is unimportant, and even rat thymocytes work well. The number of hybrid cells per well is chosen such that 30–50% of wells show no growth. At this concentration, most positive wells will consist of single clones. Each well must be assayed individually for antibody, because not all wells with growth will be active. At the first cloning, only a small minority of wells with growth may be active. Subsequent cloning will usually result in much greater efficiency. In general, cloning should be carried out at least twice.

Cloning may also be carried out by growth in soft agar (Köhler and Milstein, 1976), which prevents cell migration. Clones appear as small colonies. The author has had no experience with this method. A third possibility, which is only available to a few privileged laboratories, involves cloning by use of the fluorescence activated cell sorter (FACS) (Parks *et al.*, 1979).

E. Growth of Cells in Culture

Once the desired antibody-secreting hybrids have been identified and cloned, cultures may be expanded to obtain larger numbers of cells and larger volumes of supernatant. As mentioned previously, lymphoid cells do not grow well at low densities. It is important to expand the cultures gradually—typically the cultures may be diluted 1 : 2–1 : 4. The culture medium from the culture to be expanded may remain in the new culture.

It is very important to maintain the cells in exponential growth. If the cells run out of nutrients, the resulting selective pressure is very likely to result in loss of production of antibody. Cells should be observed every day or two under an inverted microscope, preferably one equipped with phase optics.

As soon as enough cells are available (i.e. approximately 10^7), aliquots should be frozen in liquid nitrogen (see Section III.C). This provides insurance against subsequent infection or loss of production. The importance of this step cannot be overemphasised.

Cultures may be expanded to very large sizes. Up to 200 ml cultures may be grown in flat flasks, but larger cultures are best grown in roller bottles. Typical antibody levels in the supernatant are 10–50 µg/ml. Maximum levels will be achieved by allowing the cells to overgrow. They should then be discarded.

F. Growth of Cells in Animals

Once the cells have been cloned, frozen, and expanded, they may be injected into mice, where they will produce solid tumours. Antibody levels in serum or ascitic fluid are typically 5–15 mg/ml.

Cells may be given subcutaneously or intraperitoneally. A typical cell dose is 10^7 cells, although less may suffice. The recipient mice should be histocompatible with the injected cells, in order to prevent tumour rejection. If the spleen cell donor is BALB/c and the myeloma parent is also BALB/c, then BALB/c mice are obviously used. If the spleen cell donor is C57BL (for example) and the myeloma is of BALB/c origin, then (BALB/c × C57BL)F_1 mice must be used. In general, rat × mouse hybrids will not grow in rats or mice. Occasionally, these rules may be violated successfully. Low doses of whole-body irradiation (350–500 R) may allow minor histocompatibility differences to be overcome.

Subcutaneous injection has the advantage that tumour growth is easily observed. Mice may be bled from the tail artery following a few minutes warming under a spotlight, by a gentle transverse cut under the tail with a razor blade. At each bleed, up to 1 ml blood may be obtained. Mice may be bled every 5–7 days without undue anaemia.

Intraperitoneal cell injection has the considerable advantage that tumour growth often causes the production of ascites (5–15 ml per mouse), which may easily be tapped with an 18 gauge needle. Not all mice will produce ascites, and some skill is needed to tap the fluid. Ascites production may be increased by injection of 0.5 ml pristane (2,, 6, 10, 14-tetramethylpentadecane, Aldrich Chemical Company, Inc., Milwaukee, Wisconsin 53201), intraperitoneally, 1 week prior to injection of cells. The antibody concentration in ascites is similar to that in serum.

G. Freezing of Cells

As mentioned earlier, aliquots of hybrid cells should be frozen at an early stage. It is sometimes even worth while to freeze the cells prior to cloning, as insurance against possible disasters. Cells should also be frozen from later stages. Typically, six vials are frozen, each containing 10^7 cells in a mixture of 90% foetal calf serum plus 10% dimethyl sulphoxide. The cooling rate should be around 1 °C per minute. Manufacturers of liquid nitrogen tanks supply individual instructions and apparatus.

Cells should be thawed rapidly by immersion of the vial in a 37 °C water bath, and the foetal calf serum and dimethyl sulphoxide are immediately removed by centrifugation. Cells should be cultured at high density until re-established. It is advisable to check each freezing by a test thaw of one vial. Frozen cells will remain stable for more than 6 months. However, it is advisable to thaw, regrow, test, and refreeze all lines at yearly intervals.

It is not advisable to maintain cells in culture simply as a way of maintaining them. Cells in culture should be grown for a purpose (expansion or collection of supernatants). When the cells are not in use, they should be frozen. Not to do so is to court disaster.

IV. PRACTICAL PROCEDURES

A. Stock Solutions

×100 HT solution is made by dissolving 0.039 g thymidine and 0.14 g hypoxanthine in 100 ml double distilled water (ddw) at 70–80 °C. Aliquots are sterilized by filtration, and frozen at −20 °C.

×1000 aminopterin solution is made by dissolving 17.6 mg aminopterin in 100 ml ddw and sterilizing by filtration. Aliquots are stored at −20 °C.

×50 HAT stock solution is prepared by mixing 100 ml of ×100 HT plus 10 ml ×1000 aminopterin plus 90 ml ddw. Sterilize and store as above.

Note that the aminopterin may deteriorate. It is wise to make fresh stocks from powder every 6 months. Failure of the aminopterin will result in growth of parental tumour cells and failure of HAT selection.

HAT medium is prepared by adding 4 ml of ×50 HAT to 200 ml RPMI-1640 medium containing 15% foetal calf serum (FCS).

50% polyethylene glycol (PEG) is prepared using PEG 1500 (BDH Chemicals Ltd; agents in the USA are Gallard-Schlesinger Chemical Mfg. Corp., Carle Place, New York 11514). Weigh out 50 g PEG, and sterilize by autoclaving for 20 minutes at 250–270 °F. Allow to cool. Before the PEG solidifies, add 50 ml RPMI-1640 without FCS, and mix well. Store at room temperature.

B. Fusion Protocol

The protocol described here was developed by V. T. Oi, Stanford University. Grow the tumour cells (e.g. NS-1) in two 500 ml roller flasks, or in several 200 ml rectangular bottles laid on their side. Medium should be RPMI-1640 containing 15% foetal calf serum (FCS). It is absolutely essential that the cells be in logarithmic growth when harvested. If the viability is less than 98–99% (see Parks *et al.*, 1979 for a convenient protocol), chances of success are diminished. The maximum density consistent with good viability is typically 10^5/millilitre in stationary flasks, and a little higher in roller bottles.

Harvest the tumour cells by pouring the cultures into sterile 50 ml plastic tubes. Centrifuge at 400 g for 10 minutes. Wash cells twice in RPMI-1640 without FCS, and count.

Remove spleens aseptically, and make a cell suspension by gently pressing the spleen between the frosted ends of two sterile glass slides. Wash cells twice in RPMI-1640 without FCS, and count.

Fusion is performed as follows. Mix 10^8 spleen cells with 10^8 NS-1 cells (the exact number of NS-1 cells is not critical), and centrifuge at 400 g for 10 minutes. Remove the supernatant completely, and add 1 ml PEG over a 1 minute period, using the pipette to stir the cells gently. The temperature during this and all subsequent manipulations should be held at 37 °C. Stir gently for an additional minute. Then, add 1 ml RPMI-1640 without FCS with stirring over a further 1 minute period. Stir in further 7 ml of medium lacking FCS over 2–3 minutes, and then harvest the cells by centrifugation (400 g for 10 minutes at room temperature). Gently resuspend the pellet in 30 ml RPMI plus 15% FCS (by stirring; not by pipetting), and plate out 1.0 ml into each well of three 96-well tissue culture plates. Culture at 37 °C in a well-humidified incubator (7% CO_2).

Begin HAT selection the day after fusion (day 1), by adding two drops of HAT medium to each well. On days 2, 3, 5, 8, and 11, remove half the medium in each well by suction, and add two drops of HAT medium. After a few days of HAT selection, massive cell death will be noted, and the medium will change from yellow to pink. Between 10 and 20 days after fusion, small colonies of cells should be noted. (These are most easily seen from the underside of the tray.) Most wells will show growth in a good fusion.

After day 11, add two drops of HT medium every 3 days, aspirating half the supernatant to make room. The use of HT medium assures adequate levels of hypoxanthine and thymidine while the aminopterin is being removed by dilution.

C. Assay of Supernatants

When visible colonies have begun to appear, culture supernatants should be assayed for antibody activity. Supernatants are carefully removed by sterile Pasteur pipettes (a separate pipette for each well) or using an eight channel 100 μl Titertek multichannel pipette (Flow Laboratories, Inc., Inglewood, California, catalogue number 77-844-00). Care must be taken to remove only about half the supernatant, and to avoid disturbing the cells.

The assay system obviously depends on the nature of the antigen. Speed, convenience, and reliability are crucial, while rigorous quantitation is unimportant. By far the most convenient assay is the solid phase radioimmunoassay. It should be stressed that the assay must be established *before* the hybridization is started. There will certainly be no time to iron out problems in the assay once the hybridization has commenced.

For *soluble protein* antigens, coat the plate (Cooke disposable U-bottom plates, flexible vinyl, catalogue no. 1-220-24; Dynatech Laboratories, Alexandria, Virginia 22314) with antigen at 50–200 μg/ml in phosphate buffered saline (PBS) for at least 1 hour at room temperature. Use 20–50 μl per well. The antigen solution must have no carrier protein, and detergents will inhibit binding. Remove the supernatant (which may be re-used several times), and wash ×3 with RIA buffer (PBS with 1% BSA and 0.1% sodium azide). Viruses and membrane fragments may also be adsorbed by this procedure.

For *particulate antigens*, such as lymphocytes, tumour cells or protozoan parasites, the modification of Stocker and Heusser (1979) is highly recommended. Add 50 μl cells (2×10^7/ml in phosphate buffered saline) to each well, and centrifuge the plate at 100 g for 5 minutes. Without disturbing the cell layer, gently immerse the plates in a large beaker containing 0.25% glutaraldehyde in phosphate buffered saline (PBS). After 5 minutes, remove the plate and then remove the free glutaraldehyde by flicking into the sink. Wash the plate in PBS three times, using three large beakers as above, and finally leave in RIA buffer for 1 hour to saturate any remaining binding sites on the plate. In some cased (particularly where the cells are very large), attachment via antibody may be more secure (see Stocker and Heusser, 1979).

Following coating of the tray, add 20–50 μl culture supernatant to each well. Incubate for 1 hour at room temperature. Remove supernatants by flicking, and wash ×3 in RIA buffer. Add 50 μl of ^{125}I-labelled staphylococcal protein-A (40 μCi/μg; 10,000 cpm per well; see Goding, 1978). Incubate for a further hour. Remove the radioactive supernatants by suction into a radioactive waste bottle. Wash the trays ×3 as above.

After the last wash, dry the plates under a gentle heat lamp, or by spontaneous evaporation. Take a piece of adhesive tape designed to cover the tops of the plates to prevent evaporation (individual, pre-cut, pressure sensitive acetate plate sealers, catalogue no. 1-220-30; Dynatech Laboratories, Alexandria, Virginia 22314), and place on the *bottom* of the tray. The wells are then removed by cutting with an electrically heated Nichrome wire. The wells will remain attached to the adhesive, and the tray top is discarded. Load the wells directly into the gamma counter with forceps.

The 'background' in negative wells should be 100–200 cpm, and positive wells should result in 500–5000 cpm. Providing the background is reproducible, any well with more than two or three times background may be considered positive.

Many other assay systems exist (Melchers *et al.*, 1978; Kearney *et al.*, 1979). The assay described above will not detect mouse IgG1, or IgM, or IgA. However, it many cases the convenience and simplicity of this approach compensates for missing some clones.

As soon as the positive wells have been identified, cells should be cloned. It is also a good idea to expand the uncloned cells and freeze them (Section IV.E) as insurance against loss.

D. Cloning by Limiting Dilution

Aseptically removed the thymus from mice aged 4–6 weeks (at this age, the thymus is at maximum size). Prepare a cell suspension, wash twice in RPMI-1640 plus 15% FCS, and count. Adjust the cell concentration to 10^7 per millilitre.

Remove hybridoma cells from the positive well, wash once and count. Prepare three tubes of cells, containing 10^7 thymocytes per millilitre and 50, 10, and 5 hybridoma cells per millilitre. Plate out 0.1 ml per well, into a 96-well culture plate, such that 30 wells contain five hybrid cells per well, 30 contain one hybrid cell per well, and 30 contain 0.5 hybrid cells per well.

After 7–14 days of culture, colonies should be observed. Assay the supernatants as previously. Choose a group where about half the wells are negative for growth, and select the wells with the strongest antibody activity. Clones in these wells can then be expanded.

E. Expansion of Cultures

Positive wells (whether cloned or not) should be expanded gradually. For the first 3 days after the cells have been in HAT medium, HT medium should be used.

Expansion is performed as follows. Take the cells from a positive well, and add them to a culture tray (24-well) in which each well contains 0.5 ml RPMI-1640 plus 15% FCS, plus 10^7 thymocytes. Feed with 0.5 ml medium 3 days later.

Once growth is established, cultures may be expanded to 5 ml flasks (without thymocytes), and then 20 ml flasks. Note that antibody secretion may be lost at any stage, particularly early in a hybridization. It is therefore wise to test all supernatants for activity during expansion. When the cells are growing well in

20 ml flasks, they should be frozen in liquid nitrogen as described earlier. Further expansion is usually no problem.

It is worth emphasizing that growth of hybridomas is a mixture of art and science. Perhaps the most important single point is the need to observe constantly the cells under the inverted phase microscope. With experience, it will become clear when is the best time to expand to the next step.

F. Growth of Tumours

Once the cells have cloned and expanded into stable, antibody secreting lines, they may be injected into mice. Most lines will produce tumours, typically 10–20 days after injection. It is feasible to transplant the tumours for one or two generations, but the possibility of overgrowth by non-producing cells must be constantly borne in mind. It is preferable to decide how much antibody is required, and inject the required number of mice in one or two passages. As a general rule, the longer the cells have been grown (in culture or in mice) after the last cloning, the greater the risk of loss of production. Individual mice may be assayed for antibody by serum electrophoresis. There should be a prominent 'spike' of paraprotein in the gamma globulin region, whose height may be 10–50% that of albumin.

G. Purification of Antibody

The simplest (and often the best) way to purify hybridoma antibodies is by affinity chromatography. If the antigen against which the antibody is directed is available in a suitable form, it may be coupled to cyanogen-bromide-activated Sepharose beads (see thee manufacturer's free booklet for details). Serum from tumour-bearing animals or culture fluid may be passed over the column, and eluted with a variety of deforming agents, such as acid (glycine–HCl pH 2.2–3.5), 3.5 M potassium thiocyanate, 8 M urea or 7 M guanidine hydrochloride (in order of increasing harshness). In general, the most gentle method is preferable.

Alternatively, antibodies of appropriate class (IgG2a, IgG2b, and IgG3 in the mouse) may be purified by affinity chromatography on staphylococcal protein-A–Sepharose (Goding 1978; Goding et al., 1979; Ey et al., 1978). Binding to protein-A is highly pH-dependent, and it is often worth while to explore the conditions of elution. Frequently, pH 3.5–4.0 is sufficient. Most rat immunoglobulins do not bind to protein-A. The main exception is IgG2c, which is a minor subclass (Medgyesi et al., 1978).

A third possibility is the use of Sepharose-conjugated goat or rabbit antibodies against the hybridoma immunoglobulins (e.g. goat anti-mouse immunoglobulin). In general, the columns need to be fairly large (typically 50 ml gel containing 500 mg of the globulin fraction of a strong antiserum will bind

30–50 mg). The columns should be pre-cycled with irrelevant immunoglobulin prior to use, in order to saturate high affinity antibodies whose binding will be essentially irreversible. Elution conditions are given in the beginning of this section. The columns must also be pre-cycled with the eluting buffer immediately prior to use, to remove any loosely bound material or material from previous runs. Elution is best accomplished by gentle acid buffers (pH 3.0) which minimize the risk of damage to the hybridoma protein. More harsh elution may result in higher recoveries but also higher risk of damage to the antibody.

When the starting volume is small, or when very large amounts of material must be purified, ion exchange chromatography is often the method of choice. The starting serum or culture fluid should be made 50% saturated in ammonium sulphate by addition of an equal volume of saturated ammonium sulphate (SAS). The resulting precipitate should be harvested by centrifugation (10,000 g for 5 minutes), washed once in 50% SAS, and dialysed against 0.005 M Tris, pH 8.0 overnight. (Ammonium sulphate fractionation reduces the load on the column). The column of DEAE–Sepharose or DEAE–Sephacel (Pharmacia) is equilibrated with 0.005 M Tris, pH 8.0. One ml of gel is more than sufficient for 10 mg protein. Dialysis against low salt buffers may result in precipitation of the protein. However, the precipitate may (surprisingly) be loaded on to the column with good recovery. After loading the protein, elution is accomplished by a linear gradient of 0–0.5 M NaCl in 5 mM Tris, pH 8.0. (If a gradient maker is not available, a step gradient consisting of 100 mM increases in salt is a satisfactory alternative.) Recovery of the hybridoma antibody is typically 90%, and the risk of inactivation minimal.

V. PROBLEMS

A. Foetal Calf Serum

The choice of a suitable batch of foetal calf serum is crucial to success. Before embarking on a hybridoma project, samples from several batches should be screened for activity. NS-1 myeleoma cells are plated in liquid cultures (0.1 ml wells) in RPMI-1640 containing 15% FCS. A good batch will support growth of clones from single cells without feeder cells, with close to 100% cloning efficiency. Once a good batch is identified, a large quantity should be ordered to avoid frequent testing. Only 1 in 5 to 1 in 10 batches is satisfactory.

B. Failure to Produce Antibody

With persistence and care, hybridoma antibodies may be produced against almost any antigen. Failure to produce antibody may have many reasons. It is suggested that the newcomer to hybridoma technology should try an easy hybridization first—for example, against sheep red cells or keyhole limpet haemocyanin. Success in the preliminary experiment then assures the investigator that the selection procedure is working, and allows accumulation of experience. It also assures the investigator that the chosen myeloma cell line (and subline) is suitable for fusion (not all sublines, even of good fusers, are satisfactory).

It is important that the assay procedure is worked out *before* the hybridization is commenced. A known positive serum should be included in all assays, and all assays should have appropriate negative controls. Failure to observe these rather obvious points can waste a lot of time.

It is worth while to test the serum from the immunized mouse for antibody. The presence of antibody assures that the mouse is capable of responding. There is, however, no evidence that antibody *titre* and frequency of hybrids are correlated.

If no antibody is produced, it is possible that there is simply no difference (or insufficient difference) in structure between donor and recipient. Choice of a different species (mouse versus rat) may be helpful. Within mice, there exist enormous differences in both specific and non-specific *ability to respond* to antigens. For example, SJL and 129/J mice are excellent responders. Often, responsiveness is governed by histocompatibility-linked immune response genes. A trial of different H-2 (major histocompatibility complex) types may be rewarding, especially for weak antigens.

If growth is observed, but no antibody produced, it is possible that the HAT selection is not working. It is a good idea to check the myeloma line periodically for HAT sensitivity. This will also allow verification that the aminopterin has not deteriorated.

In summary, the following questions should be asked:

(i)   Can I get the system to work for an easy antigen?
(ii) Is the HAT selection working?
(iii) Is the assay working?
(iv) Should another strain or species be used as recipient?

C. Tissue Culture Vessels

Every now and then, a 'bad' batch of tissue culture flasks or trays may be obtained. Unless this possibility is kept in mind, many weeks of fruitless effort may be spent in trying to track down the reason why the cells won't grow.

D. Infection

With good tissue culture technique, bacterial contamination should not occur. Most investigators include penicillin (100 units/ml) and streptomycin (100 µg/ml) as a safeguard, however.

Contamination with moulds can occur even with the best technique. Once a mould has been established, it tends to spread throughout the tissue culture room, the incubators, water baths, and instruments. The spores are highly resistant to heat, alcohol, and other chemical disinfectants, and are often airborne. The first culture wells to become infected are usually on the edge of the tray, and the source of infection may well be the air inside the incubator. The outer wells may be left empty, or filled with saturated $CuSO_4$.

The temptation to try to save a culture with a contaminated well is strong. In general, it is best to discard the whole culture (after wrapping it in plastic). An attempt to save the plate may be made by sucking out the infected well and filling it with 10 M NaOH. While this sometimes works, it often merely delays the spread to other wells. Treatment is more likely to succeed if contamination is caught early.

Some investigators have found that the cultures can be protected from airborne spores by wrapping them in kitchen plastic ('Glad Wrap' or 'Saran Wrap'). Evidently, sufficient gas exchange occurs through the plastic.

The use of anti-fungal agents is not recommended, because the toxic concentration is close to the therapeutic concentration. Some have found amphotericin B ('Fungizone'), 10 μg/ml, to be useful.

If an established cell line becomes infected, the infection may be cured by passaging the cells into mice, and allowing the immune system to cure the infection.

As always, prevention is better than cure. Good technique includes not touching anything which could come close to the cells, prompt cleaning of spills of media, periodic cleaning of incubators, and frequent changes of sterile water used for incubator humidification. Water baths are a potent source of infection. The number of people who enter the tissue culture room should be restricted, and if possible the tissue culture should be entrusted to a small number of people.

E. Loss of Production: Prevention and Management

Cell hybrids almost always have a tendency to lose chromosomes. Sometimes the loss is preferentially from one parental cell (Ringertz and Savage, 1976). Hybridomas are no exception. While stability of hybridomas is poorly understood, a few generalizations may be made.

It seems likely that some hybrids are inherently more stable than others. Thus, even with intensive care and repeated cloning, some lines will lose production. It is realistic to expect that 50–70% of all culture wells which are initially positive will be lost. On the other hand, it is sometimes possible, through intensive effort, to save a failing clone by recloning (up to 300 wells of cloning plates might be attempted for a particularly interesting clone). Upon recloning, a stable line may eventually be produced.

These clones which have been carried through successfully to the 20 ml culture stage will generally be stable from then on. However, the risk of loss of production never completely ceases. A few do's and dont's may help.

Do: *Maintain and replenish ample frozen stocks.*

Do: *Watch cell growth* frequently, using an inverted phase microscope.

Do: *Reclone periodically*, especially if antibody production is falling. This is a danger sign that the culture is being overgrown by non-producers.

Don't: *Let cells overgrow.* The strongest will survive, and these will usually be the non-producers.

Don't: *Maintain cultures for weeks or months without constant checking for production.*

Don't: *Maintain tumours in mice for many generations without recloning.*

ACKNOWLEDGEMENTS

I am very grateful to Leonard Herzenberg, in whose laboratory I was introduced to hybridoma technology. I am especially indebted to Vernon Oi and Jeff Ledbetter for helpful comments and suggestions.

The author is C. J. Martin Fellow of the National Health and Medical Research Council of Australia.

REFERENCES

Burnet, F. M. (1959). *The Clonal Selection Theory of Acquired Immunity.* Vanderbilt University Press, Nashville, Tennessee.

Ey, P. L., Prowse, S. J., and Jenkin, C. R. (1978). Isolation of pure IgG1, IgG2a and IgG2b immunoglobulins from mouse serum using protein A–Sepharose. *Immunochemistry*, **15**, 429–436.

Galfrè, G., Milstein, C., and Wright, B. (1979). Rat × rat hybrid myelomas and a monoclonal anti-Fd portion of mouse IgG. *Nature*, **277**, 131–133.

Goding, J. W. (1978). Use of staphylococcal protein A as in immunological reagent. *J. Immunol. Methods*, **20**, 241–253.

Goding, J. W., Oi, V. T., Jones, P. P., Herzenberg, L. A., and Herzenberg, L. A. (1979). Monoclonal antibodies to alloantigens and to immunoglobulin allotypes. In B. Pernis and H. J. Vogel (Eds.) *Cells of Immunoglobulin Synthesis*, pp. 309–331, Academic Press, New York.

Kearney, J. F., Radbruch, A., Liesengang, B., and Rajewsky, K. (1979). A new mouse myeloma cell line that has lost immunoglobulin expression but permits the construction of antibody-secreting hybrid cell lines. *J. Immunol.*, **123**, 1548–1550.

Kennett, R. H., McKearn, T. J., and Bechtol, K. (Eds) (1980). *Monoclonal Antibodies.* Plenum, New York.

Knutton, S. and Pasternak, C. A. (1979). The mechanism of cell–cell fusion. *Trends Biochem. Sci.*, **4**, 220–223.

Köhler, G., Howe, C. S., and Milstein, C. (1976). Fusion between immunoglobulin-secreting and nonsecreting myeloma cell lines. *Eur. J. Immunol.*, **6**, 292–295.

Köhler, G. and Milstein, C. (1976). Derivation of specific antibody-producing tissue culture and tumour lines by cell fusion. *Eur. J. Immunol.*, **6**, 511–519.

Ledbetter, J. A. and Herzenberg, L. A. (1979). Xenogeneic monoclonal antibodies to mouse lymphoid differentiation antigens. *Immunol. Rev.*, **47**, 63–90.

Littlefield, J. W. (1964). Selection of hybrids from matings of fibroblasts *in vitro* and their presumed recombinants. *Science*, **145**, 709–710.

Medgyesi, G. A., Füst, G., Gergely, J., and Bazin, H. (1978). Classes and subclasses of rat immunoglobulins: interaction with the complement system and with staphylococcal protein A. *Immunochemistry*, **15**, 125–129.

Melchers, F., Potter, M., and Warner, N. L. (1978). *Lymphocyte Hybridomas. Current Topics in Microbiology and Immunology*, **81**, Springer-Verlag, Berlin.

Möller, G. (1979). *Immunol. Rev.*, **47**.

Parks, D. R., Bryan, V. M., Oi, V. T., and Herzenberg, L. A. (1979). Antigen specific identification and cloning of hybridomas with a fluorescence-activated cell sorter (FACS). *Proc. Nat. Acad. Sci. USA*, **76**, 1962–1966.

Potter, M. (1977). Antigen-binding myeloma proteins of mice. *Adv. Immunol.*, **25**, 141–211.

Ringertz, N. R. and Savage, R. E. (1976). *Cell Hybrids*, Academic Press, New York.

Shulman, M., Wilde, C. D., and Köhler, G. (1978). A better cell line for making hybridomas secreting specific antibodies. *Nature*, **276**, 269–271.

Stocker, J. W. and Heusser, C. H. (1979). Methods for binding cells to plastic: application to a solid-phase radioimmunoassay for cell-surface antigens. *J. Immunol. Methods*, **26**, 87–95.

Weigert, M., Gatmaitan, L., Loh, E., Schilling, J., and Hood, L. (1978). Rearrangement of genetic information may produce immunoglobulin diversity. *Nature*, **276**, 785–790.

Specific Applications of Immunochemical and Related Techniques

Antibody as a Tool
Edited by J. J. Marchalonis and G. W. Warr
© 1982 John Wiley and Sons

Chapter 10

Immunology and the Study of Plants

R. Bruce Knox
*School of Botany, University of Melbourne,
Parkville, Victoria 3052, Australia*

I. INTRODUCTION

Defence systems need to be based on the ability to recognize self from non-self, and this property is, like cytoplasmic movement, a basic feature of all living cells. In this regard, immunology, the scientific study of immunity in animals, has contributed greatly to contemporary biological ideas and practice. This is not only because it is a twentieth-century preoccupation, but because of the uniqueness of its concepts, and the usefulness and wide applications of its techniques in the analysis of animal and plant macromolecules, both within organisms and in interactions between them. A fundamental concept is that of the antigen, the substance capable of inducing antibody formation in an animal, and reacting specifically with the antibodies raised against it (Sela, 1966). While the antigen concept is foreign to plant biology, nevertheless plant proteins, glycoproteins, and polysaccharides are usually excellent antigens. This has been known right from the historical foundations of immunology. P. Ehrlich in 1891 demonstrated that castor bean extracts could induce the production of antitoxins in animals. Plants and animals are so widely separated in evolutionary terms, that it is probably the foreign nature of plant macromolecules that makes them good antigens.

During the 1970s, the emphasis has been on molecular rather than the traditional morphological parameters in the analysis of plant function and form. Immunochemical methods have become widely used as they permit the analysis of both unknown antigen mixtures and highly purified antigens in terms of their cellular and tissue activity, sites of localization and significance in chemotaxonomy and evolution. The sensitivity of many of the methods is such that the detection of individual macromolecules of antigen within the cell is now possible by quantitative assays or by immunoelectron microscopy. In the absence of other activity, such as enzymic activity, immunochemical methods may provide the sole means for detecting a particular antigen, and for assessing

293

its relationships with similar antigens from other species. It is the purpose of this chapter to outline the significance of immunological ideas in relation to modern botanical thinking, and to review some case histories in which immunochemical tools have permitted significant advances. Antigens of flowering plants have been most widely studied and form the basis of much of this review. More recently, immunochemical methods have been applied to antigens of lower plants, which often provide simpler systems more readily amenable to experimental culture in the laboratory, and reference has been made to these studies where possible.

II. APPLICATION OF IMMUNOLOGICAL IDEAS IN PLANT BIOLOGY

Immunology has its fundamental basis in the responses of animals especially vertebrates, to foreign cells, tissues, organisms, and their products. As a defence system it has two important features: (1) phagocytosis in which cells have the ability to wall-off foreign particles; (2) the capacity to distinguish self from non-self, as seen in the ability of certain lymphocytes to recognize specific antigen and by means of cell proliferation to produce specific circulating antibodies to mediate the responses. Plants do exhibit some of the features of immunity seen in animals, but not to the extent of the antigen–antibody concept. They appear to have lost the capacity for phagocytosis at about the period in evolution of the differentiation of multicellular from unicellular life. Heterotrophic unicellular algae of the Dinophyceae are capable of phagocytosis and photosynthesis and have a specialized wall-deficient area of the cell surface for this function (Dodge and Crawford, 1970). In higher forms, it seems that the thick, rigid cell wall presents a barrier to phagotrophy. The capacity to discriminate self from non-self exists in both cellular and humoral immune systems of animals and in this section an attempt will be made to find any parallels that may exist with plants.

A. Transplantation Immunity and Tolerance

Since Medawar demonstrated the 'uniqueness of the individual' in animals, there has been enormous interest in the mechanism of acceptance or rejection in tissue and organ grafts and in the two natural situations where different tissues make contact: pregnancy and cancer. The transplantation antigens operate to ensure the morphological integrity of the body. The parallels in plants have long been known in horticultural practice, through stem grafts, though the mechanism is still obscure. Grafts between stems of different individuals and species are usually accepted, and rejection occurs when widely separated genera within a large family are grafted (Knox and Clarke, 1980). The rules of the response are thus less specific in plants, operating at the level of the species, genus, or even family.

In some cases, grafts between related species that are rejected when made between adult stems are accepted if made at the seedling stage within the first week or two from seed germination. This is analogous to immunological tolerance in animals. Skin grafts from two individuals are usually only possible in the embryonic state, in athymic individuals and between twins (Burnet, 1972).

This tolerance between individual plants within and between species is manifested not only in grafts but in chimaeras—plants which are virtual mosaics of cells of two different individuals. These can form from shoots arising at graft uions or by somatic mutation in the shoot apex—so that entire layers of cells may be genetically different (see review by Knox and Clarke, 1980). This is strikingly displayed in the case of chlorophyll or pigment mutations, which produce chimaeras showing striped and variegated leaves, flowers or fruit, as in leaves of ivy (*Hedera helix*), *Pelargonium zonale*, and in fruits of Bizzaria orange.

Tumours occur in plants, a common example being crown gall tumours of sunflower and other plants. The tumours are produced by the plant in response to infection by bacteria and plasmids. In other cases of infection, the plant can respond by walling off the infected region which withers and is lost (see Clarke and Knox, 1980). The parallels with animal pregnancy are manifested by the gametes of flowering plants which are walled off within special gametophytes. The male gametes are housed within pollen grains, two- or three-celled structures within a common, uniquely patterned wall of sporopollenin; the female gamete, the egg, within the embryo sac which is often sealed from the rest of the parental tissue by a layer of callose, a 1,3, β-glucan polymer (Rodkiewicz, 1970).

The application of immunological methods to analyse such situations in plants has provided evidence for the existence of cell, tissue, organ, and function-specific antigens in plants (see Section III.C). These appear to be analogous to the transplantation antigens of mammalian systems.

B. Hypersensitive Reactions

Environmental agents, such as pollen, may initiate the allergic response in susceptible humans. People who are allergic have an '*acquired specific, altered capacity to react*' to potential allergens (Von Pirquet, 1906) or are said to be hypersensitive to them. Pepys (1973) reviewed the essential features; *acquired* refers to previous allergen exposure needed to stimulate the immune system and develop hypersensitivity; *specific* refers to the precise molecular relationship between allergens and their specific receptors, the reaginic antibody (IgE) produced in response on mammalian cell surfaces; *altered capacity to react* describes the different response induced by the same allergen after antibodies have been produced in the body against it. Because pollen allergens are able to interact with complementary macromolecules on human cell surfaces, they may also perform a recognition function in the plant (see Section V.A).

Apart from the curious fact that the response is triggered by a plant protein or glycoprotein, hypersensitive responses are known in plants when they encounter potential pathogens (see reviews by Deverall, 1978; Clarke and Knox, 1979). In addition to the production of antagonistic substances known as phytoalexins, other metabolic changes are triggered resulting in the walling off and death of the affected tissue.

C. Immunity Against Pathogens

The history of immunological ideas began when people realized that a person with a pock-marked face did not take smallpox again (Burnet, 1972)—the Jenners' 'vaccination'. In plants there appears to be an analogy, with the elicitors of phytoalexins which are produced by the host plant in response to invasion by a potentially pathogenic fungus. The elicitors are proteins, glycoproteins, or polysaccharides. Polysaccharide elicitors are remarkably effective; they are small branched oligosaccharides containing 3-, 3,6-linked, and terminal glucosyl linkages of molecular weight 10,000. Minor structural modifications destroy their specific function. The elicitors appear to be the closest parallel to antigens known in plants but lack their specificity. The possible parallels with animals' immunization suggest that memory should be detectable in such plant responses. Phytoalexin induction can occur following infection by a non-virulent strain of pathogen which will provide a degree of protection against subsequent infection by a *virulent* strain (Deverall, 1978). In a similar way, application of polysaccharide elicitors to plant surfaces can provide the equivalent of broad spectrum antibiotic cover against later infection (Clarke and Knox, 1980).

D. Circulating Antibodies and Clonal Selection Theory

Humoral aspects of immunity are a vital feature of animal defence systems. The circulation of killer cells and specific macromolecules such as immunoglobulins able to complex with foreign antigens is unique to such systems. There are no known circulating cells in plants, analogous to those of either invertebrates or vertebrates. The defence function appears to be a property of individual cells or tissues essential to the sessile lifestyle adopted by plants, and their plastic mode of development. There is increasing evidence that callus cells, which proliferate at wounded surfaces and at graft unions (see Section II.E) may have specific roles in cell–cell interactions (Clarke and Knox, 1978; Yeoman, 1979). The vessels of the xylem and sieve tubes of the phloem may possibly contain macromolecules that could be transported within the system. A further network of secretory canals, which are usually filled with mucilage, is associated with the plant vascular system (Clarke *et al.*, 1979). They may provide a further conduit for the movement of macromolecules within the plant. These systems contribute to the bleeding sap at cut surfaces.

Antibody diversity and the clonal selection theory have no direct parallels in plants. An analogy was drawn by Linskens (1962) between the mechanism for generating diversity in the products of the S-gene which controls self-sterility (see Section IV.B) and Burnet's clonal selection theory. It seems likely that these humoral systems of animals are an adaptation to multicellular life, and represent an evolutionary option that plants have not taken up.

E. Specific Cells and Organs Associated with Immunity

The immune system of vertebrates depends for its operation on specific cells made in organs such as the spleen, thymus, and lymph nodes. Plants have no specific organs for the production of defence cells, presumably because their immobile life form has imposed a developmental plasticity for organ regeneration. When wounded, plants differentiate callus cells at the cut surface which proliferate and cover the wound, or wall off the affected organ or tissue which undergoes abscission. Such cells can be produced from almost any living cells of any organ. Thus callus cells have a special role, which extends to other situations where somatic cells interact—at graft unions and at the interface of symbiotic relationships with plant parasites (Clarke and Knox, 1980).

F. Differentiation Antigens

It is widely accepted that every diploid cell of an organism contains potentially all the genetic information present in the genome of the fertilized egg. Differentiation during embryonic and juvenile development involves a sequential expression of information-containing DNA, manifested in immunology by the differentiation of a stem cell into a variety of other cells depending on the extracellular environment. The state of differentiation of a particular cell or tissue may be determined by the gene products that are being synthesized, particularly soluble proteins and glycoproteins. Since many of these are antigens, differentiation may be visualized by observing the changes in cellular antigens during its course. In plants, differences have been detected in the suites of antigens characteristic of differentiating roots, vegetative and floral stem tissues and during seed development (see Section III.C). Furthermore, immunochemical differences between antigens, either during development of a single individual plant, or between different genera or species have been correlated with biological responses, for example, graft acceptance or rejection or ability to form hybrid seeds.

III. CHARACTERIZATION OF PLANT ANTIGENS

Research in this field has lagged considerably behind that with animal tissues, and in most cases has consisted simply in the application of methods developed for animal systems. The available techniques fall conveniently into two classes: diffusion-in-gel methods in which the antigen–antibody interaction takes place within an agar or agarose matrix which permits visualization of the precipitin patterns; and immunoprecipitation in which the antigen complexes directly with antibody and the precipitate is analysed by means of tracers covalently bound to the antigen or antibody, a procedure which often permits quantification.

Before reviewing the applications of such methods in plant immunology, it is necessary to consider whether there are specific problems associated with extraction or isolation of antigens from plant tissues.

Several kinds of antigen preparations have been used: (1) antigen extracts, which may be diffusates of whole cells or organs in aqueous buffers or detergents, or the culture filtrates of cells, containing surface macromolecules or secreted components or slurries or homogenates of organs, tissues or cells, or the soluble fraction after centrifugation; (2) antigens purified by biochemical procedures. A problem peculiar to plant tissue extracts is browning caused by polyphenol oxidases, or high levels of tyrosinases and proteases, or acidity of the sap. The released polyphenols from cell vacuoles may bind proteins and glycoproteins making them possibly inaccessible as antigens. These difficulties are especially prevalent in woody plants. They may be overcome or alleviated by addition of polyvinyl pyrollidone to the extraction medium (Loomis and Battaille, 1966), by extraction in an atmosphere of nitrogen at low temperature (Safonov and Safonova, 1968) or by adding small amounts of sulphydryl reagents such as 2-mercaptoethanol (Khavkin, *et al.*, 1977) or dithiothreitol (Chrispeels and Baumgartner, 1977) to inhibit or partially inhibit oxidation of polyphenols.

A. Diffusion-in-Gel Methods for Assessment of Antigenic Relationships

Double immunodiffusion is the classic method for analysing immunochemical relationships between phylogenetically related antigens. It is a qualitative method, and can be used for studies of both purified antigens and complex mixtures. This can be done because the precipitin lines that form in the gel exhibit characteristic patterns diagnostic of the antigenic relationships (Ouchterlony, 1949). The method has been widely used for analysis of plant antigens including common proteins found throughout the plant kingdom, little-characterized antigens which display organ specificity, and highly specific subcellular fractions or enzymes (Table 1). It has proved useful in controlling biochemical extraction procedures and has also provided evidence for phylogenetic relationships between antigens from related plant species, for

Table 1. Selected list of developmental and organ-specific antigens in flowering plants

Organ	Species	Antigen	Detection system	Reference
Leaf	*Nicotiana tabacum*	P; changes in antigens during development	ID	Boutenko and Volodarsky, 1967
			IE	Gray, 1978
	Triticum aestivum (wheat)	M; ribulose 1,5-biphosphate (RuBP) carboxylase	ID	Bourcelier and Daussant, 1973
		M; RuBP carboxylase	IE	
		M; malate dehydrogenase	ID, IE	Laurière *et al.*, 1975
	Avena sativa (barley)	M; RuBP carboxylase	ID	Kleinkopf *et al.* 1970
		M; phytochrome in coleoptile	MC	Hopkins and Butler, 1970
			ID	Pratt (1973)
			IE	Cundiff and Pratt, 1973
	Lycopersicon esculentum (tomato) *Petunia hybrida*	M; RuBP carboxylase	ID, IE	Gatenby, 1978
	Prunus avium (sweet cherry)	P; antigens with organ specificity	ID	Raff *et al.*, 1979
			IE	
Leaf Isolated chloroplasts	*Beta vulgaris* and several algae	M; ferredoxin	ID	Tel-Or *et al.*, 1978
	Nicotiana spp.	M; ferredoxin	IF	Huisman *et al.*, 1977
	Antirrhinum majus	M; RuBP carboxylase (fractional protein)	AG	Menke, 1973
		M; Ca^{2+}-dependent ATPase	AG	Kannangara *et al.*, 1970
		M; RuBP carboxylase (carboxydismutase)		Radunz *et al.*, 1971
		M; chlorophyll-containing proteins	AG	Koenig *et al.*, 1972

Table 1. *Contd.* Selected list of developmental and organ-specific antigens in flowering plants

Organ	Species	Antigen	Detection system	Reference
Roots	*Zea mays* (corn, maize)	M; various lipids and glycolipids	AG	Radunz and Berzborn, 1970 Radunz, 1971, 1972
		P; antigens common and specific to root meristem, zone of elongation and mature roots; vascular system and parenchyma tissue	ID	Misharin *et al.*, 1974
		P; meristems and mitochondria; some antigens with enzymic activity: malate dehydrogenase NAD-glutamate dehydrogenase	ID IE	Kohl *et al.*, 1974
		P; tissue-specific antigens in vascular tissue	ID, IE, CIE	Khavkin *et al.*, 1979, 1980
	Trifolium album (white clover)	M; trifolin, recognition protein for *Rhizobium* symbionts, binds to root hairs	IF	Dazzo *et al.*, 1978
Root: Isolated mitochondria	*Zea mays*	P; 12 antigens in embryonic root; 17 in mature root	ID IE, CIE	Ivanov *et al.*, 1974 Ivanov and Khavkin, 1976
Cultured callus cells	*Nicotiana tabacum*	P; expression of parental antigens	ID IE	Boutenko and Volodarsky, 1967
	Zea mays (corn, maize)	P; parental tissue antigens retained	ID IE	Khavkin *et al.*, 1978, 1979

	Species	Description	Method	Reference
Stem and shoot	*Prunus avium* (sweet cherry)	P; parental and callus cell antigens expressed	ID	Raff *et al.*, 1979
			IE	
	Zea mays	P; antigens common and specific to embryonic shoot and cotyledon	ID	Misharin *et al.*, 1974
	Prunus avium (sweet cherry)	P; tissue-specific antigen	ID, IE Abs	Raff *et al.*, 1979
	various spp.	P; phloem proteins	ID	Sabnis and Hart, 1979
	Sinapis alba	P; changes in expression of antigens at transition to flowering	ID	Pierard *et al.*, 1977
	Rudbeckia bicolor	P; vegetative and floral antigens	ID	Miliaeva *et al.*, 1979
Seeds: Period-specific proteins	*Nicotiana tabacum*	P; shoot meristem antigens	ID	Moiseeva et al., 1979
	Phaseolus vulgaris (red kidney bean)	P; expression of reserve protein antigen during seed development and germination	ID	Kloz *et al.*, 1960, 1966
			IE	
	Arachis hypogaea (peanut)	M;Gl protein	1D, 1E	Sun *et al.*, 1978
	Vicia faba (broad bean)	M; α-arachin α-conarachin	1D	Daussant *et al.*, 1969
			1E	Millerd *et al.*, 1971
			1D	Dudman and Millerd, 1975
			IE, CIE	Manteuffel *et al.*, 1976
				Lichtenfeld *et al.*, 1976
	Glycine max (soybean)	P; reserve proteins	1D, 1E	Catsimpoolas *et al.*, 1968
		M; trypsin inhibitor	1D, 1E	Freed and Ryan, 1978
	Pisum sativum and other legumes	P and M; legumin and vicilin expression during development and germination	CIE	Millerd *et al.*, 1978
				Thomson *et al.*, 1979
	Triticum aestivum (wheat)	P; gliadins—expression during development	1D 1E	Pavlov *et al.*, 1975
	Zea mays (corn, maize)	P; soluble proteins	ID, IE	Barlow *et al.*, 1973
		P; changes during development and germination in α-and β-globulins	CIE	Misharin *et al.*, 1975
				Khavkin *et al.*, 1977, 1978

Table 1. *Contd.* Selected list of developmental and organ-specific antigens in flowering plants

Organ	Species	Antigen	Detection system	Reference
	Oryza sativa (rice)	P; γ-globulin expression during seed development and germination	ID	Horikoshi and Morita, 1975
			IE	
	Hordeum vulgare (barley)	P; soluble protein antigens of aleurone layer and endosperm	ID	Jacobsen and Knox, 1974
			IE	
Period-specific enzymes	*Canavalia ensiformis*	M; urease	ID, IE, MC	Murray and Knox, 1977
	Brassica spp.	P; soluble proteins	ID, IE	Vaughan *et al.*, 1965
	Triticum aestivum (wheat)	M; α-amylase	ID	Daussant and Grabar, 1966
				Daussant and Corvazier, 1970
			IE	Olered and Jonsson, 1970
				Alexandrescu and Mihailescu, 1973
			IP	Daussant *et al.*, 1977
				Daussant, 1978a,b
				Okita *et al.*, 1978
	Hordeum vulgare	M; α-amylase	ID, IE	Jacobsen and Knox, 1973
			IP	Higgins *et al.*, 1976
	Triticale	M; α-amylase	ID	Alexandrescu and Paun, 1975
			IE	Daussant and Hill, 1979
	Vigna radiata (mung bean)	M; vicilin peptidohydrolase	ID	Baumgartner and Chrispeels, 1977
	cotyledons	M; lectin	E1	
			ID	Hankins *et al.*, 1979
Flower Pollen	*Oenothera organensis*	P; S-gene specific antigen; antigens common to other related genera	PR Abs	Lewis, 1952
			ID	Makinen and Lewis, 1962

Species	Findings	Method	References
Petunia hybrida	P; antigens common with stigma; some S-gene specificity	PR	Linskens, 1960
Brassica oleracea	P; no S-specific antigen	ID	Nasrallah and Wallace, 1967a, b; Knox *et al.*, 1975; Wodehouse, 1954, 1957
Airborne pollen species	P; common antigens between different genera	ID	King *et al.*, 1964
Ambrosia elatior (ragweed)	M; antigen E isolated as major allergen	ID	Knox, 1973; Howlett *et al.*, 1973; Hubscher and Eisen, 1972
Grasses: *Cynodon dactylon* *Dactylis glomerata* *Lolium perenne* *Phleum pratense* *Zea mays*	M; P at least 6 antigens in whole extracts; Antigen A and Group 1 allergen of *Lolium*	ID IE CIE	Augustin, 1963 Augustin *et al.*, 1971 Iwanani, 1968 Weeke and Lowenstein, 1973 Lowenstein, 1978 Marsh, 1975 Watson and Knox, 1976 Smart and Knox, 1980 Knox *et al.*, 1980
Betula verrucosa	P; antigenic nature of birch pollen allergens	ID	Belin, 1972
Populus deltoides *Cosmos bipinnatus* *Malvaviscus arboreus*	P; antigens present in pollen diffusate	ID IE	Knox *et al.*, 1972 Knox, 1973 Heslop-Harrison *et al.*, 1973 Ashford and Knox, 1980
Gladiolus gandavensis	P; one antigen shared with *Iris* pollen, others species-specific. One antigen common with stigma	ID, abs IE IP	Knox, 1971 Clarke *et al.*, 1977

Table 1. *Contd.* Selected list of developmental and organ-specific antigens in flowering plants

Organ	Species	Antigen	Detection system	Reference
	Ambrosia elatior	M; antigen E present in related genera	ID	Knox, 1973, Howlett *et al.*, 1973
	Prunus avium	P; antigens shared with cultured callus cells derived from vegetative organs, but not with the parental organs themselves; pollen expresses greater number of antigens compared with vegetative organs	IE ID IE Abs	Lee and Dickinson, 1979 Raff *et al.*, 1979
Stigma	*Petunia hybrida*	P; S-gene specific antigens present in pollen	PR	Linksens, 1960
	Brassica oleracea	P; S-gene specific antigens appear 3 days before anthesis S$_2$ antigen isolated and characterised. Abs	ID	Nasrallah and Wallace, 1967a, b Nasrallah *et al.*, 1970, 1972 Sedgley, 1974a,b Landova and Landa, 1973

Species	Description	Method	References
Iberis spp. *Brassica oleracea*	P; no common antigens with pollen	ID	Kucera and Polak, 1975 Nasrallah, 1979 Ferrari *et al.* 1981 Heslop-Harrison *et al.*, 1974
Gladiolus gandavensis	P; stigma surface antigen comon to pollen, corn, and leaf tissues	IE	Knox *et al.*, 1975
		IP	Clarke *et al.*, 1977
	M; arabinogalactan protein present at surface and in style canal mucilage	ID, IP	Gleeson and Clarke, 1979 1980
Prunus avium	P; specific and common antigens with leaf, stem and petal; S_3, S_4 antigens isolated	ID, Abs IE	Raff *et al.*, 1979, 1981
Ipomoea tricolor Petal	M; acid ribonuclease	ID, IE	Baumgartner and Matile, 1976

Explanation of abbreviations used:
M: monospecific antiserum
ID: immunodiffusion test
Abs: immunoabsorption
IE: immunoelectrophoresis
PR: micro-precipitin ring test
AG: specific agglutination

P: polyspecific antiserum
EI: Enzyme inhibition
CIE: crossed immunoelectrophoresis
IP: immunoprecipitin analysis
IF: immunofluorescence
MC: micro-complement fixation

example, the immunological relatedness between lectin antigens from various legume seeds (Hankins *et al.*, 1979).

Using antisera prepared against complex mixtures of often unknown antigens, increased resolution and simplification of patterns can be achieved by immunoabsorption. The antiserum is treated with extracts of some of the component antigens, for example, from an organ of a related species, and the common antigens are precipitated out and no longer revealed in double diffusion tests. The method has been useful in studies of antigen relationships in pollen (Lewis, 1952) in seeds of Ranunculaceae (Jensen, 1968), and in roots of corn (Misharin *et al.*, 1974).

Quantitation of the precipitin reaction has been achieved for monospecific antisera. Mancini *et al.* (1965) developed the single radial immunodiffusion method in which serial dilutions of antigens are placed in wells punched in antiserum-containing gel. The area of the diffusion ring of immunoprecipitate formed is correlated with the quantity of antigen present. This method can be made more sensitive by using radiolabelled antigen, and detecting the immunoprecipitate by autoradiography. Makinen and Lewis (1962) used the method to demonstrate quantitative differences in S-antigen of pollen of *Oenothera organensis*.

The major development of this technique has been the use of electrophoresis to separate the antigens in the gel before immunodiffusion (Grabar and Williams, 1953). This technique results in considerable simplification of precipitin patterns from polyspecific antisera and so greatly increasing the resolving power of immunodiffusion. It has been used to study a number of complex mixtures in plants including those of seeds (Kloz and Turkova, 1963), and pollen (Iwanami, 1968). Quantitation of the antigens has been achieved by electrophoresing the antigens into antiserum-containing gel. A one-dimensional method, rocket electrophoresis was introduced by Laurell (1966), and a two-dimensional technique providing enhanced resolution—crossed immunoelectrophoresis—by Clarke and Freeman (1967). These methods have been used for the study of the complex mixture of antigens in grass pollen (Weeke and Lowenstein, 1973) and seed endosperm or cotyledons (Khavkin *et al.*, 1978; Millerd *et al.*, 1978). The resolution of these methods can again be increased by using radioactively-labelled antigens or antibody and detecting labelled precipitin by autoradiography. Also some antigens retain their enzymic activity after precipitation with specific antibody, so that these immunoprecipitins can be detected using cytochemical tests for the appropriate enzyme activity. A series of mitochondrial enzymes from the roots of corn have been detected and partly characterized in this way (Kohl *et al.*, 1974) as well as two pollen enzymes (Howlett *et al.*, 1973).

Very few studies have been carried out on purified plant proteins and glycoproteins until recently (Table 1). Immunochemical tests have provided a useful guide to antigen complexity. Some highly purified proteins will produce two or more precipitin lines reflecting differences in the antigenic determinants present in the macromolecule; or the presence of multiple forms that may be separable by electrophoresis, as found for α-amylase of barley aleurone layers (Jacobsen and Knox, 1973). SDS–PAGE revealed the presence of a single band (MW 55,000) which bound specifically to the antiserum although two different precipitin arcs were each associated with two pairs of multiple electrophoretic forms of the enzyme detected by starch gel electrophoresis. In another system, chloroplast ferredoxin was shown to be denatured to apoferredoxin. This occurred during antibody formation in the rabbit and during immunodiffusion, one being ferredoxin and the other its denatured form whereas a single band was obtained with immunodiffusion at 2 °C (Huisman *et al.*, 1977). Some plant proteins have proved to be families of closely related macromolecules. A good example is to be found among the storage proteins of legume seeds (Table 1), where two major groups of globulins are present—legumin and vicilin. Legumin, after purification, produced a single precipitin band by immunodiffusion, while vicilin has proved to be a holoprotein with four different bands (Millerd *et al.*, 1978; Thomson and Doll, 1979).

B. Immunoprecipitation Analysis

This method has the advantage that it detects the antigen–antibody precipitate directly, using probes covalently conjugated to the antigen or antibody. This means that the interaction: (1) can be quantitated; (2) the antigens can be dissociated from the complex and their physicochemical constants determined; (3) the number of probes present can be estimated in various ways: radioactive labels by monitoring in a gamma or scintillation counter, by autoradiography or fluorography; enzymic activity estimated by colorimetry; fluorescent labels by fluorimetry.

The earliest immunological experiments with plant antigens employed immunoprecipitation techniques, for example, the microprecipitin ring test, in which serial dilutions of antibody are brought into contact with antigen. This test yielded the first evidence for the existence of the S-antigen in pollen of *Oenothera* (see Table 1 and Lewis, 1952). Boyden precipitin curves also provided quantitative data on antigen interactions, employing serial dilutions of antigens against antiserum, mainly to compare phylogenetically related antigen extracts. The immunoprecipitins were detected by turbidometry. For example, Jensen (1968) in Germany studied the serotaxonomy of seed proteins belonging to the family Ranunculaceae. Boyden precipitin curves obtained by testing a series of closely related antigens against one common polyspecific antiserum revealed immunochemical relationships between the seed proteins of the various genera. The results provide a quantitative assessment of the immunological distance between the genus *Adonis* and

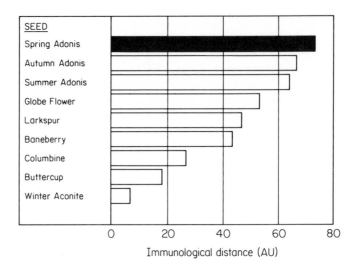

Figure 1. Immunological distance between seed antigens of *Adonis vernalis* and other species and genera within the family Ranunculaceae as revealed by Boyden precipitin curve technique using antisera raised against *A. vernalis*, and replotted from data of Jensen (1968). Spring Adonis, *A. vernalis*; autumn Adonis, *A. autumnalis*; summer Adonis, *A. aestivalis (A. annua)*; globe flower, *Trollius europaeus*; larkspur, *Delphinium consolida*; baneberry, *Actaea spicata*; columbine, *Aquilegia vulgaris*; buttercup, *Ranunculus acris*; winter aconite, *Eranthis hyemalis*

related genera of the family Ranunculaceae (Figure 1). A difficulty with this technique, however, is that differences in the antigenicity of individual proteins cannot be detected.

Immunoprecipitation by antibodies directed against enzymes can be monitored and quantitated by estimating the inhibition of enzyme activity of extracts when incubated in the presence of increasing concentrations of specific antibody; for example, a protease enzyme is involved in the breakdown of storage proteins present in germinating mung bean, *Vigna radiata*, seeds. Immunochemical studies by Chrispeels and Baumgartner (1978), showed that enzymic activity was inhibited in a linear manner. When seed extracts from closely related genera were tested the specific antibody showed reduced levels of inhibition, and no inhibition at all with extracts of kidney bean, *Phaseolus*.

One of the earliest enzymes to be detected by immunochemical methods was α-amylase, which hydrolyses starch in germinating cereal grains (Table 1). Immunoprecipitation methods have been successfully used to identify the native enzyme in germinating barley and wheat grains. Barley aleurone layers produce two distinct antigens of α-amylase (Jacobsen and Knox, 1973) and these have been shown to be synthesized *in vitro*, as the cell-free translation products of mRNA readout systems with S150 wheat germ and polysomes (Figure 2). Immunoprecipitin analysis also enabled Okita *et al.* (1979) to

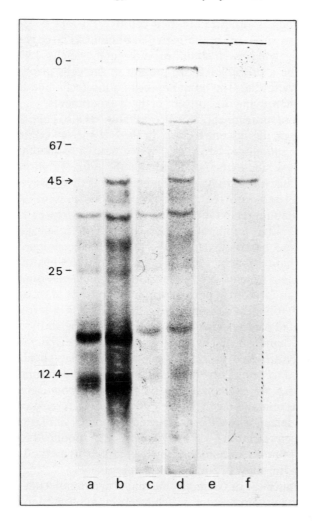

Figure 2. Synthesis of α-amylase from total and poly (A)-containing RNA extracted from barley aleurone layers in the wheat embryo cell-free protein synthesizing system as detected by immunoprecipitation and SDS–polyacrylamide gel electrophoresis of the cell-free translation products followed by fluorography. In this system, α-amylase (MW 45,000) is synthesized in response to treatment with the hormone gibberellic acid (b,d,f) and is not made in absence of the hormone (a,c,e). The proteins produced were labelled with [^{35}S]methionine. The cell-free translation products of total RNA are shown in a,b; of poly (A)-RNA in c,d; and following immunoprecipitation with specific anti-α-amylase IgG of products of total RNA in e,f. The MW markers are indicated on LHS, and O refers to the origin. The arrow indicates the position to which authentic α-amylase migrated. Reproduced with permission from Higgins *et al.* (1976)

detect two antigens synthesized in their cell-free readout system. The major antigen migrated similarly to the native enzyme in SDS–polyacrylamide gel electrophoresis, while a fraction of molecular weight 1500 larger was considered to be a precursor form, present in the cells prior to membrane transport and secretion. The immunoprecipitation technique has provided a vital means of identifying the antigens in these experiments.

Quantitation of antigen–antibody precipitates has also been approached by use of enzymic or fluorescent tracers. In the enzyme-linked immunosorbent assay (ELISA), samples of horseradish peroxidase or of alkaline phosphatase are covalently attached to the IgG fraction of the antibody before immunoprecipitation. The enzyme activity of the precipitate is then assayed colorimetrically and correlated with the amount of antibody present. An interesting example of immunoprecipitation using a fluorescent tracer is provided by applying quantitative immunofluorescence methods to antigens covalently bound to agarose beads (Dalen *et al.*, 1973). The technique has provided valuable information on the immunochemical relationships of ferredoxin, a chloroplast protein which is present in nearly all plants. Huisman *et al.* (1977) raised antisera to ferredoxin purified from chloroplasts of tobacco, *Nicotiana tabacum*. In immunodiffusion tests this cross-reacted with ferredoxin samples of other unrelated plants. However the specificity of the antibodies to tobacco ferredoxin was demonstrated by immunoabsorption. Ferredoxin preparations were covalently attached to agarose beads and batches incubated with the tobacco antisera to progressively absorb the antigenic determinants common with other species, for example, from spinach and *Nicotiana glutinosa* (Figure 3) leaving determinants specific for *N. tabacum*. A related species, *N. clevelandii* has ferredoxin with antigenic determinants similar to *N. tabacum*. The hybrid *N. clevelandii* ($♀$) × *N. glutinosa* ($♂$) produced ferredoxin with similar levels of fluorescence to the female parent. This method may provide a valuable tool in the study of antigen inheritance.

In the style mucilage of *Gladiolus* the major macromolecule is a proteoglycan, an arabinogalactan protein, which has been implicated in pollen–stigma adhesion and recognition (Clarke *et al.*, 1979). This style component has been shown to have a structure consistent with a 1→3 linked β-galactan backbone with side branches of 1→6 linked β-galactosyl residues, some of which carry terminal α-L-arabinofuranoside residues (Figure 4a) (Gleeson and Clarke, 1979). They investigated the specificity of the antiserum using immunoprecipitation with [^{3}H]arabinogalactan protein. The [^{3}H] label was introduced into the arabinogalactan protein by oxidation of the terminal galactosyl residues with galactose oxidase followed by reduction with [^{3}H]sodium borohydride. Antibody specificity was directed towards the carbohydrate component of the arabinogalactan protein. D-Galactose and L-arabinose proved the most effective hapten inhibitors of the antiserum. The antigenic features of the arabinogalactan protein were investigated by examining the

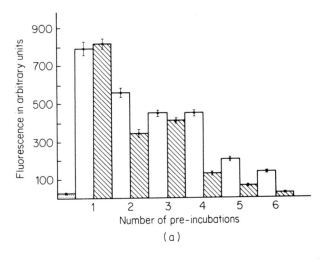

(a)

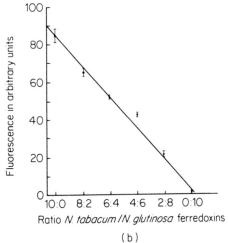

(b)

Figure 3. Use of an immunofluorescence technique with antigen conjugated to agarose beads to detect and quantitate species-specific determinants for tobacco ferredoxin. Figure 3a Preparation of specific anti-tobacco (*Nicotiana tabacum*) serum by immunoabsorption with ferredoxin beads from *N. glutinosa*. Serum samples (1 : 40 dilution in saline) were successively pre-incubated with *N. glutinosa* ferredoxin beads; open bars indicate fluorescence induced by remaining antibody determinants that bound to *N. tabacum* beads; hatched bars show fluorescence induced by remaining cross-reacting components that bound to a second sample of *N. glutinosa* beads. Control values subtracted from original values, and data are mean of 10 samples with bar showing SEM. Figure 3b Specificity of *N. glutinosa* ferredoxin absorbed antiserum for detection of *N. tabacum* ferredoxin in mixtures of the two macromolecules, as detected by the immunofluorescence method in Figure 3a. Control values subtracted from original values. Reproduced with permission of Huisman *et al.* (1977)

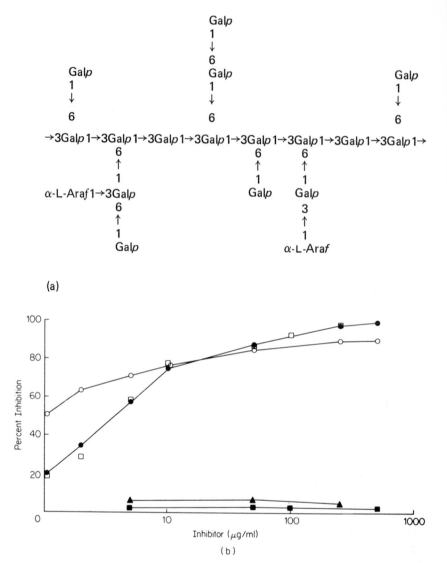

(a)

(b)

Figure 4. Nature of the antigenic determinants of a proteoglycan antigen—the stylar arabinogalactan protein from *Gladiolus* (Gleeson and Clarke, 1980). Figure 4a Proposed model of the structure of the arabinogalactan protein. Figure 4b Inhibition of the specific antiserum—[³H]arabinogalactan protein binding with enzymically and chemically modified arabinogalactan protein and arabinoxylan. Inhibition of binding of specific antiserum (dilution 1 : 4) to [³H]arabinogalactan protein (2500 d.p.s. or about 0.3 µg). The immunoprecipitation assays were carried out using a specific protein-A producing strain of *Staphylococus aureus* cells. *Symbols* (●) unlabelled arabinogalactan protein (□) galactan protein (○) oxalic acid treated arabinogalactan protein (▲) periodate oxidized arabinogalactan protein (■) arabinoxylan

interaction of the antiserum with chemically and enzymically modified antigen (Figure 4b). The dominant antigenic determinants of the arabinogalactan protein appear to be the side branches of 1,6, linked β-galactosyl residues bearing the terminal α-L-arabinosyl residues. This appears to be the first study of a proteoglycan antigen in flowering plants in which the antigenic determinants have been shown to reside in the carbohydrate side chains of the macromolecule.

C. Case History: Developmental and Organ-specific Antigens of plants

1. Organ specificity of Plant Antigens

Since W. P. Dunbar in 1910 first demonstrated the organ specificity of proteins, there has been steady progress in the characterization of antigens associated with particular organs and cell types in animals and man. This is especially true for that remarkable family of molecules, the histocompatibility or transplantation antigens which have been used to type animal cells, and play a vital role as the targets in transplant acceptance or rejection and in recognition of cell surface antigens by T lymphocytes. It appears likely that these molecules, in a similar fashion as immunoglobulins have arisen during evolution by tandem duplication as shown by the similarity in sequence of polypeptides in the constant region of the molecules. In plants it is only recently that glycoproteins have been isolated and this kind of approach has lagged far behind. Today the situation may be summed up in terms of the existence of an association between antigens and certain organs, tissues, and cells in both somatic and reproductive tissues, and some attempts are being made to isolate and localize the antigens involved and characterize them in order to approach an understanding of their functions.

The possibility that plants might have antigens involved in specific functions was first suggested by E. M. East in 1929 in connection with self-sterility between pollen and pistil of flowering plants. In many plants, the pollen is non-functional on its own stigmas but quite viable on the stigmas of another plant of the same species. He proposed that the S-gene which regulates this process produced a series of different S-antigens in the pollen which would interact in a complementary way with S-antibodies in the stigma, thus enabling discrimination of self from non-self. Lewis (1952) produced experimental evidence for East's hypothesis. Using the microprecipitin ring test, he demonstrated that the pollen of different S-genotypes of evening primrose *Oenothera organesis* contained an S-specific antigen as the major antigenic fraction; constituting at lest 20% of total pollen protein (Mäkinen and Lewis, 1962). The anthers were nearly all heterozygous for S-alleles but it was possible to prepare antisera specific for a single S-allele by immunoabsorption, and the specificity was demonstrated by double and radial immunodiffusion. In one other system, *Petunia hybrida* S-allele specificity has been detected in the pollen. In other systems, S-allele specificity could not be detected in the pollen but was clearly demonstrable in the stigma. Here the antisera against one S-genotype will cross-react with others but there is demonstrable specificity for the S-antigen after immunoabsorption (Nasrallah and Wallace, 1967a,b). The S-antigen of *Brassica campestris* stigmas has recently been isolated by lectin affinity chromatography and shown to be a glycoprotein of molecular weight 57,000 with a carbohydrate: protein ratio of 1:2. It binds to the lectin concavavalin A, perhaps indicating the presence of terminal mannosyl or glucosyl residues (Nishio and Hinata, 1978, 1979).

The S-antigen is associated with reproduction in plants—but what of the somatic antigens? Graft transplants are a standard horticultural procedure, and it might be anticipated that tissue typing using immunological methods would be well developed.This kind of approach has lagged behind, and empirical practice and the traditional morphological approach to cell typing remain pre-eminent. Some progress has come from an analysis of the relationships between somatic antigens and stem grafting success. Such an approach was first attempted by Rives (1923) who used serological tests to predict success in grafting grape vines. More recently, a quantitative evaluation has been successfully achieved by Kloz and co-workers in Czechoslavakia using the kidney bean, *Phaseolus vulgaris*. A strong correlation was obtained between the amount of immunoprecipitate formed against extracts of the hypocotyl and root from various other bean species and antiserum to extracts of one cultivar, *P. vulgaris* cv. Veltruska Saxa, and the growth rate of grafted stems on root stocks of the same cultivar. The success of grafting is of the same order as the affinity of the antibodies for the antigenic determinants. Kloz and Turkova (1963) also made an immunological analysis of the antigens in the different tissues, and found some were common and other species-specific. Seed antigens of cultivars of apple, *Malus domestica*, were examined by Dunin and Chefranova (1966) who found strong cross-reactivity between antigens of stem graft-compatible cultivars, and reduced cross-reactivity between incompatible cultivars or more distantly related forms. Similar results have been obtained by Samaan and Fadel (1979) in assessing the graft compatibility of cultivars of oranges with the various *Citrus* root stocks.

The existence of common and organ-specific antigens within a single plant species has been demonstrated in tobacco plants (Boutenko and Volodarsky, 1968); in corn roots (Misharin *et al.*, 1974; Khavkin *et al.*, 1978b); *Gladiolus* (Clarke *et al.*, 1977) and *Prunus* (Raff *et al.*, 1979). Immunoabsorption experiments demonstrated that even common antigens retained some ability to precipitate their homologous organ antigen after absorption with extracts of other organs, showing that determinants specific to the organ were present. Callus cells produced by proliferation in sterile culture on solid agar medium of explants of various plant organs retain the antigens characteristic of the organ through many subcultures. This has been shown for both callus cultures of corn, *Zea mays* (Khavkin *et al.*, 1979), and for sweet cherry, *Prunus avium* (Raff *et al.*, 1979). In the case of sweet cherry, antigens specific to callus cells were detected in calli from a number of different parental organs. In addition the calli produced from different explants were able to express a different range of antigens, and also a greater number than the parental organs (Raff *et al.*, 1979). The heterogeneity of antigen expression suggests that callus cells have the ability to produce parental antigens typical of other organs than the explant from which they were derived (Raff *et al.*, 1980). For example, the S-antigen of the cherry stigma, whose presence is correlated with the particular S-allele determining self-incompatibility, is detectable in some callus cultures derived from explants of cherry leaf by immunodiffusion and immunoelectrophoresis. The S-antigen is not detectable by these techniques in leaf extracts. An interesting feature of these experiments is that some of the antigens are secreted into the medium of liquid suspension cultures of callus cells. These results suggest that the secreted antigens may play a role in intercellular communication.

The use of antigenic determinants as specific markers for plant tissues, organs, cultivars, and species is an obvious development from such studies, particularly useful in proving cultivar identification for patent rights. Antisera to leaf extracts have been successfully used to discriminate between three cultivars of *Populus nigra* and a hybrid with *P. deltoides* (Sterba, 1975), and discrimination between different genotypes of the oat cereal has been achieved using a quantitative approach (Smith and Frey, 1970). Such tests will become increasingly useful in the future especially where the traditional morphological criteria do not reveal even quantitative differences or can be assessed only with acces to sophisticated equipment. The immunological tests are usually simple to perform and give a rapid result. Unfortunately, examples are hard to document because of the traditional secrecy of commercial practice in horticulture.

2. Developmental Antigens in Plants

The existence of antigens characteristically present at precise periods of development has been established in various animals, through immunochemical studies of extracts of the soluble proteins of amphibia, echinoderm, and insects during development (Roberts, 1971). There is evidence also for specific embryonic antigens, for example, α-fetoprotein of the mammalian embryo, and in onco-developmental systems (Fishman and Sell, 1976). In plants, changes in the suite of antigens have been associated with the self-assembly of organelles, specific enzyme synthesis, organ differentiation in leaves, shoot apical meristems and roots during development (Table 1). In the root system, there is also evidence for differences between embryonic and adult antigens. In this section, the evidence for the existence of developmental antigens in plants will be reviewed.

a. Organelle antigens   Immunochemical methods have been instrumental in providing identification and localization of the components of plant cell organelles during their biogenesis and development. This is especially true in plants for chloroplasts, which can be readily isolated, and in which specific agglutination reactions with antisera can readily be performed (Berzborn *et al.*, 1966). The chloroplast commences as a proplastid initiated in cells at a growth centre. These contain primary thylakoids as an internal membrane system that develops into the complex chlorophyll-bearing grana system (see review by Craig and Gunning, 1976). Antisera to a variety of membrane lipids, glycolipids, lipoproteins, proteins (including enzymes and chlorophyll itself) have been prepared (see Table 1) and have been used by means of sonication and agglutination to locate these components in the thylakoid membranes (see review by Menke, 1973), using both immunological assays and tests for photochemical activity. These methods have contributed significantly to our understanding of the complex processes of self-assembly of the lipids, proteins, and glycoproteins into extended membranes in both chloroplasts and mitochondria.

b. Embryonic antigens.   Differences between the antigen complements of embryonic and mature plants of corn, *Zea mays*, have been extensively investigated by E. Khavkin and co-workers at the Siberian Institute of Plant Physiology and Biochemistry, Irkutsk, USSR. They have used a double immunodiffusion technique based on an adaptation of the 'method of squares' (Abelev, 1960) in which antiserum against a different organ is used to selectively absorb common antigens as the antigen diffuses through the gel, so that only organ-specific antigens are able to precipitate with homologous antiserum (Figure 5).

Using this method, common and organ-specific antigens were detected in the roots, and even in the vascular cylinder tissue (Khavkin *et al.*, 1980) and in the cotyledons (Misharin *et al.*, 1974). In the course of developmental studies, utilizing immunoelectrophoretic techniques, the existence of three classes of embryonic antigens in corn seedlings has been established: (1) period-specific proteins, for example, the reserve globulins; (2) constitutive proteins that are persistent and may exhibit tissue or organ specificity; (3) common proteins present throughout the life cycle in most organs (Khavkin *et al.*, 1978, 1979). Embryonic antigens of class (2) were detected in developing and mature embryos but were absent from seedling shoot and root meristems. They were also expressed in proliferated callus cells in tissue culture, irrespective of the tissue or organ of the explants used to produce the callus cells. Khavkin *et al.*

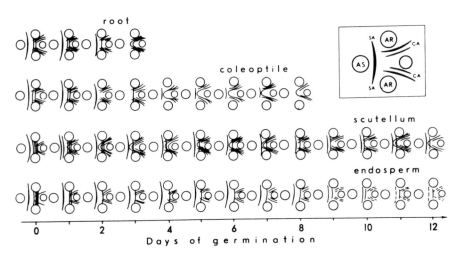

Figure 5. Period-specific antigens in the germinating grains and seedlings of corn, *Zea mays* detected by immunodiffusion by the barrier absorption test of Khavkin *et al.* (1977) reproduced with permission. The layout of the test is shown in the inset, with antigen placed in the RHS well, diffusing past the pair of absorbing antisera (AR) raised against root tips of 3-day-old seedlings with the specific antiserum (AS) on LHS raised against scutellum antigens from dry grains. Specific embryonal antigens (SA) form vertical lines towards LHS, while antigens common to dry grains and 3-day-old roots are precipitated around the absorbing antiserum wells towards RHS

(1979) have termed these 'proliferation proteins' or 'early proteins' in recognition of their occurrence in plant tissues prior to commitment to a differentiation programme. Specific antigens associated with the meristems were also detected.

The expression of a parental antigen in callus cells in tissue culture was earlier reported by Boutenko and Volodarsky (1968) working with cultured tobacco cells. The expression of a wide range of parental antigens by callus cells of sweet cherry has been recorded by Raff *et al.* (1979). This proliferation of embryonic antigens during callus cell production from adult plant tissues has been compared to events in hyperplastic and neoplastic animal tissues (Khavkin *et al.*, 1979). When tissue-specific antigens cease to be expressed in tissues, and the ratio of specific to common antigens changes drastically, the synthesis of embryonal proteins may occur (Fishman and Sell, 1976) associated with the dedifferentiation or neoplastic cell differentiation of stem cells. The stem cell concept has as yet no parallel in plants, though Khavkin *et al.* (1979) have compared it to callus cell proliferation.

In all these studies, the antigens were prepared from extracts obtained by homogenizing tissue in Tris buffer at alkaline pH in the presence of trace amounts of 2-mercaptoethanol to prevent oxidation of polyphenols. After centrifugation low molecular weight contaminants are removed by Sephadex

G25 chromatography, so that the antigen solution contains the major soluble proteins and glycoproteins of the tissue. They presumably are cytoplasmic in origin or could be in soluble wall components. They are likely to represent the major products of protein synthesis from the tissue. They may be expected to provide an excellent guide to the state of differentiation of the cells, provided the tissue cells sampled are uniform in their synthetic behaviour.

Developmental antigens have also been detected in the reproductive organs of plants. The S-antigen of stigmas of *Brassica* are present only at stigma receptivity (Nasrallah *et al.*, 1970), while the complex surface antigens associated with the walls of pollen grains may have quite different times and sites of origin during development (see review by Howlett *et al.*, 1979).

IV. LOCALIZATION OF PLANT ANTIGENS

The fluorescent antibody technique developed by Coons *et al.* (1942) was ignored by botanists for more than twenty years. Although a preliminary report of the use of fluorescent antibodies against flowering plant antigens from birch pollen was given in 1964 (Hagman, 1964), detailed immunocytochemical studies of flowering plant antigens were not published until 1970. Two groups successfully applied the method to the localization of plant antigens, the first to extracellular antigens of pollen (Knox *et al.*, 1970), and the second to intracellular antigens of bean cotyledons (Graham and Gunning, 1970). Today, immunocytochemistry is well established as a highly specific tool for the localization of proteins, glycoproteins, and polysaccharides in plant cells, tissues, organs, and surfaces.

It is the purpose of this chapter to present some of the problems that have been encountered in applying to plants immunocytochemical methods developed for animal tissues. This is particularly important in view of the availability of a wide range of fixatives in plant cytochemistry and the widespread use of modern high resolution plastic embedding techniques. Immunocytochemistry offers the possibility of localizing antigens both on cell surfaces and within cells. Plant cells, of course provide a barrier to this objective in the cell wall, which normally covers the plasma membrane except in protoplasts which have been produced by specific enzymic digestion of the wall. The primary cell wall of plants provides a potential barrier to the penetration of high molecular weight molecules. Since labelled antibodies usually have a molecular weight of 2×10^5 up to 10^6, the problems of tissue penetration are very great. Several aspects of immunocytochemistry need to be considered in the light of experience with plant cells: (1) methods for antibody detection; (2) tissue preparation to preserve both cellular fine structure and antigenic activity, and permit access of the labelled antibodies to cellular sites; (3) kinds of markers or probes conjugated to the antibody that are suitable for detection in plant tissues by light or electron microscopy.

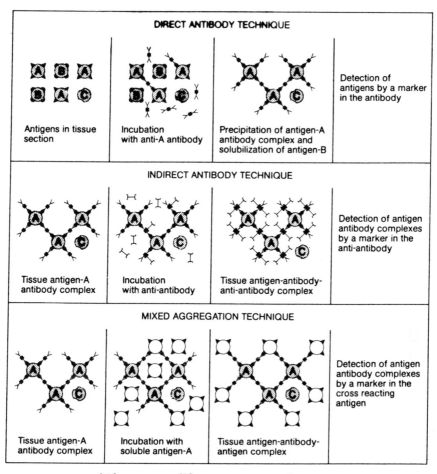

Key: soluble antigen-A [A] and antigen-B [B] ; insoluble antigen-C (C) ; hatching indicates the original antigen present in a given section; antibody directed against antigen-A >·< ; anti-antibody ⊢⊣ .

Figure 6. Schematic presentation of basic immunocytochemical assays. Reproduced with permission from Wachsmuth (1979)

1. Immunocytochemical Methods for Plant Antigens

Three kinds of antigen–antibody interactions have been utilized in immunocytochemistry (Wachsmuth, 1979; Figure 6). The direct antibody technique is a one-step procedure in which a marker is attached to the specific antibody that detects the antigen. The indirect antibody technique is a two-step procedure in which the specific antibody is attached to the antigen, and is detected by a marker in the anti-antibody, so that a sandwich of tissue antigen–antibody–antibody marker complex is formed. Finally the mixed aggregation technique is a two-step procedure in which the tissue antigen is complexed with its specific antibody, and the immunoprecipitate detected by use of labelled antigen which binds to available sites on the antibody. The direct method has the advantage of a short incubation period and greater specificity in that there is less opportunity for non-specific binding of the antibody to cellular components although it is a more time-consuming preparation since each specific antibody has to be individually conjugated to the marker by the investigator. The indirect method utilizes commercially produced antisera and results in considerable amplification of the marker, since the antibody has several antigenic determinants to which the labelled anti-antibody may bind, enhancing the resolution and sensitivity of this method. The third method is useful in cases where considerable quantities of the purified antigen, for example, an enzyme, are available for labelling with a marker, and offers the advantage of increased specificity because of the likely reduction in non-specific binding to tissue components. It has not yet been applied in a published study of plant tissue.

2. Tissue Preparation

Immunocytochemical methods depend for their success on the integrity of the antigenic determinants in their cellular sites, which bind to the labelled antibody. Pre- and post-embedding methods have been utilized. In pre-embedding staining procedures, whole cells, protoplasts, or tissue slices are incubated in labelled antibody. This method suffers from the disadvantage that in order to localize cytoplasmic antigens, antibody molecules have to diffuse into cut or whole cells. They may be unable to penetrate into uncut cells through the plasma membrane, giving false negative results.

Special methods have been developed in order to ensure that the labelled antibodies gain access to all potential sites of the antigen within the plant cell. Entry may be by diffusion into intact cells after removal of the wall by enzyme (protoplast) or by preparing 'footprints' of the protoplast membrane and washing away the cytoplasm (Lloyd *et al.*, 1979), or by the crude technique of allowing the antibodies to diffuse into sectioned cut cells or tissue injured by mechanical damage of freeze-thawing.

This method has recently been developed by Wick *et al.*, (1981) who have stabilized root tip cells of onion to localize tubulin in cells at different stages of the cell cycle. Paraformaldehyde fixation is first carried out in the presence of the chelating agent EGTA, which improves structural preservation so that the cells retain their characteristic polyhedral shape. The tissue is then incubated in a cellulose preparation then squashed to separate the cells which are ready for immunocytochemistry. Antibody penetration is improved by treatment with methanol at $-10\,°C$. The native organization of microtubule arrays can be detected, without the artefacts of random orientation seen in studies using isolated protoplasts. This method involving the pre-embedding staining technique offers considerable potential for studies of developmental problems involving membrane-bound antigens.

Alternatively, the post embedding method may provide a more satisfactory solution. The tissue is embedded and sectioned to ensure entry of antibodies to cut cell surfaces. However, depending on the supporting matrix, binding may occur only at the surface of the section. Plant tissues have recently been infiltrated and embedded in plastic resins for immunocytochemistry, a technique which permits antibody access to all cut surfaces in the thin 0.5–1 µm sections. Two main problems have been encountered in animal and plant studies: (1) denaturation of antigenic determinants during embedding procedures (Striker *et al.*, 1966) has been partially overcome by use of plastic resins that do not require heat for polymerization and are more water soluble, thus allowing increased antibody access to the tissues; (2) non-specific binding of labelled antibodies to the surface of the plastic section (Striker *et al.*, 1966; Sternberger, 1974; Shahrabadi and Yamamoto, 1971), problems that have been largely solved by purification of the resin (e.g. Tippett and O'Brien, 1976) or by more thorough washing procedures after incubation.

The specificity of immunocytochemical reactions may be questioned because of a number of non-specific interactions that may occur with certain components of plant cells. Certain lectins, common components of plant cells, especially in legume seeds, may bind IgG (see Clarke *et al.*, 1975). Most immunocytochemical studies of seed antigens have required considerable antibody purification, and consequent reduction of total IgG levels (Graham and Guning, 1970; Baumgartner *et al.*, 1978; Craig *et al.*, 1979). Non-specific binding to secondary-thickened cell walls, especially those of xylem vessels of vascular tissue is often encountered in immunofluorescence studies of plant tissues, and is presumably caused by binding of the antibody or probe to phenolic components which also bind basic dyes in histochemical studies. These non-specific interactions point to the importance of an adequate set of controls in the experimental design, which should include both normal (pre-immune) IgG and another standard protein such as albumin.

Aldehyde fixatives, such as formaldehyde and glutaraldehyde, are efficient cross-linkers of proteins, and may be expected to have a deleterious effect on the antigen–antibody interaction, reducing the binding of antibody in animal cell studies (Nakane, 1973). Attempts to demonstrate the effects of fixatives on the antigen–antibody interaction are not easy; Craig *et al.* (1979) have used double immunodiffusion to assess the effects of aldehyde fixatives on a plant antigen *in vitro*, and found it retained its ability to form a precipitin line after similar fixation treatment given to tissues, Such experiments may not necessarily throw light on the *in vivo* situation, where the antigen may be closely associated with other cell components, and may be affected differently by fixation. Both formaldehyde and glutaraldehyde are known to alter the structure of plant glycoproteins; for example, pollen allergens are modified to 'allergoids' which are immunologically different (Marsh, 1975). It is obviously essential that the effects of fixation are monitored in immunocytochemical reactions, just as the effects of fixation on enzyme activity are estimated in enzyme cytochemistry.

A quantitative approach to this problem has recently been developed for animal tissue antigens by Kraehenbuhl (1979). He coupled the antigen to Sepharose beads, and demonstrated the effects of fixation on the immunocytochemical reactions of fixed beads. He found that even concentrations of glutaraldehyde as low as 0.5% were almost completely inhibitory to the immunological reaction in times as short as 15 minutes. He recommends the use of even lower concentrations of glutaraldehyde for short periods. In a recent study of the effects of fixation on plant glycoproteins, Howlett *et al.* (1981) showed that fixation in 2.5% glutaraldehyde for 1 h at 4 °C depressed antibody-binding ability by 15%, whilst paraformaldehyde had no effect. These studies made use of a novel radioimmunoassay method involving the binding of antigen to the wells of PVC microtitre trays, exposure to the fixative, antibody-binding and detection of bound antibody by $[^{125}I]$Protein A. Paraformaldehyde has been widely used in plant studies where chemical fixation has been employed, though there is a tendency for use of low temperature and minimum incubation periods. Aldehyde fixatives are directed against proteins rather than carbohydrates and thus denature most antigens. Possibilities exist for designing a fixative which is directed against lipid and carbohydrate components of the cell structure, with less interaction with protein components. Some success for animal antigens has been achieved with a periodate:lysine:paraformaldehyde fixative, which has been useful for relatively weak antigens which have been localized in apparently well preserved tissue (Nakane, 1973). *p*-Benzoquinone and diimidoesters are chemical fixatives that have also still to be explored for plant tissues (Pearse and Polak, 1975). Some of these have been partially successful in preserving the antigenicity of peptide antigens of animal tissues but none could match the ultrastructural preservation obtained with glutaraldehyde. The possibilities offered by freeze-substitution and modern methods of freeze-drying (Edelmann, 1978) are especially important for soluble antigens, and those that are sensitive to chemical fixation.

3. Detection of Bound Antibody

Suitable antibody markers for the light microscope include fluorescein isothiocyanate (FITC), lissamine rhodamine B (LRB) tetramethyl rhodamine isothiocyanate (TRITC), and stilbene isothiocyanate (SITC). For fluorescence microscopy, it is essential that the best filter combinations be used (Cornelisse and Ploem 1976). FITC gives an intense green fluorescence with blue or violet excitation (365–405 nm) but autofluorescence of tissue components may be minimized by using short pass filters with emission at a higher wavelength between 485 and 500 nm. LRB provides more stable conjugates than TRITC and has an advantage over FITC in giving less fading problems and reduced autofluorescence of tissue components at its higher excitation wavelength. Stilbene is a relatively new probe, gives a blue emission by excitation at 365–405 nm, and should be useful in double labelling techniques. These fluorescent markers have the advantage of giving the highest possible resolution in the light microscope, since the colours are viewed against a dark background. Epi-illumination systems are now widely available for fluorescence microscopy and these provide the additional advantage of being suitable for the study of markers attached to uneven plant or cell surfaces, or in interacting cells or surfaces. Following conjugation, it is important to check the affinity of the labelled antibody for its original antigen by immunodiffusion.

Immunofluorescence methods have greater sensitivity in antigen detection than diffusion-in-gel methods because they involve direct immunoprecipitation, visualized by the fluorescent tracer, rather than extensive precipitates in a gel matrix. On animal cell surfaces, the limit of detection has been estimated at between 100 and 1000 FITC molecules per cell surface by immunofluorescence (Cornelisse and Ploem, 1976), and the amount of binding has been shown to be quantitatively related to the number of antigen molecules or their concentration and also to that of the antibody in the incubation medium. Soluble antigens can be effectively fixed by interaction with high concentrations of high affinity antibody—a technique that has been used to fix pollen antigens on the stigma during pollination (Knox and Heslop-Harrison, 1971; Knox, 1973).

Quantitative estimates of the concentration of two different fluorescent markers, such as in double-labelling experiments with FITC and TRITC, may be achieved by the two-wavelength excitation method of Cornelisse and Ploem (1976). The fluorescence of the tissue is measured using a microscope fluorometer, first with lower wavelength blue excitation which causes both fluorochromes to fluoresce, and second with green excitation when only the red fluorescence is estimated. The values for green fluorescence are obtained by subtraction. In a semi-quantitative study with rhodamine-labelled antibody, Pierard *et al.* (1981) followed the appearance and disappearance of three antigenic proteins during the transition to flowering in the shoot apex of *Sinapis*. They measured the specific fluorescence of cores of tissue, which is computed by deducting values from control sections treated with pre-immune IgG.

Other light microscope markers include enzymes such as horseradish peroxidase or acid phosphatase, which may be conjugated to the antibody, and their presence revealed by cytochemical simultaneous coupling procedures. Thus, the antibody is detected by the enzyme activity as a coloured reaction product. This has the disadvantage that the colours are more difficult to detect in low concentration by bright field microscopy and also that native enzymes present in the tissue must be inhibited prior to antigen detection. However, they have the advantage of quantitation by microdensitometry rather than the more sophisiticated equipment needed for microfluorometry.

In order to be visualized in the transmission electron microscope, antibody markers must possess electron opacity—a characteristic of metal atoms. For immuno-electron microscopy, antibody may be labelled with ferritin, a marker which is electron-dense because of its high content of iron atoms. Each ferritin molecule contains approximately 3,000 iron atoms, in the form of ferric hydroxide micelles of 6 nm diameter with a protein shell of 12 nm diameter, giving a molecular weight of 550,000. When covalently conjugated to IgG the molecular weight of the complex is $\sim 10^6$. An example of an antigen detected using ferritin-labelled antibodies is the enzyme cellulase in epicotyls of pea, *Pisum savitum* (Bal *et al.*, 1976). This study, and a succeeding one from members of the same group who have localized leghaemoglobin, a protein produced by root cells in response to bacterial symbiosis (Verma *et al.*, 1978) have both been carried out by the pre-embedding staining technique. The post-embedding technique has proved successful in two cases for immunoelectron microscopy. Coleman and Pratt (1974) used polyethylene glycol to embed and section oat coleoptile, and peroxidase-labelled antibody to locate phytochrome by the indirect method. Knox *et al.* (1980) have used plastic-resin embedded sections and ferritin-labelled antibodies to locate two antigens of ryegrass pollen also by the indirect method.

The problems involved in immunolectron microscopy have been reviewed by Knox and Clarke (1979). They include a number of interpretative difficulties: (1) the need for sufficient antibody binding for the marker to be detectable in an ultra-thin section; (2) heterogeneity and false negative results in the pre- or post-embedding technique in sections of cut cells as the field of view moves away from the cut surface; (3) the difficulties of assessing the absence of binding in control sections when very little tissue can actually be surveyed in each field or even section. These, however, are basic problems of transmission electron microscopy, and point to the need for detailed and thorough preliminary immunofluorescence studies of antigen localization.

A. Localization of Intracellular Antigens

One of the major problems in attempting to localize intracellular antigens, is to ensure access of the antibodies to the sites of the antigen. This has now been tackled in a variety of ways from the use of sophisticated sectioning procedures to exposure of whole cells treated with enzymes to increase permeability. The following three case histories illustrate the potentialities and difficulties involved.

1. Enzymes and Storage Proteins of Seeds

A feature of these cases is the sophistication in techniques revealed even in the first study by Graham and Gunning (1970). Antigen affinity chromatography was used to fractionate the antiserum so that only specific IgG antibodies were employed for localization of two storage protein antigens, legumin and vicilin, in the cotyledon cells of broad bean, *Vicia faba*. Specificity for legumin or vicilin was obtained by immunoabsorption of FITC-labelled IgG preparations. Frozen sections 10 μm in thickness were used for immunofluorescence by the direct method, after fixation in 2.5% glutaraldehyde. The sections were incubated for a minimum of 1 h at 37 °C, and specific fluorescence was associated with the protein bodies in the cytoplasm. Similar results were recently obtained by Craig *et al.* (1979) in a study of legumin localization in the cotyledons of the pea, *Pisum sativum*, using the post-embedding staining method. In initial experiments, rhodamine-labelled antibodies were employed, with the tissue embedded in glycol-methacrylate (Craig *et al.*, 1979). In a more recent work, gold-conjugated Protein A has been used to visualize antibody-binding by transmission electron microscopy in ultra-thin sections of tissue embedded in glycomethacrylate or Spurr's resin (Craig and Millerd, 1981). An advantage of this method is that double-labelling experiments could be performed because the gold particles can be produced in small or large sizes permitting the localization of two different antigens simultaneously.

The necessity for adequate control tests in immunocytochemical studies of legume seeds was pointed out by Clarke *et al.* (1975) who found that rabbit IgG bound most effectively to the lectin concanavalin A in sections of cotyledons of jack bean, *Canavalia ensiformis*. The lectin was able to bind to the carbohydrate chains of the IgG. The problem of adequate control becomes acute in immuno-electron microscopy. In a recent study Craig and Millerd (1981) carried out eight different controls to establish the validity of their immunocytochemical staining with antibody detected by gold-labelled Protein A. Some gold deposition occurred in a dilution-dependent fashion following incubation with pre-immune IgG, although no binding occurred using antibody absorbed with excess antigen.

Of especial interest is a developmental immunofluorescence study by Chrispeels and Baumgartner (1978) of a proteolytic enzyme which hydrolyses the major protein reserve in mung bean seeds. A unique feature of this study is the use of ultracryotomy. Small pieces of tissue were fixed in 4% paraformaldehyde in sodium phosphate buffer a pH 7.5, containing 0.14 M NaCl, 0.1 M sucrose, and 0.02% sodium azide, for 12 h at 3°C, then transferred to the fixative in 0.9 M sucrose for 5 h, before the blocks were frozen in liquid nitrogen on copper rods, and sections 0.2–5 μm in thickness cut with glass knives in the cryokit bowl of an ultramicrotome. Sections were picked up on a small wire loop in a semi-frozen drop of fixative in 2.3 M sucrose, brought to room temperature and mounted on slides pre-coated with 1% silicone. Reactive groups of the aldehyde fixative were bound to 0.01 M glycine in phosphate-buffered saline before indirect immunofluorescence staining with monospecific antibodies for 8–10 minutes, washed and incubated with the anti-antibody labelled with lissamine rhodamine B for 7 minutes at a concentration of 0.3 mg/ml. Sections were washed and mounted in 90% glycerol and viewed by incident fluorescence microscopy using a green excitation filter.

The results of the immunofluorescence study precisely matched those of biochemical analyses. In ungerminated seeds, and on the first day of germination no enzyme activity could be detected (Figure 7A). By day 3, specific fluorescence was present in discrete areas of the cytoplasm, (Figure 7B), and only one day later was present in the protein bodies in addition to the cytoplasmic sites (Figure 7C).

The combination of thin sections and specific IgG antibodies not only enhanced immunological specificity, but greatly reduced incubation times to a total of 15 minutes compared with a minimum of 60 minutes in previous studies. The use of an immune serum control on day 1 tissue (in absence of the enzyme) is a particularly striking feature of these results. Chrispeels and Baumgartner (1978) record that non-specific binding had been a problem when whole antiserum was used containing high concentrations of IgG. This is presumably due to the presence of lectins (Clarke *et al.*, 1975). These methods do offer the real possibility of obtaining precise antigen localization within plant cells as the sectioning overcomes some of the difficulties of penetration through the walls and plasma membrane.

2. Antigens Associated with Cytoskeletal Elements of Plant Cells

Cytoplasmic streaming is a feature of living plant cells and it has been studied in cell models in which the plasma membrane or the tonoplast surrounding the cytoplasm has been removed. Williamson and Toh (1979) have reviewed work on a cell model they have developed of the giant internodal cells of characean algae. In this system, the tonoplast was removed by rapid vacuolar perfusion, to give a model in which streaming can be reactivated, and is associated with subcortical fibrils. They have demonstrated by indirect immunofluorescence that these fibrils stain with anti-actin antibodies from human smooth muscle. This antibody preparation cross-reacts with a wide variety of cytoplasmic actins in many types of animal cells (Toh *et al.*, 1976). The antibody preparation was introduced into the living cell model by slow perfusion over 30 minutes. The specific fluorescence was associated with cortical fibrils of indefinite length, and was clearly distinguishable from the red autofluorescence of the chloroplasts. An interesting feature of these experiments is that perfusion provided a suitable method of washing out unreacted labelled antibody from the cell to give good specificity of staining. This study appears to be the first application of immunofluorescence to living plant cells.

The fibrillar cytoskeleton of plant cells, composed of microtubules and microfilaments, has been investigated by immunofluorescence by two groups who have also made use of the cross-reactivity of antisera raised against another animal antigen, tubulin. Mammalian anti-tubulin antibodies have been shown by Franke and co-workers (1977) to bind to the mitotic spindle fibres of dividing endosperm cells of *Leucojum*, the March cup flower. More recently Lloyd and co-workers (1979) used carrot callus cells to demonstrate indirect immunofluorescence binding of mammalian anti-tubulin antibodies to cytoplasmic fibrils associated with the plasma membrane in cellulose-treated suspension cultured cells or in isolated protoplasts. The cells were attached to polylysine-treated coverslips before being extracted in isotonic microtubule-stabilizing buffer containing the detergent Triton X-100 followed by brief fixation in formaldehyde. Elongated cells showed a pattern of fibrils at right angles to the long axis of the cells (Figure 8). The fluorescent images obtained are consistent with the cross-bridged state of plant microtubules, which were visualized as interconnected transverse loops. These experiments have been used to study the role of microtubules in the control of cell shape and the cell cycle (Wick *et al.* 1981).

B. Localization of Extracellular Antigens Associated with the Pollen–Stigma Interaction

The first immunocytochemical studies of flowering plant antigens were made on the proteins diffusing from pollen grains, when they were shown to be located in wall sites (Knox *et al.*, 1970). In subsequent studies, it has become clear that the intricate sculpturing of the outer exine layer of the pollen wall may be an adaptation for the storage of these wall proteins and glycoproteins revealed by immunofluorescence. Immunofluorescence methods both with freeze-sectioned pollen and with 'pollen-prints', the impressions left on a thin agarose film when antigens diffuse from grains pressed against the film for periods of 5 seconds–15 minutes, reveal the sites of storage within the wall and the routes and kinetics of emission (Heslop-Harrison *et al.*, 1973; Belin and Rowley, 1971; Howlett *et al.*, 1973; Heslop-Harrison, 1975a,b).

Pollen interactions with the stigma surface have also been revealed by use of immunofluorescence methods. The exine antigens make initial contact with the stigma surface (Knox and Heslop-Harrison, 1971) and pollen antigens are released and bind to the adjacent stigma surface during pollination, and are present on the surface of the pollen tube that transports the gametes to the egg cell (Knox and Heslop-Harrison, 1971; Knox *et al.*, 1972; Knox, 1973).

The S-antigen that regulates self-incompatibility reactions between pollen and stigma has been shown to diffuse readily from stigmas of cabbage, *Brassica oleracea* (Nasrallah and Wallace 1967a,b), and stigma antigens of *Brassica*

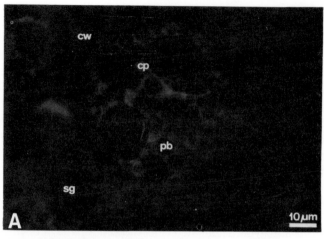

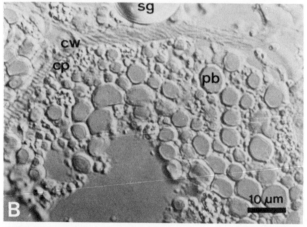

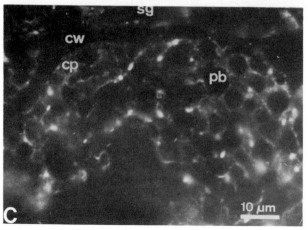

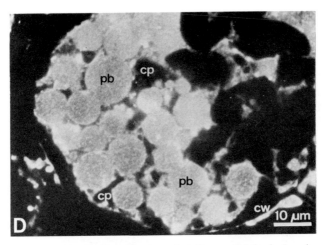

Figure 7. Immunocytochemical localization of vicilin peptidohydrolase in germinating cotyledons of mung bean, *Vigna radiata* using frozen sections 0.5 μm in thickness and the indirect method with goat anti-rabbit IgG labelled with lissamine rhodamine B. Reproduced with permission from Baumgartner *et al.*, 1978. Figure 7A day 1 seedling, specific IgG, only faint background fluorescence associated with cytoplasm; Figures 7B and 7C 3-day-old seedling cotyledon, specific IgG, fluorescence present in distinct foci in the cytoplasm but absent from protein bodies and cell walls: (B) Nomarski DIC optics; (C) Epifluorescence illumination; (D) 4-day-old seedling cotyledon, fluorescence present both in cytoplasm and protein bodies (cp, cytoplasm; cw, cell wall; pb, protein body; sg, starch grain)

have been located on the surface of the receptive cells (Helsop-Harrison *et al.*, 1975) where they are secreted to provide both for pollen adhesion and for the early events of pollination. Recently, progress has been made in the localization of S-allele specific antigens in sweet cherry, *Prunus avium*, where the S-antigen has been identified by immunoelectrophoresis, and been shown to be present both in the stigma cells and in the transmitting tissue that provides both a route and nutrition for the pollen tube (Raff *et al.*, 1980).

The allergens of ragweed pollen were localized by immunofluorescence in both the inner intine and outer exine layers of the pollen wall, like the other antigens present (Knox *et al.*, 1970; Knox and Heslop-Harrison 1971; Howlett *et al.*, 1973). The allergens of grass pollen especially Group 1 allergen, have proved much more intractable to locate in mature pollen, and the freeze-sectioning methods used for the ragweed studies failed to provide a convincing localization in the wall sites, with very rapid diffusion to the outer surface in even the briefest exposure to aqueous media. Recently, a combination of anhydrous processing and the post-embedding technique using the plastic resin JB-4 has resulted in precise location of the allergen both by immunofluores-

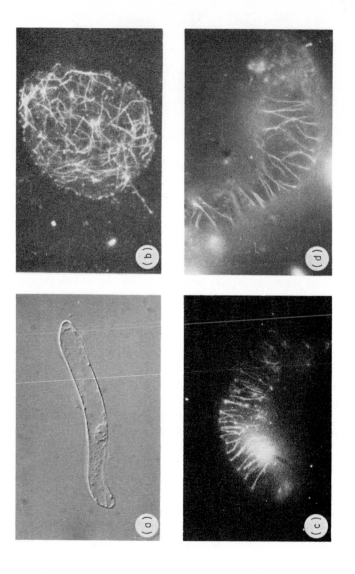

Figure 8. Immunofluorescent localization of tubulin in microtubule-like structures in cultured callus cells and protoplasts of carrot, *Daucus carota*, using the indirect technique and FITC-labelled goat anti-rabbit IgG. Reproduced with permission from Lloyd *et al*. (1979). (a) Appearance of elongate carrot cell, Nomarski DIC optics ($\times$ 300); (b) 'Footprint' or unravelled fibrils fluorescing in a cell converted into a protoplast by 60 minute cellulase treatment ($\times$ 740); (c) and (d) Fluorescence in elongated cells after only 30 minutes cellulase treatment showing fluorescent fibrils running in interconnected hoops transversely around the elongate cells ($\times$ 740). b,c,d, Fluorescence illumination

cence and immunoelectron microscopy. In mature grains, ferritin-labelled antibodies raised against Group 1 allergen or Antigen A were detected in the outer wall cavities and on the surface of the grains (Knox *et al.*, 1980; Vithanage *et al.*, 1982). The route for release is through small microchannels on both inner and outer surfaces of the exine wall layer. Immunofluorescence alone did not provide sufficient resolution to determine the precise wall location of the antigens, and this was provided by the ferritin-labelled antibodies in the transmission electron microscope.

V. INTERACTIONS OF IgE ANTIBODY AND PLANT ALLERGENS

Environmental agents, such as pollen, may initiate the allergic response in susceptible humans. People who are allergic have an altered capacity to react to potential allergens or are said to be hypersensitive to them. Pollens have been implicated in several allergic diseases, including asthma (allergic lung disease), hay fever (allergic rhinitis), together with several eye, skin, and respiratory disorders. As early as 1831, Elliotson observed that the worst of catarrh symptoms accompanied the maturing of the grasses during the haymaking season. Later Blackley (1873) demonstrated the role of pollen in initiating allergic disease and the presence of the allergenic pollens in the atmosphere. Kammann (1903) and later Noon (1911) found that protein extracts of grass pollen produced skin reactions in sensitive patients. Since then considerable efforts have been made to understand more about the nature of these proteins and glycoproteins, which are termed allergens because they are capable of eliciting the formation of specific skin-sensitizing or reaginic antibodies, Immunoglobulin E (IgE), in susceptible humans. Ishizaka and co-workers (1966) demonstrated that when certain genetically predisposed individuals become exposed to allergens, specific IgE is formed and may bind to pairs of adjacent IgE molecules on the surface of the mast cells, resulting in degranulation and the release of histamine and other substances causing contraction of smooth muscle of bronchioles, vasoconstriction, and other symptoms of allergic disease.

A. Nature of Plant Allergens

Pollen types that may act as sources of allergens are generally those that utilize air currents for pollination rather than animal vectors. There are three main classes: (1) tree pollen which is released in late winter and early spring in temperate climates, and includes conifers, such as cypress, birch, and alder; (2) grass pollen which is released in spring and early summer in temperate climates, especially cocksfoot, timothy, ryegrass and bermuda grass; (3) weeds and other herbs, released in summer and fall, including various chenopods, amaranths and ragweeds.

Pollen allergens are proteins or glycoproteins, and have been purified and characterized for ragweed and grass pollens. T. P. King and co-workers at the Rockefeller University in New York isolated and purified the allergens from ragweed pollen in 1964, naming the two most potent Antigens E and K. They have proved to be acidic proteins comprising two subunits, an α chain of molecular weight 21,800 and a β chain of molecular weight 15,700, giving a total molecular weight of 38,000. The two chains are readily dissociated by heat, are linked by covalent bonds, and when separated, have very little allergenic or antigenic activity. Several other chemical modifications have been carried out (see review by King, 1976). Antigen E is present in four different forms, that are all immunologically similar but differ in isoelectric points. Atigens E and K contain less than 1% carbohydrate, account for 6% and 3%, respectively, of the soluble pollen protein, and show partial immunological identity. Three other basic protein allergens have been isolated from ragweed pollen: Antigen Ra3 (Underdown and Goodfriend, 1969), Ra5 (Lapkoff and Goodfriend, 1974), and Ra4 or BPA-R (Griffiths and Brunet, 1971; Roebber *et al.*, 1975). The amino acid sequence of Antigen Ra5 has been determined and consists of 45 amino acids, 8 of which are cysteine (Mole *et al.*, 1975). At the terminal end of the polypeptide three of the five amino acids are lysine, making this region very alkaline.

The allergens of grass pollen are equally complex, and three groups of heat-stable glycoproteins are the principal allergens. The two major groups of allergens of ryegrass, *Lolium perenne*, named groups I and II by Johnson and Marsh (1965) have molecular weights of 30,000 and 10,000 and each have several isoallergens differing in isoelectric point. The Group I allergens appear to differ in amino acid composition only in the ration of glutamate to glutamine. Groups III and IV allergens are basic with molecular weights of 11,000 and 50,000 respectively (Marsh, 1975). Augustin and co-workers (1959, 1963, 1971) isolated a series of allergens from cocksfoot (*Dactylis glomerata*) and timothy (*Phleum pratense*) pollen, called the I antigens. Each of the allergens proved to be antigenic in rabbits. The major antigen, Antigen A, however, proved to have much less allergenic activity than the I antigens.

In northern Europe, the pollen of birch, *Betula verrucosa*, and alder, *Alnus glutinosa*, are equally important as the grasses. Birch pollen contains an acidic protein allergen, molecular weight 20,000, which has been partially purified (Belin, 1972). This antigen cross-reacts immunologically with the alder allergen (Herbestson *et al.*, 1978).

B. Detection of Pollen Allergens

Pollen allergens may be detected in sensitized individuals by a number of *in vivo* tests, for example, direct skin testing using a small sample of the suspected allergen usually in a buffered saline extract, which is pricked intradermally on the forearm, giving a swollen red wheal in allergic patients. This can be compared with a histamine control to give an indication of the allergenicity of the sample. Similarly, bronchial provocation tests provide an indication of lung sensitivity. *In vitro* tests include the ability of allergens to release histamine from sensitized leukocytes. However, the affinity of IgE in the sera of allergic subjects for its specific allergen provides the basis of the radioallergosorbent test (RAST), a relatively simple and highly specific means of measuring the concentration of IgE in the serum of normal healthy people and in allergic individuals. Since IgE is present at much lower concentrations than IgG, probably by a factor of 500,000 times less, it cannot be detected by immunodiffusion methods. Instead, use is made of its affinity for specific allergen, which is insolubilized to a solid phase, such as a filter paper disk (Figure 9). For testing, the allergen-coated disk is first incubated with a drop of the patient's serum which contains the IgE to be estimated, and after several hours, it is washed to remove unbound proteins that will not interact with the allergen molecules. The specific IgE on the disk is detected by its interaction with ^{125}I-labelled antiserum raised in a sheep against human IgE. The amount of radioactivity present is estimated with a gamma counter, and is computed in units of IgE in relation to a standard control serum used in the test. Results show that healthy people have, in general, a low level of IgE, around 14 units per millilitre of serum, while in allergic patients, levels rise in excess of 100 units per millilitre. The test has been in laboratory use since 1969 and provides a high degree of discrimination between allergic and non-allergic individuals.

IgE antibody concentrations in serum are not constant, and will increase with challenge by an allergen. In hay fever patients, Johansson (1974) in Sweden has found that the lowest levels occur in the 2 weeks before onset of the pollen season. There can be a two- or threefold increase in IgE levels during the pollen season, followed by a gradual decrease back to pre-seasonal levels. Results with tree, grass, and ragweed pollens as allergens with proven pollen-sensitive patients have demonstrated that RAST reactivity is in good agreement with the other methods of testing.

RAST inhibition is a test in which the ability of the solid phase allergen to bind to IgE in allergic sera is tested in the presence of competing soluble allergens from other species with allergenic pollen. The soluble phase allergens act as an inhibitor of IgE binding to the solid phase allergen in proportion to the similarity of its allergenic determinants. In experiments with various ragweed and grass species, Gleich *et al.* (1975) demonstrated the immunological distance between the pollen allergens (Figure 9). The most closely related ragweeds and grasses showed inhibition with low levels of pollen allergens as inhibitors, while other species showed little inhibitory effect.

Binding of pollen allergens to specific IgE has provided a unique means of detecting the allergens within complex mixtures, and has been utilized to detect specific IgE-binding antigens by crossed-radioimmunoelectrophoresis in

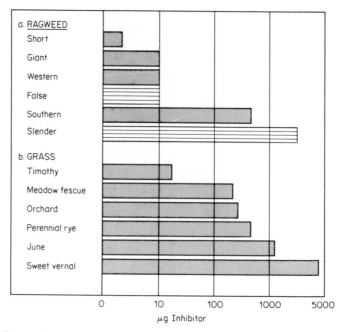

Figure 9. Comparison of the cross-reactivity of allergens from pollen of ragweeds (a) or grasses (b) determined by RAST inhibition. The test gives a measure of the immunological distance of the allergenic determinants. In (a) the solid phase allergen was an extract of short ragweed, *Ambrosia elatior*, and the peaks indicate the concentration of competing pollen extracts from other species required to produce 50% inhibition in the RAST. Giant ragweed, *Ambrosia trifida*; western, *A. coronopifolia*; false, *Franseria acanthicarpa*; slender, *F. tenuifulia*; southern *A. bidentata*. In (b) the solid phase allergen was timothy pollen extract, *Phleum pratense*, and the competing fluid phase extracts were of meadow fescue, *Festuca pratensis*; five grass, *Poa pratensis*; orchard grass, *Dactylis glomerata*; perennial ryegrass, *Lolium perenne*; and sweet vernal grass, *Anthoxanthum odoratum*. Data replotted from Gleich *et al.* (1975)

various grass pollens (Weeke *et al.*, 1973; Lowenstein, 1978). In pollen of ryegrass, radioimmunoelectrophoresis was used in conjunction with biochemical extraction procedures to characterize the Group I allergens (Smart and Knox, 1979). A feature of these results was that specific IgE from ryegrass-sensitive patients had an affinity not only for the two Group I allergen precipitin arcs, but for Antigen A, a cathodal-migrating antigen of low allergenic activity.

Affinity for specific IgE has not yet been used as a means of localizing allergens within pollen grains by cytochemical methods. This is probably because of the low levels of IgE in allergic sera, and the unavailability of commercial preparations. Instead, rabbit antisera raised to purified allergens have been used to localize allergens from ragweed, grass and birch pollen by immunocytochemistry (see Section IV.B).

VI. CONCLUSIONS AND FUTURE DEVELOPMENTS

Immunochemistry has been a valuable tool in plant biology, where its applications have closely followed technical developments in animal cell biology. The concept of the antigen and antibody is one that is foreign to plant cell biology because of the lack of circulating cells in plants, although circulating macromolecules may exist. Movement of macromolecules in plants has been demonstrated only in the bleeding sap which exudes from a wounded surface.

Organ and species specificity of plant antigens has been demonstrated in several systems; antigens have been considered to be markers of tissue, organ and cellular identity, and differentiation. Quantitative differences in cross-reactivity between antigens of different individual genotypes, cultivars, species or genera have been correlated with several biological responses of the organs, tissues, or cells which contain them; for example, the grafting ability of stems or the production of viable hybrid seeds. Molecular differences detected by the immune system of the experimental animal are mirrored by response of the cells containing the antigens. It is in this area that immunochemistry has made its greatest contribution to plant biology.

In addition, immunochemistry has proved invaluable in monitoring the isolation and purification of plant proteins and glycoproteins. Several purified plant glycoproteins with no demonstrable enzymic activity have now been successfully isolated and characterized. The unique specificity and sensitivity of immunochemical methods have also enabled the synthesis of a few of these macromolecules to be followed by *in vitro* cell-free translation systems.

Immunocytochemistry is now widely used in plant cell biology, at both the light and electron microscopic levels. Both the pre-embedding and post-embedding staining procedures have been used. Suitable antibody markers include the range of fluorescent probes which provide the highest resolution by light microscopy, and ferritin, gold or enzymic markers such as horseradish peroxidase at the ultrastructural level.

A future development of considerable importance is likely to be the application of monoclonal antibodies to the immunochemical characterization and localization of plant antigens. This powerful technique greatly increases the antibody specificity so that individual or smaller groups of antigenic determinants may be detected. The method is likely to be particularly useful in detecting differences in antigens of closely related species, cultivars or individual plants and in immunochemical studies of cellular proteins and glycoproteins of common occurrence in plant cells.

Immunocytochemistry offers the possibility of studying interactions between plant cell and organ surfaces, for example, in stem transplants plant interactions with symbionts and pathogens, and during sexual reproduction. The availability of a range of probes for light and electron microscopic applications will provide renewed impetus for the study of cell–cell interactions in plants.

REFERENCES

Abelev, G. I. (1960). Modification of the agar precipitin method for comparing two antigen–antiserum systems. *Folia Biol.*, **6**, 56–58.

Alexandrescu, V. and Mihailescu, F. (1973). Immunochemical investigations on germinated seed endosperm α-amylase of some cereals. *Rev. Roum. Biochim.*, **10**, 89–94.

Alexandrescu, V. and Paun, L. (1975). Amylases in the endosperms of wheat, rye and triticale germinated seeds. I. Electrophoretic and immuno-electrophoretic investigations. *Rev. Roum. Biochim.*, **12**, 3–5.

Ashford, A. E. and Knox, R. B. (1980). Characteristics of pollen diffusates and pollen-wall cytochemistry in poplars. *J. Cell Sci.* (in press).

Augustin, R. (1963). Antigens and other allergens of grass pollens. *Proc. 5th Eur. Congr. Allergy, Basle* (Sellostverlag der Schweizerischen Allergie-Gesellschaft). 137–146.

Augustin, R., O'Sullivan, S., and Davies, E. (1971). Isolation of grass pollen antigens failing to induce IgE reagin formation though capable of inducing IgG antibody formation. *Int. Archs Allergy*, **41**, 144–147.

Badley, R. A., Lloyd, C. W., Woods, A., Carruthers, L., Allvack, C., and Rees, D. A. (1978). Mechanisms of cellular adhesion III. Preparation and preliminary characterization of adhesions. *Exp. Cell Res.*, **117**, 231–244.

Bal, W. K., Verma, D. P. S., Byrne, H. and Maclachlan, G. A. (1976). Subcellular localization of cellulases in auxin-treated pea. *J. Cell Biol.*, **69**, 97–105.

Barlow, K. K., Simmonds, D. H., and Kenrick, K. G. (1973). The localization of water-soluble proteins in the wheat endosperm as revealed by fluorescent antibody techniques. *Experientia (Basel)*, **29**, 229–231.

Baumgartner, B. and Matile, Ph. (1976). Immunocytochemical localization of acid ribonuclease in morning glory flower tissue. *Biochem Physiol. Pflanzen*, **170**, 279–285.

Baumgartner, B., Tokuyasu, K. T., and Chrispeels, M. J. (1978). Localization of vicilin peptidohydrolase in the cotyledons of mung bean seedlings by immuno-fluorescence microscopy. *J. Cell. Biol.*, **79**, 10–9.

Belin, L. (1972). Separation and characterisation of birch pollen antigens with special reference to the allergenic components. *Int. Archs. Allergy. Appl. Immun.*, **42**, 329–342.

Belin, L. and Rowley, J. R. (1971). Demonstration of birch pollen allergen from isolated pollen grains using immunofluorescence and a single radial immunodiffusion technique. *Int. Arch. Allergy Appl. Immunol.*, **40**, 754–769.

Berzborn, R. (1969). Untersuchungen uber die Oberflachenstruktur des Thylakoidsystems der Chloroplasten mit Hilfe von Antikorpen gegen die Ferredoxin-NADP-Reduktase, *Z. Naturforsch.*, **24b**, 436–446.

Berzborn, R., Menke, W., Trebst, A., and Pistorius, E. (1966). Uber die Hemmung photosynthetischer Reaktionen isolierter Chloroplasten durch Chloroplasten-Antikorper. *Z. Naturforsch.*, **21b**, 230–235.

Blackley, C. H. (1873). *Experimental Researches on the Cause and Nature of Catarrhus aestivus.* Bailiere, Tindall and Cox, London.

Bonner, W. M. and R. A. Laskey. (1974). A film detection method for tritium-labelled proteins and nucleic acids in polyacrylamide gels. *Euro, J. Biochem.*, **46**, 83–88.

Bourcelier, C. and Daussant, J. (1973). La fraction I protéique du limbe de Blé: purification et caractérisation immunochimique préliminaire. *C.R. Acad. Sc.*, **276**, série D, 2525–2528.

Boutenko, R. G. and Volodarsky, A. D. (1968). Analyse immunochimique de la différenciation cellulaire dans les cultures de tissus de tabac. *Physiol. Veg.*, **6**, 299–306.

Burnet, F. M. (1972). *Self and Not Self.* Melbourne University Press.

Catsimpoolas, N., Campbell, T. G., and Mayer, E. W. (1968). Immunochemical study on changes in reserve proteins of germinating soybean seeds. *Plant Physiol.*, **43**, 799–805.

Chrispeels, M. J. and Baumgartner, B. (1977). Trypsin inhibitor in mung bean cotyledons, purification, characteristics, sub-cellular localization and metabolism. *Plant Physiol.*, **61**, 617–623.

Chrispeels, M. J. and Baumgartner, B. (1978). Serological evidence confirming the assignment of *Phaseolus aureus* and *P. mungo* to the genus *Vigna. Phytochem.*, **17**, 125–126.

Clarke, A. E., Gleeson, P. A., Jermyn, M. A., and Knox, R. B. (1979). Characterization and localization of β-lectins in lower and higher plants. *Aust. J. Plant Physiol.*, **5**, 707–722.

Clarke, A. E. and Knox, R. B. (1978). Cell recognition in plants. *Q. Rev. Biol.*, **53**, 3–28.

Clarke, A. E. and Knox, R. B. (1980). Plants and immunity. *Devel. Comp. Immunol* **3**, 571–589 and **4**, 379–382.

Clarke, A. E., Knox, R. B., Harrison, S., Raff, J., and Marchalonis, J. (1977). Common antigens and male-female recognition in plants. *Nature (Lond.)*, **265**, 161–163.

Clarke, A. E., Knox, R. B., and Jermyn, M. A. (1975). Localization of lectins in legume cotyledons. *J. Cell. Sci.*, **19**, 157–167.

Clarke, H. G. M. and Freeman, T. A. (1967). A quantitative immunoelectrophoresis method (Laurell electrophoresis). In Peeters, *Prot. Biol. Fluids*, **14**, 503–509, Elsevier, Amsterdam.

Coons, A. H., Creech, H. J., Jones, R. N., and Berliner, E. (1942). The demonstration of pneumococcal antigens in tissues by the use of fluorescent antibody. *J. Immunol.*, **45**, 159–170.

Cornelisse, C. J. and Ploem, J. S. (1976). A new type of two-colour fluorescence staining for cytology specimens. *J. Histochem. Cytochem.*, **24**, 72–81.

Craig, I. W. and Gunning, B. E. S. (1976). *Organelle Development* In C. Graham and P. F. Wareing (Eds) *Developmental Biology of Plants and Animals*, pp. 270–301. Blackwell, Oxford.

Craig, S., Goodchild, D., and Millerd, A. (1979). Immunofluorescent localization of pea storage proteins in glycol-methacrylate embedded tissue. *J. Histochem. Cytochem.*

Craig, S. and Millerd, A. (1981). Pea seed storage proteins—immunocytochemical localization with Protein A–Goldin electron microscopy. *Protoplasma*, **105**, 333–339.

Coleman, R. A. and Pratt, L. H. (1974). Electron microscopic localization of phytochrome in plants using an indirect antibody-labelling technique. *J. Histochem. Cytochem.*, **22**, 1039–1046.

Cundiff, S. C. and Pratt, L. H. (1973). Immunological determination of the relationship between large and small sizes of phytochrome. *Plant Physiol.*, **51**, 210–216.

Dalen, van J. P. R., Knapp, W., and Ploem, J. S. (1973). Microfluorometry on antigen–antibody interaction in immunofluorescence using antigens covalently bound to agarose beads. *J. Immunol. Methods*, **2**, 383–392.

Daussant, J. (1978a). Immunochemical characterization of α-amylases in wheat seeds at different ontogenical steps. *Ann. Immunol. (Paris)*, **129** (213), 215–232.

Daussant, J. (1978b). Caractérisation immunochimique d'α-amylases de grain de blé à différents stades ontogéniques. *Ann. Immunol. (Inst. Pasteur Paris)*, **129** C, 215–232.

Daussant, J. and Corvazier, P. (1970). Biosynthesis and modifications of α- and β-amylases in germinating wheat seeds. *FEBS Lett.*, **7**, 191–194.

Daussant, J. and Grabar, P. (1966). Comparaison immunologique des α-amylases extraites des céréales. *Ann. Inst. Pasteur (Paris)*, **110**, 79–83.

Daussant, J. and Hill, R. D. (1979). Immunochemical identification of α-amylases in developing, mature and germinated *Triticale* seeds. *Physiol. Plant*, **45**, 255–59.

Daussant, J., Lauriere, C., Carfantan, N., and Skakoun, A. (1977). Immunochemical approaches to questions concerning enzyme regulation in plants. In H. Smith (Ed.) *Regulation of Enzyme Synthesis and Activity in Higher Plants*, pp. 197–223. Academic Press, New York, and London.

Daussant, J., Nevcere, N. J., and Yatsu, L. Y. (1969). Immunochemical studies on *Arachis hypogaea* proteins with particular reference to the reserve proteins. 1. Characterization, distribution, and properties of α-arachin and α-conavachin. *Plant Physiol.*, **44**, 471–479.

Davies, H., Taylor, J. E., White, D. J. G., Binn, S. R. M. (1978). Major transplantation antigens of lung, kidney and liver. Comparisons between the whole organs and their parenchymal constituents. *Transplantation*, **25**, 290–295.

Dazzo, Frank, B., Yanke, William, E., and Brill, Winston, J. (1978). Trifoliin: A *Rhizobium* recognition protein from white clover. *Biochem. Biophys. Acta*, **539** (3), 276–286.

Deverall, B. (1978). *Defence Mechanisms of Plants. Monographs in Exp. Biol.*, **19**. 110pp. Cambridge University Press, Cambridge.

Dodge, J. D. and Crawford, R. M. (1970). The morphology and fine structure of *Ceratium hirundenella* (Dinophyceae). *J. Phycol.*, **6**, 137–145.

Dudman, W. F. and Millerd, A. (1975). Immunochemical behaviour of legumin and vicilin from *Vicia faba*: survey of related proteins in the Leguminosae subfamily Faboideae. *Biochem. Syst. Ecol.*, **3**, 25–33.

Dunin, M. C., Abd-El-Rehim, M. A., and Vinitskaya, O. P. (1966). Serological relations between feeding horse bean plants and the causal agent of fusariosis. *J. Biol. Nauk.*, **1**, 265.

Dunin, M. S. and Chefranova, L. I. (1966). *Rev. Roum. Biol. ser. Bot.*, **11**, 61.

Edelmann, L. (1979). Gefriertrocknung von chemisch nicht fixiertem biologischem Material für die Elektronenmikroskopie Mikroskopie **35**, 31–36.

Ferrari, T. E., Bruns, D and Wallace, D. H. (1981) Isolation of a plant glycoprotein involved with control of intercellular recognition. Plant Physiol. **67**, 270–277.

Fishman, W. and Sell, S. (1976). Regulation of gene expression in development and neoplasia. *Cancer Res.*, **36**, 4201–4331.

Franke, W. W., Seib, E., Osborn, M., Weber, K., Herth, W., and Falk, H. (1977). Tubulin-containing structures in the anastral nutotic apparatus of endosperm cells of the plant *Leucojum aestivum* as revealed by immunofluorescence microscopy. *Cytobiologie*, **15**, 24–48.

Freed, R. C. and Ryan, D. S. (1978). Changes in Kunitz trypsin inhibitor during germination of soybean. An immunoelectrophoresis assay system. *J. Food Sci.*, **43** (4), 1316–1319.

Gatenby, A. A. (1978). A comparison of the polypeptide isoelectric points and antigenic determinant sites of the large subunit of fraction 1 protein from *Lycopersicum esculentum*, *Nicotiana tabacum* and *Petunia hybrida*. *Biochim Biophys Acta*, **534** (1), 169–172.

Gell, P. G., Hawkes, J. G., and Wright, S. T. C. (1960). The application of immunological methods to the taxonomy of species within the genus *Solanum. Proc. R. Soc.*, **B 151**, 364–383.

Gillis, T. P. *et al.* (1978). Quantitative fluorescent immunoassay of antibodies to, and surface antigens of, *Actinomyces viscosus. J. Clin. Microbiol.*, **7**, 202–8.

Gleeson, P. A. and Clarke, A. E. (1980a). Antigenic determinants of a plant proteoglycan, the *Gladiolus* style arabinogalactan protein. *Biochem. J.* (in press).

Gleeson, P. A. and Clarke, A. E. (1980b). Arabinogalactans of sexual and somatic tissues. *Phytochem.* (in press).

Gleich, G. J., Larson, J. B., Jones, R. T. and Baer, H. (1974). Measurement of the potency of allergen extracts by their inhibitory capacities in the radioallergosorbent test. *J. Allergy*, **53**, 158–169.

Goding, J. W. (1976). Conjugation of antibodies with fluorochrome modifications to the standard methods. *J. Immunol. Methods*, **12**, 81–9.

Grabar, P. and Daussant, J. (1964). Study of barley and malt amylases by immuno-chemical methods. *Cereal Chem.*, **41**, 523–532.

Grabar, P. and Williams, C. A. (1953). Méthode permettant l'étude conjuguée de propriétés électrophoréteques et immunochimiques d'un mélange de protéines: application au sérum sanguin. *Biochem. Biophys. Acta*, **10**, 193–194.

Graham, T. A. and Gunning, B. E. S. (1970). Localization of legumin and vicilin in bean cotyledon cells using fluorescent antibodies. *Nature (Lond.)*, **228**, 81–82.

Gray, J. C. (1978). Serological reactions of fraction I proteins from interspecific hybrids in the genus *Nicotiana. Plant Syst. Evol.*, **129** (3), 177–184.

Griffiths, B. W. and Brunet, R. (1971). Isolation of a basic protein antigen of low ragweed pollen. *Can. J. Biochem.*, **49**, 396–400.

Hagman, R. (1964). The use of disc electrophoresis and serological reactions in the study of pollen and style relationships. In H. F. Linskens (Ed) *Pollen Physiology and Fertilization*, pp. 244–250. North Holland.

Hall, O. (1959). Immunoelectrophoretic analyses of allopolyploid ryewheat and its parental species. *Hereditas*, **45**, 495–504.

Hankins, C. N., Kindinger, J. I., and Shannon, L. M. (1979). Legume lectins 1. Immunological cross-reactions between the enzymic lectin from mung beans and other wall characterized legume lectins. *Plant Physiol.*, **64**, 104–107.

Herbestson, S., Porath, J., and Colldahl, H. (1978). Allergens from alder pollen. *Acta Chem. Scand.*, **12**, 737–747.

Heslop-Harrison, J. (1975a). Physiology of the pollen-grain surface. *Proc. R. Soc.*, **B**, **190**, 275–299.

Heslop-Harrison, J. (1975b). Incompatibility and the pollen–stigma interaction A. *Rev. Pl. Physiol.* **26**, 403–425.

Heslop-Harrison, J., Heslop-Harrison, Y., Knox, R. B., and Howlett, B. (1973). Pollen-wall proteins: 'gametophytic' and 'sporophytic' fractions in the pollen walls of Malvaceae. *Ann. Bot.*, **37**, 402–412.

Hiedemann-Van Wyk, D. and Kannangara, C. G. (1971). Localization of ferredoxin in the thylakoid membrane with immunological methods. *Z. Naturforsch.*, **26 b**, 46–50.

Higgins, T. J. V., Zwar, J. A., and Jacobsen, J. V. (1976). Gibberellic acid enhances the level of translatable mRNA for α-amylase in barley aleurone layers. *Nature*, **260**, 166–169.

Hinata, T. and Nishio, K. (1978). S-allele specificity of stigma proteins in *Brassica oleracea* and *B. campestris. Heredity*, **41**, 93–100.

Hopkins, D. W. and Butler, W. L. (1970). Immunochemical and spectroscopic evidence for protein conformational changes in phytochrome transformations. *Plant Physiol.*, **45**, 457–70.

Horikoshi, M. and Morita, Y. (1975). Localization of γ-globulin in rice seed and changes in γ-globulin content during seed development and germination. *Agr. Biol. Chem.*, **39**, 2309–2314.

Howlett, B. J., Knox, R. B., and Heslop-Harrison, J. (1973). Pollen-wall proteins: release of the allergen Antigen E from intine and exine sites in the pollen grains of ragweed and *Cosmos*. *J. Cell Sci.*, **13**, 603–619.

Howlett, B. J., Vithanage, H. I. M. V. and Knox, R. B. (1979). Pollen antigens, allergens and enzymes. *Curr. Adv. Plant. Sci.*, **35**, 1–17.

Howlett, B. J., Vithanage, H. I. M. V. and Knox, R. B. (1981). Immunofluorescent localization of two water-soluble glycoproteins including the major allergen from the pollen of ryegrass, *Lolium perenne*. *Histochem. J.*, **13**, 461–480.

Hubscher, T. and Eisen, A. H. (1972). Localization of ragweed antigens in the intact ragweed pollen grain. *Int. Arch. Allergy*, **42**, 466–473.

Huisman, J. G., Bernards, A., Liebregts, P., Gebbink, M. G. T., and Stegwee, D. (1977). Qualitative and quantitative immunofluorescence studies of chloroplast ferredoxin. *Planta*, **137**, 279–286.

Ishizaka, K., Ishizaka, T., and Hornbrook, M. M. (1966). Physico-chemical properties of reaginic antibody: IV Presence of a unique immunoglobulin as a carrier of reaginic activity. *J. Immunol.*, **97**, 75–85.

Ivanov, V. N. and Khavkin, E. E. (1976). Protein patterns of developing mitochondria at the onset of germination in maize (*Zea mays L.*) *FEBS Letters*, **65**, 383–385.

Ivanov, V. N., Misharin, S. E., Reimers, F. E., and Khavkin, E. E. (1974). Changes of mitochondrial and cytoplasmic antigens in growing and mature cells of maize roots (in Russian). *Dokl. Akad. Nauk SSR*, **218**, 1229–1232.

Iwanami, Y. (1968). Physiological researches of pollen. *19* Studies on the antigen substances in the pollen grains by immunoelectrophoresis. *J. Yokohama City Univ.*, **184**; *CC-59 Biol.*, **26**, 1–17.

Jacobsen, J. V. and Knox, R. B. (1973). Cytochemical localization and antigenicity of α-amylase in barley aleurone tissue. *Planta*, **112**, 213–224.

Jacobsen, J. V. and Knox, R. B. (1974). The proteins released by isolated barley aleurone layers before and after gibberellic acid treatment. *Planta Berl.*, **115**, 193–206.

Jensen, V. (1968). Serologische Beitrage zur Systematik der Ranunculaceae. *Bot. Jb.*, **88**, 204–268.

Johansson, S. O. (1974). Determination of IgE and IgE antibody by RAST. In R. Evans (Ed) *Advances in Diagnosis of Allergy: RAST*. 7–16 Symposia Specialists, Miami.

Johnson, P. and Marsh, D. G. (1965). The isolation and characterisation of allergens from the pollen of rye grass (*Lolium perenne*). *Europ. Polymer J.*, **1**, 63–77.

Kahlem, G. (1975). A specific and general biochemical marker of stamen morphogenesis in higher plants: anodic peroxidases. *Z. Pflanzenphysiol.*, **76**, 80–85.

Kahlem, G. (1976). Isolation and localization by histo-immunology of isoperoxidases specific for male flowers of the dioecious species. *Devel. Biol.*, **50**, 58–76.

Kamann, O. (1903). Zur kenntnis des Roggen-Pollens und des darin enthaltenen Heufiebergiftes. *Beitr. Chem. Physiol. Path.*, **5**, 346–354.

Kannangara, C. G., Van Wik, D., and Menke, W. (1970). Immunological evidence for the presence of latent Ca^{2+} dependent ATPase and carboxydismutase on the thylakoid surface. *Z. Naturforsch.*, **25 b**, 613–618.

Khavkin, E. E., Markov, E. Y., and Misharin, S. I. (1980). Evidence for proteins specific for vascular elements in intact and cultured tissues and cells of maize. *Planta* **148**, 116–123.

Khavkin, E. E., Misharin, S. I., Ivanov, V. N., and Danovich, K. N. (1977). Embryonal antigens in maize caryopses: the temporal order of antigen accumulation during embryogenesis. *Planta*, **135**, 225–231.

Khavkin, E. E., Misharin, S. I., Markov, Y. Y., and Peshkova, A. A. (1978a). Identification of embryonal antigens of maize: globulins as primary reserve proteins of the embryo. *Planta*, **143**, 11–20.

Khavkin, E. E., Misharin, S. I., Monastyreva, L. E., Polkarpochkina, R. T., and Sukhorzhevskaia, T. B. (1978b). Specific proteins maitained in maize callus cultures. *Z. Pflanzenphysiol.*, **86**, 273–277.

Khavkin, E. E., Misharin, S. I., and Polikarpochkina, R. T. (1979). Identical embryonal proteins in intact and isolated tissues of maize (*Zea mays* L). *Planta*, **145**, 245–251.

King, T. P. (1976). Chemical and biological properties of some atopic allergens. *Adv. Immunol.*, **23**, 77–105.

King T. P., Norman, P. S., and Tao, N. (1974). Chemical modifications of the major allergen of ragweed pollen, antigen E. *Immunochemistry*, **11**, 83–92.

Klenkopf, G. E., Huffaker, R. C., and Matheson, A. (1970). A simplified purification and some properties of ribulose 1,5-diphosphate carboxylase from barley. *Plant Physiol.*, **46**, 204–207.

Kloz, J. and Turkova, V. (1963). Graft affinity and serodiagnostical relationships. *Serological Museum Bull.*, **29**, 8.

Kloz, J., Turkova, V., and Klozova, E. (1960). Serological investigation of the taxonomic specificity of proteins in various organs in some taxons of the family Viciaceae. *Biol. Plant*, **2**, 126–137.

Kloz, J., Turková, V., and Klozová, E. (1966). Proteins found during maturation and germination of *Phaseolus vulgaris* L. *Biol. Plant*, **8**, 164–173.

Knox, R. B. (1971). Pollen-wall proteins: localization, enzymic and antigenic activity during development in *Gladiolus* (Iridaceae). *J. Cell. Sci.*, **9**, 209–237.

Knox, R. B. (1973). Pollen-wall proteins: cytochemical observations of pollen–stigma interactions in ragweed and *Cosmos* (Compositae). *J. Cell Sci.*, **12**, 421–443.

Knox, R. B. and Clarke, A. E. (1979). Localization of proteins and glycoproteins by binding to labelled antibodies and lectins. In J. L. Hall (Ed) *Electron Microscopy and Cytochemistry of Plant Cells*, pp. 149–185. Elsevier-North Holland Biomedical Press, Amsterdam.

Knox, R. B. and Clarke, A. E. (1980). Discrimination of self and non-self in plants. *Contemp. Topics in Immunobiol.*, **9**, 1–36.

Knox, R. B. and Heslop-Harrison, J. (1971). Pollen-wall proteins: fate of intine-held antigens in compatible and incompatible pollinations of *Phalaris tuberosa* L. *J. Cell. Sci.*, **9**, 239–251.

Knox, R. B., Heslop-Harrison, J., and Heslop-Harrison, Y. (1975). Pollen-wall proteins. In J. G. Duckett and P. A. Racey (Eds) *The Biology of the Male Gamete*, pp. 177–187, Academic Press, London, and New York.

Knox, R. B., Heslop-Harrison, J., and Reed, C. E. (1970). Localization of antigens associated with the pollen grain wall by immunofluorescence. *Nature (Lond.)*, **225**, 1066–1068.

Knox, R. B., Howlett, B. J., and Vithanage, H. I. M. V. (1980). Botanical immunocytochemistry, a review with special reference to pollen antigens and allergens. *Histochem. J.* **12**, 247–272.

Knox, R. B., Willing, R., and Ashford, A. E. (1972). Role of pollen-wall proteins as recognition substances in interspecific hybridization in poplars. *Nature*, **237**, 381–383.

Koenig, F., Menke, W., Craubner, H., Schmid, G. H., and Radunz, A. (1972). Photochemically active chlorophyll-containing proteins from chloroplasts and their localization in the thylakoid membrane. *Z. Naturforsch.*, **27 b**, 1225–1238.

Kohl, J. G., Misharin, S. I., Ivanov, W. N., and Khavkin, E. E. (1974). Enzymatische Identifikation der Antigene in den Wachsenden Zellen der Wurzel von *Zea mays*. L. 355–362. In G. Hoffmann (Ed) *2nd Int. Symp. Ecology and Physiology of Root Growth*. Akademie Verlag, Berlin.

Kraehenbuhl, J. P. (1979). Quantitative immunocytochemistry in the electron microscope.

Lapkoff, C. B. and Goodfriend, L. (1974). Isolation of a low molecular weight pollen allergen Ra5. *Int. Archs. Allergy. Appl. Immun.*, **46**, 215–229.

Laskey, R. A. and Mills, A. D. (1975). Quantitative film detection of ^{3}H and ^{14}C in polyacrylamide gels by flurography. *Eur. J. Biochem.*, **56**, 335–341.

Laurell, C. B. (1966). Quantitative estimation of proteins by electrophoresis in agarose gel containing antibodies. *Analyt. Biochem.*, **15**, 45–52.

Laurière, C., Skakoun, A., and Daussant, J. (1975). Adaptation de méthodes immunochimiques à l'étude de l'evolution ontogenique de protéines: fractional protéique et malate déshydrogénase des feuilles de Blé en voie de sénescence. *Physiol. Veg.*, **13**, 467–478.

Lee, Y. S. and Dickinson, D. B. (1979). Characterisation of pollen antigens from Ambrosia L. (Compositae) and related taxa by immunoelectrophoresis and radial immunodiffusion. *Am. J. Bot.*, **66**, 245–252.

Lewis, D. (1952). Serological reactions of pollen incompatibility substances. *Proc. R. Soc. B.*, **140**, 127–

Lichtenfeld, C., Manteuffel, R., Muntz, K., Neumann, D., Scholz, G., and Weber, E. (1979). Protein degradation and proteolytic activities in germinating field beans (*Vicia faba* L. var minor). *Biochem. Physiol. Pflanzen*, **174**, 255–274.

Linskens, H. F. (1960). Zur Frage der Abwehrkorper der Inkompatibilitats reaktion von Petunia III. *Z. Bot.*, **48**, 126–135.

Linskens, H. F. (1962). Die Anwendung der 'Clonal Selection Theory' auf erscheinungess der Selbsinkompatibilität bei der Befruchtung der Blütenpflanzen. Portugal. *Acta Biol.*, **6**, 232–238.

Lloyd, C. W., Slabas, A. R., Powell, A. J., Macdonald, G., and Badley, R. A. (1979). Cytoplasmic microtubules of higher plant cells visualized with anti-tubulin antibodies. *Nature*, **279**, 239–241.

Loomis, W. D. and Battaille, J. (1966). Plant phenolic compounds and the isolation of plant enzymes. *Phytochem.*, **5**, 423–428.

Lowenstein, H. (1978). Quantitative immunoelectrophoretic methods as a tool for the analysis and isolation of allergens. *Prog. Allergy*, **25**, 1–62.

Makinen, Y. and Lewis, D. (1962). Immunological analysis of incompatibility proteins and of cross-reacting material in a self-compatible mutant of *Oenothera organensis*. *Genet. Res.*, **3**, 352–363.

Mancini, G., Carbonara, A. O., and Heremans, J. F. (1965). Immunochemical quantitation of antigens by single radial immunodiffusion. *Immunochemistry*, **2**, 235–254.

Manteuffel, R., Muntz, K., Puchel, M., and Scholz, G. (1976). Phase dependent changes of DNA, RNA and protein accumulation during the ontogenesis of broad bean fruits. *Biochem. Physiol. Pflanzen*, **169**, 595–605.

Marsh, D. G. (1975). Allergens and the genetics of allergy. In M. Sela (Ed) *The Antigens*, volume 3, pp. 271–359. Academic Press, London.

Menke, W. (1973). Proteins of the thylakoid membrane, properties and functions. *Physiol. Vég.*, **11**, 231–238.

Miliaeva, E. L., Kovaleva, L. V., Lobova, N. V., and Chalakhyan, M. K. (1979). Changes in protein spectra of two-colour *Rudbeckia* stem apices upon transition from vegetative to generative state (in Russian). *Dokl. Akad. Nauk. SSSR*, **245**, 269–272. *Trans. in Doklady Botanical Sciences*, **245**, 21–23.

Millerd, A., Simon, M., and Stern, H. (1971). Legumin synthesis in developing cotyledons of *Vicia faba*. *Plant Physiol.*, **48**, 419–425.

Millerd, A., Thomson, J. A., and Schroeder, H. E. (1978). Cotyledon storage proteins in *Pisium Sativum*. III Patterns of accumulation during development. *Aust. J. Plant Physiol.*, **5**, 519–534.

Misharin, S. I., Antipina, A. I., Ivanov, V. N., Danovich, K. N., Reimers, F. E., and Khavkin, E. E. (1975). Transient antigens in the developing and germinating maize seeds (in Russian). *Dokl. Akad. Nauk. SSSR*, **223**, 479–482.

Misharin, S. I., Antipina, A. I., Reimers, F. E., and Khavkin, E. E. (1974). Phase, tissue and organ-specific proteins of corn germ plants. *Dokl. Akad. Nauk. SSSR*, **219**, 473–476. *Trans. in Doklady Biol. Sciences*, 516–518.

Moiseeva, N. A., Volodarsky, A. D., and Butenko, R. G. (1979). Detection of antigen markers in tobacco stem meristem (in Russian). *Fiziol. Rast.*, **26**, 479–484.

Mole, L. E., Goodfriend, L., Lapkoff, C. B., Kehoe, J. M., and Capra, J. D. (1975). The amino acid sequence of ragweed pollen allergen Ra5. *Biochemistry N.Y.*, **14**, 1216–1220.

Murray, D. R. and Knox, R. B. (1977). Localization and antigenicity of urease in the cotyledons of jack bean, *Canavalia ensiformis*. *J. Cell Sci.*, **26**, 9–18.

Nakane, P. K. (1973). Ultrastructural localization of tissue antigens with the peroxidase-labelled antibody method. In E. Wisse, W. Th. Daems, I. Molenaar, and P. van Duijn (Eds) *Electron Microscopy and Cytochemistry*, pp. 129–143. North-Holland Pubishing Co. Amsterdam, Holland.

Nasrallah, M. E. (1979). Self-incompatibility antigens and S-gene expression in *Brassica*. *Heredity*, **43** (in press).

Nasrallah, M. E., Barber, J., and Wallace, D. H. (1970). Self-incompatibility proteins in plants: detection, genetics and possible mode of action. *Heredity*, **25**, 23–

Nasrallah, M. E. and Wallace, D. (1967a). Immunogenetics of self-incompatibility in *Prassica oleracea* L. *Heredity*, **22**, 519–

Nasrallah, M. E. and Wallace, D. (1967b). Immunochemical detection of antigens in self-compatibility genotypes of cabbage. *Nature (Lond.)*, **213**, 700–701.

Nishio, T. and Hinata, K. (1979). Purification of an S-specific glycoprotein in self-incompatible *Brassica campestris* L. *Jap. J. Genetics*, **54**, 307–311.

Noon, L. (1911). Prophylactic inoculation against hay fever. *Lancet*, **1**, 1972.

Okita, T. W., Decaleya, R. and Rappaport, L. (1979). Synthesis of a possible precursor of α-amylase in wheat aleurone cells. *Pl. Phys.* **63**, 195–200.

Olered, R. and Jonsson, G. (1970). Electrophoretic studies of α-amylase in wheat. *J. Sci. Food Agric.*, **21**, 385–392.

Ouchterlony, O. (1949). Antigen–antibody reactions in gels. *Acta Pathol. Microbiol. Scand.*, **26**, 507–515.

Pavlov, A. N., Konarev, V. G., Kolesnik, T. I. and Shaiakhmetov, I. F. (1975). Gliadins of wheat caryopsis in the course of its development (in Russian). *Fisiol. Rastenii*, **22**, 80–83.

Pearse, A. G. E. and Polak, J. M. (1975). Bifunctional reagents as vapour and liquid-phase fixatives for immunohistochemistry. *Histochem. J.*, **7**, 179–186.

Pepys, J. (1973). Types of allergic reaction. *Clin. Allergy*, **3**, Suppl. 491–509.

Pfenninger, M. F. M. and Jamieson, J. D. (1979). Distribution of cell surface saccharides on pancreatic cells. I. General method for preparation and purification of lectins and lectin–ferritin conjugates. *J. Cell Biol.*, **80**, 69–76.

Pierard, D., Jacqmard, A., and Bernier, G. (1977). Changes in the protein composition of the shoot apical bud of *Sinapis alba* in transition to flowering. *Physiol. Plant*, **41**, 254–258.

Pierard, D., Jacqmard, A., and Bernier, G. (1979). Changements de la composition en protéines des differentes parties du bougeon apical de *Sinapis alba* au cours de sa mise à fleurs. *C.R. Acad. Sci. (Paris)*, **289**, 761–763.

Pierard, D., Jacqmard, A., Bernier, G., and Salmon, J. (1981). Appearance and disappearance of proteins in the shoot apical meristem of *Sinapis alba* in transition to flowering, *Planta*, **150**, 397–405.

Pratt, C. H. (1973). Comparative immunochemistry of phytochrome. *Plant Physiol.*, **51**, 203–212.

Pratt, L. H. and Coleman, R. A. (1971). Immunocytochemical localization of phytochrome. *Proc. Natl. Acad. Sci. USA*, **68**, 2431–2439.

Pratt, L. H. and Coleman, R. A. (1974). Phytochrome distribution in etiolated grass seedlings as assayed by an indirect antibody-labelling method. *Amer. J. Bot.*, **61**, 195–202.

Radunz, A., (1971). Phosphatidylglycerin-Antiserum und seine Reaktionen mit Chloroplasten. *Z. Naturforsch*, **26b**, 916–919.

Radunz A. (1972). Lokaliesierung des Monogalaktosyldiglcerids in Thylakoidmembranen mit serologischen Methoden. *Z. Naturforsch*, **27b**, 822–826.

Radunz, A. and Berzborn (1970). Antibodies against sulphoquinovosyl-diacyl glycerol and their reactions with chloroplasts. *Z. Naturforsch*, **25b** 412–419.

Radunz, A., Schmid, G. H., and Menke, W. (1971). Anitbodies to chlorophyll and their reactions with chloroplast preparations. *Z. Naturforsch*, **26b**, 435–446.

Raff, J. W., Hutchinson, J. F., Knox, R. B., and Clarke, A. E. (1979). Cell recognition: antigenic determinants of plant organs and their cultured callus cells. *Differentiation*, **12**, 179–186.

Raff, J. W., Knox, R. B. and Clarke A. E. (1981). Style and S-allele-associated antigens of *Prunus avium*. *Planta*, **153**, 124–129.

Rives, L. (1923). Sur l'emploi du serodiagnostic pour la détermination de l'affinité au greffage des hybrides de vigne. *C.r. hebd. Séanc. Acad. Agric. Fr.* **9**, 43–47.

Roberts, D. B. (1971). Antigens of developing *Drosophila melanogaster*. *Nature*, **233**, 394–397.

Rodkiewicz, B. (1970). Callose in cell walls during megasporogenesis in angiosperms. *Planta*, **93**, 39–47.

Roebber, M., Marsh, D. G . and Goodfriend, L. (1975). An improved procedure for the isolation of ragweed pollen allergen Ra5. *J. Immunol.*, **115**, 303–304.

Sabnis, D. D. and Hart, J. W. (1979). Heterogeneity in phloem protein complements from different species. Consequences to hypotheses concerned with P-protein function. *Planta*, **145**, 459–466.

Safonov, V. I. and Safonova, M. P. (1968). Isolation of soluble protein preparations from the vegetative organs of plants for electrophoretic investigation (in Russian). *Fiziol. Rastenii*, **16**, 161–166.

Samaan, L. G. and Fadel, F. M. (1979). Determination of compatible graft combinations in certain *Citrus* species by serological methods. *Egypt. J. Hort.*, 31–34.

Scotto, J. (1977). Immunofluorescence of resin-embedded material. *Histopathology*, **1** (5), 371–374.

Sela, M. (1966). Immunological studies with synthetic polypeptides. In F. J. Dixon and J. H. Humphrey (Eds). *Advanc. Immunol.* **5**, 29–130.

Sexton, R., Durbin, M. L., Lewis, L. N., and Thomson, M. W. (1980). Use of cellulase antibodies to study leaf abscission. *Nature*, **283**, 873–874.

Shahrabadi, M. S. and Yamamoto, T. (1971). A method for staining intracellular antigens in thin sections with ferritin-labelled antibody. *J. Cell. Biol.*, **50**, 246–250.

Skeete, M. V. *et al* (1977). The evaluation of a special liquid fixative for direct immunofluorescence. *Clin Exp. Dermatol.*, **2** (1), 49–56.

Smart, I. J. and Knox, R. B. (1980). Rapid batch fractionation of ryegrass pollen allergens. *Int. Arch. Allergy Appl. Immunol.* **62**, 179–87.

Smith, R. L. and Frey, K. J. (1970). Use of quantitative serology in predicting the genotypic relationships of oat cultivars. *Euphytica*, **19**, 447–000.

Sterba, S. (1975). Prispevek ke studiu vlastnosti extraktu topoloveho listu. Pr. Vyzk. Ustavu Lesn. Hospod. *Myslivosti*, **46**, 45–000.

Sternberger, L. A. (1974). *Immunocytochemistry*. Prentice-Hall, New Jersey.

Striker, G. E., Donati, E. J., Petrali, J. P., nd Sternberger, L. A. (1966). Postembedding staining for electron microscopy with ferritin-antibody conjugates. *Exp. Mol. Pathol.*, Suppl. 3,52.

Sun, S. S., Mutschler, M. A., Bless, F. A., and Hall, T. C. (1978). Protein synthesis and assimilation in bean cotyledons during growth. *Plant Physiol.*, **61**, 918–923.

Tel-or, E., Cammack, R., Rao, K. K., Rogers, L. J., Stewart, W. D. P., and Hall, D. O. (1978). Comparative immunochemistry of bacterial algal and plant ferredoxins. *Biochim Biophys Acta*, **490** (1), 120–131.

Thomson, J. A. and Doll, H. (1979). Genetics and evolution of seed storage proteins. In *Seed Protein Improvement in Cereals and Grain Legumes*, pp. 109–124. IAEA, Vienna.

Thomson, J. A., Millerd, A., and Schroeder, H. E. (1979). Genotype-dependent patterns of accumulation of seed storage proteins in *Pisum*. In *Seed Protein Improvement in Cereals and Grain Legumes*, volume 1, pp. 231–240. IAEA, Vienna.

Tippett, J. T. and O'Brien, T. P. (1975). A simple procedure for purifying 2-hydroxy ethyl methacrylate and some methods for using it impure in plant histology. *Lab. Practice*, **24**, 239–245.

Toh, B. H., Gallichio, H. A., Jeffrey, P. L., Livett, B. G., Muller, H. K., Cavchi, M. N., and Clarke, F. M. (1976). Anti-actin stains synapses. *Nature*, **265**, 648–650.

Underdown, B. J. and Goodfriend, L. (1969). Isolation and characterization of a protein allergen from ragweed pollen. *Biochemistry NY*, **8**, 980–989.

Vaughan, J. G., Waite, A., Boulter, D., and Walters, S. (1965). Taxonomic investigation of several *Brassica* species using serology and the separation of proteins by electrophoresis on acrylamide gels. *Nature*, **208**, 704–000.

Verma, D. P. S., Kazazian, V., Zogbi, V. and Bal, A. K. (1978). Isolation and characterization of the membrane envelope enclosing the bacteroids in soybean root nodules. *J. Cell. Biol.*, **78**, 919–936.

Vithanage, H. I. M. V., Howlett, B. J., Jobson, S. and Knox, R. B. (1982). Immunocytochemical localization of water soluble glycoproteins, including Group 1 allergen, in pollen of ryegrass, *Loliun perenne* using ferritin-labelled antibody. Histochem. J. (in press).

Wachsmuth, E. D. (1979). Principles of immunocytochemical assays. *Proc. Roy. Micr. Soc.*, **14**, 252–255.

Weeke, B. and Lowenstein, H. (1973). Allergens identified in crossed-immunoelectrophoresis. *Scand. J. Immunol.*, **2**,Suppl. 1, 149–153.

Weeke, B., Lowenstein, H., and Nielsen, L. (1974). Allergens in timothy pollen identified by crossed-radio immuno-electrophoresis (CRIE). *Allergy*, **29**, 402–417.

Weinstien, W. M. *et al.* (1977). A restaining method to restore fluorescence in faded preparations of tissues treated with the indirect immunofluorescence technique. *J. Immunol Methods*, **17** (3–4), 375–378.

Wick, S. M., Seagull, R. W., Osborn, M., Weber, K. and Gunning, B. E. S. (1981). Immunofluorescence microscopy of organized microtubules in structurally-stabilized meristematic plant cells. *J. Cell Biol.* (in press).

Williamson, R. E. and Toh, B. H. (1979). Motile models of plant cells and the immunofluorescent localization of actin in a motile *Chara* cell model. In S. Hataro,

H. Ishikawa and H. Sato, (Eds) *Cell Motility: molecules and organization.* Univ. Tokyo Press, Tokyo.

Wodehouse, R. P. (1954). Antigenic analysis by gel diffusion. I. Ragweed. *Int. Archs Allergy Appl. Immun.*, **5**, 425–433.

Wodehouse, R. P. (1957). Antigenic analysis by gel diffusion. III. Pollens of the Amaranth-Chenopod group. *Ann. Allergy*, **15**, 527–536.

Yeoman, M. M., Kilpatrick, D. C., Miedzybrodzka, M. B., and Gould, A. R. (1978). Cellular interactions during graft formation in plants, a recognition phenomenon? In Cell–Cell Recognition in Plants. *Symp. Soc. Exp. Biol.*, **32**, 139–60.

Chapter 11

The use of Lectins in the Study of Glycoproteins

A. E. Clarke and R. M. Hoggart

Plant Cell Biology Centre
School of Botany, University of Melbourne,
Parkville, Victoria 3052, Australia

I. INTRODUCTION

Lectins are a group of proteins and glycoproteins of non-immune origin which agglutinate cells and/or precipitate glycoconjugates (Goldstein *et al.*, 1980.) The specificity of individual lectins for carbohydrate is usually directed to a single monosaccharide, for example D-mannose or L-fucose, but some lectins have a broader specificity which extends to several structurally related monosaccharides, or to a sequence or series of monosaccharides; on the other hand they may have a more restricted specificity so that they will only interact with a monosaccharide in a particular sequence of a complex oligosaccharide. In most cases, though, lectins bind to their complementary monosaccharides whether they occur as free sugars, or as terminal groups in oligosaccharides or complex carbohydrates such as membrane glycoproteins or glycolipids.

Another characteristic feature of lectins is their subunit structure: they usually have two, four, or more subunits, each with a carbohydrate-combining site. This allows the lectins to act as effective cross-linking agents and to interact with saccharide-containing macromolecules such as polysaccharides and glycoproteins in solution, to give insoluble aggregates. Usually these reactions can be inhibited and often reversed by the presence of specific monosaccharides at the appropriate concentration. Lectins are also able to cross-link cells by interacting with their membrane glycoproteins and glycolipids causing agglutination. It was their ability to agglutinate red blood cells which led to their discovery almost a century ago (Stillmark, 1886), and the original term 'phytohaemagglutinins' was used to describe these molecules of plant origin which could agglutinate red blood cells. Stillmark used an extract of castor bean seeds to demonstrate erythrocyte agglutination and this observation was the basis of a study by Ehrlich on the inhibition of lectin-induced erythrocyte agglutination by antisera raised to castor bean extracts (Ehrlich, 1891a,b). His experiments with the castor bean lectin laid the foundations of modern immunology, and since then lectins have continued to be an important tool for immunologists. Historically, their next major role was in establishing the molecular basis of blood group specificity. Boyd and Reguera (1949) tested a range of seed types for their capacity to agglutinate red blood cells and noted that some extracts showed blood group specificity; later, in 1952, Watkins and Morgan used blood group specific agglutination by lectins, and its inhibition by monosaccharides to establish the monosaccharide determinants of the ABO blood groups. There was then a lull in interest in lectins until, in 1960, Nowell discovered that extracts of kidney bean were mitogenic, and stimulated division of lymphocytes. Soon after, lectins became a significant tool in cancer research when Aub and co-workers (Aub *et al.*, 1963, 1965) established that some transformed cells were preferentially agglutinated by the wheat germ agglutinin. The following period of intense interest in the basis of interaction of lectins with cells has coincided with a revived interest in the role and distribution of lectins in plants, by plant cell biologists. Although the lectins were first discovered in plants, especially in seeds, macromolecules with remarkably similar properties have now been found in lower plants, micro-organisms and more recently, in animals, both vertebrates and invertebrates. Interactions between these lectins and their complementary carbohydrate ligands are now believed to form the basis of many cellular recognition and communication reactions. The widespread implications for fields as diverse as medicine and plant pathology have led to an enormous interest in lectin–carbohydrate interactions. A result of this interest has been the development of a whole 'lectin technology' which includes techniques for detecting both lectins and their carbohydrate receptors in tissues and cells at the light and electron microscope levels, and techniques for extraction and isolation of the lectins and their receptors.

This chapter is concerned with the application of this technology to the detection, isolation, and investigation of functional properties of glycoproteins both in tissue fluids and in whole cells. Similar techniques have recently been used in investigations on the form and function of glycolipids and reference to these studies is also made in the text. Comprehensive coverage of the huge literature has not been attempted here, but rather an outline of the main ideas and methods which are in current use is given. Practical details for the methods discussed are given in the Appendix. For a more detailed view of the chemistry, biochemistry, and biology of lectins, the reader is referred to the recent excellent and exhaustive reviews of Barondes (1981), Lis and Sharon (1980), Kauss (1980), Goldstein and Hayes (1978), Brown and Hunt (1978), Lis and Sharon (1977), Liener (1976), earlier reviews of Lis and Sharon (1973) and Sharon and Lis (1972, 1975).

Abbreviations

Sugars Glc, D-glucose
Man, D-mannose
Fuc, L-fucose
Gal, D-galactose
GlcNAc, *N*-acetyl-D-glucosamine
GalNAc, *N*-acetyl-D-galactosamine
NANA, *N*-acetyl-D-neuraminic acid; (sialic acid);
(Glc NAc)$_2$, chitobiose, a 1,4-β-disaccharide of *N*-acetylglycosamine

Lectins Con A, Concanavalin A
RCA, castor bean (*Ricinus communis*) lectin
PHA, phytohaemagglutinin lectin from red kidney bean *Phaseolus vulgaris*
WGA, wheat germ agglutinin
SBA, soybean agglutinin

FITC Fluorescein isothiocyanate
RITC Rhodamine isothiocyanate
PBS Phosphate-buffered saline
(0.43 g NaH$_2$PO$_4$, 1.48 g Na$_2$HPO$_4$, 7.2 g/l NaCl, pH 7.2)

II. THE LECTINS

Lectins are available which bind each of the monosaccharides found in animal glycoproteins: glucose, galactose, mannose, fucose, *N*-acetylglucosamine, *N*-acetylgalactosamine, and sialic acid. The utility of the lectins as tools in biological research has been recognized by the major chemical supply houses which now offer a range of lectins in purified form. They are also available fluorescent-labelled for microscopic work, ferritin-labelled for electron microscopic observations, and in some cases radiochemically-labelled for general use in cell biology. Many lectins are also available as affinity reagents, that is, coupled to a support such as Sepharose, for use in the chromatographic isolation of glycoproteins.

The lectins can themselves be readily purified by affinity chromatography; thus Sephadex (a cross-linked dextran derivative with predominantly 1,6-α-glucopyranosyl linkages) and Sepharose (a galactose, anhydrogalactose, derivative) are ideal affinity reagents for the preparation of lectins specific for glucosyl and galactosyl residues, respectively. Adsorbents for lectins with other carbohydrate specificities can be prepared by coupling carbohydrate ligands to an insoluble matrix (See Appendix 1A). The range of affinity supports used in lectin purification are listed by Lis and Sharon (1977), along with other techniques which have been used successfully for lectin isolation. Of the hundreds of lectins detected in tissue extracts, about fifty have been isolated and characterized. Extensive lists of purified and partially purified lectins have been assembled by Lis and Sharon (1973), Gold and Balding (1975), Lis and Sharon (1977), Liener (1976), and Goldstein and Hayes (1978).

The sugar specificity of lectins is usually established by hapten inhibition tests in cell agglutination assays. For a few lectins, oligosaccharide and glycopeptide inhibitors have been used, as well as the range of simple monosaccharides; these tests have revealed differences in the detailed specificity requirements of lectins which have the same monosaccharide-binding properties. A list of lectins which are commercially available is given is Table 1—these are lectins which can be purchased in purified form, insolubilized for affinity chromatography, fluorescent-labelled for microscopy, and ferritin-labelled for electron microscopy. Other lectins are available in a more restricted range of derivatives. The lectins are grouped according to their carbohydrate binding specificity: Con A, pea, and lentil lectins for D-mannose; peanut, castor bean and *Bandeiraea simplicifolia* lectins for D-galactose; lima bean, soybean, *Dolichos biflorus*, and *Sophora japonica* lectins for N-acetyl-D-galactosamine; wheat germ agglutinin for N-acetyl-D-glucosamine; *Lotus tetragonolobus* and gorse lectins for L-fucose, and the horse shoe crab lectin for sialic acid. Within these groups, individual lectins, while having similar overall sugar specificities may have subtle differences in their detailed requirements for binding to complex oligosaccharides and their effects on cell systems; these fine differences maybe useful when considering which of the available lectins to use for a particular experimental procedure. The notes on the individual lectins are relevant to these properties only; descriptions of the isolation, physical and chemical properties of the lectins as well as detailed discussions of their carbohydrate-binding properties are given by Goldstein and Hayes (1978).

Of all the lectins listed here and described elsewhere, there are none available which will bind to monosaccharides such as xylose and arabinose, which do occur in glycoproteins but which are not components of the erythrocyte surface glycoproteins. This is a reflection of the method of screening of materials for lectin activity, usually the ability of an extract to agglutinate erythrocytes.

A. Notes on Individual Lectins

1. Concanavalin A

This lectin was the first to be isolated and the first to be offered for sale as a commercial product. It is readily extracted from ground seed of the jack bean *Canavalia ensiformis* and purified by affinity chromatography on Sephadex G-50.

It is unusual in being a protein, rather ithan a glycoprotein. The amino acid sequence (Cunningham *et al.*, 1975) and its three-dimensional structure

---

The specificity of a number of lectins for glycopeptides and oligosaccharides derived from glycoproteins containing the N-glycosylamine linkage has recently been established in a detailed study by Debray *et al.* (1981).

Table 1. Lectins available commercially: purified, insolubilized, and labelled for fluorescence and electron microscopy

Lectin	Source	Inhibitory saccharides	Associated metal ions	Mitogenic activity	Notes
Concanavalin A (Con A)	Jack bean (*Canavalia ensiformis*)	α-Man, α-Glc, GlcNAc, 2-substituted mannosyl residues	Mn^{2+} Ca^{2+}	+	Succinyl Con A also available in labelled forms. Also available with metal and radioactive labels: Con A–Mn, Con A–Co, Con A–Zn, Con A–^{63}Ni
Garden pea lectin (PSA)	Garden pea (*Pisum sativum*)	Man, Glc, 3-substituted mannosyl residues	Mn^{2+} Ca^{2+}	+	
Lentil lectin (LcH)	Lentil (*Lens culinaris*)	α-Man, α-Glc, GlcNAc 2-substituted mannosyl residues (Low binding constants)	Mn^{2+} Ca^{2+}	+	Available in three forms: LcH A + B, LcH A, LcH B
Bandeiraea simplicifolia lectin (BSL)	*Bandeiraea simplicifolia*	α-Gal	Mg^{2+} Ca^{2+}	–	
Peanut agglutinin (PNA)	Peanut (*Arachis hypogaea*)	Galβ1,3 GalNAc α-Gal, GalNH$_2$		?	
Castor bean lectin (RCA) RCA$_1$ RCA$_{11}$	Castor bean (*Ricinus communis*):	β-Gal β-GalNAc	No apparent metal ion requirements	–	Available in three forms: RCA$_1$ + RCA$_{11}$ mixture RCA$_1$ (RCA$_{120}$)—the non-toxic agglutinin RCA$_{11}$ (RCA$_{60}$)—the non-agglutinating toxin

Table 1. *Contd.* Lectins available commercially: purified, insolubilized, and labelled for fluorescence and electron microscopy

Lectin	Source	Inhibitory saccharides	Associated metal ions	Mitogenic activity	Notes
Sophora japonica agglutinin (SJA)	Japanese pagoda tree (*Sophora japonica*)	β-GalNAc β-Gal		?	Anti A + B lectin
Soybean agglutinin (SBA)	Soybean (*Glycine max*)	β-GalNAc	Mn^{2+} Ca^{2+}	±	
Bauhinia purpurea agglutinin (BPA)	*Bauhinia purpurea*	β-GalNAc GalNAc			
Dolichos biflorus lectin	Horse gram (*Dolichos biflorus*)	GalNAc		–	Anti A lectin
Lima bean agglutinin (LBA)	Lima bean (*Phaseolus lunatus*)	GalNAc	Mn^{2+} Ca^{2+}	+	Anti A lectin
Phytohaemagglutinin (PHA)	Red kidney bean (*Phaseolus vulgaris*): PHA-E PHA-L	GalNAc		+	Available in four forms: PHA-E, the erythroagglutinin PHA-L, the leucoagglutinin PHA-Ls, lymphocyte stimulating—non-erythroagglutinating PHA-LsE, lymphocyte stimulating erythroagglutinating The PHA-Ls and PHA-LsE are available only in the purified and FITC and RITC-labelled forms
Wistaria floribunda agglutinin (WFA)	*Wistaria floribunda*	Gal NAc		–	
Fucose binding lectin	*Lotus tetragonolobus*	α-L-fuc		+	Available in three forms, A, B, and C

Lectin	Source	Sugar specificity	Cations required		Availability
Ulex europaeus lectin (UEA)	Gorse seed (Ulex europaeus): UEA₁ UEA₁₁	L-Fuc, di-N-acetyl-chitobiose	Mn²⁺ Ca²⁺	±	Available in three forms: UEA₁ and UEA₁₁ mixture UEA₁ UEA₁₁
Limulus polyphemus agglutinin (LPA) (Limulin)	Horse shoe crab heamolymph (Limulus polyphemus)	Sialic acid	Ca²⁺	−	
Wheat germ agglutinin (WGA)	Wheat (Triticum aestivum)	GlcNAc and its oligosaccharides with sialic acid also present			
Poke weed mitogen (PWM)	Poke weed (Phytolacca americana)	unknown		+	

The lectins listed are those which are available commercially in each of the following forms: purified; insolubilized for affinity chromatography; FITC- and RITC-labelled for fluorescent microscopy; and ferritin- and peroxidase-labelled for electron microscopy.

The following companies supply lectins:

Boehringer Mannheim GmbH, PO Box 310120, D-6800 Mannheim 31, West Germany.
Calbiochem, PO Box 12087, San Diego, California, 92112, USA.
EY Laboratories, PO Box 1787, San Mateo, California 94401, USA.
L'Industrie Biologique Française (IBF), 16 Boulevard du general Leclerc, 92115 Clichy, France.
Miles Laboratories Inc., PO Box 272, Kankakee, Illinois 60901, USA.
Pharmacia Fine Chemicals, 800 Centennial Avenue, Piscataway, New Jersey 08854, USA.
PL Biochemicals Inc., 1037 W. McKinley Avenue, Milwaukee, Wisconsin 53205, USA.
Vector Laboratories, 3-H Hamilton Drive, Novato, California 94947, USA.

The lectins are usually supplied as lyophilized powders, but in some cases are available in buffered solution. The insolubilized forms are either on agarose (EY Laboratories, Miles Laboratories, PL Biochemicals, Vector Laboratories), Sepharose (Pharmacia), or ultrogel (IBF). A wide range of both FITC- and RITC-labelled lectins are offered by EY Laboratories, IBF, Miles Laboratories, and Vector Laboratories. In addition EY Laboratories have a range of lectins labelled with ferritin or peroxidase for electron microscopy. Other lectins are available in a more restricted range of forms and the seed sources of many other lectins are also offered (PL Biochemicals).

This list is given as a guide for access of investigators to the products, but does not necessarily include all sources.

(Edelman *et al.*, 1972; Reeke *et al.*, 1975) have been established. Solutions of Con A usually contain a mixture of subunit forms and often subunit fragments as well, even in freshly prepared samples. At pH 7.0 it exists in the tetrameric form and below pH 5.6, the dimer is predominant. Each subunit has one saccharide binding site and one binding site for each of two metal ions, Mn^{2+} and Ca^{2+}.

The sugar binding requirements of Con A have been established by Goldstein and co-workers (1974). The binding site for each subunit is complementary to mannopyranose and related sugars which are not modified at C-3, C-4, or C-6. Arabinofuranosides and fructofuranosides are also bound, but less effectively. The α-glycosides of the complementary sugars are apparently also bound through the glycosidic oxygen. Apart from these simple sugars, Con A also binds 1,2α-linked mannosyl residues either in terminal or non-terminal positions in oligosaccharides. This is important in view of the frequency with which 1,2-linked mannosyl residues are found in glycoproteins, including the membrane glycoproteins (see Section III). Because of its ready availability and its saccharide specificity, it has been extremely useful for the isolation of glycoproteins both from membrane preparations and other sources, for cell surface studies, and as a model for physicochemical studies of the carbohydrate–protein binding interaction. Many of the techniques used in these types of investigations were first developed using Con A as the model (Chowdhury and Weiss, 1975; Bittiger and Schnebli, 1976), and subsequently similar studies were carried out with other lectins. Thus Con A occupies a special place in the lectin literature.

2. Pea *(Pisum sativum)* lectin

The two isolectins which have been isolated from garden pea (Entlicher *et al.*, 1970) resemble Con A in that they are mitogens as well as agglutinins; they are proteins with a requirement for Ca^{2+} and Mn^{2+} for activity and they have a similar specificity for mannose and glucose α-glycosides. However, the detailed specificity requirements are somewhat different in that the pea lectin will interact with 3-*O*-substituted but not 2-*O*-substituted sugars, in contrast to Con A, which interacts with 2-*O*-substituted but not 3-*O*-substituted sugars (Van Wauwe *et al.*, 1975).

3. Lentil *(Lens culinaris)* lectin

The lectin isolated from lentil meal, either by classical fractionation or affinity chromatography on Sephadex, consists of two proteins (LcHA and LcHB) which can be separated electrophoretically. The two lectins have the same molecular weight, metal ion requirements, sugar specificity, haemagglutinating properties, and immunochemical reactions; the electrophoretic differences apparently reside in minor differences in amino acid sequences in both of the two subunits (Howard *et al.*, 1971).

The sugar specificity is similar to that of Con A and pea lectin in being directed primarily to α-D-mannopyranosyl residues; D-glucose, *N*-acetyl-D-glucosamine and their methyl glycosides are effective inhibitors of haemagglutination and the lentil lectin also binds to internal 2-*O*-substituted α-D-mannopyranosyl units (Kaifu *et al.*, 1975). However, a major difference between the lentil lectin and Con A is the extremely low binding constants for these sugars [$K_a = 2.3 \times 10^2$ M^{-1} for the lentil lectin–D-mannose association (Stein *et al.*, 1971), compared with K_a 2.06×10^4 M^{-1} for the Con A–methyl-α-D-mannopyranoside interaction (So and Goldstein, 1968)]. Consequently, the lentil lectin is not as effective as Con A in precipitating dextrans and gives a different pattern of interaction with a number of glycopeptides (Young *et al.*, 1971). The relatively low affinity of the lentil lectin for its complementary sugars has been useful in the separation of membrane glycoproteins which bind strongly to Con A and are difficult to recover from Con A affinity columns (Hayman and Crumpton, 1972).

4. Castor Bean Lectin

Extracts of the castor bean are both extremely toxic and are powerful agglutinins. These activities are due to two different components which have been separated: both are glycoproteins, and both are available commercially. The agglutinin RCA I is non-toxic, has two non-identical subunits, and does not have any apparent metal ion-binding requirement. The sugar specificity is primarily for D-galactopyranose and D-galactopyranosides such as lactose. The β-configuration is preferred but α-galactosides are also bound. Neither *N*-acetyl-D-galactosamine nor *N*-acetyl-D-galactosides are inhibitors of agglutination (Irimura *et al.*, 1975). The toxin RCA II, or ricin, also consists of two subunits; it exerts its toxic effects by binding of one subunit to the plasma membrane of a cell; this is followed by ingestion of the other chain which then effectively inhibits protein synthesis. It has a similar carbohydrate specificity to that of the agglutinin, except that in contrast to the agglutinin the toxin binds *N*-acetyl-D-galactosamine (Nicholson *et al.*, 1974).

5. Peanut Agglutinin

This lectin, like Con A, is a protein and has no covalently associated carbohydrate. Its sugar specificity is generally directed to D-galactose, and both α and β-galactosides. D-Galactosamine also fulfils the binding requirements but *N*-acetyl-D-galactosamine does not. The most useful property of this lectin in glycoprotein research is that, apart from binding α- and β-galactosides, it has a high affinity for the disaccharide Gal-β-1,3-GalNAc (2-acetamido-2-

deoxy-3-0-β-galactopyranosyl-D-galactose) (Pereira *et al.*, 1976). This is a common sequence of glycoproteins (see Section III); however, it is often sialylated and the lectin will only bind after removal of the sialic acid residues; this is related to the observation that red blood cells of group A, B, and O are only agglutinated after neuraminidase treatment (Lotan *et al.*, 1975a).

6. *Bandeiraea simplicifolia* lectin

Bandeiraea simplicifolia seeds contain multiple lectins of which one, BSLI, is particularly useful as it preferentially binds α-D-linked galactopyranosides; β-linked galactopyranosides are less effectively bound although aromatic β-galactosides are good inhibitors of the precipitation reaction between the lectin and a galactomannan (Iyer *et al.*, 1976). This specificity is reflected in its blood group specificity: B and AB erythrocytes are strongly agglutinated, A cells weakly and A_2 and O cells are not agglutinated at all (Judd *et al.*, 1976). It has a requirement for Ca^{2+} and Mg^{2+} ions.

7. *Sophora japonica* agglutinin

The seeds of *Sophora japonica* contain a lectin which preferentially binds *N*-acetyl-D-galactosaminyl residues in the β-configuration. It will also bind β-D-galactopyranoside effectively and α-D-galactopyranosides less effectively.

8. Soybean agglutinin

The carbohydrate binding specificity of this lectin is directed to terminal α- or β-linked *N*-acetyl-D-galactosamine residues (Lis *et al.*, 1970). In contrast to Con A and WGA, it does not bind internal residues effectively —furthermore, branching or substitution of the penultimate sugar has blocking effect on the binding of lectin to terminal *N*-acety-D-galactosamine residues (Pereira *et al.*, 1974).

9. *Dolichos biflorus* lectin

This lectin is similar to the lima bean (*Phaseolus lunatus*) lectin in that they both specifically agglutinate type A erythocytes and the carbohydrate specificity is directed to terminal *N*-acetyl-D-galactosaminyl groups. (Etzler and Kabat, 1970).

10. *Phaseolus vulgaris* (red kidney bean) lectin

Extracts of the red kidney bean contain haemagglutinating, leucoagglutinating, and mitogenic activities. The active principle is known as phytohaemagglutinin, PHA, and it can be fractionated into L-PHA which is mitogenic and agglutinates only leucocytes, and E(or H)-PHA which has an erythrocyte binding site. The E and L subunits occur as a series of isolectins, E_4, E_3L_1, E_2L_2, E_1L_3, and L_4. Monosaccharides are generally poor inhibitors of both the agglutinating and mitogenic activity, but N-acetylgalactosamine is effective at high concentrations, and erythrocyte surface glycopeptides containing the sugar sequence Gal $\rightarrow$ GlcNAc $\rightarrow$ Man $\rightarrow$ at lower concentrations (Kornfeld and Kornfeld, 1974).

11. Lotus tetragonolobus (asparagus pea) lectin

Extracts of *Lotus tetragonolobus* seeds contain three related L-fucose binding proteins. They are all glycoproteins and powerful haemagglutinins. The activity is inhibited by methyl α-L-fucopyranoside, L-fucose, a series of α-L-fucosides, and to a lesser extent β-L-fucosides. Inhibition studies established that the lectin required fucose to be in the pyranose form, to be unsubstituted at C-4 and to have an oxygen atom at C-2 and C-3, for binding. By virtue of these binding properties, the *Lotus* lectin precipitated blood group H substance particularly with the unsubstituted Type 2 oligosaccharide of blood group H substance (Springer and Williams, 1962; Pereira and Kabat, 1974).

12. Ulex europaeus (Gorse) lectin

Ulex seed extracts contain two distinct lectins, one (*Ulex* I) which binds α-L-fucosides and one (*Ulex* II) which binds β-D-glucosides. *Ulex* I has been purified and contains two closely similar species, molecular weight 31,000 and 32,000. The haemagglutinating activity is inhibited by α-L-fucosides and by A, B, and H blood group substances (Osawa and Matsumoto, 1972).

13. Limulus polyphemus (horse shoe crab) agglutinin

The haemolymph of the horseshoe crab contains a sialic-acid-binding lectin which has been isolated (molecular weight 400,000) and shown to contain about 18–20 glycoprotein subunits held non-covalently in a ring structure. The lectin requires Ca^{2+}, is mitogenic, and effectively agglutinates cells such as erythrocytes, leucocytes, and platelets which have surface components with terminal sialic acid residues. The haemagglutination is inhibited by sialic acid and D-glucuronic acid (Nowak and Barondes, 1975).

14. Wheat germ agglutinin

Like Con A, this lectin is protein rather than glycoprotein in nature. Interest in this lectin stemmed from the observations of Aub and co-workers (Aub *et al.*,

1963, 1965) that wheat germ lipase preparations were contaminated with a protein which preferentially agglutinated malignant cells. The agglutinin has been purified and shown to exist as the dimer at neutral pH, and below pH 3.5 as the monomer. Each subunit has two binding sites for *N*-acetylglucosamine and its β-1, 4-linked oligosaccharides. The affinity of the oligosaccharides for WGA is greater than that of the monosaccharide and increases from the di- to the tri- and tetrasaccharides. The essential features of the monosaccharide for binding are the α-acetamido group and a free hydroxyl group at C-3; the anomeric configuration of the glycosidic linkage is apparently not important as both α- and β-glycosides are effective inhibitors of WGA-induced haemagglutination (Goldstein *et al* 1975). There is no blood group specificity in the reaction.

Wheat germ agglutinin can bind to terminal GlcNAc residues of glycoproteins (Montreuil, 1975) and also to the GlcNAc-β-1,4-GlcNAc sequence which commonly occurs in the core region of the carbohydrate component of asparagine-linked glycoproteins. An unusual feature of the binding of WGA to glycoproteins is the influence of sialic acid residues: for example, the effectiveness of a glycopeptide from human erythrocyte membranes as an inhibitor of WGA haemagglutinating activity is lost if the terminal sialic acid residues of the glycoprotein are removed (Adair and Kornfeld, 1974). The effect of sialic acid on WGA binding to glycoproteins is also seen in the loss of agglutinability of WGA of certain transformed cells after enzymic removal of sialic acid (Burger and Goldberg, 1967). Recently, evidence in favour of a direct, specific interaction between sialic acid of glycoproteins and WGA has been presented (Bhavanandan and Katlic, 1979) which may be based on the similar configurations of *N*-acetylneuraminic acid and *N*-acetylglucosamine at the points of contact in the WGA binding site.

15. Pokeweed mitogen

Extracts of the roots and leaves of pokeweed, *Phytolacca americana,* contain a powerful mitogen. The mitogenic activity is due to five different glycoproteins which have different activities. One (Pa-1) is a polymer of subunits molecular weight 22,000, the other are monomers in the molecular weight range 19,000 to 31,000. Pa-1 is mitogenic for both T and B lymphocytes whereas the other fractions are mitogenic for T lymphocytes only, as indeed are other mitogenic lectins (Waxdal, 1974). The sugar specificity of the lectins has not yet been defined.

16. Myeloma proteins

A number of IgA myeloma proteins bind carbohydrates in a highly specific manner, for example IgA produced by the mouse myeloma J539 specifically binds β 1,6-galactosyl residues and that from the myeloma J558 specifically binds α 1,3-linked glucose residues. Detailed lists of mouse myeloma proteins and their specifities are given by Glaudemans (1975). These proteins can be used for detecting saccharides in the same way as lectins.

It is remarkable that while both the lectins and the myeloma proteins bind carbohydrates in a highly specific manner, the *raison d'être* for the high concentrations of lectins in plant tissues or for the binding properties of the IgA myeloma proteins is not apparent.

III. THE GLYCOPROTEINS

Glycoproteins are found in all mammalian tissues, either as membrane components or in the tissue fluids and secretions. For example, most plasma proteins, including the immunoglobulins, are glycoproteins: all mucous secretions contain a major glycoprotein component and many enzymes and hormones are glycoproteins. Within this group of macromolecules there is enormous diversity both of form and function—for example the carbohydrate component may account for up to 85% of the total weight of secreted blood group substance or less than 1% of the total weight of some enzymes. A similar diversity is seen in the form of membrane glycoproteins. All mammalian cells have surface glycoproteins inserted asymmetrically into the lipid bilayer with the carbohydrate concentrated at the extracellular face of the membrane. Apart from glycoproteins, membranes also contain some carbohydrate in the form of glycolipids which are also inserted into the lipid bilayer. Recently there has been an enormous interest in these membrane glycoconjugates because their carbohydrate components are now considered to play a role in defining the identity of a cell surface, by variation in nature and arrangement of their monosaccharide units. Furthermore, a number of instances in which these carbohydrate components are apparently involved in specific intercellular recognition reactions have been reported. In these cases the interaction is mediated by specific binding between a cell surface carbohydrate and a complementary protein receptor, which may be located on the surface of another cell.

The major structural features of the carbohydrate components of glycoproteins will now be briefly reviewed. More detailed discussions of glycoprotein structure are given by Gottschalk (1972); Marshall (1972); Kornfeld and Kornfeld (1976); Lennarz (1980), and Hubbard and Ivatt (1981). Several books on membrane glycoproteins are also available (Hughes, 1976; Maddy and Dunn, 1976; Glick and Flowers, 1978).

In the broadest sense glycoproteins are macromolecules containing carbohydrate and protein in covalent linkage. There are two distinct groups of these glycoconjugates: the glycoproteins and the proteoglycans. The glycoproteins are characterized by having one or more heterosaccharide units which are

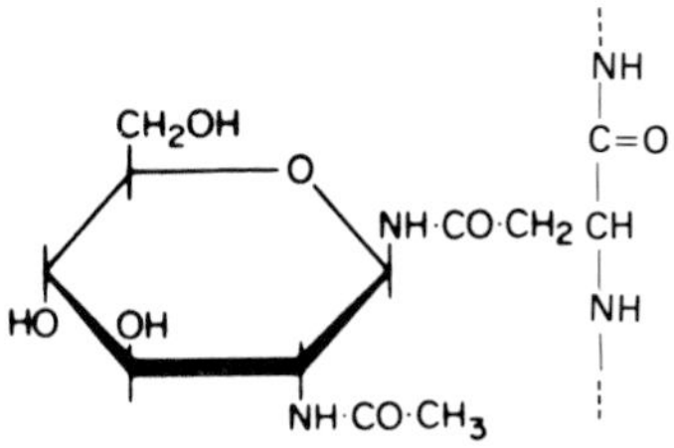

N-Acetyl glucosaminyl–asparagine linkage

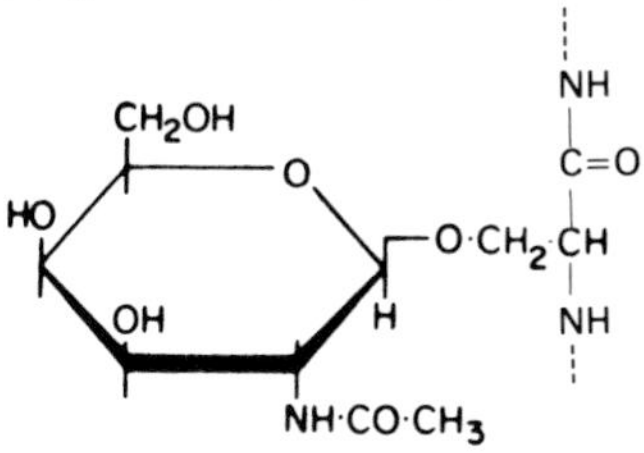

N-Acetyl galactosaminyl–serine (threonine) linkage

Figure 1. The major types of linkage between carbohydrate and protein in glycoproteins

usually branched and each heterosaccharide has a relatively small number of sugar residues which are not arranged in a repeating unit (Gottschalk, 1972). In contrast, the proteoglycans characteristically have a linear saccharide component, often containing a repeating unit, and a relatively high number of sugar residues per chain. Animal protoeglycans also characteristically contain sulphated sugars and uronic acids.

In this chapter we will discuss primarily mammalian glycoproteins; however, glycoconjugates having similar properties are also found in viruses, micro-organisms, and plants and can be examined by techniques similar to those described for the mammalian glycoproteins.

The oligosaccharide unit of animal glycoproteins usually contains only a few monosaccharides: D-mannose, D-galactose, L-fucose, N-acetyl-D-glucosamine, N-acetyl-D-galactosamine, and sialic acid. Of these units, sialic acid and fucose are found only in terminal positions. Glucose and xylose are also found in a relatively small group of glycoproteins.

There are two major types of linkage between the carbohydrate and protein components of glycoproteins: O-glycosidic linkages from the N-acetylgalactosamine of the oligosaccharide component to the serine or threonine of the peptide component and N-glycosidic linkages between N-acetylglucosamine and the amide nitrogen of asparagine (see Figure 1).

A. O-Glycosidic Linkages

This type of linkage is found in mucous and other secreted glycoproteins such as blood group substances, immunoglobulins, and fetuin. In order to study the oligosaccharide component of glycoproteins the linkage must be cleaved by

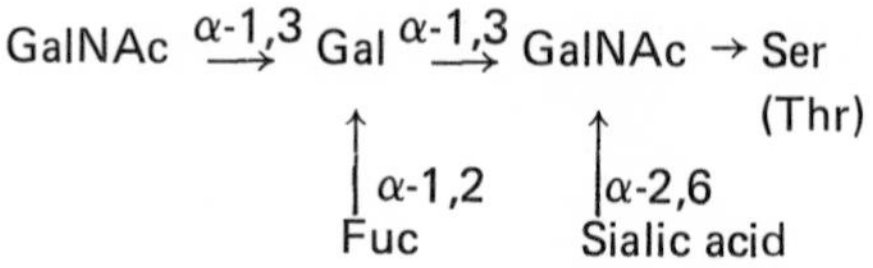

$$\text{GalNAc} \xrightarrow{\alpha\text{-1,3}} \text{Gal} \xrightarrow{\alpha\text{-1,3}} \text{GalNAc} \rightarrow \text{Ser}$$

$$\text{(Thr)}$$

$$\uparrow \alpha\text{-1,2} \qquad \uparrow \alpha\text{-2,6}$$

$$\text{Fuc} \qquad \text{Sialic acid}$$

Figure 2. Structure of a glycopeptide from porcine submaxillary mucin (Carlson, 1968)

alkali treatment, which releases the saccharide component by β-elimination and the linkage sugar is converted to the corresponding alcohol in the presence of borohydride.

The glycoproteins of this group have a number of structural features in common. They have a core disaccharide [$\text{Gal} \xrightarrow{\beta\text{-1,3}} \text{GalNAc} \rightarrow \text{Ser (Thr)}$] which is identical for most glycopeptides with the exception of the submaxillary mucins, which have the structure $\text{NANA} \xrightarrow{\alpha\text{-2,6}} \text{GalNAc} \rightarrow \text{Ser (Thr)}$.

The linkage of sialic acid residues to the oligosaccharide component is always α 2,6 to *N*-acetylgalactosamine and fucose is always linked α 1,2 to galactose (see Figure 2). However, individuality of the glycoproteins is given by variations of the peripheral sugar residues and linkages, e.g. the sialic acid may be α 2,3-linked to galactose.

Other sugars have been shown to be involved in *O*-glycosidic linkages. In yeast and fungal glycoproteins it is common to find mannose linked *O*-glycosidically to serine or threonine. There may be from one to four mannose residues in the oligosaccharide chain along with glucose and galactose (Rosenthal and Nordin, 1975). The cutical collagen of the earthwork was shown by Muir and Lee (1969, 1970) to have galactose linked *O*-glycosidically to serine (threonine) and it has been reported that a fucose–threonine linkage occurs in human urine (Hallgren *et al.*, 1975) and in rat tissue (Larriba *et al.*, 1977).

Collagen and basement membranes have another type of glycoprotein linkage in which galactose or glycosylgalactose is linked *O*-glycosidically to the hydroxyl group of hydroxylysine (Hyl) of the peptide. This type of linkage was first detected by Butler and Cunningham (1966) and was shown by Spiro (1967) to be $\text{Glc} \xrightarrow{\beta\text{-1,2}} \text{Gal} \rightarrow \text{Hyl}$.

Extensin, a hydroxyproline-rich glycoprotein from plant cell walls, has been shown to contain arabinose linked covalently to the hydroxyl group of hydroxyproline (Lamport, 1969; Heath and Northcote, 1971), and galactose covalently linked to the serine residues of the peptide (Lamport *et al.*, 1973).

B. *N*-Glycosidic Linkages

There are two main types of oligosaccharides involved in these linkages: the simple or 'high-mannose' type which contain only mannose and *N*-acetylglu-

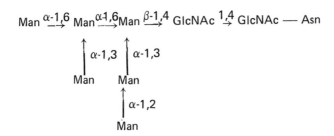

Figure 3. Structure of ovalbumin glycopeptide (Tai *et al.*, 1975)

cosamine, and the complex type, which contain mannose, N-acetylglucosamine, sialic acid, galactose, and fucose. The core structure of both types is: Man $\overset{\beta\rightarrow^4}{}$ GlcNAc $\overset{\beta\rightarrow^4}{}$ GlcNAc $\rightarrow$ Asn i.e. mannosyl di$N$-acetylchitobiose. The 'high-mannose' type oligosaccharides all have this core but vary in the number and linkages of outer mannosyl residues. The mannose of the core is always branched to mannose residues in α 1,3- and α 1,6-linkages. Outer chain branching is always confined to a mannose residue linked to C-6 of the core mannosyl residue (see Figure 3).

Variation in this core structure is given by further mannosyl residues in the peripheral region in a pattern which may involve multiple branched mannosyl chains.

The consistent arrangement of the core region of these 'high-mannose' type oligosaccharides suggests a common pathway of biosynthesis. However, there are some unusual 'high-mannose' type oligosaccharides which have the same core structure but differ in their side chain. A glycopeptide from lima bean lectin has been shown by Misaki and Goldstein (1977) to have a fucose residue linked to the N-acetylglucosamine in the core and the linkage of the terminal mannose to the β-mannosyl of the core is via C-2. Pineapple stem bromelain is also unusual in that it has a xylose residue β 1,2- or 1,6-linked to the core β-mannose residue and a fucose residue α 1,3-linked to the core N-acetylglucosamine (Fukuda *et al.*, 1976).

The complex type of oligosaccharide chain has the same core structure as the 'high-mannose' type but in addition it has two extra mannose residues attached to the mannosyl di-N-acetylchitobiose unit, i.e.

Man $\overset{\alpha\rightarrow^6}{}$ Man $\overset{\beta\rightarrow^4}{}$ GlcNAc $\overset{1,4}{\rightarrow}$ GlcNAc $\rightarrow$ Asn
Man$\overset{\alpha\ 1,3}{}$

To this core are attached a variable number of outer chains which are usually NANA $\overset{\alpha\ 2,3\ \text{or}\ \alpha\ 2,6}{\longrightarrow}$ Gal $\overset{\beta\rightarrow^4}{}$ GlcNAc.

Individuality of the glycopeptides results from variation in the sialic acid–galactose linkage from α 2,3 to α 2,6, substitution of N-acetylglucosa-

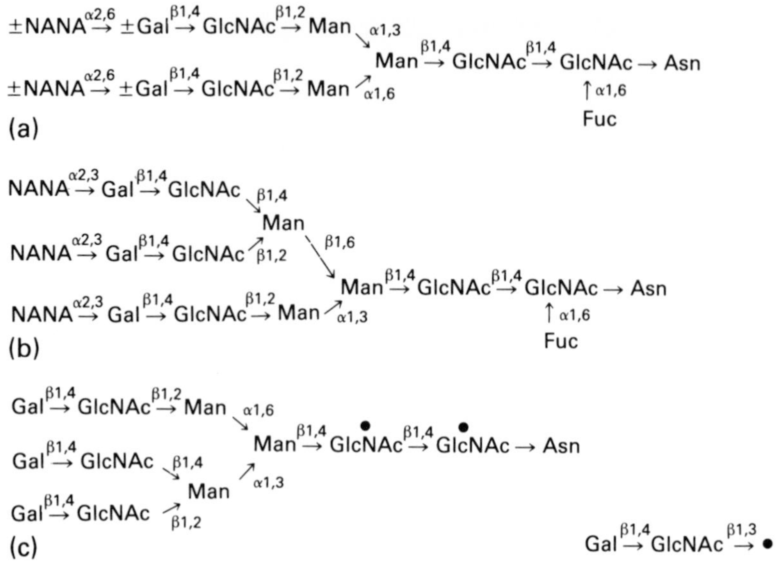

$\pm$NANA $\overset{\alpha2,6}{\to}$ $\pm$Gal $\overset{\beta1,4}{\to}$ GlcNAc $\overset{\beta1,2}{\to}$ Man $\searrow^{\alpha1,3}$

$\pm$NANA $\overset{\alpha2,6}{\to}$ $\pm$Gal $\overset{\beta1,4}{\to}$ GlcNAc $\overset{\beta1,2}{\to}$ Man $\nearrow_{\alpha1,6}$

Man $\overset{\beta1,4}{\to}$ GlcNAc $\overset{\beta1,4}{\to}$ GlcNAc $\to$ Asn

$\uparrow\alpha1,6$

Fuc

(a)

NANA $\overset{\alpha2,3}{\to}$ Gal $\overset{\beta1,4}{\to}$ GlcNAc $\searrow_{\beta1,4}$

NANA $\overset{\alpha2,3}{\to}$ Gal $\overset{\beta1,4}{\to}$ GlcNAc $\nearrow_{\beta1,2}$ Man $\searrow^{\beta1,6}$

Man $\overset{\beta1,4}{\to}$ GlcNAc $\overset{\beta1,4}{\to}$ GlcNAc $\to$ Asn

NANA $\overset{\alpha2,3}{\to}$ Gal $\overset{\beta1,4}{\to}$ GlcNAc $\overset{\beta1,2}{\to}$ Man $\nearrow_{\alpha1,3}$

$\uparrow\alpha1,6$

Fuc

(b)

Gal $\overset{\beta1,4}{\to}$ GlcNAc $\overset{\beta1,2}{\to}$ Man $\searrow_{\alpha1,6}$

Gal $\overset{\beta1,4}{\to}$ GlcNAc $\searrow_{\beta1,4}$

Man $\overset{\beta1,4}{\to}$ GlcNAc $\overset{\beta1,4}{\to}$ GlcNAc $\to$ Asn

Gal $\overset{\beta1,4}{\to}$ GlcNAc $\nearrow_{\beta1,2}$ Man $\nearrow^{\alpha1,3}$

Gal $\overset{\beta1,4}{\to}$ GlcNAc $\overset{\beta1,3}{\to}$ $\bullet$

(c)

Figure 4. Structure of glycopeptides of complex oligosaccharides of: (a) Human IgG, IgE, and IgA. (From Kornfeld and Kornfeld, 1976) (b) Fetuin (From Baenziger and Fiete, 1979), and (c) desialized α_1,-acid glycoprotein (Schwarzmann *et al.*, 1978)

mine with fucose in the outer regions, variation in the number of branches, and variation in the number of branches terminated by sialic acid residues.

The branching pattern of the side chain varies from two branches as in human IgG, IgE, and IgA (Kornfeld and Kornfeld, 1976) to three outer chains linked to one of the α-mannosyl residues as in fetuin, vesicular stomatitis virus glycoprotein, and porcine thyroglobulin β (Reading *et al.*, 1978); other molecules can have four outer chains with an additional one linked to one of the *N*-acetylglucosamine residues as in desialized α_1-acid glycoprotein (Schwarzmann *et al.*, 1978) and glycopeptide B-3 from calf thymocyte membranes (Kornfeld, 1978) (see Figure 4). These molecules are known as bi-, tri- and tetraantennary, respectively.

There are some atypical complex *N*-glycosidically linked oligosaccharides which can vary from short unbranched molecules not containing mannose, e.g. glycopeptides from human urine (Sugahara *et al.*, 1976),to highly branched molecules that lack the typical complex core structure and have low levels of mannose, e.g. glycopeptide I from rabbit liver membrane glycoprotein (Kawasaki and Ashwell, 1976).

Glycoproteins often contain only one linkage type, but both glycoprotein and immunoglobulin G, for example, contain oligosaccharide units attached by the two different major linkage types. Analysis of glycoproteins and understanding the principles of organization of the monosaccharide units in individual glycoproteins has been complicated by the 'microheterogeneity' usually encountered, that is, the equivalent carbohydrate units of individual molecules from the same source may be very similar, but not necessarily identical, probably as a result of incomplete processing during biosynthesis or variable degradation during isolation.

Not only may an individual glycoprotein contain both *O*- and *N*-glycosidically linked chains, but both complex and 'high-mannose' oligosaccharide chains may be present on the same glycoprotein (e.g. thyroglobulin and IgM) (Chapman and Kornfeld, 1979).

Glycoproteins can be classified according to this scheme whether they are soluble or membrane bound. Information regarding the structure of membrane glycoproteins is more difficult to obtain, mainly because of the problem of obtaining enough material for analysis. Two major approaches have been adopted: firstly, peripheral fragments of the membrane glycoprotein are either cleaved enzymically from the intact cell or dissociated from the membrane by, for example, mild detergent. In these cases, the carbohydrate component of the released fragments can be examined by the same techniques used for investigation of soluble glycoproteins. Secondly, the presence and arrangement of cell surface carbohydrate can be inferred by the interaction of whole cells with lectins, lectin derivatives, and other cell surface probes.

The arrangement of individual monosaccharide components of a glycoprotein will dictate its potential for interaction with a particular lectin: the linkage position, anomeric configuration, degree of branching, and proximity of other residues are all important in determining whether a particular residue or sequence will comply with the specificity requirements of a particular lectin. Thus Con A will bind to the internal α 1,2-linked or terminal mannosyl residues; the castor bean lectin will bind β-linked galactosyl residues in terminal (non-sialylated) positions. For other lectins a sequence or combination of monosaccharides in the chain may influence the binding; for example binding of wheat germ agglutinin involves both internal *N*-acetylglucosamine and sialic acid residues, phytohaemagglutinin (E-PHA) binding can depend on the presence of both galactosyl and core mannose residues. The other lectins listed in Table 1 might be expected to bind to glycoproteins where a monosaccharide or saccharide sequence which fulfils the binding requirements of the lectin is displayed in a situation accessible to the lectin. Some potential lectin binding sites of a model 'complex' glycoprotein are shown in Figure 5. The interaction of glycolipids with lectins has been considered by Williams *et al.*, (1979).

The techniques by which the potential of both membrane-bound and soluble glycoproteins for lectin binding can be used for study of their structure and function will now be considered.

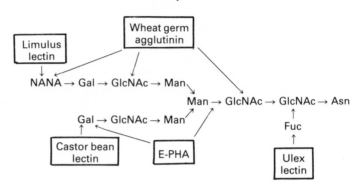

Figure 5. Some potential lectin binding sites in a hypothetical 'complex' type glycoprotein

IV. STUDY OF SOLUBLE GLYCOPROTEINS USING LECTINS

A. Detection of Soluble Glycoproteins

One of the simplest ways to screen an extract for a glycoprotein containing a particular saccharide residue is to test its capacity to react with a lectin complementary for that saccharide. The reaction can be carried out in solid or liquid media and is dependent on the concentration of both lectin and glycoprotein. In this respect, and in its specificity, the reaction resembles the antigen–antibody precipitin reaction. Double diffusion using lectins and tissue extracts at various concentrations in opposite wells is a convenient method to detect glycoproteins in solution (Appendix I.B.1). The reaction between glycoprotein and lectin can be seen in the agar gel by formation of a precipitin band, and the sensitivity of detection can be enhanced by staining the dried gel. Alternatively, a radiochemical label on either the lectin or glycoprotein can be used and the precipitin band detected by autoradiography. This reaction can be quantitated by following the precipitation from liquid media. In this case information regarding the saccharide component of the glycoprotrein, gained from its interaction with a lectin of known specificity, can be confirmed by specific inhibition of precipitate formation by defined saccharides (Appendix I.B.2).

Glycoproteins can also be detected and some information about the nature of their saccharide component can be obtained by their ability to inhibit the agglutination reaction between erythrocytes and a particular lectin (Appendix I.B.3).

Another useful method of detecting glycoproteins is by their reaction with lectins after electrophoretic separation. The method is applicable to any kind of electrophoretic separation, but is most easily handled in gels. For example, if electrophoresis of a glycoprotein is carried out in a standard immunoelectrophoresis gel, a lectin solution can be placed in the well and a precipitin arc will form between the lectin and a glycoprotein carrying an appropriate saccharide determinant. Alternatively, glycoproteins can be separated in SDS–polyacrylamide gels and immersed or overlaid with a solution of a lectin which has previously been labelled with either ^{125}I or a fluorescent marker (Furlan *et al.*, 1979). The lectin can also be detected in the gel by its binding to a glycoprotein enzyme such as peroxidase, which is then detected by its reaction products. Glycoproteins can also be detected by a technique analogous to rocket immunoelectrophoresis: in this method the electrophoresis is into a gel-containing dissolved lectin (Appendix I.B.5).

Recently methods have been developed for the transfer of proteins and glycoproteins after SDS–gel electrophoresis to derivatized or activated cellulose [e.g. diazobenzyloxymethylcellulose (DBM paper) or nitrocellulose paper]. Originally the method involved cleavage of the polyacrylamide linkages with periodic acid or ammonium hydroxide to facilitate transfer of the proteins and glycoproteins which was achieved by blotting techniques requiring buffer flow under pressure through the gel for approximately 10 hours (Renart *et al.*, 1979). This method has been improved by Bittner *et al.* (1980) and Towbin *et al.* (1979). They achieved transfer of the proteins and glycoproteins from polyacrylamide gels to activated cellulose by electrophoresis. This has the advantages that it is relatively quick (*ca.* 1 hour), does not require degradation of the cross-linked polyacrylamide gel, requires no mechanical stress (e.g. pressure), and is highly reproducible. Once immobilized on the paper, the proteins and glycoproteins can be detected using immunological procedures or by using radio-, FITC- or peroxidase-labelled specific ligands (e.g. lectins). Alternatively, the specific ligand can be coupled to the derivatized, activated paper and the gels containing the separated proteins and glycoproteins are then laid on this matrix under pressure. The proteins and glycoproteins that interact with the affinity ligand are specifically transferred from the gel to the matrix, they are then detected by autoradiography or by immunological techniques (Erlich *et al.*, 1979).

Another recently developed method which could be used for the detection of soluble glycoproteins involved the immobilization of the glycoproteins on polyvinyl chloride microtitre plates (Howlett and Clarke, 1981). The glycoprotein being examined is adsorbed into the wells of the plate and its ability to bind radiolabelled lectins is measured. This method is cheap, quick, and requires only microgram quantities of the glycoprotein. The lectin binding is extremely sensitive and a wide range of lectins can be screened in a short period of time.

B. Isolation of Soluble Glycoproteins

The mose useful method for glycoprotein isolation is affinity chromatography using immobilized lectins. The glycoprotein containing extract is applied to a column of the immobilized lectin: glycoproteins having the arrangement of saccharide units complementary to the lectin are bound to the column. After extensive washing of the column, the bound glycoprotein can usually be eluted by a solution of the appropriate monosaccharide or oligosaccharide, which is subsequently separated from the glycoprotein. If the lectin-binding capacity is dependent on metal ions, it is possible for the glycoprotein to be bound in buffer containing the metal ion and eluted by buffer lacking the metal ion (Gleeson *et al.*, 1979); in this case there is no need for a final separation of glycoprotein from eluting saccharide. As many lectins are active in the presence of low concentrations of detergent (Lotan *et al.*, 1977) the same procedure can be applied to glycoproteins extracted from membranes with detergent.

Lectins specific for all the monosaccharides of animal glycoproteins are commercially available in insolubilized forms (Table 1). Alternatively, affinity columns can be prepared quite simply from cyanogen-bromide-activated Sepharose (Appendix I.E).

These methods have been applied to the isolation of many serum glycoproteins, for example, immunoglobulins (Hrkal and Vodrazka, 1977; Uhlenbruck *et al.*, 1978), fetuin (Lootan *et al.*, 1977), blood group substances (Pereira and Kabat, 1976), and many enzymes and other glycoproteins. (For review, see Kornfeld and Kornfeld, 1978; Dulaney, 1979.)

Some of these glycoproteins can be isolated using an affinity column which involves binding of the terminal sialic acid residues such as Sepharose–WGA or Sepharose–*Limulus* agglutinin. After isolation, the terminal sialic residues can be specifically removed by neuraminidase treatment, exposing the penultimate sugars. Where several sialyl glycoproteins were isolated on the basis of their binding of terminal sialyl residues, fractionation could be achieved on the basis of the different lectin affinities of the variety of exposed subterminal sugars (Adair and Kornfeld, 1974; Lotan *et al.*, 1977). Other methods by which fractionation of mixtures of glycoproteins can be achieved are elution of adsorbed material with a concentration gradient of eluting saccharide, or preferential adsorption of the components with the highest affinity for the lectin by deliberate sequential overloading of the affinity column (Kristiansen, 1974).

LECTINS IN THE STUDY OF MEMBRANE-BOUND GLYCOPROTEINS

A. Detection of Membrane-Bound Glycoproteins

1. Detection by Physiological Effects

If a lectin exerts an observable effect on a cell system, the presence of surface saccharide receptor for that lectin, usually a glycoprotein or glycolipid, is implied. Agglutination of cells is one of the most studied effects and a number of different cell types apart from red blood cells are agglutinated by lectins, for example vertebrate and invertebrate, egg and sperm cells (for review, see Oppenheimer, 1977), and plant protoplasts (Larkin, 1978). Lectins cause a wide range of other effects on animal cells such as mitogenic stimulation of lymphocytes, inhibition of adhesion, phagocytosis and fertilization, inhibition of growth of tumour cells, induction of platelet release reaction, and an insulin-like effect on fat cells (for a review and more extensive lists of effects, see Lis and Sharon, 1977; Goldstein and Hayes, 1978; Kornfeld and Kornfeld, 1978). They are also useful probes in investigating the nature of plant cell surfaces: the normally naked cells such as the algal gametes are particularly amenable to investigation and gametes of the unicellular green alga *Chlamydomonas* (McLean and Brown, 1974) and of the brown alga *Fucus* (Bolwell *et al.*, 1979) both bind Con A, a treatment which effectively blocks fertilization in these systems. Lectins also bind to fungal cell walls (Barkai and Sharon, 1978) and may inhibit mycelial growth (Mirelman *et al.*, 1975). Their use is more restricted for investigation of higher plants because of the presence of the cellulosic cell wall; however, they have been shown to stimulate pollen germination (Southworth, 1975).

Any one of these lectin-induced effects which is inhibited by a particular monosaccharide is presumptive evidence for the presence of that monosaccharide or a related monosaccharide at the cell surface; however, unequivocal proof requires isolation and chemical analysis of the surface receptor, a procedure which has been performed in only a few instances.

In many instances, specific cellular interactions have been shown to be mediated by binding between particular cell surface carbohydrate sequences and cell surface proteins or glycoproteins. These protein or glycoprotein receptors would then be lectins or lectin-like molecules in having the ability to bind to specific carbohydrate residues; thus specific recognition of compatible mating partners in yeasts and the unicellular green alga *Chlamydomonas* and attachment of microorganisms to their host tissue such as *Escherichia coli* to intestinal mucosa, zoospores of a plant pathogen to slime on the host root surface (Hinch and Clarke, 1980), and *Rhizobium* to plant root surfaces, are apparently dependent on this type of reaction. Influenza virus is known to have a surface haemagglutinin or lectin which binds the sialic acid residues of the major erythrocyte glycoprotein, glycophorin. For review of these interactions see Callow (1977), Curtis (1978), Hughes and Sharon (1978), Simpson *et al.* (1978), Williams (1978), Frazier and Glaser (1978), Pierce *et al.* (1980), Bauer (1981), and Barondes (1981).

A theoretical basis for this type of interaction has been presented by Roseman (1970): this theory proposes that, the carbohydrate binding protein is actually a glycosyl transferase; adhesion of cells occurs by an enzyme substrate interaction between a glycosyl transferase on one cell surface and its substrate exposed at the surface of another cell. The state of adhesion rests on the availability of the appropriate nucleotide sugar; if it is available the enzymic reaction is completed and the enzyme and modified substrate are released, if it is absent the enzyme and substrate remain bound and the cells adhere. This theory has neither been proved nor disproved, but recently the aggregation of sponges has been interpreted on a basis which embodies part of Roseman's theory. The sponge cells have glucuronic acid containing surface receptors and surface-located glucuronidases; the extracellular aggregation factor has associated glucuronyl transferase activity: aggregation may be mediated by glucuronylation of cell surface aggregation receptors (Müller *et al.*, 1979). These observations are of particular interest in view of the finding that some lectins are enzymically active (Shannon and Hankins, 1981; Horejsi, 1979).

The appearance of lectins on the surface of slime moulds during their aggregation phase has also suggested the involvement of this type of interaction in cell adhesion and differentiation. The findings that a mutant defective for lectin production was non-cohesive and that the mutant developed normally when mixed with wild-type cells (Ray *et al.*, 1979) strongly support this suggestion and the concept that the interaction is mediated by a complementary binding of cell surface molecules.

Recently, carbohydrate-binding proteins have also been found on mammalian cell surfaces; for example, hepatocytes contain a carbohydrate-binding protein specific for galactosyl units, which is able to withdraw circulating glycoproteins, if the normally penultimate galactose residues are exposed by removal of terminal sialic acid residues (Ashwell and Morell, 1978). The same cells have a receptor which specifically binds glycoproteins through a fucosyl α 1,3-*N*-acetylglucosamine group (Prieels *et al.*, 1978), and sinusoidal cells in the liver have a receptor for mannose-terminated glycoproteins (Steer *et al.*, 1979).

Moreover, developmentally regulated lectins have been found on the surface of a number of embryonic chick tissues (Kobiler *et al.*, 1978), and in cells of the reticuloendothelial system. These findings, and the notion that the role of the surface glycoproteins may be informational, have generated considerable interest both in glycoprotein structure and in the detailed specificity requirements of their complementary lectins. The evidence that cell surface glycolipids may also mediate cell–cell interactions in a similar way has been reviewed by Critchley *et al.* (1979).

2. Detection by Binding of Radiochemically Labelled Lectins

The extent of lectin binding to cell surfaces can be quantitated by incubating cells with radiochemically labelled lectins (Appendix I.D.1). By using this technique a measurement of the number of receptor sites on the cell and their binding constants can be obtained. In cases in which a particular lectin is found to bind to a particular cell type, the binding is usually in a simple saturation pattern and is dependent on such factors as lectin concentration, pH, and temperature. The association constants for lectin–cell interactions are usually higher than for lectin–monosaccharide binding, suggesting that the affinity of the lectin for the complex saccharide sequences of the surface receptors may be higher than that for the simple sugars. These techniques and their application have been reviewed by Nicolson (1974), Lis and Sharon (1977), and Hubbard and Cohn (1976).

Some insight into the monosaccharide composition and sequence of surface glycoproteins can be obtained by comparing the ability of the cell to bind a variety of lectins before and after removal of terminal sialic acid and fucosyl residues (Nicolson, 1973). Studies of the influence of one lectin bound to a cell surface, on the ability of a second lectin to bind, give some ideas of the spatial arrangement of carbohydrate receptors on the cell surface. However, interpretation of these experiments is often difficult because, among other things, of the possibility of lectin–lectin interactions.

3. Detection by Binding of Fluorescent- or Ferritin-Labelled Lectins

Lectins can be used as probes to examine the nature and distribution of cell surface saccharides both in isolated cells and in sections of whole tissues. They can be visualized by attaching a fluorescent marker and examining their binding to cells by fluorescence microscopy or by attaching an electron-dense marker and examining the cells by electron microscopy. The procedures for fluorescent, ferritin, or radioactively labelling the lectins are simple and can be carried out in the laboratory. Details of method are given in Appendix I.C; alternatively, commercially labelled lectins are available. One of the major pitfalls in using these modified lectins is that carbohydrate-binding specificity may be altered during the labelling procedure, and it is important that the sugar specificity of the labelled product be checked before it is used as a probe. The fluorescent markers most commonly used are fluorescein isothiocyanate (yellow-green) and tetramethyl rhodamine isothiocyanate (red). The cell preparation is allowed to bind to the cell under defined conditions of temperature, time, and lectin concentration, and control experiments are performed by incubating the cells with the lectin in the presence of its complementary receptor. This technique has been most useful in the study of the nature and distribution of receptors over the cell surface.

The lectin receptors of many cell types, such as the immunoglobulins of lymphocyte surfaces, are able to undergo lateral movement within the plane of the membrane to form patches and caps: initially there is an even distribution which rapidly changes to a patchy distribution at 37 °C. The effect is not observed at 4 °C. Under some conditions, the patches may aggregate to form caps at one pole of the cell. The capping process is apparently energy dependent while the patching may be due to a simple diffusion (Nicolson, 1976a,b). The mobility of a particular lectin receptor is in many cases

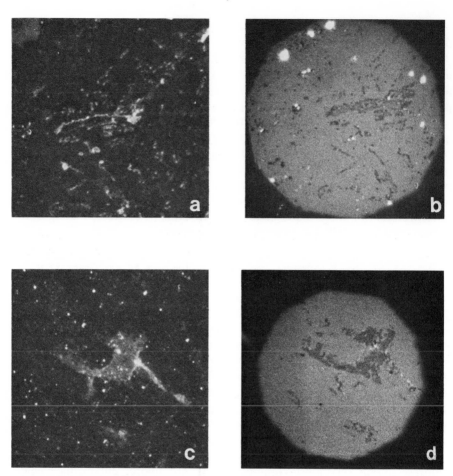

Figure 6. Examination of adhesive material from rat dermal fibroblasts by treatment with fluorescent-labelled lectins. Cells were grown on coverslips for 24 hours, washed off with Dulbeccos medium, and the remaining cell adhesions examined by interference microscopy or after binding to FITC-labelled lectins. (a) FITC-ricin viewed by fluorescence microscopy. (b) Same area viewed by interference microscopy. (c) FITC-Con A viewed by fluorescence microscopy. (d) Same area viewed by interference microscopy (10 μm). (From Badley *et al.*, 1978)

independent of that of receptors for other lectins and antibodies, as in the case of the surface immunogolublins of lymphocytes (Inbar *et al.*, 1973; Karnovsky and Unanue, 1973). However, under certain experimental conditions such as high lectin concentrations, Con A may inhibit anti-IgG induced cap formation (Yahara and Edelman, 1973).

There is evidence that at least some of the receptors involved are connected in some way with the underlying components of the cytoskeletal system, the microtubules, and microfilaments (Edelman, 1976; Rees *et al.*, 1977). The relationship between the cell surface and the cytoskeleton in rat fibroblasts has recently been examined by a combination of fluorescent labelled antibodies and lectins (Badley *et al.*, 1978) (Figure 6). The pattern of staining indicated that material derived from the cytoplasmic face contains the major components of both the actomyosin and tonofilament systems as well as ricin receptor sites. Adhesions derived from the extracellular face can be identified by either binding to Con A and to antibodies raised to the cell surface. This combination of lectins and antibodies is a very powerful cell surface probe.

The distribution of lectin receptor sites on the surfaces of a number of different cell types has been examined by binding to fluorescent-labelled lectins: for animal systems the most common are erythrocytes, lymphocytes, sperm and egg cells, and rod cells (Bridges and Fong, 1979); for lower plants, several algal (Bolwell *et al.*, 1979) and fungal (Mirelman *et al.*, 1975) systems have been used and for higher plants, root slime (Hinch and Clarke, 1980) (see Figure 7), female sexual tissues (Knox *et al.*, 1976; Clarke *et al.*, 1979), pollen grain walls, and isolated protoplasts. In some cases lectin binding could only be observed after alteration of the surface either by glutaraldyde fixation or trypsinization. Studies by this technique also indicate that lectin receptor sites may alter during a particular biological process such as cell contact, fertilization, and differentiation (Monroy *et al.*, 1973). Binding of fluorescent lectins is not restricted to cell surface studies, but can also be applied to the examination of the nature of surfaces of isolated cellular components—for example FITC-Con A binds specifically to puffs in polytene chromosomes (Critchley *et al.*, 1979). These kinds of effects can be followed at the ultrastructural level by using ferritin-labelled lectins to detect surface receptors: in this case the complex is examined in the electron microscope and the ferritin is recognized by its electron-dense iron oxide core (5.5 nm). Ferritin can be coupled to the lectin with glutaraldyde or lectin–ferritin conjugates can be obtained commercially. The conjugate is then applied directly to the cell suspension under defined conditions of temperature, time, and concentration, and the cells subsequently embedded and sectioned by the usual procedures. Alternatively, plasma membranes from cells such as erythrocytes can be lysed at an air–water interface, collected directly on to EM grids and treated with the lectin–ferritin conjugate on the grid. A detailed description of the techniques used and a critical discussion of the applications to animal cells have been published (Nicolson, 1978); the applications and potential of this technique for investigation of plant cells has been discussed (Knox and Clarke, 1978).

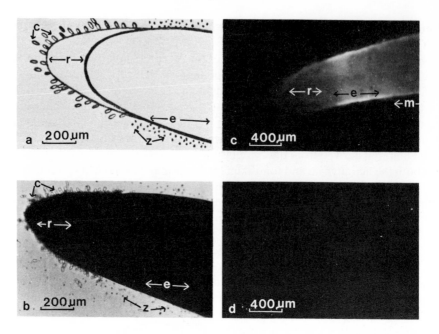

Figure 7. Localization of fucose-containing root slime in the zone of elongation of *Zea mays*. Fluorescent micrographs of: (a) Diagram and (b) light micrograph of root showing capasea (r) and zone of elongation (e): (c) root treated with FITC-*Ulex* lectin; (d) root treated with FITC-*Ulex* lectin in the presence of 0.2 M fucose. The lectin binds preferentially to the zone of elongation (e) rather than the cap region (r) = 10 μm. (From Hinch and Clarke, 1980)

The major drawbacks are that the covalent coupling leads to a mixture of molecules of which the ideal conjugate with equimolar ratios of lectin and label is found only in low yield. Also, the resulting complex has a high molecular weight and there may be steric hindrance to its binding to a cell surface. However, the value of this type of study can be seen, for example, in the recent elegant work of Pfenninger and Jamieson (1979b), who have examined the distribution of surface saccharides on pancreatic acinar, centroacinar, and endocrine cells by their binding to ferritin-labelled lectins and shown that the three cell types could be distinguished on the basis of their differential lectin binding. Acinar cells bound all lectin conjugates tested, but endocrine and centroacinar cells preferentially bound Con A, *Lens culinaris*, wheat germ, and castor bean RCA$_I$ lectins. Centroacinar, but not endocrine cells, bound RCA$_{II}$, and had few receptors for *Lotus, Ulex*, or soybean lectins (Figure 8). Thus there are apparently differences in cell surface saccharide composition in different cells of the same organ. Furthermore, there were differences in distribution of the receptors: the Con A and *Lens culinaris* lectin receptors

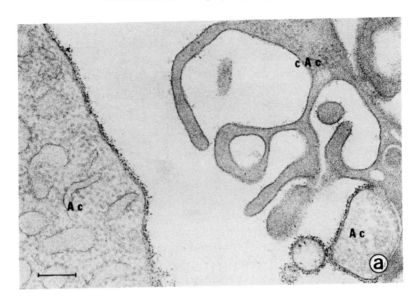

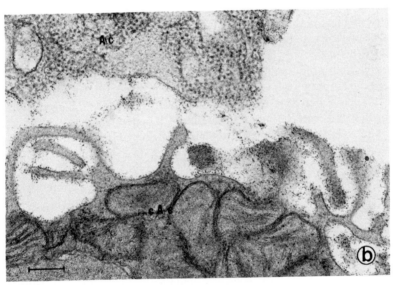

Figure 8. Localization of pancreatic cell surface receptors using ferritin-labelled lectins. (a) Electron micrograph showing part of an acinar cell (Ac) and a centroacinar cell (cAc) labelled with *Lotus* lectin–ferritin conjugate. The acinar cell surface binds the lectin strongly while the centroacinar cell surface does not. (× 42,700) (b) Electron micrograph showing part of an acinar cell (Ac) and a centroacinar cell (cAc) labelled with RCA–II–ferritin conjugate. Both cell surfaces bind this lectin. Bar 0.2 μm (× 40,600). (From Pfenninger and Jamieson, 1979b)

were in distinct patches on the cell surface, while those for all other lectins tested were homogeneously distributed. Some understanding of the nature of the receptor sites was also obtained by the use of this technique in conjuction with enzymic and solvent treatment. Freeze-etch electron microscopy of cells after binding of ferritin-labelled lectins has been successfully used to establish the relationship between lectin receptors at the cell surface and intramembranous particles (Pinto da Silva and Nicolson, 1974).

Recently a range of glycosylated derivatives of both peroxidase and ferritin have been used to detect lectin receptors. These derivatives can be prepared by coupling diazotized *p*-nitrophenyl sugar derivatives to the protein or they are available commercially (IBF). They are used in a two-step reaction—initially the lectin is bound to the cell surface and then the marker, either ferritin or peroxidase covalently coupled to the appropriate sugar, is bound to the free saccharide binding sites of the multivalent lectin (Kieda *et al.*, 1977). This technique partially overcomes one of the major difficulties associated with the use of covalently coupled lectin–marker conjugates, that is the low diffusion rate of the high molecular weight conjugates. This technique has also been adapted for fluorescent visualization of membrane-bound lectins, in this case a protein such as bovine serum albumin is coupled to the diazotized *p*-nitrophenyl sugar and the complex is labelled with FITC. The fluoroseinyl-glycosylated protein can then be used directly as a cell-surface probe (Kieda *et al.*, 1977, 1979).

Other methods of visualizing lectins at the electron microscope level are also used, for example enzymes which catalyse the formation of electron-dense products such as peroxidase may be bound to the lectin. As the peroxidase is a glycoprotein, it can be bound to Con-A-labelled cells by virtue of its 2-*O*-mannosyl residues in a two-step labelling procedure. However, for other lectins the peroxidase must be covalently coupled to the lectin, usually with glutaraldehyde. To visualize the peroxidase labelling the cell–lectin–peroxidase complex is allowed to react with peroxide and 3,3'-diaminobenzidine tetrahydrochloride or with 1-chloronaphthol to give an insoluble, coloured product which can be seen in the light microscope. Alternatively, the preparation can be treated with osmium tetroxide and examined by electron microscopy. This method has the advantage that as a single molecule of peroxidase generates a number of molecules of product, and it is this product which is detected, being more sensitive than the direct binding of ferritin-labelled lectin. Also, its molecular weight (40,000 daltons) is low compared with that of ferritin (molecular weight 750,000 daltons) and it is considered to be a more suitable label for detection of intracellular receptors than ferritin. A comprehensive discussion giving details of this method and its application has been published (Gonatas and Avrameas, 1977). A summary of these methods is given schematically in Figure 9.

Cell surface lectin receptors may also be viewed directly in the scanning electron microscope, and in this case the lectin is usually labelled with a marker which has a distinct and readily recognizable shape: for example, haemocyanin a cylindrical molecule (length 35 nm) which is a glycoprotein and like peroxidase can be used to detect Con A bound to cell surfaces by virtue of its saccharide residues. Gold markers have also been used successfully (Horisberger and Rosset, 1977). This technique can be used to quantitate the number of receptors over a relatively large surface area. The many hazards in the use of this technique, both experimental and interpretive, are discussed in detail by Brown and Revel (1978).

Other methods of visualizing cell surface receptors for lectins are by their binding to specific antibodies or to mannan–iron complexes. Details of the methods used, their applications and their advantages and disadvantages have been considered by Sharon and Lis (1975), Hubbard and Cohn (1976). Knox and Clarke (1978), and Nicolson (1978).

B. Isolation of Membrane-Bound Glycoproteins

One of the major problems of isolating membrane glycoproteins is the small quantity of material available. Generally the carbohydrate of the membrane represents only 1–5% of the total mass of the membrane, so that usually only microgram quantities of the individual components are available for analysis. Lectin affinity chromatography has been extremely useful in the separation of membrane glycoproteins. The same techniques employed for the separation of soluble glycoproteins apply, the major problem being to select a method for their solubilization which does not significantly alter the carbohydrate binding properties of the lectin.

Detergents such as sodium deoxycholate (1%) (Allan *et al.*, 1972), sodium dodecylsulphate, Triton X-100 (0.5%)(Cuatrecasas, 1972; Adair and Kornfeld, 1974), and a non-ionic detergent Nonidet NP40 (Schwartz *et al.*, 1973) have been successfully used. These detergents break hydrophobic and ionic bonds and cause dissociation of the extracted material into subunits. A major drawback of this technique is the difficulty of removing the detergent from the glycoprotein, so that all the subsequent analytical procedures must be carried out in the presence of the detergent. A careful study of the effect of detergents on saccharide-binding properties of lectins has been made by Lotan *et al.* (1977), which is an extremely useful reference for designing experimental procedures for preparation and analysis of membrane glycoproteins. The difficulty of associated detergent has been partly overcome by the use of lithium diiodosalicylate (Marchesi, 1972) which acts as a detergent but can be effectively removed from the glycoprotein. Proteins and glycoproteins can also be solubilized from intact membranes with organic solvents and salts such as 3 M KCl and guanidine hydrochloride (for a review see Maddy and Dunn, 1976).

Light microscope level
   1. Direct binding of FITC- or RITC-labelled lectin.

Cell + fluorescent – labelled lectin

   2. *Two-step binding of lectin peroxidase

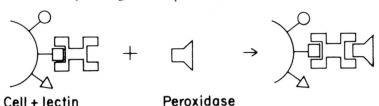

Cell + lectin   **Peroxidase**

                              Cell – lectin – peroxidase
                                     complex

   3. Direct binding of covalent lectin-peroxidase.

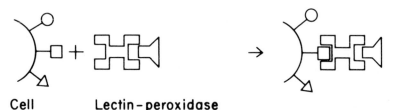

Cell   **Lectin – peroxidase**

                              Cell – lectin – peroxidase
                                     complex

   The other major method of obtaining preparations of membrane glycoproteins is by surface digestion of intact cells by proteolytic enzymes, for example
by pronase or papain. This method releases glycopeptides derived from the
intact glycoproteins and it may be difficult to relate subsequent analyses of the
glycopeptide to its parent glycoprotein. Details of these procedures are given
by Maddy and Dunn (1976) and Hughes (1976).
   In many cases, fractionation of membrane components is carried out on cell
preparations which have been surface labelled either with ^{125}I by the
lactoperoxidase technique (Marchalonis, 1969) or with tritium by oxidation
with galactose oxidase followed by reduction with tritiated borohydride

Electron microscope level
1. Direct binding of covalent lectin–ferritin complex.

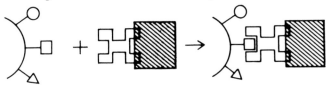

Cell   **Lectin-ferritin complex**   **Cell-lectin-ferritin complex**

2. Two-step binding of lectin to glycosylated ferritin.

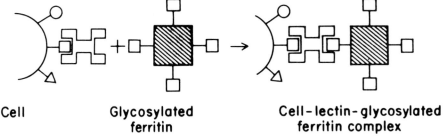

Cell   **Glycosylated ferritin**   **Cell-lectin-glycosylated ferritin complex**

Figure 9. Detection of cell surface saccharides with labelled lectin.

*The reaction is detected by the enzymic products of the peroxidase reaction in either the light or electron microscope.

(Gahmberg, 1978). Another method of introducing a label in the cell surface is by oxidation with dilute sodium metaperiodate followed by reduction with tritiated borohydride. Under controlled conditions the acyclic group of sialic acid residues is selectively oxidized (Blumenfeld *et al.*, 1972).

C. Lectin Binding to Whole Cells

Binding of lectins to cell surfaces can also be used to fractionate whole cells as well as their isolated membrane components. For example, thymocytes can be separated from erythrocytes by their preferential binding to low concentrations of Con A bound to nylon fibres (Edelman *et al.*, 1971). Separation on Con A–Sepharose columns is not usually successful because of the high affinity of the lectin cell binding and the difficulty of recovering the cells from the column. However, successful fractionation of lymphocytes on *Helix pomatia* haemagglutinin–Sepharose has been achieved (Hellstrom *et al.*, 1976). Changes in membrane carbohydrates can be detected during the cell cycle by following the ability of lectins to bind to the cell surface: more lectin molecules are bound at mitosis than at interphase (Noonan *et al.*, 1973).

It is also possible to select for resistance to lectin toxicity from particular cell lines. Some lectins such as ricin and wheat germ agglutinin are powerful cytotoxic agents at extremely low concentrations; other lectins such as Con A are mitogenic at low concentrations but may exert cytotoxic effects at higher concentrations. Cells which are resistant to toxic lectins are believed to have lost the capacity to bind the lectin because of some alteration in the surface saccharides: thus the complementary residue may be absent or masked by an additional saccharide residue or may be prevented from binding because of steric factors resulting from altered arrangement in the display of carbohydrate groups at the cell surface.

These effects can be explained in terms of the biosynthetic pathway for the glycoproteins. Biosynthesis of the asparagine-linked carbohydrate chains involves transfer of a precursor unit consisting of nine mannose, two or three glucose, and two N-acetylglucosamine residues from a lipid intermediate to the nascent glycoprotein in the rough endoplasmic reticulum. As the glycoprotein passes through the endomembrane system it is modified by enzymatic removal of the glucose and part of the mannose to give a pentamannose-di-N-acetylglucosamine core. This structure is then modified by attachment of N-acetylglucosamine which then signals further hydrolytic removal of the two remaining mannose residues on the branch. This step is followed by transfer of N-acetylglucosamine to the same branch, then galactose and sialic acid residues to both branches (Schacter, 1978). Lectin-resistant cell lines may lack one or more of the transferases resulting in an accumulation of partially formed oligosaccharide sequences lacking the saccharide units complementary to the toxic lectin; hence these cells do not bind the lectin and are resistant to its toxic effects. For example, WGA-resistant Chinese hamster ovary cells have surface glycoproteins deficient in terminal sialic acid but with a concomitantly high proportion of terminal galactosyl units; they are thus less able to bind the toxic lectin WGA (which depends on the presence of both sialic acid residues and N-acetylglucosamine residues) and more able to bind to the galactose-specific lectin, ricin. Defects in other cell surface glycoproteins synthesized by lectin-resistant cells have been listed by Lis and Sharon (1977) and Briles and Kornfeld (1978) The availability of such lectin-resistant cell lines and the amazing range of physiological effects induced by binding of lectins to surfaces of different cell types (Section V.A.1) offer a powerful experimental approach to understanding the form and function of membrane saccharide components and their relationship to cytoplasmic structures and metabolic events.

APPENDIX I

A. Lectin Purification

Many lectins can be purified from tissue extracts by affinity chromatography. The lectin-containing solution is allowed to absorb to an affinity column and the column extensively buffer-washed. The lectin is then eluted with a solution of the complementary sugar or a low pH buffer, the sugar is removed by dialysis, and the purified product freeze-dried or concentrated. The same approach can be used for purification of lectins after modification, as for example after labelling. Several polysaccharide gel preparations suitable as affinity reagents for purification of some lectins are commercially available. In some cases gels with either a glycoprotein or oligosaccharide containing a complementary saccharide, and covalently coupled to an insoluble support, have been used successfully. A useful list of methods for modification for both glycoproteins and carbohydrates to prepare affinity supports is given by Kennedy (1977).

A multipurpose 'universal' affinity column of hog gastric mucin coupled to agarose has been described by Pfenninger and Jamieson (1979a). The range of mono- and oligosaccharides of the hog gastric mucin provides binding sites for a number of lectins, each of which could be specifically eluted by its hapten sugar. In this way Con A, wheat germ, castor bean, soybean, *Lotus, Ulex,* and *Limulus* lectins have been purified from extracts of source material and also after ferritin labelling.

Where the lectin is itself a glycoprotein, it may be purified by chromatography on the basis of the affinity of its saccharide component for another lectin—for example, the glycoprotein lectins phytohaemagglutinin, soybean lectin, and *Dolichos bifloris* lectin have all been purified by affinity chromatography on Con A-Sepharose and elution with α-methyl-D-mannoside (Goldstein *et al.*, 1973). Examples of these procedures are summarized in Table 2.

Where affinity methods are not available, conventional methods for protein fractionation such as salt precipitation, ion exchange and gel chromatography, etc., have been used. Details of many methods of this type are given in *Methods in Enzymology,* Volumes 28 and 50.

B. Detection of Lectins and Glycoproteins

1. Double Diffusion

An agar plate (1% in PBS and 0.02% sodium azide) is prepared and solutions of lectin (1–10 mg/ml) and test material (containing about 1.0 mg/ml carbohydrate) placed in opposite wells. The plates are incubated for 24 hours at 37 °C in a moist chamber and examined for the presence of precipitin bands. The sensitivity of the procedure may be enhanced by drying the gel and staining it for protein, for example with Coomassie Brilliant Blue. A convenient method is to immerse the stained gel in 0.1% Coomassie Brilliant Blue in water : methanol : acetic acid (5 : 5 : 1 by volume) for 15 minutes, then to de-stain in five washes of 7.5% acetic acid, 7.5% methanol in water.

2. Quantitative Precipitin Assay

The lectin is incubated with a series of concentrations of glycoprotein, the resulting precipitates are centrifuged, washed, and their nitrogen content

Table 2. Examples of lectin purification by affinity chromatography

Lectin	Affinity adsorbent	Supplier	Eluant	Reference
Commercially available adsorbents				
Con A	Sephadex G-50	Pharmacia	Glucose	Agrawal and Goldstein (1967)
Lentil lectin	Sephadex G-1000	Pharmacia	Glucose	Howard et al. (1971)
Garden pea lectin	Sephadex G-150	Pharmacia	Glycine–HCl	Entlicher et al. (1970)
Castor bean lectin	Sepharose 4B	Pharmacia	Galactose	Tomita et al. (1972)
	Biogel A	Bio-Rad	Galactose/or Lactose	Nicolson et al. (1972)
Tridacna maxima lectin	Sepharose 4B		Ca²⁺-free buffer	Gleeson et al. (1979)
Wheat germ agglutinin	Chitin	Pharmacia	?	Bloch and Burger (1974a)
Adsorbents prepared by coupling a glycoprotein to an insoluble support				
Phytohaemaglutinin	Thyroglobulin–Sepharose		Glycine–HCl	Matsumoto and Osawa (1972)
Wheat germ agglutinin	Ovomucoid–Sepharose		Acetic acid	Le Vine et al., (1972)
Limulus polyphemus lectin and others	Fetuin			Sela et al. (1975)
Con A, wheat germ agglutinin,	Hog gastric mucin 'Universal'		Hapten sugar	Pfenninger and Jamieson (1979a)

Lectin	Adsorbent / affinity column	Eluent	Reference
castor bean, Lotus, Ulex, lima bean, and Limulus lectins	affinity column		

Adsorbents prepared by coupling saccharides to an insoluble support

Lectin	Adsorbent	Eluent	Reference
Ulex europaeus lectin	L-Fucose–starch	Glycine–HCl	Matsumoto and Osawa (1972)
Soybean agglutinin	N-Acetylglucosamine epoxy-activated Sepharose		Vretblad (1976)
Wheat germ agglutinin	N-Acetylgalactosamine epoxy-activated Sepharose		Vretblad (1976)
Lotus tetragonolobus lectin	N-(ε-Aminocaproyl)-β-glycosylamine of fucose		Bloch and Burger (1974b)
Wheat germ agglutinin	N-Acetylglucosamine		
Soybean lectin	Galactose		

Purification on Con A–Sepharose

Lectin	Adsorbent	Eluent	Reference
Phytohaemagglutinin	Con A–Sepharose	α-Methyl mannoside	Bessler and Goldstein (1973)
Dolichos biflorus lectin	Con A–Sepharose	α-Methyl mannoside	Bessler and Goldstein (1973)
Soybean lectin	Con A–Sepharose	α-Methyl mannoside	Bessler and Goldstein (1973)

More extensive lists of lectin purification procedures are given in Lis and Sharon (1977) and Brown and Hunt (1978), and details of procedures are given in *Methods in Enzymology*, Vols. 28 and 50.

measured. Two incubation schedules are commonly used: 48 hours at 25 °C (So and Goldstein, 1967) or 1 hour at 37 °C followed by 1 week at 4 °C (Schiffman *et al.*, 1964). This reaction is conveniently carried out in plastic tubes which are centrifuged in a Beckman microfuge. For hapten inhibition studies of this reaction, conditions are chosen which give maximum precipitation; lectin at this concentration is incubated with a range of sugar inhibitors, for 30 minutes, before addition of the glycoprotein and measurement of the nitrogen content of the precipitate.

3. Haemagglutination Assay

Blood is obtained freshly from a donor and transferred to a heparinized tube (100 units/ml). A thumb prick will readily yield 0.5 ml of blood which is sufficient for many assays. The blood group of the donor may be relevant to the test and should be considered in the experimental design. The erythrocytes are collected by centrifugation (3 minutes at 2000 g) and washed three times with PBS. The packed cells are diluted to give a 3% v/v suspension in the same buffer. Serial two-fold dilutions of the lectin are made in a microtitre test tray and an equal volume of the cell suspension is added, the tray rocked to mix, and the wells are examined for agglutination after incubation for 1 hour at room temperature. The titre is the reciprocal of the highest dilution showing agglutination. This assay is extremely sensitive and lectin levels as low as 10 ng/ml can be detected, but the reproducibility is limited by the two-fold dilution procedure. The sensitivity of the assay can be increased by using trypsinized cells, but cells treated in this way do not retain their blood group specificity.

Diluted cells are trypsinized by incubation with 0.1% trypsin (Bacto-trypsin 1 : 250 in PBS) (9 ml cells + 1 ml 1% trypsin) at 37 °C for 1 hour. The cells are then washed with PBS five times and resuspended to give a 2% suspension.

Formalinized erythrocytes are also used and these cells can be used to assay tissue extracts containing detergents. They are also relatively stable and can be stored for several months. Washed cells are made to an 8% (v/v) suspension which is mixed with an equal volume of fresh 3% formaldehyde in PBS, adjusted to pH 7.4 with 1 M NaOH just before use. The mixture is incubated for 18 hours at 37 °C with gentle shaking. The cells are then washed repeatedly with PBS (five times), stored as a 10% suspension in PBS and diluted with PBS to 3.3% prior to use in an assay (Butler, 1963).

For detection of a glycoprotein or other saccharide-containing inhibitors of the reaction, a set of conditions are chosen from the haemagglutination assay outlined, which give complete agglutination. The lectin, at the concentration selected, is then incubated with a range of concentrations of inhibitor for 30 minutes at room temperature, and then mixed with an equal volume of prepared cells, incubated for 1 hour,and the reaction is examined for haemagglutination. The concentration at which the inhibitor is effective can then be calculated. Both the haemagglutination assay and its inhibition can be more precisely quantitated by using a spectrophotometric method or an electronic particle counting technique (Köhle and Kauss, 1980) for estimating the extent of haemagglutination (Liener, 1955).

4. Radioimmuneassay

Lectins are generally antigenic and antisera can be raised to them in rabbits; if the lectin is toxic, extremely low doses in the initial challenge should be used. When both purified lectin and specific antiserum are available, the amount of lectin present in a tissue extract can be measured by a radioimmune assay (Pueppke *et al.*, 1978). One set of experimental conditions which have been used are 250 µl of rabbit antiserum (diluted so that 90% of counts of a 50 µl aliquot of [^{125}I]soybean lectin at 40,000 cpm/ml containing 20 ng lectin were precipitated) was incubated with a 50 µl aliquot of [^{125}I]soybean lectin containing 20 ng lectin at 40,000 cpm/ml, and 100 µl of the test sample containing 0.1 to 1.0 µl of lectin. The mixture was incubated for 1 hour at 4 °C then 20 µl of goat anti-rabbit IgG was added and the mixture incubated for 24 hours at 5 °C. The immunoprecipitate was then collected by centrifugation and the amount of [^{125}I]lectin in the supernatant and the precipitate determined. The relationship between the number of counts precipitated and amount of lectin present in the sample was calculated from a standard curve.

5. Detection of Glycoproteins in Gels by their Binding to Labelled Lectins

Glycoproteins can be detected after separation by gel electrophoresis by their binding to a lectin labelled with either a radioactive isotope, fluorescent marker, or an enzyme.

After electrophoresis, the gels are fixed either with water : methanol : acetic acid 5: 1 by volume) or for low molecular weight material with glutaraldehdye. The gels may then be stained with Coomassie Brilliant Blue, 0.1% in water : methanol : acetic acid (5 : 5 :1 (v/v/v)); this procedure should be used cautiously or avoided if possible as it may block the binding of certain lectins or give non-specific binding of some gel bands. After either fixing and or staining, the gels are treated with several changes of a solution of 7.5% methanol, 7.5% acetic acid in water and then equilibrated in PBS by immersion in several changes of buffer. The gel may then be treated with the labelled lectin, either by total immersion or by overlaying one surface of the gel (Hoffman and McMahon, 1978; Burridge, 1978). After incubation for a suitable period (1–20 hours); the gels were washed with PBS over an extended period (2 days) and examined. Bound ^{125}I-labelled lectins are detected by autoradiography, fluorescent-labelled lectins are detected by examination in UV light, and enzyme-labelled lectins are detected by insoluble, coloured products formed on application of a suitable substrate (Gonatas and Avrameas, 1977).

Alternatively, the polyacrylamide gels can be incubated with 2% periodic acid or 0.25 M ammonium hydroxide for 30 minutes to break down the cross-linkages, and washed three times with buffer. The gels are then placed in contact with freshly prepared DBM paper (Alwine *et al.*, 1977) and the proteins are transferred to it by blotting under pressure overnight at room temperature. The remaining active sites on the paper are then blocked with 0.1 M Tris–HCl (pH 9.0)-ethanolamine–gelatin. The proteins are now fixed to the paper and can be detected using radio-, fluorescent-, and peroxidase-labelled lectins or immunological techniques (Renart *et al.*, 1979).

A better technique for protein transfer to derivatized and activated paper has been developed by Bittner *et al.* (1980) and Towbin *et al.* (1979). They both use electrophoretic techniques to facilitate protein transfer. The polyacrylamide gels are washed and equilibrated with buffer. Either freshly prepared DBM-paper or nitrocellulose paper which has been equilibrated with buffer is placed in direct contact with the gels. The gel-transfer sheet assemblage is then placed between buffer equilibrated supports (e.g. filter paper or scouring pads) and the 'sandwich' is placed in an electrophoresis tank which allows uniform distribution of an electrical field over the entire gel surface. The gels are run at *ca*. 6 V/cm for 1 hour, after which time the remaining active sites on the paper are blocked using bovine serum albumin (3%). The proteins are now covalently linked to the paper and can be detected using radio-, fluorescent-, or peroxidase-labelled affinity ligands (e.g. lectins) or by using immunological techniques.

The reverse procedure can also be used: the lectin is coupled to the paper and used to detect electrophoretically separated glycoproteins (Erlich *et al.*, 1979). The freshly diazotized paper is incubated with Con A (or other lectins) at 2 mg/ml in 25 mM phosphate buffer (pH 6.5) for 12 hours at 4 °C with gentle agitation. The remaining unreacted active sites are blocked with bovine serum albumin (1%) for 3 to 5 hours at 37 °C with gentle shaking. The polyacrylamide gels are treated to remove any detergent before placing them in contact with the affinity ligand–paper matrix. Filter papers and a weight, to maintain pressure, are placed on the gels which are then left undisturbed for 1–2 hours at room temperature. After this time, sufficient transfer of glycoproteins to the support for their detection by radiochemical or immunological techniques is achieved.

Another useful technique is electrophoresis of glycoproteins into gels containing lectins: it is analogous to rocket immunoelectrophoresis and can be used to quantitate the separated glycoproteins (Bøg-Hansen *et al.*, 1977).

6. *Lectin Binding to Immobilized Glycoproteins*

A method similar to the radioimmunoassay has been developed by Howlett and Clarke (1981). In this method, the wells of a polyvinyl chloride microtitre plate are coated with the glycoprotein to be examined. This is simply achieved by placing an aqueous solution of the glycoprotein (40 μl, 16 mg/ml) into the wells of the tray and leaving it to incubate for 3 hours at 20 °C. After this time, the solution is removed and any unreacted active sites are blocked with 1% bovine serum albumin. The wells are extensively washed, drained and left to air dry. The binding of radiochemically labelled lectins by the glycoprotein can now be studied. The labelled lectin (specific activity 10^8 cpm/μg) is added to the wells of the tray and left to incubate for 6 hours at 20 °C. The wells are again washed extensively, dried and the individual wells are counted to determine the saccharide residues present on the glycoprotein and the amount of lectin bound to the glycoprotein. Control experiments in which the lectin is pre-incubated for 30 minutes at 20 °C with its complementary hapten should also be performed to determine the level of non-specific binding.

C. Lectin Labelling

It is important to remember that in all manipulations with lectins there may be ion depletion, which will result in loss of specificity in the binding reaction. The buffers in which the lectins are used should be maintained at 0.5 mM for the essential ions. Wherever possible, the specificity of lectin binding should be confirmed by demonstrating specific inhibitions of the reaction with simple saccharides before use. Repurification of the labelled lectins is often worthwhile and can usually be simply achieved by affinity chromatography (Appendix I. A).

1. Labelling with Radioactive Tracers

Lectins may be iodinated either by the chloramine-T method (Hunter and Greenwood, 1962), by the lactoperoxidase method (Marchalonis, 1969; Philipps *et al.*, 1974) or by the Iodogen method (Fraker and Speck, 1978). A convenient and stable iodination of lectins has been achieved (Briles *et al.*, 1979) using [^{125}I]*N*-succinimidyl-3-(4-hydroxyphenyl) propionate (Bolton and Hunter, 1973. Often the labelling is performed in the presence of the complementary sugar, in order to protect the binding site. The method described by Phillips *et al* (1974) involves labelling Con A while bound to a column of Sephadex G-75. This allows ready removal of reactants from the labelled Con A, protection of the binding sites during labelling and results in a product with high specific activity. A tritium label can be introduced by acetylating the lectin protein with [^{3}H]acetic anhydride by the procedure described by Ostrowski *et al.* (1970) or, if the lectin is a glycoprotein, by galactose oxidase or periodate oxidation followed by reduction with sodium

[³H]borohydride (Lotan   *et al.*, 1975b). Galactose oxidase will oxidize terminal galactosyl residues, while periodate treatment preferentially oxidizes sialic acid residues (Gahmberg, 1978).

Procedure for iodination of lectins. (a) Lacto-peroxidase method: Lectin (100 mg) is incubated (1 hour at 37 °C) with 0.1 M glucose, 0.05 M hapten sugar, 0.30 U lactoperoxidase, 0.3 U glucose oxidase, 2 nM KI and 1 mCi Na¹²⁵I in a volume of 10 ml. The reaction mixture is then dialysed exhaustively to remove unreacted ¹²⁵I and hapten sugar. The iodinated lectin is then repurified by affinity chromatography (Marchalonis, 1969; Hubbard and Cohen, 1972; Pfenninger and Jamieson, 1979a). (b) Iodogen method. Iodogen (1,3,4,6-tetrachloro-3a,6a-diphenylglycoluril) is sparingly soluble and can be coated on to a reaction vessel in which it acts as a solid phase that when in contact with an aqueous mixture of iodine-125 and protein results in the labelling of the protein. A small amount of Iodogen (1-2 mg) is dissolved in chloroform and is plated in a thin film on to the reaction vessel by evaporation under nitrogen (to ensure a high efficiency of labelling, the film should be completely dry). When the reaction vial has been prepared, an aqueous solution of the protein (e.g. lectin) (40–100 μl) is added together with 4–10 μl of iodine-125 (specific activity 17 mCi ¹²⁵I/μg iodine). The solution is left in contact with the Iodogen film for 30 to 45 minutes at room temperature, after which time the reaction is terminated by removal of the solution from the vial. The labelled protein is separated from the free iodine by passage down a Bio-Gel P-2 column (1 × 5 cm) (Fraker and Speck, 1978).

2. Fluorescent Labelling of Lectins

Labelling of lectins with either fluorescein or rhodamine can be simply achieved by the diffusion method: lectin (1–25 mg) in 0.15 M NaCl, 0.05 M sodium carbonate buffer (pH 9.5), is placed in a dialysis sac and dialysed overnight against a solution of FITC (0.1 mg/ml) in the same buffer at 4 °C. The excess FITC is then removed on a Bio-Gel P6 column. The ratio of FITC to protein can be calculated from the absorbance of the labelled material at 280 and 493 nm (Goldman, 1968).

3. Ferritin Labelling of Lectins

The procedure most often used is glutaraldehyde conjugation of ferritin to lectin as described by Avrameas (1969); modifications are given by Nicolson (1978) and Pfenninger and Jamieson (1979a). The ferritin must be either elec-tron-microscopic grade (e.g. Sigma Chemical Co.) or should be recrystallized from 5% sodium sulphate and further purified by centrifugation (85,000 *g*,

3 hours, 5 °C) and filtration on Bio-Gel A5m to remove polymeric material. For ease of monitoring the coupling procedure, the lectin may first be radioiodinated. The following procedure is that used by Pfenninger and Jamieson (1979a). Lectin $(2 \times 10^{-5}$ M) and ferritin $(2 \times 10^{-5}$ M) in PBS containing 0.1 M hapten sugar are stirred with glutaraldehyde $(200 \times$ molar excess) for 1 hour at room temperature. The reaction is stopped by addition of 0.1 M $NaBH_4$ for 15 minutes to quench unreacted aldehyde groups. The conjugates are purified by dialysis and affinity chromatography. Monomeric lectin–ferritin conjugates were obtained by chromatography on Bio-Gel A5m.

This conjugation procedure does not significantly alter the binding properties of the lectins. Nicolson (1978) has given a detailed practical description of this type of coupling as well as alternative coupling and labelling procedures and this work should be consulted before initiating investigations of this type.

D. Detection of Cell Surface Receptors by Binding to Labelled Lectins

1. Binding of Radioactivly-labelled Lectins to Cells

The cells are incubated with the labelled lectin in a suitable buffer for periods of about 30–90 minutes with gentle rotation to ensure contact. After incubation, the cells are collected by centrifugation, washed, and counted. Control experiments in the presence of complementary sugars are important to establish the extent of non-specific binding; additional control experiments in which the cells are incubated with non-labelled lectin before the labelled lectin, to confirm the specificity of the reaction should also be performed. The precise conditions will depend on such factors as the nature of the cell, the number of receptors present, and the particular lectin under consideration. One set of conditions used are: erythrocytes $(5 \times 10^7$ cells/ml) in 1 ml of PBS were added to serial dilutions of ^{125}I-labelled lectin $(6–12 \times 10^3$ cpm/μg), and incubated for 90 minutes at room temperature. The cells were collected, washed once by centrifugation, and counted. The binding of soybean lectin to erythrocytes determined by this procedure followed a simple saturation curve (Reisner *et al.*, 1976).

2. Binding of Fluorescent-labelled Lectins to Cells

Usually the cells are incubated directly with the FITC- or RITC-labelled lectin for period of 10–60 minutes at a defined temperature, the cells are washed with an appropriate buffer, and viewed by fluorescent microscopy. Lectin concentrations of about 0.5 mg/ml are used. Control experiments in which the hapten sugar is included in the incubation mixture are run. Untreated cells should also be viewed to establish whether there is autofluorescence: this is a real problem for certain types of plant cells.

3. Binding of Ferritin-Lectin Conjugates to Cell Surfaces

Typically cells are incubated with radioiodinated lectin–ferritin conjugates at 4 °C; labelling at higher temperatures induces redistribution of lectin binding sites. Short incubation periods (5–30 minutes) are also used to minimize receptor redistribution. The cells may be fresh and suspended in buffer in which case 2×10^7 cells/ml and lectin–ferritin conjugate (0.5 mg/ml in PBS) would be a typical reaction mixture. Inclusion of 1% BSA and 0.2 M hapten sugar in the incubation mixture reduced the non-specific binding from 38% to 5% of total binding.

4. Preparation of Cells for Electron Microscopy

After incubation with lectin conjugate, cells are washed, fixed with glutaraldehyde, post-fixed with osmium tetroxide and thin sections stained before observation.

The procedure used by Pfenninger and Jamieson (1979b) involved fixing the cells with an equal volume of 4% glutaraldehyde in 0.2 M Na cacodylate buffer (pH 7.4) for 1 hour at 25 °C, or overnight at 4 °C. Cell pellets were collected by centrifugation, post-fixed with 1% OsO_4 in the same buffer for 1 hour at 4 °C, washed, and stained for 1 hour at 23 °C with 0.5% magnesium cinamylacetate in 0.15 M NaCl. The pellets were dehydrated in ethanol and propylene oxide and embedded in Epon before sectioning and stained with bismuth subnitrate before viewing. Other practical details are given by Nicolson (1978).

E. Glycoprotein Isolation by Lectin Affinity Chromatography

Lectin affinity supports may be purchased commercially, or prepared by mixing cyanogen-bromide-activated Sepharose 4B (2g) with the lectin (20 mg) in 0.1 M $NaHCO_3$, 0.5 M NaCl. The complementary saccharide (10 mM) is often included in the reaction mixture to protect the binding sites (Axen *et al*, 1970).

The lectin–gel is then packed into a column and equilibrated with buffer. The buffer or detergent solution of the glycoprotein is then applied and the column washed with at least five bed volumes of the same buffer. The bound material is then eluted with either a solution or a concentration gradient of the complementary saccharide. This is the principle of the method, but the precise choice of conditions depends on the particular system under consideration.

For example, the capacity of a lectin affinity column will vary for different glycoproteins, and figures are rarely quoted. However, from the available data (for review see Dulaney, 1979) it would seem that a ten-fold excess of lectin to glycoprotein on a weight basis would be a guide for a pilot experiment. The composition of the buffer must also be chosen with regard to the particular system: a pH in the range 6–8 is usually satisfactory; in some cases NaCl in concentrations up to 1 M is added to the buffer to minimize non-specific binding. Metal ions are also included if they are essential to the binding of saccharide by the particular lectin being used. The concentration of eluting glycoside is another parameter which must be established for each system, and may be up to 1 M. Most procedures of this type are run slowly at room temperature. In general best results are obtained when the sample is both added to and eluted from the column over a period of several hours. The best approach to a choice of all these variables is to establish the most favourable conditions for binding and elution on a small scale and then to apply these conditions to a subsequent preparative-scale experiment.

Fractionation of membrane glycoproteins released by detergent treatment on lectin affinity columns is often possible as many lectins are active in the presence of low detergent concentrations. The affinity column must be washed extensively with the detergent solution before use to ensure removal of any non-covalently bound lectin. The detergent extract of membrane is applied to the column and eluted with a solution of monosaccharide or glycoside complementary to the lectin. Membrane fractions obtained in this way are electrophoretically heterogeneous, but are enriched in carbohydrate and are powerful inhibitors of the corresponding lectin activity (Allan *et al.*, 1972; Jansons and Burger, 1973). Glycopeptides released by enzymic digestion of intact cells can also be fractionated on lectin affinity columns.

REFERENCES

Adair, W. L., and Kornfeld, S. (1974). Isolation of receptors for wheat germ agglutinin and the *Ricinus communis* lectins from human erythrocytes using affinity chromatography. *J. Biol. Chem.*, **249**, 4696–4704.

Agrawal, B. B. C., and Goldstein, I. J. (1967). Protein–carbohydrate interaction. VI. Isolation of concanavalin A by specific adsorption on cross-linked dextran gels. *Biochim Biophys. Acta*, **147**, 262–271.

Allan, D., Avgar, J., and Crumpton, M. J. (1972). Glycoprotein receptors for concanavalin A isolated from pig lymphocyte plasma membrane by affinity chromatography in sodium deoxycholate, *Nature (Lond.).*, **236**, 23–25.

Alwine, J. C., Kemp, D., and Stark, G. (1977). Method for detection of specific RNAs in agarose gels by transfer to diazobenzyloxymethyl–paper and hybridization with DNA probes. *Proc. Nat. Acad. Sci. USA.*, **74**, 5350–5354.

Ashwell, G., and Morell, A. G. (1978). Signals for degradation of glycoproteins. In Horowitz and Pigman (Eds) *The Glycoconjugates*, volume II, Academic Press, New York.

Aub, J. C., Stanford, B. H., and Cote, M. N. (1965). Studies on reactivity of tumor and normal cells to a wheat germ agglutinin. *Proc. nat. Acad. Sci. USA.*, **54**, 396.

Aub, J. C., Tieslau, C., and Lankester, A. (1963). Reactions of normal and neoplastic cell surfaces to enzymes. I. Wheat germ lipase and associated mucopolysaccharides. *Proc. Nat. Acad. Sci. USA.*, **50**, 613–619.

Avrameas, S. (1969). Coupling of enzymes to proteins with glutaraldehyde. Use of the conjugates for the detection of antigens and antibodies. *Immunochemistry*, **6**, 43–52.

Axen, R., Porath, J., and Ernback, S. (1970). Chemical coupling of peptides and proteins to polysaccharides by means of cyanogen halides. *Nature (Lond.).*, **214**, 1302.

Badley, R. A., Lloyd, C. W., Woods, A., Carruther, S., Allcock, C., and Rees, D. A. (1978). Mechanisms of cellular adhesion. III. Preparation and preliminary characteristics of adhesions. *Exp. Cell Ress.*, **117**, 231–244.

Baenziger, J. U., and Fiete, D. (1979). Structure of the complex oligosaccharides of fetuin. *J. Biol. Chem.*, **254**, 789–795.

Barkai, R., and Sharon, N. (1978). Lectins as a tool for the study of yeast cell walls. *Exp. Mycol.*, **2**, 110–113.

Barondes, S. H. (1981). Lectins: their multiple endogenous cellular function. *Ann. Rev. Biochem.*, **50**, 207–231.

Bauer, W. D. (1981). Infection of legumes by rhizobia. *Ann. Rev. Plant Physiol.*, **32**, 407–449.

Bessler, W., and Goldstein, I. J. (1973). Phytohaemagglutinin purification: a general method involving affinity and gel chromatography. *FEBS Lett.*, **34**, 58–62.

Bhavanandan, V. P., and Katlic, A. W. (1979). The interaction of wheat germ agglutinin with sialoglycoproteins. *J. Biol. Chem.*, **254**, 4000–4008.

Bittiger, H., and Schnebli, H. P. (1976). *Concanavalin A as a Tool*. Wiley, New York.

Bittner, M., Kupferer, P., and Morris, C. F. (1980). Electrophoretic transfer of proteins and nucleic acids from sheets. *Anal. Biochem.*, **102**, 459–471.

Bloch, R., and Burger, M. M. (1974a). Purification of wheat germ agglutinin using affinity chromatography on chitin. *Biochem. Biophys. Res, Commun.*, **58**, 13–19.

Bloch, R., and Burger, M. M. (1974b). A rapid procedure for derivatizing agarose with a variety of carbohydrates: its use for affinity chromatography of lectins. *FEBS Lett.*, **44**, 286–289.

Blumenfeld, O. O., Gallop, P. M., and Liao, T. H. (1972). Modification and introduction of a specific radioactive label into the erythrocyte membrane sialoglycoproteins, *Biochem. Biophys. Res. Commun.*, **48**, 242–251.

Bøg-Hansen, T. C., Bjerrum, V. J., and Brogren, C. H. (1977). Identification and quantification of glycoproteins by affinity electrophoresis. *Anal. Biochem.*, **81**, 78–87.

Bolton, A. E., and Hunter, W. M. (1973). The labelling of proteins to high specific activities by conjugation to a ^{125}I-containing acylating agent. *Biochem. 'J.*, **133**, 529–539.

Bolwell, G. P., Callow, J. A., Callow, M. E., and Evans, L. V. (1979). Fertilization in brown algae. II. Evidence for lectin-sensitive complementary receptors involved in gamete recognition in *Fucus serratus*. *J Cell. Sci.*, **36**, 19–30.

Boyd, W. C., and Reguera, R. M. (1949). Haemagglutinating substances for human cells in various plants. *J. Immunol.*, **62**, 333–339.

Bridges, C. D. B., and Fong, S.-L. (1979). Different receptors for distribution of peanut and ricin agglutinins between inner and outer segments of rod cells. *Nature (Lond.)*, **282**, 513–514.

Briles, E. B., and Kornfeld, S. (1978). Lectin-resistant cell surface variants of eukaryotic cells. *Trends Biochem. Sci.*, **3**, 223–227.

Briles, E. B., Gregory, W., Fletcher, P., and Kornfeld, S., (1979). Comparison of properties of β-galactoside-binding lectins from tissue of calf and chicken. *J. Cell Biol.*, **81**, 528–537.

Brown, J. C., and Hunt, R. C. (1978). Lectins. *Int. Rev. Cytol.*, **52**, 277–349.

Brown, S. S., and Revel, J.-P. (1978). Cell surface labelling for the scanning electron microscope. In J. K. Koehler, (Ed.) *Advanced Techniques in Biological Electron Microscopy*, volume II. Springer-Verlag, Berlin.

Burger, M. M., and Goldberg, A. R. (1967). Identification of a tumor specific determinant on neoplastic cell surfaces. *Proc. Nat, Acad. Sci. USA.*, **57**, 359–366.

Burridge, K. (1978). Direct identification of specific glycoproteins and antigens in sodium dodecyl sulphate gels. In V. Ginsburg (Ed.) (Gen. Eds. S. P. Colowick and N. O. Kaplan) *Methods in Enzymology*, volume L. *Complex Carbohydrates*, Part C. Academic Press, New York.

Butler, W. T. (1963). Hemagglutinations studies with formalinized erythrocytes. Effect of bis-diazobenzidine and tannic acid treatment on sensitization by soluble antigen. *J. Immunol.*, **90**, 663–671.

Butler, W. T., and Cunningham L. W. (1966). Evidence for the linkage of a disaccharide to hydroxylysine in tropocollagen. *J. Biol. Chem.*, **241**, 3882.

Callow, J. A. (1977). Recognition, resistance and the role of plant lectins in host parasite interactions. *Adv. Bot. Res.*, **4**, 1–49.

Carlson, D. (1968). Structures and immunochemical properties of oligosaccharides isolated from pig submaxillary mucins. *J. Biol. Chem.*, **243**, 616–626.

Chapman, A., and Kornfeld, R. (1979). Structure of the high mannose oligosaccharides of a human IgM myeloma protein. *J. Biol. Chem.*, **254**, 816–823.

Chowdhury, T. K., and Weiss, A. K. (1975). *Concanavalin A*. Plenum Press, New York.

Clarke, A. E., Gleeson, P., Harrison, S., and Knox, R. B. (1979). Cell recognition in plants: characterization of pollen and stigma surface determinants. *Proc. Nat. Acad. Sci. USA*, **76**, 3358.

Critchley, D. R., Ansell, S., and Dilks, S. (1979). Glycolipids: a class of membrane receptors. *Biochem. Soc. Trans.*, **7**, 314–319.

Cuatrecasas, P. (1972). Properties of the insulin receptor isolated from liver and fat cell membranes. *J. Biol. Chem.*, **247**, 1980.

Cunningham, B. A., Wang, J. L., Waxdal, M. J., and Edelman, G. M. (1975). The covalent and three-dimensional structure of Concanavalin A. *J. Biol. Chem.*, **250**, 1503–1512.

Curtis, A. (Ed.) (1978). Cell–cell recognition. *Symp. Soc. Exp. Biol.*, **32**, Cambridge University Press, Cambridge.

Debray, H., Decout, D., Strecker, G., Spi., G. and Montreuil, J. (1981). Specificity of twelve lectins towards oliogosaccharides and glycopeptides related to N-glycosyl proteins. *Eur. J. Biochem.* **117**, 41–55.

Dulaney, J. T. (1979). Binding interaction of glycoproteins with lectins. *Mol. Cell. Biochem.*, **21**, 43–62.

Edelman, G. M., Cunningham, B. A., Reeke, G. N., Becker, J. W., Waxdal, M., and Wang, J. L. (1972). The covalent and three dimensional structure of Concanavalin A. *Proc. Nat. Acad. Sci. USA*, **69**, 2580–2584.

Edelman, G. M. (1976). Surface modulation in cell recognition and cell growth. *Science*, **192**, 218–226.

Edelman, G. M., Rutishauser, V., and Millette, C. F. (1971). Cell fractionation and arrangement on fibres, beads and surfaces. *Proc. Nat. Acad. Sci. USA*, **68**, 2153–2157.

Ehrlich, P. (1891a). Experimentelle Untersuchungen über Immunität. I. Veber Ricin. *Wochens Chr.*, **17**, 976–979.

Ehrlich, P. (1891b). Experimentelle Untersuchungen über Immunität. II. Veber Abrin. *Wochens Chr.,* **17,** 1218–1219.

Entlicher, G., Kostin, J. V., and Kocourek, J. (1970). Studies on phytohaemagglutinins. III. Isolation and characterization of haemagglutinins from the pea (*Pisum sativum* L.). *Biochim. Biophys. Acta,* **221,** 272–281.

Erlich, H. A., Levinson, J. R., Cohens, N., and McDevitt, H. O. (1979). Filter affinity transfer. *J. Biol. Chem.,* **254,** 12240–12241.

Etzler, M. E., and Kabat, E. A. (1970). Purification and characterization of a lectin (plant haemagglutinin) with blood group A sensitivity from *Dolichos bifloris. Biochemistry,* **9,** 869–877.

Fraker, P. J., and Speck, J. C. (1978). Protein and cell membrane iodinations with a sparingly soluble chloroamide, 1,3,4,6-tetrachloro-3*a*,6a-diphenylglycoluril. *Biochem. Biophys. Res. Commun.,* **80,** 849–857.

Frazier, W., and Glaser, L. (1979). Surface components and cell recognition. *Ann. Rev. Biochem.,* **48,** 491–523.

Fukuda, M., Kondo, T., and Osawa, T. (1976). Studies on the hydrazinolysis of glycoproteins, core structures of oligosaccharides obtained from porcine thyroglobulin and pineapple stem bromelain. *J. Biochem., Tokyo,* **80,** 1223.

Furlan, M., Perret, B. A., and Beck, E. A. (1979). Staining of glycoprotein polyacrylamide and agarose gels with fluorescent lectins. *Anal. Biochem.,* **96,** 208–214.

Gahmberg, C. G. (1978). Tritium labelling of cell surface glycoproteins and glycolipids using galactose oxidase. In V. Ginsberg (Ed.) *Methods in Enzymology,* volume L, Part C, p. 204. Academic Press, New York.

Glaudemans, C. P. J. (1975). The interaction of homogeneous, murine myeloma immunoglobulins with polysaccharide antigens. *Adv. Carbohydr. Chem Biochem.,* **31,** 313–346.

Gleeson, P. A., Jermyn, M. A., and Clarke, A. E. (1979). Isolation of an arabinogalactan-protein by lectin affinity chromatography on Tridacnin-Sepharose 4B. *Anal. Biochem.,* **92,** 41–45.

Glick, M. C., and Flowers, H. (1978). Surface membranes. In M. I. Horowitz and W. Pigman (Eds) *The Glycoconjugates,* Volume II. pp. 337–384. Academic Press, New York.

Gold, E. R., and Balding, P. (1975). *Receptor-Specific Proteins, Plant and Animal Lectins.* Elsevier, New York.

Goldman, M. (1968). *Flourescent Antibody Methods.* Academic Press, New York.

Goldstein, I. J., Hammarström, S., and Sundblad, G. (1975). Precipitation and carbohydrate-binding specificity studies on wheat germ agglutinin. *Biochim. Biophys. Acta,* **405,** 53–61.

Goldstein, I. J., and Hayes, C. E. (1978). The lectins: carbohydrate binding proteins of plants and animals. *Adv. Carbohydr. Chem. Biochem.,* 128–340.

Goldstein, I. J., Hughes, R. C., Monsigny, M., Osawa, T., and Sharon, N. (1980). What should be called a lectin? *Nature (Lond.).* **285,** 66.

Goldstein, I. J., Reichart, C. M., Misaki, A., and Gorin, P. A. J. (1973). An 'extension' of the carbohydrates binding specificity of Concanavalin A. *Biochim. Biophys. Acta.* **317,** 500–504.

Goldstein, I. J., Reichart, C. M., and Misaki, A. (1974). Interaction of Concanavalin A with model substrates. *Ann. N.Y. Acad. Sci.,* **234,** 283–295.

Gonatas, N. K. and Avrameas, S. (1977). Detection of carbohydrates with lectin–peroxidase conjugates. *Methods Cell Biol.,* **15,** 387–404.

Gottschalk, A. (Ed.) (.1972). *Glycoproteins,* 2nd edn. Elsevier, Amsterdam.

Hallgren, P., Lundblad, A., and Svensson, S. (1975). A new type of carbohdyrate–protein linkage in a glycopeptide from normal human urine. *J. Biol. Chem.,* **250,** 5312.

Hayman, M. J., and Crumpton, M. J. (1972). Isolation of glycoproteins from pig lymphocyte plasma membrane using *Lens culinaris* phytohaemagglutinin. *Biochem. Biophys. Res. Coomun., 47*, 923–930.

Heath, M. F., and Northcote, D. H. (1971). Glycoprotein from the wall of sycamore tissue culture cells. *Biochem J., 125*, 952.

Hellstrom, U., Hammastrom, S., Dillner, M.-L., Perlman, H., and Perlman, P. (1976). Fractionation of human blood lymphocytes on *Helix pomatia*. A haemagglutinin coupled to sepharose beads. *Scand. J. Immunol., 5*, Suppl. 5, 45–55.

Hinch, J., and Clarke, A. E. (1980). Adhesion of fungal zoospores to root surfaces is mediated by carbohydrates of the root slime. *Physiol. Plant Pathol., 16*, 303–307.

Hoffman, S., and McMahon, D. (1978). Defective glycoproteins in the plasma membrane of an aggregation minus mutant of *Dictyostelium discoideum* with abnormal cellular interactions. *J. Biol. Chem., 253*, 278–287.

Horejsi, V. (1979). Galactose oxidase: with lectin properties. *Biochim. Biophys. Acta, 577*, 383–388.

Horisberger, M., and Rosset, J. (1977). Colloidal gold, a useful marker for transmission and scanning electron microscopy. *J. Histochem. Cytochem., 25*, 295–305.

Howard, I. K., Sage, H. J., Stein, M. D., Young, N. M., Leon, M. A., and Dyckes, D. F. (1971). Studies on a phytohaemagglutinin from the lentil. II. Multiple forms of *Lens culinaris* haemagglutinin. *J. Biol. Chem., 246*, 1590–1595.

Howlett, B. J., and Clarke, A. E. (1981). Detection of lectin binding to glycoconjugates immobilized on polyvinyl chloride microtitre plates. *Biochem. Int., 2*, 553–560.

Hrkal, Z., and Vodrazka, Z. (1977). Isolation of serum albumin and immunoglobulins by chromatography on Con A–Sepharose and Sephadex G-150. *J. Chromatogr., 135*, 193–195.

Hubbard, A. L., and Cohn, Z. A. (1976). Specific labels for cell surfaces. In A. H. Maddy (Ed.) *Biochemical Analyses of Membranes*, p. 427. Wiley, New York.

Hubbard, S. C., and Ivatt, R. J. (1981). Synthesis and processing of asparagine linked oligosaccharides. *Ann. Rev. Biochem., 50*, 555–583.

Hughes, R. C. (1976). *Membrane Glycoproteins*. Butterworths, London.

Hughes, R. C., and Sharon, N. (1978). Carbohydrates in recognition. *Trends Biochem. Sci., 3*, 275.

Hunter, W. M., and Greenwood, F. C. (1962). Preparation of iodine-131 labelled human growth hormone of high specific activity. *Nature (Lond.), 194*, 495.

Inbar, M., Ben-Bassat, H., and Sachs, L. (1973). Difference in the mobility of lectins sites on the surface membrane of normal lymphocytes and malignant cells. *Int. J. Cancer, 12*, 93–99.

Irimura, T., Kawaguchi, T., Terao, T., and Osawa, T. (1975). Carbohydrate-binding specificity of so-called galactose-specific phytohaemagglutinins. *Carbohydr. Res., 39*, 317–327.

Iyer, P. N., Wilkinson, K. D., and Goldstein, I. J. (1976). An *N*-acetyl-D-glucosamine binding lectin from *Bandeiraea simplicifolia* seeds. *Arch. Biochem. Biophys., 177*, 330–333.

Jansons, V. K., and Burger, M. M. (1973). Isolation and characterization of agglutinin receptor sites. II. Isolation and partial purification of a surface membrane receptor for wheat germ agglutinin. *Biochim. Biophys. Acta, 291*, 127–135.

Judd, W. J., Steiner, E. A., Friedman, B. A., Hayes, C. E., and Goldstein, I. J. (1976). Serological studies on an α-D-galactosyl-binding lectin isolated from *Bandeiraea simplicifolia* seeds. *Vox Sang., 30*, 216–267.

Kaifu, R., Osawa, T., and Jeanloz, R. W. (1975). Synthesis of 2-*O*-(2-acetamido-2-deoxy-β-D-gluco-pyranosyl)-D-mannose, and its interaction with D-mannose specific lectins. *Carbohydr. Res., 40*, 111–117.

Karnovsky, M. J., and Unanue, E. R. (1973). Mapping and migration of lymphocyte surface macrolecules. *Fed. Proc. Am. Soc. Exp. Biol., 32*, 55–59.

Kauss, H. (1980). Lectins and their physiological role in slime moulds and in higher plants. In *Encyclopedia of Plant Physiology. New Series. Plant Carbohydrates,* volume II. Springer-Verlag, Berlin.

Kawaski, T., and Ashwell, G. (1976). Carbohydrate structure of glycopeptides isolated from an hepatic membrane-binding protein specific for asialoglycoproteins. *J. Biol. Chem., 251*, 5292.

Kennedy, J. F. (1977). Chemical synthesis and modification of oligosaccharides, polysaccharides, glycoproteins, enzymes and glycolipids. *Carbohydr. Chem., 9*, 412–462.

Kieda, C., Delmotte, F., and Monsigny, M. (1977). Preparation and properties of glycosylated cytochemical markers. *FEBS Lett., 76*, 257–261.

Kieda, C., Roche, A.-C., Delmotte, F., and Monsigny, M. (1979). Lymphocyte membrane lectins: direct visualization by the use of fluoresceinyl-glycosylated cytochemical markers. *FEBS Lett.* 99, 329–332.

Köhle, H., and Kauss, H. (1980). Improved analysis of haemagglutination assays for quantitation of lectin activity. *Anal. Biochem.* (in press).

Knox, R. B., and Clarke, A. E. (1978). Localization of proteins and glycoproteins by binding to labelled antibodies and lectins. In J. L. Hall (Ed.) *Electron Microscopy and Cytochemistry of Plant Cells,* pp. 150–185. Elsevier, North-Holland, Amsterdam.

Knox, R. B., Clarke, A. E., Harrison, E., Smith, P., and Marchalonis, J. J. (1976). Cell recognition in plants: determinants of the stigma surface and their pollen interactions. *Proc. Nat. Acad. Sci. USA., 73*, 2788–2792.

Kobiler, D., Beyer, E. C., and Barondes, S. H. (1978). Developmentally regulated lectins from chick muscle, brain and liver have similar chemical and immunological properties. *Dev. Biol., 64*, 265–272.

Kornfeld, R., (1978). Structure of the oligosaccharides of three glycopeptides from calf thymus plasma membranes. *Biochemistry, 17*, 1415.

Kornfeld, R., and Kornfeld, S. (1974). Structure of membrane receptors for plant lectins. *Ann N.Y. Acad. Sci., 234*, 276–282.

Kornfeld, R., and Kornfeld, S. (1976). Comparative aspects of glycoprotein structure. *Ann. Rev. Biochem., 45*, 217–237.

Kornfeld, S., and Kornfeld, R. (1978). Use of lectins in the study of mammalian glycoproteins. In M. I. Horowitz and W. Pigman (Eds) *The Glycoconjugates,* volume II. Academic Press, New York.

Kristiansen, T. (1974). Studies on blood group substances. III. Biospecific affinity chromatography of blood group substance A on *Vicia cracca* phytohaemagglutinin–agarose. *Biochim. Biophys. Acta, 338*, 246–253.

Lamport, D. T. A. (1969). The isolation and partial characterization of hydroxyproline-rich glycopeptides obtained by enzymatic degradation of primary cell walls. *Biochemistry, 8*, 1155.

Lamport, D. T. A., Katona, L., and Roerig, S. (1973). Galactosylserine in extensin. *Biochem. J., 135*, 125.

Larkin, P. (1978). Plant protoplast agglutination by lectins. *Plant Physiol., 61*, 626–629.

Larriba, G., Klinger, M., Sramek, S., and Steiner, S. (1977). Novel fucose-containing components from rat tissues. *Biochem. Biophys. Res. Commun., 77*, 79.

Lennarz, W. J. (1980). *The Biochemistry of Glycoproteins and Proteoglycans.* Plenum Press, New York.

LeVine, D., Kaplan, M. K. J., and Greenaway, P. J. (1972). The purification and characterization of wheat-germ agglutinin. *Biochem. J., 129*, 847–856.

Liener, I. E. (1955). The photometric determination of the haemagglutinating activity of soyin and crude soybean extracts. *Arch. Biochem. Biophys.*, **54**, 223–231.

Leiner, I. E. (1976). Phytohaemagglutinins (Phytolectins). *Ann. Rev. Plant Physiol.*, **27**, 291–319.

Lis, H., Sela, A., Sachs, L., and Sharon, N. (1970). Specific inhibition by *N*-acetyl-D-galactosamine of the interaction between soybean agglutinin and animal cell surfaces. *Biochim. Biophys. Acta,* **211**, 582–585.

Lis, H., and Sharon, N. (1973). The biochemistry of plant lectins (phytohaemagglutinins). *Ann. Rev. Biochem.*, **42**, 541–574.

Lis, H., and Sharon, N. (1977). Lectins: their chemistry and application to immunology. In M. Sela (Ed.) *The Antigens* IV. pp. 429–529, Academic Press, New York.

Lis, H., and Sharon, N. (1980). Lectins in higher plants. In Stumpf, R. K., Con, E. E. (Eds) *The Biochemistry of Plants*. Academic Press, New York, Vol. VI.

Lotan, R. H., Beattie, G., Hubbell, W., and Nicolson, G. L. (1977). Activities of lectins and their immobilized derivatives in detergent solutions. Implications on the use of lectin affinity chromatography for the purification of membrane glycoproteins. *Biochemistry,* **16**, 1787–1794.

Lotan, R. H., Debray, M., Cacan, M., Cacan, R., and Sharon, N. (1975b). Labelling of soybean agglutinin by oxidation with sodium peroxidase followed by reduction with sodium [^{3}H]borohydride. *J. Biol. Chem.*, **250**, 1955–1957.

Lotan, R., Skutelsky, E., Danon, D., and Sharon, N. (1975a). The purification, composition and specificity of the Anti-T lectin from peanut (*Arachis hypogaea*). *J. Biol. Chem.*, **250**, 8518–8523.

Maddy, A. H., and Dunn, M. J. (1976). The solubilization of membranes. In A. H. Maddy (Ed.) *Biochemical Analysis of Membranes*. Wiley, New York.

Marchalonis, J. J. (1969). An enzymic method for the trace iodination of immunoglobulins and other proteins. *Biochem. J.*, **113**, 299–305.

Marchesi, V. T. (1972). Isolation of membrane bound glycoproteins with lithium diiodosalicylate. In V. Ginsburg (Ed.) *Enzymology,* pp. 282–254. Academic Press, New York, London.

Marshall, R. D. (1972). Glycoproteins. *Ann. Rev. Biochem.*, **41**, 673–702.

Matsumoto, I., and Osawa, T. (1972). The specific purification of various carbohydrate-binding haemagglutinins. *Biochem. Biophys. Res. Commun.*, **46**, 1810–1815.

Mirelman, D., Galun, E., Sharon, N., and Lotan, R. (1975). Inhibition of fungal growth by wheat germ agglutinin, *Nature (Lond.)*, **256**, 414–416.

Misaki, A., and Goldstein, I. J. (1977). Glycosyl moiety of lima bean lectin. *J. Biol. Chem.*, **252**, 6995.

Monroy, A., Ortolani, G., O'Dell, D., and Millonig, G. (1973). Binding of Concanavalin A to the surface of unfertilized ascidian eggs. *Nature (Lond.)*, **242**, 409–410.

Montreuil, J. (1975). Recent data on the structure of the carbohydrate moiety of glycoproteins, metabolic and biological implications. *Pure Appl. Chem.*, **42**, 431–477

Muir, L., and Lee, Y. C. (1970). Glycopeptides from earthworm cuticle collagen. *J. Biol. Chem.*, **245**, 502.

Muir, L., and Lee, Y. C. (1969). Structures of D-galactose oligosaccharides from earthworm cutile collagen. *J. Biol. Chem.*, **244**, 2343.

Müller, W. E. G., Zahn, R. K., Kurelec, B., Müller, I., Uhlenbruck, G., and Vaith, P. (1979). Aggregation of sponge cells: a novel mechanism of controlled intercellular adhesion basing on the interrelation between glycosyl transferases and glycosidases. *J. Biol. Chem.*, **254**, 1280–1287.

McLean, R. J., and Brown, R. M. (1974). Cell surface differentiation of *Chlamydomonas* during gametogenesis. *Dev. Biol.*, **36**, 279–285.

Nicolson, G. L. (1973). Neuraminidase 'unmasking'and failure of trypsin to 'unmask' β-D-galactose-like sites on erythrocyte, lymphoma, and normal and virus-transformed fibroblast cell membranes. *J. Nat. Cancer Inst.*, **50**, 1443–1451.

Nicolson, G. L. (1974). Interaction of lectins with animal cell surfaces. *Int. Rev. Cytol.*, **39**, 89–190.

Nicolson, G. L. (1976a). Transmembrane control of the receptors on normal and tumor cells. I. Cytoplasmic influence over cell surface components. *Biochim. Biophys Acta.* **457**, 57–108.

Nicolson, G. L. (1976b). Trans-membrane control of the receptors on normal and tumor cells. II. Surface changes associated with transformation and malignancy. *Biochim. Biophys. Acta*, **458**, 1–72.

Nicolson, G. L. (1978). Ultrastructual localization of lectin receptors. In J. K. Koehler (Ed.) *Advanced Techniques in Biological Electron Microscopy*. Springer-Verlag, Berlin.

Nicolson, G. L., and Blaustein, J. (1972). The interaction of *Ricinis communis* agglutinin with normal and tumor cell surfaces. *Biochim. Biophys. Acta*, **266**, 543–547.

Nicolson, G. L., Blaustein J., and Etzler, M. (1974).Characterization of two plant lectins from *Ricinus communis* and their interaction with a murine lymphoma. *Biochemistry*, **13**, 196–204.

Noonan, K. D., Levine, A. J., and Burger, M. M. (1973). Cell cycle changes in the surface membrane as detected with ^{3}H-Concanavalin A, *J. Cell Biol.*, **58**, 491–497.

Nowak, T. P., and Barondes, S. H. (1975). Agglutinin from *Limulus polyphemus*. Purification with formalinized horse erythrocytes as the affinity adsorbent. *Biochim Biophys. Acta*, **393**, 115–123.

Nowell, P. C. (1960). Phytohaemagglutinin: an initiator of mitosis in cultures of normal human leukocytes. *Cancer Res.*, **20**, 462–466.

Oppenheimer, S. B. (1977). Interactions of lectins with embryonic cell surfaces. *Curr. Topics Dev. Biol.*, **11**, 1–14.

Osawa, T., and Matsumoto, I. (1972). Gorse (*Ulex europaeus*) phytohameagglutinins. *Methods Enzymol.*, **28**, Part B, 323–327.

Ostrowski, K., Barnard, E. A., Sawicki, W., Chorzelski, T., Langer, A., and Mikulski, A. (1970). Autoradiographic detection in cells using tritium-labelled antibodies. *J. Histochem. Cytochem.*, **18**, 490–497.

Pereira, M. E. A., and Kabat, E. A. (1974). Specificity of purified haemagglutinin (lectin) from *Lotus tetragonolobus*. *Biochemistry*, **13**, 3184–3192.

Pereira, M. E. A., Kabat, E. A., and Sharon, N. (1974). Immunochemical studies on the specificity of soybean agglutinin. *Carbohydr. Res.*, **37**, 89–102.

Pereira, M. E. A., and Kabat, E. A. (1976). Immunochemical studies on blood groups. LXII. Fractionation of hog and human A, H and AH blood group active substance on insoluble immunoadsorbents of *Dolichos* and *Lotus* lectins. *J. Exp. Med.*, **143**, 422–436.

Pereira, M. E. A., Kabat, E. A., Lotan, R., and Sharon, N. (1976). Immunochemical studies on the specificity of the peanut (*Arachis hypogaea*) agglutinin. *Carbohydr. Res.*, **51**, 107–118.

Pfenninger, M.-F. M., and Jamieson, J. D. (1979a). Distribution of cell surface saccharides on pancreatic cells. I. General method for preparation and purification of lectins and lectin–ferritin conjugates. *J. Cell Biol.*, **80**, 69–76.

Pfenninger, M.-F. M., and Jamieson, J. D. (1979b). Distribution of cell surface saccharides on pancreatic cells. II. Lectin labelling patterns on mature guinea pig and rat pancreatic cells. *J. Cell Biol.*, **80**, 77–95.

Phillips, P. G., Furmanski, P., and Lubin, M. (1974). Cell surface interaction with

Concanavalin A—location of bound radiolabelled lectin. *Expt. Cell Res.*, **86**, 301–308.

Pierce, M., Turley, E. A., and Roth, S. (1980). Cell surface glycosyl transferase activities. *Int. Rev. Cytol.*, **65**, 2–47.

Pinto da Silva, P., and Nicolson, G. L. (1974). Freeze-etch localization of Concanavalin A receptors to the membrane intercalated particles on human erythrocyte membranes. *Biochim Biophys. Acta*, **383**, 311–319.

Prieels, J.-P., Pizzo, S. V., Glasgow, L. R., Paulson, J. C., and Hill, R. (1978). Hepatic receptor that specifically binds oligosaccharides containing fucosyl α 1,3-*N*-acetylglucosamine linkages. *Proc. Nat. Acad. Sci. USA*, **75**, 2215–2219.

Pueppke, S. G., Bauer, W. D., Keegstra, K., and Ferguson, A. L. (1978). Role of lectins in plant microorganism interactions. II. Distribution of soybean lectin in tissues of *Glycine max*. *Plant Physiol.*, **61**, 779–784.

Ray, J., Shinnick, T., and Lerner, R. (1979). A mutation altering the function of a carbohydrate binding protein block cell-wall cohesion in developing *Dictostelium discoideum*. *Nature (Lond.)*, **279**, 215–221.

Reading, C. L., Penhoet, E. E., and Ballou, C. E. (1978). Carbohydrate structure of vesicular somatitis virus glycoprotein. *J. Biol. Chem.*, **253**, 5600.

Reeke, G. N., Becker, J. W., and Edelman, G. M. (1975). The covalent and three-dimensional structure of Concanavalin A. *J. Biol. Chem.*, **250**, 1525–1547.

Rees, D. A., Lloyd, C. W., and Thom, D. (1977). Control of grip and stick in cell adhesion through lateral relationships of membrane glycoproteins. *Nature (Lond.)*, **267**, 124–128.

Reisner, Y., Lis, H., and Sharon, N. (1976). On the importance of the binding of lectins to cell surface receptors at low lectin concentrations. *Expt. Cell Res.*, **97**, 445–447.

Renart, J., Reiser, J., and Stark, G. (1979). Transfer of proteins from gels to diazobenzyloxymethyl paper and detection with antisera. A method for studying antibody specificity and antigen structure. *Proc. Nat. Acad. Sci. USA.*, **76**, 3116–3120.

Roseman, S. (1970). The synthesis of complex carbohydrates by multiglycosyl transferase systems and their potential function in intercellular adhesions. *Chem. Phys. Lipids*, **5**, 270–297.

Rosenthal, A. L., and Nordin, J. H. (1975). Enzymes that hydrolyze fungal cell wall polysaccharides. *J. Biol. Chem.*, **250**, 5295.

Schacter, H. (1978). Glycoproteins biosynthesis. In M. I. Horowitz and W. Pigman (Eds) *The Glycoconjugates*, volume II,pp.86–168. Academic Press, New York.

Schiffman, G., Kabat, E. A., and Thomson, W. (1964). Immunochemical studies on blood groups. XXX. Cleavage of A, B and H blood group substances by alkali. *Biochemistry*, **3**, 113–120.

Schwartz, B. D., Kato, K., Cullen, S. E., and Nathenson, S. G. (1973). H-2 histocompatibility alloantigens. Some biochemical properties of the molecules solubilized by NP-40 detergent. *Biochemistry*, **12**, 2157–2164.

Schwarzmann, G., Hatcher, V. B., and Jeanloz, R. W. (1978). Purification and structural elucidation of several carbohydrate side chains from αl-acid glycoprotein. *J. Biol. Chem.*, **253**, 6983.

Sela, B. A., Wang, J. L., and Edelman, G. M. (1975). Isolation of lectins of different specifities on a single affinity adsorbent. *J. Biol. Chem.*, **250**, 7535–7538.

Shannon, L. M., and Hankins, C. N. (1981). Enzymic properties of phytohaemagglutinins. *Recent Adv. Phytochem.*, **15**, 93–114.

Sharon, N., and Lis, H. (1972). Lectins: cell agglutinating and sugar specific proteins. *Science*, **177**, 949–959.

Sharon, N., and Lis, H. (1975). Use of lectins for the study of membranes. In E. Korn

(Ed.) *Methods of Membrane Biology*, volume 3. Plenum Press, New York, London.

Simpson, D. L., Thorne, D. R., and Loh, H. H. (1978). Lectins: endogenous carbohydrate binding proteins from vertebrate tissues: functional role in recognition processes? *Life Sci., 22*, 727.

So, L. L., and Goldstein, I. J. (1967). Protein–carbohydrate interaction. IV. Application of the quantitative precipitin method to polysaccharide–Concanavalin A interactions. *J. Biol. Chem., 242*, 1617–1622.

So, L. L., and Goldstein, I. J. (1968). Protein–carbohydrate interaction. XX. On a number of combining sites of Con A, the phytohaemagglutinin of jack bean. *Biochim. Biophys. Acta, 165*, 398–404.

Southworth, D. (1975). Lectins stimulate pollen germination. *Nature (Lond.), 258*, 600–602.

Spiro, R. G. (1967). The structure of the disaccharide unit of the renal glomerular basement membrane. *J. Biol. Chem., 242*, 4813.

Springer, G. F., and Williams, P. (1962). Immunochemical significance of L- and D-fucose derivatives. *Biochem. J., 282*–291.

Stein, M. D., Howard, I. K., and Sage, H. J. (1971). Studies on a phytohaemagglutinin from the lentil. IV Direct binding studies of *Lens culinaris* haemagglutinin with simple saccharides. *Arch. Biochem. Biophys., 146*, 353–355.

Stillmark, H. (1886). Uber Ricin, in *Arbeiten des pharmakologischen Institutes zu Dorpot* (ed. R. Kobert), p. 57.

Sugahara, K., Funakoshi, S., Funalcoshi, I., Aula, P., and Yamashira, I., (1976). Characterization of one neutral and two acidic glycoasparagines isolated from the urine of patients with aspartylglycosylaminuria. *J. Biochem., Tokyo, 80*, 195.

Tai, T., Yamashita, K., Ogata-Arakawa, M., Koidle, N., Muramatsu, T., Iwashita, S., Inoue, Y., and Kobata, A. (1975). Structural studies of two ovalbumin glycopeptides in relation to the endo-β-*N*-acetylglucosaminidase specificity. *J. Biol. Chem., 250*, 8569–8575.

Tomita, M., Kurokawa, T., Onozaki, K., Ichiki, N., Osawa, T., and Ukita, T. (1972). Purification of galactose-binding phytoagglutinins and phytotoxin by affinity column chromatography using Sepharose. *Experientia, 28*, 84.

Towbin, H., Staehelin, T., and Gordon, J. (1979). Electrophoretic transfer of proteins from polyacrylamide gels to nitrocellulose sheets: procedure and some applications. *Proc. Nat. Acad. Sci. USA., 76*, 4350–4354.

Uhlenbruck, G., Baldo, B. A., Steinhausen, G., Schwick, H. G., Chatterjee, B.P., Horejsi, V., Krajhanzl, A., and Kocourek, J., (1978). Additional precipitation reactions of lectins with human serum glycoproteins. *J. Clin. Chem. Clin. Biochem., 16*, 19–23.

Van Wauwe, J. P., Loonteins, F. G., and Debruyne, C. K. (1975). Carbohydrate binding specificity of the lectin from the pea *(Pisum sativum)*. *Biochim. Biophys. Acta, 379*, 456–461.

Vretbald, P. (1976). Purification of lectins by biospecific affinity chromatography. *Biochim. Biophys. Acta, 434*, 169–176.

Watkins, W. M., and Morgan, W. T. J. (1952). Neutralization of the anti-H agglutinin in eel serum by simple sugars. *Nature (Lond.), 169*, 825–826.

Waxdal, N. J. (1974). Isolation, characterization and biological activities of five mitogens from pokeweed. *Biochemistry, 13*, 3671–3677.

Williams, A. F. (1978). Membrane glycoproteins in recognition. *Biochem. Soc. Trans., 6*, 490–494.

Williams, T. J., Plessas, N. R., Goldstein, J., and Lönngren, J. (1979). A new class of model glycolipids: synthesis, characterisation and interaction with lectins. *Arch. Biochem. Biophys., 195*, 145–151.

Yahara, I. and Edelman, G. M. (1973). The effects of Concanavalin A on the mobility of lymphocyte surface receptors. *Exp. Cell Res.*, **81**, 143–155.

Young, N. M., Leon, M. A., Takahash, I., Howard, I. K., and Sage, H. J. (1971). Studies on a phytohaemagglutinin from the lentil. III. Reaction of *Lens culinaris* haemagglutinin with polysaccharides, glycoproteins and lymphocytes. *J. Biol. Chem.*, **246**, 1596–1601.

Chapter 12

Immunochemical Approaches in Developmental and Reproductive Biology

E. J. JENKINSON
*Department of Anatomy, The University of Birmingham,
Medical School, Birmingham, UK*

and

R. F. SEARLE
*Department of Pathology, University of Bristol,
Bristol Royal Infirmary, Bristol, UK.*

I. INTRODUCTION

The use of immunological techniques in the study of developmental and reproductive biology has already made a considerable contribution to the understanding of these biologically complex processes. In the analysis of development, antibody probes provide the opportunity to examine the changing pattern of cell surface phenotype during differentiation, to identify antigens as markers of gene activity, to investigate the functional role of cell membrane components during embryogenesis and organogenesis and to monitor the appearance of cell products specific to particular tissues or phases of development. Immunological procedures also provide powerful tools for the isolation, identification, and characterization of hormones and other products associated with the reproductive process and have played an important part in elucidating the foeto–maternal interactions consequent upon the viviparous state in mammals. In addition, the rapid development of immunological techniques for the separation and selection of viable cells offers considerable potential for the isolation and experimental manipulation of embryonic cell populations in a way that should facilitate a better understanding of the interactions required to ensure normal development.

As may be expected much of the information on the application of immunology to studies on reproduction and development relates to the mammal, although many of the approaches are applicable to non-mammalian species. Before considering examples of the information obtained by the use of immunological procedures, however, it is pertinent to consider some of the techniques and assays which have made these investigations feasible.

II. ASSAYS

The basic requirement in the majority of immunochemical procedures is the production of an antiserum able to recognize the cell product or cell surface determinant under investigation. Where immunization is carried out between individuals of the same species alloantisera may be produced when the antigen under investigation is sufficiently polymorphic to differ from one individual to another. Similarly, antisera may be raised within a species if the immunizing antigen, although not necessarily polymorphic, is normally unavailable to the adult immune system as in the case of the F-9 antigen of teratoma cells (Section III. A.3). Alternatively, xenoantisera may be produced by immunizing one species with the appropriate tissues or products from another to produce, for example, antisera to organ and tissue-specific antigens or to hormones. Such antisera when raised against tissues or entire cells require considerable absorption against other tissues of the immunizing species to render them specific. More recently the advent of techniques for monoclonal antibody production, where a single clone of cells synthesizing antibodies of a single class against a desired specificity is isolated and allowed to produce relatively large quantities of antibodies, has provided a new approach for the production of highly specific antisera without the need for exhaustive absorption. This technique is dealt with in Chapter 9 while the principles of antigen presentation and antibody production are considered more fully in Chapters 1, 2, and 3.

A. Immunolabelling

In the detection of cell associated components a useful facility is the ability to visualize antibody binding in order that reactivity can be related to a particular cell type or developing structure. In this section examples of techniques which are applicable to studies on reproduction and development will be outlined and their advantages and disadvantages discussed. Detailed accounts of the practical aspects of immunofluorescence and immunoelectron microscopical techniques, are also given in Chapters 6 and 7.

1. Molecular Antibody Labels

Since the development of fluorescein as a label for the visualization of antibody binding to target antigens a variety of molecular labels including rhodamine, ferritin, haemocyanin, heavy metals, enzymes, and radiolabels have been employed (Andres *et al*, 1978; Johnson *et al.*, 1978). Most techniques fall into two categories, direct tests in which the label is coupled directly to the antibody recognizing the target antigen and the more sensitive indirect test in which the first antibody is unlabelled and is visualized by the addition of labelled anti-immunoglobulin prepared in another species.

Antibodies labelled with fluorescent compounds have been widely employed and provide a fairly rapid technique which has the advantage that the entire procedure can be carried out on either fixed or living cells thus allowing dynamic studies on membrane components (Taylor *et al.*, 1971). The availability of fluorescein- or rhodamine-conjugated antibodies allows also double labelling to be carried out on the same cell. Disadvantages are the relative impermanence of the preparations, background autofluorescence, quenching of the label, and limited resolution in the light microscope. Immunofluorescence is also relatively insensitive although recent reports show that sensitivity can be increased by loading the first antibody with hapten and using a high purified fluorescein-conjugated anti-hapten antibody as the second reagent (Lamm *et al.*, 1972; Cammisuli and Wofsy, 1976).

Enzymes, of which the most widely used is horseradish peroxidase, can allow antigen tracing in both the light microscope and the electron microscope with the greater resolution the latter confers. Development of the reaction product of the enzyme also provides a degree of amplification while the use of soluble peroxidase–anti-peroxidase complexes in a triple bridge technique can provide a degree of sensitivity 100–1000-fold higher than immunofluorescence (Sternberger, 1972; Burns, 1975). In general enzyme labelling has been considered superior to other markers in terms of sensitivity and specificity (Berquist *et al.*, 1976; Bellon *et al.*, 1978) and because it excludes autofluorescence and the preparations are long-lasting (Feteanu, 1978).

Coupling antibodies with electron-dense markers such as ferritin and haemocyanin has also been used for antigen localization at the fine structural level and, since the variability of enzyme–substrate interaction is avoided, can be useful where a degree of quantitation is required. Haemocyanin has been primarily used for cell surface labelling, its molecular size inhibiting penetration into cells. Ferritin, on the other hand, can also be used for localizing intracellular antigens (Wagner, 1973; Andres *et al.*, 1978; Feteanu, 1978). Labelling with hybrid antibodies with dual specificities (see Figure 1) one of which recognizes ferritin has however been reported to give more uniform labelling than conventional methods employing ferritin (Hammerling *et al.*, 1968; Andres *et al.*, 1978; Feteanu, 1978).

With cells in suspension or in tissue culture, labelling of living material is usually preferred to avoid fixative-induced antigen denaturation. The possibility of antibody-induced redistribution or internalization of antigens mobile in the plane of the membrane on living cells should however be borne in mind and minimized by the addition of sodium azide and incubation at lower

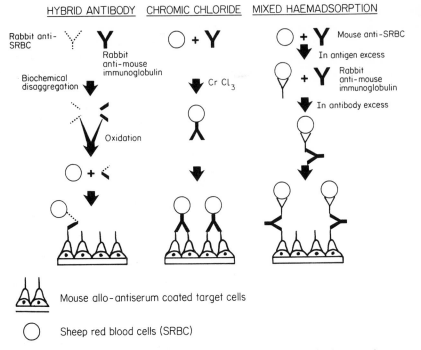

Figure 1. Methods for detecting surface antigens using particulate markers

temperatures or by the use of Fab monomers (Taylor *et al.*, 1971). Where intracellular antigens or antigen distribution within a tissue is being sought, fixation and/or sectioning are necessary to allow antibody access. Choice of fixative is usually a compromise between adequate tissue preservation and preservation of the antigen under examination (Feteanu, 1978). Care must also be taken to minimize the diffusion of hydro-soluble antigens where lightly fixed or unfixed frozen material is employed.

Tissue sections for use with immunolabelling have been obtained using paraffin or polyester wax embedded material as well as cryostat sectioning of snap-frozen tissue (Feteanu, 1978). Techniques are now available which allow post-embedding labelling of ultra-thin plastic sections for examination in the electron microscope (Kawarai and Nakane, 1970; Sternberger and Petrale, 1976). Direct labelling of ultra-thin sections of mildly fixed or frozen tissue cut using a cryoultramicrotome also permits localisation of intracellular antigens at the fine structural level (Andres *et al.*, 1978). Again choice of technique depends on the stability of the antigen involved.

2. Particulate Antibody Labels

In addition to the molecular antibody labels, antibody binding to target cells can be followed by the use of particulate markers such as red cells which can be readily detected in a conventional light microscope.

In the mixed haemadsorption assay (MHA) based on the technique developed by Coombs *et al.* (1956) and subsequently adapted for use on cell monolayers (Fagraeus and Espmark, 1961; Fagraeus *et al.*, 1965), immunoglobulin coated indicator sheep red blood cells (SRBC) are treated with anti-immunoglobulin in excess in such a way that one Fab element of the anti-immunoglobulin molecule remains free as indicated in Figure 1, which shows a system for the detection of mouse alloantigens (see also Hausman and Palm, 1973; Reddy *et al.*, 1977; Sellens *et al.*, 1978, for applications). Several variants of this procedure have also been developed which avoid the need to build up two antibody layers on the indicator cells. Hybrid antibodies have been synthesized in which one element recognizes determinants on the SRBC (or other marker such as virus) while the other element is an anti-immunoglobulin (Hammerling *et al.*, 1973; Wachtel *et al.*, 1975). Chromic chloride can also be used to couple anti-immunoglobulin directly to RBC (Coombs *et al.*, 1977; Parish and McKenzie, 1978) avoiding the somewhat specialized procedures for hybrid antibody preparation. Protein-A, which will bind to the Fc region of IgG from a variety of species can also be coupled to RBC with chromic chloride producing a more universal reagent (Sandrin *et al*., 1978).

In assays of this type target cells, either handled in suspension or grown as monolayers on coverslips or in the wells of disposable plastic culture plates, are first incubated with alloantibody and then exposed to the sensitized indicator cells. A positive reaction is indicated by adherence of the indicator red cells to the target monolayers which can be examined in the living state or fixed and stained as a permanent record (see Figure 2a and b). Less subjective assessment of labelling has also been achieved by the use of radiolabelled RBC (Wood and Barth, 1975). As with the other assays appropriate controls to ensure the specificity of the reaction are required including substitution of normal serum for the antiserum used on the target cells, exposure of target cells to sensitized indicators without pre-exposure to antibody and where appropriate, testing of the first antiserum on inappropriate targets, e.g. cells of a different haplotype in the case of alloantisera.

Apart from the ready visibility of the indicator particles in the conventional light microscope, the primary advantage of the conventional MHA assay is the high degree of sensitivity it can provide, a useful feature when attempts are being made to detect antigens likely to be present at low levels. Comparative tests have shown that the MHA can be 10–100 times more sensitive than complement-mediated lysis in the detection of rat and human cell surface antigens (Reddy *et al.*, 1977; Rosenberg *et al.*, 1977) and 500–1000 times more sensitive than indirect immunofluorescence using murine H-2 alloantisera (Wood and Barth, 1975). On the other hand, the MHA assay suffers the disadvantage that many types of target cells must be grown as monolayers

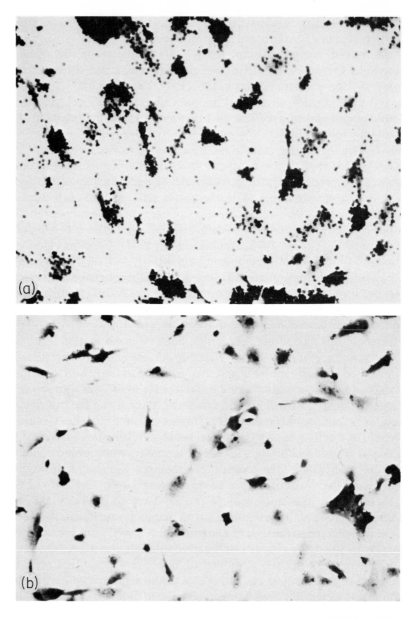

Figure 2(a). Mixed haemadsorption assay on monolayer culture of 14-day-old mouse embryo cells treated with anti-H-2 antiserum followed by anti-immunoglobulin-coated sheep red cells. Note adherence of red cells to monolayer indicating presence of antigen. Fixed 2.5% glutaraldehyde, stained Giemsa. (× 70) (b). Control culture treated with normal serum before exposure to indicator red cells. Note absence of red cell binding to monolayer. (× 70)

making it more difficult to relate the cells examined to organized structures *in vivo* as well as raising the possibility that surface antigen arrays may be modified by the disaggregation procedures employed or by *in vitro* conditions.

As an alternative to RBC a number of other particulate markers are now available. As mentioned previously virus particles have been used with hybrid antibodies and in conjunction with scanning electron microscopy have proved valuable in relating antigen distribution to surface topography (Koo *et al.*, 1977). Polyacrylamide beads the size of RBC (Ammann *et al.*, 1977) and polymeric microspheres of varying sizes conjugated with anti-immunoglobulin can also be prepared and used for visualization by light, scanning and/or transmission electron microscopy (see Roth, 1977 for review and detailed bibliography). As yet these have not been widely applied to developmental studies but their potential seems considerable.

B. Cytotoxicity and Absorption

A well established technique for the detection of cell surface antigens is based on the ability of antibody to lyse antigen-bearing cells in the presence of complement. Assessment of the proportion of cells killed is usually based on dye exclusion, release of previously incorporated radiolabel or incorporation of labelled precursors into surviving cells. These techniques are described in detail in the literature and will not be considered further here (see Boyse *et al.*, 1964; Gotze and Ferrone, 1972; Welsh and Batchelor, 1978). It should be noted however that embryonic material can be particularly sensitive to the deleterious effects of some batches of complement necessitating careful screening and/or absorption on target tissues (Goldberg *et al.*, 1971) or on agarose (Douglas, 1972) prior to use.

Where direct cytotoxic testing is not feasible the antigenic status of tissues can be assessed by using them to absorb antisera which is then tested for residual activity on a convenient cell suspension, usually lymphocytes. Using known amounts of antibody and absorbing tissue the selective absorptive capacity, and therefore antigenic content of different tissues, can be assessed (Edidin, 1964, 1972). As a further refinement, absorption using purified plasma membranes rather than whole cells can be carried out (Goodfellow *et al.*, 1976).

C. Immunoprecipitation

Investigation of antigen production and expression can be achieved by immunoprecipitation of radiolabelled antigen from cell extracts. Direct labelling by radioiodination can be carried out in the case of externally exposed membrane antigens (Delovitch and McDevitt, 1975) while labelling of both membrane and intracellular proteins is accomplished by incorporation of radiolabelled amino acids into living cells (Vitetta *et al.*, 1975; Delovitch *et al.*, 1978). Subsequent to either of these processes the cells are extracted, incubated with antiserum and the resultant complexes precipitated by the appropriate anti-immunoglobulin or by staphylococcal protein-A (Cullen and Schwartz, 1976). Products of immunoprecipitation obtained in this way can then be counted to determine the presence and relative amount of antigen which can then be further characterized by gel electrophoresis and compared with other known antigens if required.

D. Radioimmunoassay

The development of radioimmunoassays (RIA), in which the presence of a particular antigen is detected by measuring its ability to compete with a fixed amount of radiolabelled antigen for a limiting amount of antibody, has provided a precise and highly sensitive technique for the detection of hormones and other products associated with reproduction such as the embryonic proteins AFP and CEA (Section III. A.3) in biological fluids. A reversal of the RIA system involves the radiolabelling of antibody instead of antigen in the immunoradiometric assay (Miles and Hales, 1968). The main advantage of these assays lies in their quantitative aspects and their ability to handle large numbers of samples in a semi-automatic manner thus facilitating longitudinal studies. A detailed account of the principles and applications of RIA is given in Chapter 6.

Enzyme immunoassays (EIA) and enzyme-linked immunosorbent assays (ELISA) are also based on competition between a particular antigen and a labelled antigen for a limited amount of antibody but enzymes such as alkaline phosphatase and horseradish peroxidase are used as the label rather than radioisotopes (Engvall and Carlsson, 1976; Weemen and Schuurs, 1976; Feteanu, 1978; Grant, 1978; Hunter, 1978). The enzymes catalyse a colour reaction which can be easily and cheaply quantified by a simple colorimeter unlike RIAs which require sophisticated equipment to measure the radioactivity. Both assays, with their high degree of sensitivity and specificity, can be used as alternatives to RIA and antigens quantified include α-foetoprotein, pregnancy-associated macroglobulin, carcinoembryonic antigen, oestrogens and human chorionic gonadotropin (see Weeman and Schuurs, 1976).

III. APPLICATIONS

A. Antibodies as Probes of Molecular Events in Differentiation

The ability to identify various antigenic specificities in the embryo offers the possibility of examining the differentiation of structure and organization at the macromolecular level in the cell membrane and in the internal and external cellular environments. Labelled antibodies can also be used for investigation of the dynamic properties of the cell membrane (Taylor *et al.*, 1971) and it seems likely that studies on changes in the mobility of membrane components during development, e.g. fertilization and blastocyst implantation (see Johnson, 1975a,b) will be extended to a variety of situations where changes in organization could play an important part in cellular interactions. In addition, the correlation of cell surface products with genetic loci known to have a specific effect on development should give a better understanding of the role of the cell surface in such events. The tracing of antigenic specificities with a restricted distribution may also be useful in the construction of fate maps and in the elucidation of cell lineage as differentiation proceeds. Furthermore, there is the possibility of using antibodies as markers when cells of two different genotypes are experimentally mixed as in the case of rat/mouse embryo fusion chimaeras where anti-species antibodies have been used to follow the distribution of tissues from each partner in the fusion (Gardner and Johnson, 1973).

While most of these approaches are still to be fully exploited, sufficient information is available to illustrate the principles involved. For convenience, examples of the various antigen systems which have been examined are considered under the following headings although the allocation of certain antigens to a particular group is necessarily arbitrary.

1. Histocompatibility Antigens

These represent one of the most widely studied groups of surface antigens and can be divided into two broad categories, the major histocompatibility complex (MHC) antigens which are highly polymorphic and readily give rise to antibody production when tissues are exchanged between genetically differing individuals, and the so-called weak or minor histocompatibility antigens (non-MHC) which are much less well defined. Of the various MHC systems, the mouse H-2 complex has been particularly well studied owing to the ready availability of inbred congenic and recombinant strains (see Klein, 1975; Snell, 1966). Although originally thought to be a simple genetic locus, whose products played a primary role in eliciting antibody production and cell-mediated graft rejection, the H-2 system is now known to be a complex consisting of several regions and subregions each containing at least one gene (see Klein, 1975 and Klein, 1979 for review).

As well defined surface products MHC antigens provide a handle with which to study general principles of cell surface differentiation in relation to morphological development and with which changes affecting the behaviour of membrane macromolecules may also be probed. There is also some speculation that the MHC may play a general role in cellular interactions

(Bodmer, 1972) and it has been suggested that its products may serve as general linking sites in the membrane for the anchorage of a variety of other membrane proteins which direct organogenesis and cell differentiation (Ohno, 1977). More specifically, MHC antigens provide important markers with which to follow the ontogeny of the immune system in which they play a central role, while the analysis of their expression throughout development is fundamental to the assessment of the status of the foetus as a potential allograft within the pregnant uterus. Both MHC and non-MHC antigens, having a wide tissue distribution, also fulfil some of the criteria for useful biological markers and may provide an adjunct to the enzyme markers used in the analysis of clonal growth and cell mixing in inter-strain mouse embryo chimaeras (West, 1978).

Only limited information is available to suggest that MHC products are expressed on the unfertilized ovum (Edidin *et al.*, 1974) and it has recently been reported that there is a differential expression of MHC antigens on unfertilized and fertilized mouse eggs (Heyner and Hunziker, 1979). The MHC status of spermatozoa and cells of the male germ line has been more extensively investigated but has led to conflicting results which serve to highlight some of the problems faced in assessing the antigens of any tissue (see Erickson, 1977). The balance of evidence from immunolabelling (Erickson, 1972; Vojtiskova and Pokorna, 1972; Vojtiskova *et al.*, 1974), absorption (Vojitskova and Pokorna, 1972), and cytotoxicity tests (Goldberg *et al.*, 1970; Johnson and Edidin, 1972) is, however, in favour of MHC antigen expression on spermatozoa in both the mouse and man (see Fellous and Dausset, 1973 and Halim *et al.*, 1974), although probably at much lower levels than those present on lymphocytes (Erickson, 1972). In the mouse at least, it would also appear that products of the K, D, and I regions of the MHC are present (Hammerling *et al.*, 1974; Erickson *et al.*, 1977). Whether these antigens are produced post-meiotically or simply persist from earlier stages which are known to express H-2 antigens from the primary spermatocyte stage onwards is unresolved (see Erickson, 1977).

The expression of minor histocompatibility antigens on the pre-implantation embryo of the mouse has been amply demonstrated by a number of investigators (see Billington and Jenkinson, 1975; Jenkinson and Billington, 1977 for review). The possible functional significance of these antigens is not clear but the expression of such antigens of paternal origin in heterozygous embryos has been useful in tracing the onset of embryonic gene activity in relation to cell surface products and indicate an early activation (by the 6–8 cell stage) comparable to that seen with paternally inherited enzyme variants as markers (Chapman *et al.*, 1977). In contrast, identification of MHC antigens on the pre-implantation period has proved controversial and several investigators have failed to demonstrate their presence using either transplantation, immunofluorescence, or cytotoxicity assays with alloantisera (see Jenkinson and Billington, 1977). Xenoantisera raised against the core of the murine H-2 molecule also fail to label either morulae or blastocysts when used in indirect immunofluorescence tests (Morello *et al.*, 1978). The labelling of the outer trophectoderm surface of the blastocyst with alloantiserum produced in congenic mice has, however, been reported when isotope antiglobulin (Håkansson *et al.*, 1975) and immunoelectron microscopical (Searle *et al.*, 1976) procedures have been employed, possibly reflecting the greater sensitivity of these techniques. A recent report also indicates that MHC antigens can be detected as early as the eight cell stage using a complement-dependent cytotoxicity assay (Krco and Goldberg, 1977). These findings thus serve to highlight the variability between assays, particularly when low levels of antigen expression are involved. It should also be noted in this context that some murine antisera are now known to contain antibodies to murine leukaemia virus (Nowinksi and Klein, 1975). The extent to which these contribute to the observed labelling of various embryonic stages with anti-MHC antisera requires further investigation and is a factor to bear in mind with any antiserum used in investigations of embryonic material where expression of viral antigen is a possibility. Whatever the precise nature of the alloantigens expressed on the outer trophectoderm layer of the mouse blastocyst, with the onset of implantation, their detectability decreases dramatically, disappearing in the case of reactivity to H-2 antisera (Håkansson *et al.*, 1975). Interestingly, these changes in membrane organization, indicated by antibody probes, take place at a time when the trophoblast appears to undergo functional changes enabling it to attach to, and invade, the uterine wall. Further investigation of the role of the surface changes in implantation may be possible by assessing the effects of various antisera on this process *in vivo* and *in vitro*. In any event, it would seem that the decrease in surface antigen expression, especially of H-2, should enable the embryo to present an antigenically neutral front to the maternal immune system at the time when it first makes tissue contact with the mother.

In the context of foeto–maternal immunological interactions, it is significant that the trophoblast giant cells surrounding the post-implantation mouse *conceptus* are also deficient in MHC expression (Searle *et al.*, 1976; Sellens, 1977). With the appearance of several trophoblast subpopulations in the definitive placenta, however, MHC-positive cells can be detected in trophoblast cultures (Sellens *et al.*, 1978) and in freshly prepared placental cell suspensions (Chatterjee-Hasrouni and Lala, 1979), and appear to be derived from the spongio-trophoblast elements of the placenta (Jenkinson and Owen—unpublished observations). Mechanisms other than simple lack of antigen therefore need to be considered to explain the survival of the placental graft in an immunologically hostile maternal environment (see Billington, 1976 for discussion). In man MHC antigens have not been detected on the syncytio-trophoblast clothing the villi which make up the bulk of the absorptive surface (Seigler and Metzger, 1970; Goodfellow *et al.*, 1976; Faulk *et al.*, 1977).

It is presently not known whether or not there are MHC-expressing trophoblastic components in other parts of the human placenta, as in the mouse.

In addition to the trophectoderm and its derivatives, the ontogeny of MHC antigens during the differentiation of the blastocyst inner cell mass (icm) into the embryo proper has also been examined in the mouse. MHC expression on the icm is first detectable around the time of implantation (Heyner, 1973; Searle *et al.*, 1976; Webb *et al.*, 1977) when differentiation of the primitive endoderm is also proceeding. By day 7½ MHC antigens are readily detectable on the intact egg cylinder (see Jenkinson and Billington, 1977) and are probably confined to the endoderm, the comparatively unspecialized embryonic ectoderm lacking MHC antigens (Searle and Jenkinson—unpublished observations) which do not become detectable on this tissue until after day 9 and the onset of organogenesis (Edidin, 1972; Jacob, 1977). Whether there is any causal relationship between the expression of MHC antigens and differentiation is not yet known. In the light of the previously mentioned proposals that the MHC may be involved in cellular interactions and organogenesis it is, however, noteworthy that their appearance parallels, to a degree, the emergence of differentiated structures.

Subsequent to day 9, H-2 expression on tissue preparations from the whole embryonic body shows a continuing increase, although with a few exceptions (Schlesinger, 1964; Klein, 1965, 1975; Edidin, 1972; Hausman and Palm, 1973) its progress in different organs has not been extensively examined. The ontogeny of H-2 I region products (Ia antigens) which are restricted to a few cell types in the adult, notably B lymphocytes, has however been traced in relation to those organs involved in the genesis of the immune system (Delovitch *et al.*, 1978) and provides an example of the use of MHC product to determine the history of a particular cell type.

Some indication of the way in which genetic controls may operate on cell surface components has come from studies showing that the onset of H-2 expression on murine RBC is strain dependent. Thus, C57BL(H-2^b) RBC are agglutinable at birth, while those of A strain (H-2^a) do not become so until 3 days later (Moller and Moller, 1962). B10.A mice which have been bred to produce the H-2^a haplotype on a C57BL background, behave as early expressers like the C57BL type rather than following the later pattern normally seen with H-2^a. This has led to the conclusion that there is a gene controlling erythrocyte H-2 expression which is not actually part of the H-2 complex although normally linked to it (Boubelik *et al.*, 1975). The operation of this type of control in other tissues and at earlier stages has not yet been investigated, nor is it clear whether the appearance of H-2 determinants occurs at the same rate since most antisera employed in studies of development have been polyspecific. Using oligospecific antisera on later embryonic tissues Pizzaro *et al.* (1961) have obtained evidence of coordinate H-2 gene product appearance. On the other hand, H-2 antigen expression on mouse blastocyst derived cell tissues is only partial as indicated by the detectability in cytotoxicity tests of some determinants but not others (presumably on the same polypeptide) of a given haplotype. Apart from incomplete synthesis, this could suggest that the availability of a particular macromolecule can be masked to varying degrees of association with other components. Alternatively, interaction with antibody may be restricted by changes in membrane fluidity such that the antigens may not assume the close proximity necessary for complement fixation and consequent cytolysis (see Edidin, 1976). Evidently, the control of H-2 expression is far from resolved. The well defined antigen system offered by the MHC does, however, offer interesting possibilities in terms of analysing the genetic and epigenetic factors determining cell surface phenotype.

2. Cell- and Tissue-Specific Antigens

A number of antigens have now been identified which are tissue specific or which at least show a restricted distribution. Various attempts have been made to examine such antigens during development either to establish their history as indicators of the molecular changes accompanying differentiation or in the hope that they may provide useful markers in determining cell lineage. The latter is of particular value in the study of complex organs composed of cells of potentially diverse origin which often assume their final positions as a result of complex migrations. In addition, as mentioned for MHC antigens, the ability to trace specific cell products may also provide valuable markers of gene activity during development. In this section selected examples of cell- or tissue-associated antigens which have been examined at different stages of development will be considered.

a. Cellular antigens   At the earliest stages of development in the mammal, absorbed antiserum prepared in rabbits against mouse placental cells has been shown to label mouse embryos throughout the pre-implantation period, being detectable on both inner cell mass and trophoblast (Wiley and Calarco, 1975). This would suggest that these particular placental-specific molecules do not become segregated to the trophoblast until some time after the blastocyst stage. More recently, absorbed rabbit antiserum to mouse ectoplacental cone, which provides a relatively uncontaminated trophoblastic population, has been shown to give a pattern of labelling on pre- and early post-implantation embryos which closely parallels the appearance of the trophectoderm and its immediate derivatives as defined by experimental and morphological studies (Searle and Jenkinson, 1978). Thus the emergence of the trophectoderm appears to be associated with molecular specialization of the cell membrane which is maintained in its primary products. Whether the surface molecules recognized by this antiserum have any functional significance in the biological activities of the trophoblast is not known but might be assessed by the effect of the antiserum on trophoblast development and behaviour *in vitro* (see Section III.B). In man, a number of trophoblast-specific products have been identified, including a cell membrane antigen (Faulk *et al.*, 1978) and the placental specific proteins SP-1 and PP-5 (Bohn, 1976) which offer trophoblast markers for normal or pathological trophoblasts as well as potential targets for fertility regulation.

Much of the basic information on morphogenetic movements and germ layer interactions, especially at gastrulation, has been obtained in non-mammalian species such as the chick, amphibian, or sea-urchin where embryonic material is more readily available or more accessible to manipulation. These studies have relied mainly upon tracing the fate of cell populations marked by the localized application of dyes or on the use of transplantation techniques which may in themselves alter the normal pattern of development. The availability of antibody labels, for specific cells or tissue types, which can be applied retrospectively and without the use of invasive techniques, could thus be of considerable value as an adjunct to the traditional methods. Attempts have been made to immunize rabbits with germ layer components of the chick embryo (Wolk and Eyat-Giladi, 1977) and have resulted in antisera recognizing a variety of components appearing at different times in germ layer formation and some of which are germ-layer specific. Using antisera to hypoblast-specific antigen, it has been shown that cells characterized by this antigen do not contribute to the head process, a finding contrary to that obtained with carbon-marking experiments. On the other hand, the observation that cells from the primitive streak invade the hypoblast, from which they can be distinguished by their lack of hypoblast-specific antigen, and contribute to the secondary hypoblast or entoderm is in agreement with studies using tritiated thymidine-labelled transplants. Further studies are required to establish the general applicability of this approach but it is of interest that germ-layer-specific antigens may also be present in the sea-urchin embryo (McClay and Chambers, 1978). Germ-layer-specific antigens have not yet been identified in mammalian embryos but as described below cell products such as fibronectin (this section), AFP (Section III.A.3) and some of the teratoma-defined antigens (Section III.A.3) may be operationally germ layer specific during the early phases of embryogenesis. Furthermore, with the advent of techniques for the separation of the components of the pre-implantation embryo (see Section III.C) and of the germ layers in the early post-implantation mouse embryo (Rossant, 1977) it should now be possible to raise specific antisera which may discriminate between cell populations during early embryogenesis.

In later development the formation of the central nervous system presents a particularly challenging problem in understanding cell relationships and lineage. One approach to this problem has been the preparation of antisera in rabbits to newborn mouse brain which have served to define a series of antigens designated NS-1, NS-2, etc. (see Chaffee and Schacner, 1978a,b). Of these antigens one (NS-6) is present on an undifferentiated neural tumour, on many cell types in the adult brain and as early as day 9 of gestation, and is considered to represent a component of pluripotential neural progenitor cells which is passed on to both neural and glial progeny. In contrast, antigen NS-1 appears to be specific to glial cells (Schacner, 1974) and could be useful in tracing their history in the developing brain. The labelling pattern seen in the embryo with some of the NS antigens shows, however, that these are present on many non-central-nervous tissue cells in the early embryo and become restricted to neural tissues (and in some cases kidney and sperm) at different stages of development. Antigen NS-4 for example, can be detected on the cleavage stage embryo and on the trophectoderm and inner cell mass of the blastocyst but is restricted to neural structures by day 12 of gestation (Solter and Schacner, 1976). It should prove interesting to determine how this restriction comes about in relation to the formation of the ectoderm and subsequently the neurectoderm from which the nervous system is derived.

A system paralleling that of the nervous system in the complexity of its interacting components is also seen in those cells and tissues responsible for immunological functions. In this area too, many advances have arisen from the availability of antigen markers for different lymphoid populations and subpopulations. Antigens such as Thy-1 characteristic of T lymphocytes and the Ly series of antigens defining various T cell subsets have been particularly useful in identifying cells in heterogeneous populations and in tracing lymphocyte differentiation from precursor pools in the adult (Cantor and Boyse, 1977). With the exception of Thy-1 however, these have not been extensively investigated during embryonic life (see Owen, 1979). Also within the lymphoid system, immunoglobulin recognized by anti-immunoglobulin antisera has proved a useful marker in studying B cell development. In combination with *in vitro* culture immunoglobulin labelling has enabled the detection of the sites of primary B cell production and has shown that pre-B cells expressing cytoplasmic but not surface immunoglobulin are present in the foetal liver as early as day 12 of gestation. Subsequently these cells appear in other sites of foetal and adult haemopoiesis and appear to give the small surface IgM-positive B lymphocytes which are not detectable by immunofluorescence in the embryo until days 16–17 of gestation (Owen, 1979).

Outside the lymphoid and nervous systems the use of antisera in tracing cell lineage in organogenesis is illustrated by recent studies on the mouse lung (Ten Have-Opbroek, 1979). Heterologous antiserum to adult mouse lung, suitably absorbed, labels cells which appear at day 14 of gestation. These may be the stem cells of the alveolar epithelium which also labels, unlike the prospective bronchial epithelium suggesting that this has a different origin.

In contrast to most of the foregoing which represents cell membrane antigens, specific antisera may also be employed in the detection of intracellular products. Perhaps the best example of this is provided by the proteins of the developing lens which has been widely studied as a model system. The pattern of appearance of the characteristic lens proteins α-, β-, and γ-crystallins has been investigated by antibody labelling during development in various species including amphibia and birds (Zwaan, 1968; Brahma and McDevitt, 1974). In the rat the pattern of crystallin production has been shown to change sequentially from α-crystallin alone to production of all three types during the conversion of proliferating lens epithelium cells into non-dividing elongating lens fibres (McAvoy, 1978). Sequential activation of the crystallin gene thus seems to occur during fibre formation, possibly as a result of exposure to the different microenvironments as the cells change position within the lens. Antisera to lens crystallins have also been of value in assessing the potential of retinal pigment cells for transdifferentiation into lens fibres under various experimental conditions, a system which provides a model for exploration of the stability of the differentiated state (Eguchi, 1979). Similarly, immunolabelling of crystallins in mouse and chick has been used in *in vitro* studies to demonstrate the ability of isolated presumptive lens ectoderm to form differentiated lens products under permissive conditions and the ability of the optic cup to induce lens-type differentiation in ectoderm from other regions (Karkinen-Jaaskelainen, 1978).

b. Extracellular antigens   The role of the extracellular matrix in tissue and organ modelling is the subject of continuing debate, interest having centred upon collagen and fibronectin (or LETS) a high molecular weight cell-surface associated glycoprotein which is a major component of connective tissue matrix and basement membranes and may also have a role in cell adhesion (Stenman and Vakeri, 1978). Although not strictly tissue specific these proteins do show a somewhat restricted distribution during development and immunolabelling studies have indicated major changes in their localization in association with morphogenetic events. In the early mouse embryo, fibronectin becomes detectable by immunofluorescence at the blastocyst stage and has been reported to be associated with the differentiation of the primitive endoderm (Wartiovaara *et al.*, 1979) although a conflicting report suggests that only cells of the embryonic ectoderm are able to synthesize fibronectin during early development (Zetter and Martin, 1979). With the formation of the mesoderm layer, fibronectin appears in the cytoplasm of the mesoderm cells, possibly producing a useful marker in the study of mesoderm segregation. This cytoplasmic staining soon disappears, however, although fibronectin can be found intracellularly in the region of the expanding mesoderm (Wartiovaara *et al.*, 1979). This programmed loss of mesodermal cytoplasmic fibronectin and its restriction to basement membranes can be observed by imunofluorescence on tissue sections in the development of various organs. In the developing tooth germ, for example, fibronectin disappears from the mesenchyme differentiating into odontoblasts and accumulates at the epithelio–mesenchymal interface where it could be important in shaping tooth morphology and as a mediator in the contact-dependent inductive interactions between the mesenchyme and the dental epithelium (Thesleff *et al.*, 1979).

A changing pattern of collagen distribution in the mesenchyme, similar to that of fibronectin, has also been observed in the tooth germ (Thesleff *et al.*, 1979) and it seems likely that a similar pattern occurs in the development of other organs. During the formation of the mouse extraembryonic membranes collagen formation, as detected by biochemical analysis and immunoperoxidase labelling, has also identified different collagen types associated with different endoderm populations (Adamson and Ayers, 1979). The parietal endoderm throughout development and the visceral endoderm of the early post-implantation embryo appear to produce Type IV collagen. In contrast the visceral endoderm of the definitive yolk sac produces only Type I implying a switch in collagen gene expression if these cells are in fact derived from the earlier visceral endoderm. Such changes in collagen synthesis and distribution as revealed by labelling studies may reflect the need for different types of collagen at different stages of development. Given the likely role of basement membranes in organizing tissue architecture and the identification of at least five genes controlling the different collagen types, these studies offer one approach to the analysis of the genetic control of tissue modelling.

3. Developmental Antigens

In the course of development there is a changing pattern of synthetic activity, presumably reflecting changes in gene expression leading to the appearance of products characteristic of a particular phase of development (see Schultz and Church, 1975; Van Blerkom and Manes, 1977; Ibsen and Fishman, 1979). With appropriate immunization (see Section II) some of these products can be recognized as antigens which can be termed developmental or stage (phase) specific antigens. Normally, these disappear as development proceeds but may persist when development is arrested. Such arrest appears to occur naturally in the case of teratocarcinoma cells or may be induced by the irradiation of embryonic cells or their explantation into culture at the appropriate stage (Ying *et al.*, 1978).

a. Antigens recognized by immunization with embryonic tissue   Stage-specific antigens have been identified at several points in the development of the frog (*Rana temporaria*) (Romanovsky, 1964a,b) by immunizing rabbits with frog embryos of different ages. In the mammal some attempts have been made to raise antisera directly against early embryos, although the amount of material available for this purpose can be limiting. Antisera from guinea pigs immunized with unfertilized mouse eggs detect an antigen present on the pre-implantation embryo and on SV-40 transformed adult cells, but absent from normal adult cells, disappearing from the embryo shortly after implantation (Baranska *et al.*, 1970; Moskalewski and Koprowski, 1972). Similarly, rabbit anti-mouse blastocyst antiserum detects an antigen, showing peak expression on the cleavage stages, which disappears after implantation (Wiley and Calarco, 1975). Stage-specific antigens of the larger mid-gestation embryo are more easily studied when direct immunization with embryonic tissues is to be employed (Coggin *et al.*, 1971) and can be detected by isologous antisera and by antibodies elicited by pregnancy in the rat and mouse, presumably as a result of exposure to embryonic antigens (Baldwin and Vose, 1974). Interest in these antigens has centred on their re-expression on adult cells during tissue regeneration (Abelev, 1974) or following malignant transformation occurring spontaneously or induced by chemical or viral agents (Coggin and Anderson, 1974; Baldwin *et al.*, 1974). It seems probable that some of these antigens are controlled by genes which are not expressed after a particular stage except under certain conditions. The level at which the control of expression takes place is uncertain but it has been argued that it is primarily at the post-transcriptional level (Ibsen and Fishman, 1979). Studies on the effect of various inhibitors on antigen expression may be helpful in this regard. Alternatively, in some cases lack of expression in the adult may be due to the production of a masking substance by normal adult cells (Rogan *et al.*, 1973).

Despite the interest they have aroused little is known of the precise ontogeny, tissue distribution or relationship the various developmental antigens share with one another and with virus-determined antigens. Detailed mapping and tissue distribution studies are required to elucidate these points. In two cases, however, information of this type is available. Carcinoembryonic antigen (CEA) represents a stage-specific antigen of the foetal digestive tract in man which is not present in the adult except in association with colonic and rectal tumours (Terry *et al.*, 1974). Similarly, α-foetoprotein (AFP) is known to be produced by the yolk sac and foetal liver but is found in the adult only under conditions which may reflect a reversion to the embryonic state as in liver regeneration or when teratomas or hepatomas are present (see Abelev, 1974). Recently it has been shown, using immunoperoxidase labelling, that AFP is first produced by day 7 of gestation of the mouse, synthesis at this stage being confined to the embyronic region of the visceral endoderm for which it thus provides a marker (Dziadek, 1978). This localized expression of AFP has also proved a useful marker in the study of tissue interaction. Thus, although normally confined to the visceral embryonic endoderm, immunolabelling studies have demonstrated that AFP can also be produced by the extraembryonic visceral endoderm when this is separated from the underlying extraembryonic ectoderm. Conversely, combination of the embryonic visceral endoderm with extraembryonic ectoderm results in the inhibition of AFP synthesis by this tissue (Dziadek and Adamson, 1978). These findings provide direct evidence for the modulating effect of one tissue on the synthetic activity of another and raise the possibility that it is breakdown of such regulatory influences that lead to re-expression of AFP in the adult.

b. Teratoma defined antigens More precise information in terms of ontogeny and localization, has been obtained using antisera prepared by immunization with mouse teratocarcinomas. These arise spontaneously in the gonads of certain strains or may be induced by the ectopic transplantation of genital ridges or early embryos (Stevens, 1967, 1970). In particular, the stem cell-like embryonal carcinoma (EC) cells present in these tumours, which have been likened to the multipotential cells of the early embryo, have proved a valuable source of cells which can be cloned *in vitro* to provide relatively large amounts of homogeneous material maintaining the otherwise transient properties of normal embryonic cells (see Jacob, 1977; Gachelin, 1978 for detailed reviews).

Unlike most of the stage-specific antigens described above, the teratocarcinoma-defined antigens are not present on transformed adult cells and seem to be mainly confined to multipotential stem cell-like populations. Most widely studied has been the F-9 antigen raised by syngeneic immunization of 129/Sv mice with nullipotential F-9 EC cells. Anti-F-9 antisera have been found to label the pre-implantation embryo, the antigens first appearing shortly after fertilization and being present on both inner cell mass and trophectoderm of the blastocyst. This labelling pattern confirms the view that the EC cells and early embryos have some shared surface features. Since F-9 antigen cannot be found on an adult somatic cell, its time of disappearance during embryogenesis has also been examined. The antigen persists on cells of the embryo proper until around day 9 probably being confined to the embryonic ectoderm which is still considered to be multipotential. Subsequent to this time with the rapid differentiation of embryonic ectoderm and its concomitant loss of multipotentiality (Diwan and Stevens, 1976) F-9 antigen is no longer detectable (Jacob, 1977; Buc-Caron *et al.*, 1978). As indicated in Section III.A.1 H-2 antigens do not appear on the progeny of the embryonic ectoderm until around day 9 in the normal embryo suggesting a reciprocal relationship between F-9 and H-2 expression. This also seems to be the case for EC cells themselves which express F-9 and lack H-2 until they begin to differentiate when the situation is reversed (Gachelin, 1978). An exception to this reciprocal relationship is provided by sperm which appear to express both H-2 and F-9 antigens (Gachelin *et al.*, 1976). In fact, in contrast to adult somatic cells, F-9 appears to be present on all male germ-line cells (Gachelin *et al.*, 1976) an observation which has led to the speculation that it may in some way contribute to the sorting out of the germinal cells (Jacob, 1977).

In contrast to the results obtained by immunization with nullipotential F-9 cells, syngeneic immunization with multipotential PCC4 EC cells has given a different pattern (Gachelin *et al.*, 1977). After appropriate absorption to remove anti-F-9-like activity anti-PCC4 antiserum still labels PCC4 and other multipotential cells as well as spermatozoa. Unlike anti-F-9 sera however it does not label the cleavage stage embryo nor the trophectoderm or inner cell mass of the pre-implantation blastocyst. In the late blastocyst around the time of implantation PCC4 antigen can be detected on the inner cell mass. Thus, while its history in the older embryo has still to be traced, this antigen does appear to provide a differentiation marker for inner cell mass as opposed to trophectoderm although not unfortunately at the earliest states of trophoblast/ inner cell mass segregation.

A somewhat different approach to the use of teratomas as immunogens to provide antisera to probe development has been employed by Edidin and his co-workers (Gooding and Edidin, 1974; Edidin, 1976). In these experiments heteroantisera raised in rabbits against teratoma 402-AX, with appropriate absorption, has been found to define a group of antigens (antigens I, II, III). Again there appears to be a reciprocal relationship between the expression of teratoma antigens (particularly antigen I) and H-2 expression. This has led to the speculation that there may be a precursor relationship between these two sets of surface products especially as antigen I has been shown by co-capping experiments to be in close physical association with H-2 in a cultured cell line which expresses both these products. The relationship, if any, between the various antigens defined by heteroantisera and isoantisera against EC cells remains to be clarified.

Although much of the foregoing strongly suggests that certain phases of development are associated with the presence of particular surface structures it is necessary to establish whether these components have any functional role if such observations are to lead to an interpretation of the mechanisms of embryogenesis. Considerable interest was therefore aroused by the suggestion that F-9 antigen might represent a product of the *T/t* locus (Artzt *et al.*, 1974). Mutant *T/t* locus haplotypes show arrested embryonic development at specific stages in the homozygous state and each haplotype also appears to specify a particular set of antigens detectable on the surface of spermatozoa (Yanagisawa *et al.*, 1974). Thus it seemed possible that these antigens represented the abnormal equivalent of surface products of wild type genes involved in cellular interactions at sequential stages of normal development (Bennett, 1975). In particular, the pattern of F-9 labelling on embryos and sperm and absorption studies on spermatozoa of various genotypes indicated that the F-9 antigen might represent the product of the wild type equivalent of the tw^{32} gene (Artzt *et al.*, 1974). Subsequent studies in which the various t antigens present on the sperm have been sought directly on appropriate pre-implantation embryos have indeed indicated the presence of these antigens. However, all the antigens tested were found to be present on the cleavage stages implying that they are not expressed sequentially as might be expected if they were to correlate with the sequence of lethal effects caused by haplotypes in homozygous embryos (Kemler *et al.*, 1976). More information is clearly needed to determine whether lethal *t*-mutations are in any way due to failures to produce appropriate surface molecules or whether *t*-mutants are more general cell lethals (Sherman and Wudl, 1977). If nothing else, however, the search for *T/t*-locus determined surface products has served to focus attention on the possibility of associating altered surface phenotype with specific failures in embryonic organization as a means of identifying the role of the cell surface in developmental events.

B. Antibodies in the Study of Cellular Interactions

The cell surface is considered to play a direct role in morphogenesis and there is considerable interest in the identification of these components mediating the cellular interactions underlying this process. Both protein and carbohydrate components have been considered important and have been investigated by a variety of biochemical and histochemical techiques (Winzler, 1970; Bretscher and Raff, 1975; Marchesi *et al.*, 1978). In recent years the increased availability of plant lectins with specificity for various sugars has greatly facilitated the study of surface carbohydrates both *in situ* and in membrane extracts (see Chapter 10). Similarly, antibodies provide probes of protein/glycoprotein arrays on the membrane while carbohydrate-specific antibodies raised against microbial carbohydrate structures have also been applied to the study of mammalian cells in a comparable manner to lectins (Trenker and Sarker, 1978).

Apart from the demonstration of surface-located compounds as described in preceding sections, immunological approaches to cellular interactions have been based on the premise that inhibition of cellular interactions by antibody may indicate a functional role for the particular antigen(s) recognized. There is, however, a reservation in the interpretation of such findings arising from the possibility of steric hindrance of the function of one receptor by antibody binding to another whether these are on two different parts of the same macromolecule or on separate components closely adjacent on the cell surface. Furthermore, extensive cross-linking of one type of antigen on the cell surface may trap or inhibit the mobility of other components so interfering indirectly with their function. These problems may be reduced by the use of monovalent Fab antibody fragments which, while retaining their specificity, are smaller and unable to induce cross-linking.

The slime moulds have provided useful models in the morphological and biochemical analysis of cellular interactions. Recent studies have demonstrated the presence of lectin-like (carbohydrate-binding) proteins on the cells of these organisms and it has been suggested that these may serve as cellular adhesion molecules by binding to oligosaccharide receptors. Support for this view has come from the demonstration that monovalent antibody (Fab) to these proteins can inhibit the aggregation phase of development in *Polysphondylium pallidum* under conditions called 'permissive' (Rosen *et al.*, 1977). In optimally aggregating cells under normal conditions, however, the anti-lectin-like protein Fab failed to inhibit appreciably cell aggregation (Bozzaro and Gerisch, 1978). The role of carbohydrate binding lectin-like proteins in cell adhesion has therefore been recently questioned (see Muller and Gerisch, 1978). In normal conditions cellular aggregation can be completely inhibited by monovalent antibody directed against other membrane antigens, called contact sites. Similarly, inhibition of aggregation in *Dictyostelium discoidum* by rabbit antiserum selectively absorbed on different stages has indicated that there are two different membrane components or contact sites mediating end-to-end and side-to-side contact of aggregating cells (Beug *et al.*, 1970, 1973), suggesting one way in which some organization may be imposed. In *P. pallidum*, as well as in *D. discoideum* the principal target antigens of the adhesion-blocking antibody appear to be different from the carbohydrate-binding lectin-like proteins and, in the case of the end-to-end type of cellular aggregation, involves a lectin (Concanavalin A)-binding glycoprotein on the cell surface (Muller and Gerisch, 1978). Models of cell adhesion have been proposed which involve a three component system in which the lectin-binding glycoproteins or contact sites may have a regulatory role in cell adhesion.

There is also some evidence that lectin-like molecules are present in the tissues of the developing chick, preliminary studies with labelled anti-lectin antibodies indicating their location on the cell surface (Barondes, 1978). It will be important to determine whether such carbohydrate-binding membrane components are present in tissues of a variety of species and if so whether cellular interaction is affected by addition of monovalent antibody raised against them.

Changes in the behaviour of cells during morphogenesis have also been extensively studied in the sea urchin (Gustafson and Wolpert, 1967) and immunological probes are now being applied to the investigation of the molecular basis of these changes. Thus the appearance of new antigens at gastrulation shows a temporal correlation with changes in adhesive specificity while cellular aggregation at the gastrula stage can be blocked by antibody, again indicating a likely functional role for some of these antigens (McClay *et al.*, 1977).

In vertebrate systems heterologous antisera to the zona pellucida of the mammalian ovum are able to prevent attachment to, and penetration of, the zona by spermatozoa (Shivers, 1974). Such antisera may be blocking specific receptor sites for sperm on the zona and with refinement may enable the isolation and identification of the receptors. Similarly, antisera recognizing plasma membrane antigens of eggs and sperm may also be of use in elucidating gamete membrane interaction and fusion. During pre-implantation development in the mouse certain antigens including the F-9 antigen (see Section III.A1) and the developmental antigen recognized by a rabbit anti-mouse blastocyst antiserum (see Section III.A3) appear to achieve maximal expression at the early morula stage. It is at this stage that the first morphological events involving changes in cell contact and adhesion take place, the embryo undergoing a process of 'compaction' with the formation of tight and gap junctions at the periphery of the morula as a prelude to blastocyst formation (Ducibella, 1977). It seems possible that some of the surface antigens may be involved in these events especially as it has now been shown that Fab fragments of the rabbit anti-F-9 antiserum are able to induce reversible inhibition of compaction (Kemler *et al.*, 1977). This may be due to a direct effect on a surface component involved in adhesion, or may be more indirect, for example, by interference with moieties involved in the uptake of calcium which is a known requirement for compaction and junction formation (Ducibella, 1977). Similarly the rabbit anti-mouse blastocyst antiserum prevents embryo development (Wiley and Calarco, 1975) although it is not known whether the effect of antibody in this case is reversible.

During organogenesis the ways in which cells are directed to form ordered structures are still largely unknown although some hypotheses have been developed from the application of immunological techniques to this problem. The ability of mixed cell suspensions to sort out in a histiotypic fashion is well known (Moscona, 1965) and the possibility that there are tissue-specific surface molecules which could be used in the mutual recognition of cells has been indicated by the demonstration that antisera can be raised against selected tissues and can selectively inhibit the reaggregation of dispersed cells from such tissues (Goldschneider and Moscona, 1972; Moscona and Moscona, 1962). The existence of specific organogenesis directing molecules has also been predicted from studies of the mouse H-Y antigen. This model, based originally on indirect evidence, proposes that the immunologically defined H-Y antigen on the surface of male gonadal cells causes them to form a testis-like structure, while in the absence of this antigen an ovary is formed (Ohno, 1977). Recently some experimental support for this hypothesis has been obtained with the demonstration that the reaggregation of dispersed testis cells to form tubules is prevented by exposure of the cells to anti-H-Y antibody, an ovary-like structure being formed instead (Ohno *et al.*, 1978; Zenzes *et al.*, 1978). It will be interesting to see how widely this model can be applied to other organizing systems.

Antibodies have also been prepared to a cell adhesion molecule (CAM) associated with the cell membrane of chick retinal and neural cells (Rutishauser *et al.*, 1978a,b). Anti-CAM Fab fragments are able to disrupt the organization that occurs in cultures of aggregating retinal cells and can inhibit the side-to-side adhesions between neurites apparently involved in the production of nerve bundles suggesting that this molecule may be important in ordering cell relationships in nervous tissue. Similarly, inhibition of tissue organization *in vitro* by antibodies to certain surface carbohydrates has been reported for mouse cerebellum (Trenker, 1979). Thus, given a suitable culture system, or even *in vivo* administration, reagents of this type may ultimately prove useful in determining how recognition capable of giving rise to a precise pattern of cell contacts is established within the nervous system.

It is evident from the foregoing that there are various situations during development where antibodies may be employed to probe cellular interactions. While most of these are still in the stage where careful experimentation is required to separate direct and indirect effects the eventual availability of antisera known to identify components involved in surface interactions justifies such efforts. Thus, such antibodies could be used in immunoprecipitation (see Section II.C) or immobilized on columns in preparative techniques for the isolation of surface molecules from membrane preparations. In this way, in combination with biochemical analysis and lectin-binding techniques, it may be possible to gain a better understanding of the molecular basis of cell recognition.

C. Antibodies in Cell Selection and Sorting

In addition to molecular separation of cell extracts mentioned in previous sections, separation and sorting of viable cells using antibody is also feasible. To date, these techniques have been employed mainly in studies on the adult immune system. There is no reason, however, why this approach cannot be applied to cell populations in the developing embryo or in the endocrine and reproductive organs of the adult, given the increasing numbers of antibodies recognizing markers with a restricted distribution. Thus it may be possible to separate hormone-producing cells and other cells for biochemical and functional analysis as well as embryonic cell populations for examination of their normal fate and potential *in vitro* and, following transfer to another embryo, *in vivo*.

A range of techniques are now available which have potential in this regard. Where the deletion of a particular cell population is required, treatment with specific antibody and complement can be employed (see Section II.B). Cells in suspension which have bound specific antibody can be separated, in a viable state, from those which have not by incubation with anti-immunoglobulin-coated red cells (see Section II.A.2) to form rosettes which can be separated from non-rosetting cells by centrifugation (Parish and Hayward, 1974). Separation of antibody-labelled cell suspensions has also been achieved by incubation on anti-immunoglobulin-coated petri dishes to which the labelled cells adhere, to be dislodged subsequently by gentle pipetting (Mage *et al.*, 1977). Similarly, passage through columns of glass or agarose beads coated with anti-immunoglobulin (Dalianus *et al.*, 1977) or the immunoglobulin- binding protein-A (Ghetie *et al.*, 1978) as well as lectins (see Chapter 10) will also retain antibody-labelled cells which can be recovered. The development of the fluorescence-activated cell sorter (FACS) which is capable of sorting living cells on the basis of size and the presence of bound antibodies conjugated with a fluorochrome (Herzenberg and Herzenberg, 1978) is also proving a powerful tool in immunological research and should have wider application in sorting any cell populations that can be obtained in suspension.

An example of the use of immunological separation techniques which is of considerable interest in reproductive biology, is the possibility of separating mammalian X and Y chromosome bearing spermatozoa by virtue of differences in their expression of the male-specific H-Y antigen. There are suggestions of an alteration of the sex ratio in the mouse following artificial insemination with sperm treated with anti-H-Y antibody and complement (Bennett and Boyse, 1973) and technically, separation of both X and Y bearing sperm of adequate viability by rosetting or FACS may be possible. The question as to whether there is haploid expression of H-Y on Y chromosome bearing sperm is still contentious however, and there is also the possibility that H-Y antigen may persist on X chromosome bearing sperm from the pre-meiotic stages hindering a clear-cut distinction between X and Y populations (see Koo *et al.*, 1977; Erickson, 1977). Recent indications that the H-Y antigen is expressed as early as the eight-cell stage in the mouse (Krco and Goldberg, 1976), do however raise the possibility of sexing pre-implantation embryos using fluorescence or rosetting techniques compatible with embryo survival, prior to re-transfer to a foster mother.

In addition to the separation techniques based on those derived from studies of the immune system a novel use of antibodies for cell separation has also been devised for the micro-dissection of the early mouse embryo (Solter and Knowles, 1975; Handyside and Barton, 1977). This immunosurgical procedure relies on the fact that the exposure of the blastocyst to rabbit anti-mouse antiserum results in antibody binding only to the outer exposed surface of the trophectoderm cells which have tight junctions preventing antibody access to the inner cell mass. After washing, antibody-treated blastocysts are exposed to complement resulting in lysis of the trophectoderm which can be pipetted away leaving an isolated, viable inner cell mass. In this way considerable numbers of inner cell masses can be obtained in a relatively short time. The technique has also been used sequentially on the developing embryo being applied to remove the outer endoderm layer which forms around isolated inner cell masses in culture (Strickland *et al.*, 1976). Using the appropriate anti-species antibody, the method would seem to have potential for the micro-dissection of any structure in embryos of various species where an outer, antibody impermeable, layer encloses an inner component(s).

D. Antibodies in the Study of Foeto–Maternal Relationships

Pregnancy in the mammal involves the establishment of an intimate relationship between mother and foetus involving both physiological and immunological interactions some of which are amenable to study by immunochemical techniques. In addition to studies on histocompatibility and tissue-specific antigens, heteroantisera to a wide variety of human proteins have been used in immunofluorescence assays to investigate the molecular composition of the human placenta in order to further the understanding of its physiological function (Faulk *et al.*, 1974; Faulk and Johnson, 1977). This has shown the presence of abundant actin in the syncytiotrophoblast cells possibly reflecting the role of microfilaments in the specialized transport functions of this tissue. Transferrin is also readily detectable in the apical regions of the trophoblast cells and could be considered to have an important role in the iron economy of pregnancy. Both C1q within the walls of foetal stem vessels of the human placenta (Faulk and Johnson, 1977) and Fc receptors on placental stem vessel endothelium (Johnson *et al.*, 1976) have been detected by immunofluorescence and rosetting techniques and it has been suggested that these may serve as a mechanism to precipitate or trap immune complexes before they enter the foetal circulation. Similarly, rosetting techniques employing antibody-coated SRBC have been employed to demonstrate the presence of receptors for the Fc portion of the IgG molecule on the surface of mouse (Elson *et al.*, 1975) and rabbit (Wild and Dawson, 1977) yolk sac endoderm cells in suspension and on human placental trophoblast cells in suspension (Jenkinson *et al.*, 1976) and in frozen sections (Matre *et al.*, 1975; Matre and Johnson, 1977). These receptors have also been investigated by following the transport of radiolabelled immunoglobulin fragments *in vivo* and may play an important part in the transfer of passive immunity from mother to young (Brambell, 1970; Hemmings, 1976).

As well as the possibility of antigenic silence of the trophoblast (see Section II. A. 1) various other mechanisms have been considered to contribute to the protection of the foetus from adverse maternal immune responses (see Billington, 1976; Bernard, 1977). Factors capable of blocking cell-mediated attack directed against maternal alloantigens or embryonic antigens have been demonstrated in murine pregnancy sera (Hellstrom and Hellstrom, 1974; Smith, 1979) and the use of anti-immunoglobulin immunoabsorbent columns has suggested that, in at least one system, IgG2a and IgG2b but not IgG1 are involved (Tamerius *et al.*, 1975). In the same study, heterologous antiserum to mouse embryos was also found to neutralize the blocking activity of the pregnancy serum implying that antigen/antibody complexes may be responsible. In man, pregnancy serum or placental eluates contain factors capable of blocking the mixed lymphocyte response, macrophage migration and mitogen stimulation and, although the specificity of these effects is not clear, in some cases IgG does appear to be involved (see Youtananukorn and Matangkasombut, 1973; Faulk and Jeannet, 1976; Rocklin *et al.*, 1976; Revillard *et al.*, 1976; McIntyre and Faulk, 1978. In the mouse, IgG obtained by acid elution of the placenta will protect paternal strain allografts suggesting that this may play a similar role in the protection of the *conceptus* (Voisin and Chaouat, 1974). A role for the placenta as an immunoabsorbent removing deleterious antibody before it reaches the embryo proper has also been suggested. Experimental support for this concept has come from the injection of females pregnant by males of a different strain with immunabsorbent purified radiolabelled anti-paternal antibody which is found to localize within the placenta (Wegman *et al.*, 1979).

Interest in the role of maternal immunoglobulins in the foeto–maternal relationship has also lead to studies on their distribution in the pregnant uterus. Prior to implantation it would appear that immunoglobulins are not detectable by immunofluorescence within the cleavage stage mouse embryo although they are present in the uterine and tubal stroma, the block to transfer possibly residing in the epithelial lining of the reproductive tract (Glass and Hanson, 1976). Immunoglobulin can be detected by immunoperoxidase labelling in the uterine glands and lumen at implantation and can be found in and around the trophectoderm and in the endoderm and blastocoele of the implanted embryo. Subsequently it is apparent in all the embryonic cavities being particularly noticeable in the endoderm of the yolk sac and gut (Bernard, 1977; Bernard *et al.*, 1977). Thus immunoglobulin is intimately associated with the trophoblastic and other surfaces of the embryo and is in a position to contribute to its protection against maternal immune responses. Cells located in the metrial gland of the pregnant rat uterus have also been shown to contain immunoglobulin. While the source of this immunoglobulin is not clear it has been suggested that these cells are B lymphocyte derived and may be acting as local producers of blocking antibody for the protection of the *conceptus* (Bulmer and Peel, 1977).

Apart from immunoglobulins the uterine environment contains a variety of macromolecules which may be important for the developing embryo (Aitken, 1977a,b). Under the influence of progesterone, changes have been observed in the contents of the uterine fluid among which blastokinin or uteroglobulin, a protein first described in a rabbit, has been most widely studied (Beier, 1976, 1977). Interest in this protein has centred on its possible role in the synchronization of early embryonic development with uterine receptivity, its usefulness as a model to study the endocrine regulation of the uterine environment, and its potential as a target for the immunological regulation of fertility (see Johnson, 1974). Antisera recognizing this protein have allowed quantitative scanning by immunodiffusion during the reproductive cycle, tissue localization by immunofluorescence (Kirchner, 1972), and precise quantitation by radioimmunoassay (Johnson, 1976). As a result of these investigations it has been shown that uteroglobulin is synthesized and stored in epithelial cells of the uterine crypts during oestrus and is progressively synthesized and released under the influence of progesterone following coitus until the time of implantation when there is a switch off of intracellular production.

Elucidation of the history of other uterine products by immunological means (Joshi and Murray, 1974; Johnson *et al.*, 1975) also promises to be a valuable adjunct to biochemical analyses of the uterine fluid. In addition, the use of immobilized antisera on immunoabsorbent columns should facilitate the isolation and purification of uterine molecules for subsequent analysis of their composition and biological activity.

E. Antibodies in the Study of Reproductive Endocrinology

The application of immunological assays has made a substantial contribution to the analysis of the hormonal regulation of reproductive processes. In addition to protein hormones, with the development of techniques for producing antibody responses to non-immunogenic steroids and small peptides by coupling to a suitable carrier, the whole range of hormone activity has become accessible to immunological investigation. Further improvements in technique have also been achieved by immunization with hormone subunits, fragments or synthetic analogues to avoid cross-reactivity due to structural homology between different hormones as in the case of the α subunit of the gonadotrophins LH, FSH, and hCG (Canfield *et al.*, 1971). There is now a considerable literature in this field (see Nieschlag, 1975; Edwards and Johnson, 1976; Talwar, 1979) and only the general areas of application with a few selected examples will be considered here.

1. Hormone Monitoring

The development of RIA and more recently ELISA (see Section II. D) based on hormone-specific antibodies has greatly facilitated quantitative studies on the changing pattern of hormonal secretion. One of the most notable examples of this is the detection of chorionic gonadotrophin (hCG), produced by the human *conceptus*, in maternal serum or urine as an indicator of pregnancy and its progression. In particular the use of antibodies to the β subunit of hCG in a radioimmunoassay has enabled detection of production by the human embryo at a very early stage close to the time of implantation when other non-specific assays could not have distinguished it from a rise in pituitary gonadotrophins (Braunstein *et al.*, 1973; Mishell *et al.*, 1973; Kosasa *et al.*, 1974). At present, however, the suggestion that hCG-like substances may be produced by the pre-implantation embryo in the rabbit, mouse, and man remains controversial (Saxena *et al.*, 1974; Wiley, 1974; Catt *et al.*, 1975; Lee and Ryan, 1975; Sundaram *et al.*, 1975; Edwards, 1976; Channing *et al.*, 1978).

2. Physiological Function of Hormones

Apart from their use in the measurement of hormone levels, anti-hormone antibodies have also proved useful in investigating the physiological function of hormones in the control of gonadal activity. *In vitro*, antibodies to follicle stimulating hormone (FSH), luteinizing hormone (LH), and prolactin have been used to neutralize selectively these hormones in human serum before assaying its effect on cultures of granulosa cells (McNatty *et al.*, 1976). The findings provide support for the concept that these hormones form a luteotrophic complex needed to maintain steroidogenesis by the corpus luteum. *In vivo*, immunization (either active or passive) against steroids (Scaramuzzi, 1976; Hillier and Cameron, 1976) and gonadotrophin hormones (Setchell and Edwards, 1976; Raj, 1976) has enabled neutralization of individual hormones without resort to the removal of the hormone-producing organs. In all these studies the possibility of incomplete neutralization, depending on the relative affinity of antibody and hormone receptors for the hormone as well as feedback effects eliciting the release of more gonadotrophins when steroids are mopped up by antibody, is an important consideration. Immunity to the gonadotrophin-releasing hormone, LH-RH has also been valuable in the analysis of the neuroendocrine control of gonadal activity and offers the possibility of blocking gonadotrophin release at the central level thus allowing assessment of the action of individual gonadotrophins using replacement therapy (Jeffcoate *et al.*, 1976; Fraser, 1976). Furthermore, immunological blocking of LH-RH activity also provides a possible mechanism for fertility control (Hodges and Hearn, 1979).

In terms of fertility control most attention has been given to immunization against hCG. While this has met with some success it is still not clear whether immunization has a direct effect on the embryo preventing implantation or serves primarily to neutralize gonadotrophin support of the corpus luteum (Hearn, 1979). It is now also realized that cross-reaction with other hormones, particularly those of the pituitary needs to be avoided, as mentioned earlier, while reports of hCG production in non-pregnant animals suggest that the possibility of side effects in other tissues needs careful scrutiny (see Talwar *et al.*, 1979 for review).

3. Localization of Hormones and Hormone Receptors

Antibodies to hormones can be used in immunolabelling assays to localize hormone synthesis and hormone-binding sites at the cellular level, thereby enabling the identification of the involved cell types within the heterogeneous population of a complex organ. In these studies immunofluorescence and immunoperoxidase labelling of either paraffin wax or cryostat sections of tissue, where the problem of hormone diffusion needs to be considered, and post-embedding immunoperoxidase labelling of ultrathin plastic sections (Moriarty *et al.*, 1973) have been employed.

In the human placenta antisera to human chorionic somatomammotrophin (HCS) and hCG have enabled localization of both these hormones to the trophoblast (Ikonicoff and Cedard, 1973) while studies at the electron microscope level confirm that the syncytiotrophoblast rather than the cytotrophoblast is the primary site of production (Dreskin *et al.*, 1970; Ikonicoff, 1974). Similarly, labelling with antisera to ovine placental lactogen has shown that this hormone is produced by binucleate epithelial cells of the chorionic villi and uninucleate cells of the trophoblast in the sheep placenta (Reddy and Watkins, 1978). Human chorionic gonadotrophin or LH-like molecules have been detected on the surface of pre-implantation mouse morulae using immunofluorescence techniques on intact embryos cultured from the two-cell stage to reduce the likelihood of uptake from maternal fluids (Wiley, 1974). Furthermore, receptors for these hormones have also been reported to be present on the pre-implantation embryo (Sen Gupta *et al.*, 1978) adding to the speculation that gonadotrophins could be directly involved in the signalling between mother and embryo. In this context, reports, based on histochemical investigation, that the pre-implantation embryo is also capable of steroidogenesis (Dickman *et al.*, 1976) remain controversial and here too the application of immunolabelling with antibodies to steroids may prove useful.

Steroid hormones have been localized in the testis by post-embedding immunolabelling (Gardner, 1975) and, at the central level, adjacent ultrathin sections have been used to determine whether the same secretory cell contains more than one type of hormone granule. This method has also been employed to detect receptors for the gonadotrophin-releasing hormone LH-RH in the anterior pituitary by exposing one section to LH-RH followed by antiserum to LH-RH while an adjacent section is exposed to antisera to LH or FSH (Sternberger and Petrali, 1976). In this way, it has been shown that only gonadotrophic cells (i.e. containing LH and FSH) have releasing hormone receptors. In addition, these studies have provided some evidence for the pathway of action of this hormone on its target cell showing that after the receptor has interacted with LH-RH on the plasma membrane it is translocated to the secretory granules where it mediates secretion of preformed gonadotrophins.

IV. CONCLUSION

The ability to produce antibodies to a variety of cellular and extracellular products is providing the basis for an increasing array of tools with application in reproductive and developmental biology. In all these applications success depends both on the ability to produce antibody and on the specificity which can be achieved. In this respect one of the most exciting developments in the use of antibody as tool is the development of techniques for the production of monoclonal antibodies with the high degree of specificity and standardization which these confer (see Chapter 9). Monoclonal reagents to a variety of MHC antigens are now available and are beginning to be applied to the embryo. Recently, the application of monoclonal antibody techniques has revealed the presence of two new antigens on the surface of the pre-implantation mouse embryo (Solter and Knowles, 1978; Willison and Stern, 1978) and with increasing application it seems likely that a new range of monoclonal antibody probes will become available. Finally, the production of monoclonal reagents recognizing hormonal products offers not only the possibility of a high degree of specificity but, with the perpetuation of antibody-producing clones, a long-term supply of standard reagents available for widespread distribution.

REFERENCES

Abelev, G. I. (1974). α-Fetoprotein as a marker of embryo specific differentiation in normal and tumour tissues. *Transplant. Rev.*, **20**, 3–37.

Adamson, E. D. and Ayers. S. E. (1979). The localisation and synthesis of some collagen types in developing mouse embryos. *Cell*, **16**, 953–965.

Aitken, R. J. (1977a). Changes in protein content of mouse uterine flushings during normal pregnancy and delayed implantation and after ovariectomy and oestrogen administration. *J. Reprod. Fertil.*, **50**. 29–36.

Aitken, R. J. (1977b). Embryonic diapause. In M. H. Johnson (Ed.) *Development in Mammals*, volume 3, pp. 307–359. North Holland, Amsterdam.

Ammann, A. J., Borg, D., Kondo, L., and Wara, D. W. (1977). Quantitation of B cells in peripheral blood by polyacrylamide beads coated with anti-human chain antibody. *J. Immunol. Meth.*, **17**, 365–371.

Andres, G. A., Hsu, K. C., and Seegal, B. C. (1978) Immunologic techniques for the identification of antigens or antibodies by electron microscopy. In D. M. Weir (Ed.) *Handbook of Experimental Immunology*, 3rd edn. pp. 37.1–37.54. Blackwell Scientific Publications, London.

Artzt, K., Bennett, D., and Jacob, F. (1974). Primitive teratocarcinoma cells express a differentiation antigen specified by a gene at the T-locus in the mouse. *Proc. Natl. Acad. Sci. USA*,**71**, 811–814.

Baldwin, R. W., Embleton, M. J., Price, M. R., and Vose, B. M. (1974). Embryonic antigen expression on experimental rat tumours. *Transplant. Rev.*, **20**, 77–99.

Baldwin, R. W. and Vose, B. M. (1974). The expression of phase-specific foetal antigens on rat embryo cells. *Transplantation*, **18**, 525–530.

Baranska, W., Koldovsky, P., and Koprowski, H. (1970). Antigenic study of unfertilized mouse eggs: cross reactivity with SV-40 induced antigens. *Proc. Natl. Acad. Sci. USA.*,**67**, 193–199.

Barondes, S. H. (1978). Regulated lectins in cellular slime mold and embryonic chick tissues. *Prog. Clin. Biolog. Res.*, **23**, 633–636.

Beier, H. M. (1976). Uteroglobin and related biochemical changes in the reproductive tract during early pregnancy in the rabbit. *J. Reprod. Fertil. Suppl.*.,**25**, 53–69.

Beier, H. M. (1977). Physiology of uteroglobin. In C. H. Spilman and J. W. Wilk (Eds) *Novel Aspects of Reproductive Physiology Proceedings of the 7th Brook Lodge*

Workshop on Problems of Reproductive Physiology, pp. 219–245, Spectrum Publications, New York.

Bellon, B., Sapin, C., and Druet, P. (1978). Comparison de la sensibilité des techniques d'immunofluorescence et d'immunoperoxidase en methodes directe et indirect. *Ann. Immunol. Inst. Past.*, **126C** 15–22.

Bennett, D. (1975). The T locus of the mouse. *Cell*, **6**, 441–454.

Bennett, D. and Boyse, E. A. (1973). Sex ratio in progeny mice inseminated with sperm treated with H-Y antiserum. *Nature*, **246**, 308–309.

Bergquist, N. S., Carlsson, J., and Huldt, G. (1976). Comparative studies of fluorochrome and enzyme-labelled antibodies. In F. Feldmann, P. Druet, J. Bignon, and S. Avrameas (Eds) *1st International Symposium on Immunoenzymatic Techniques*, pp. 37–41. North-Holland/American Elsevier, Amsterdam.

Bernard, O. (1977). Possible protecting role of maternal immunoglobulins on embryonic development in mammals. *Immunogenetics*, **5**, 1–15.

Bernard, O., Ripoche, M.-A., and Bennett, D. (1977). Distribution of maternal immunoglobulins in the mouse uterus and embryo in the days after implantation. *J. Exp. Med.*, **145**, 58–75.

Beug, H., Gerisch, G., Kempff, S., Riedel, V., and Cremer, G. (1970). Specific inhibition of cell contact formation in *Dictyostelium* by univalent antibodies. *Exp. Cell Res.*, **63**, 147–158.

Beug, H., Katz, F. E., and Gerisch, G. (1973). Dynamics of antigenic membrane sites relating to cell aggregation in *Dictyostelium discoidium*. *J. Cell Biol.*, **56**, 647–658.

Billington, W. D. (1976). The immunobiology of trophoblast. In J. S. Scott and W. R. Jones (Eds) *Immunology of Human Reproduction*, pp. 81–102. Academic Press, London.

Billington, W. D. and Jenkinson, E. J. (1975). Antigen expression during early mouse development. In M. Balls and A. E. Wild (Eds) *The Early Development of Mammals*, pp. 219–232. Cambridge University Press, London.

Bodmer, W. F. (1972). Evolutionary significance of the HL-A system. *Nature*, **237**, 139–145.

Bohn, H., (1976). The protein antigens of human placenta as a basis for the development of contraceptive vaccine. In *Development of Vaccines for Fertility Regulation*, WHO Session: Third International Symposium on Immunology of Reproduction, pp. 111–125, Scriptor, Copenhagen.

Boubelik, M., Lengerova, A., Bailey, D. W., and Matousek, V. (1975). A model for genetic analysis of programmed gene expression as reflected in the development of membrane antigens. *Devel. Biol.*, **47**, 206–214.

Boyse, E. A., Old, L. J., and Chouroulinkov, I. (1964). Cytotoxic test for demonstration of mouse antibody. *Meth. Med. Res.*, **10**, 39–47.

Bozzaro, S. and Gerisch, G. (1978) Contact sites in aggregating cells of *Polysphondylium pallidium*. *J. Molec. Biol.*, **20**, 265–279.

Brahma, J. K. and McDevitt, D. S. (1974). Ontogeny and localisation of gamma-crystallins in *Rana temporaria*, *Amblystoma* and *Pleucodeles watti* normal lens development. *Exp. Cell Res.*, **19**, 379–387.

Brambell, F. W. R. (1970). *The Transmission of Immunity from Mother to Young*, Elsevier/North Holland, Amsterdam.

Braunstein, G. D., Grodin, J. M., Vaitukaitas, J., and Ross, G. T. (1973). Secretory rates of human chorionic gonadotrophin by normal trophoblast. *Amer. J. Obstet. Gynaec.*, **115**, 447-450.

Bretscher, M. S. and Raff, M. C. (1975). Mammalian plasma membranes. *Nature*, **258**, 43–49.

Buc-Caron, M. H., Condamine, H., and Jacob, F. (1978). The presence of F-9 antigen on the surface of mouse embryonic cells until day 8 of embryogenesis. *J. Embryol. Exp. Morphol.*, **47**, 149–160.

Bulmer, D. and Peel, S. (1977). The demonstration of immunoglobulin in the metrial gland of the rat placenta. *J. Reprod. Fertil.*, **49**, 143–145.

Burns, J. (1975). Background staining and sensitivity of the unlabelled antibody-enzyme (PAP) method. Comparison with the peroxidase labelled antibody sandwich method using formalin-fixed paraffin embedded material. *Histochemistry*, **43**, 291–294.

Cammisuli, S. and Wofsy, L. (1976). III Bifunctional reagents for immunospecific labelling of cell surface antigens. *J. Immunol.*, **117**, 1695–1704.

Canfield, R. E., Morgan, F. J., Kammerman, S., Bell, J. J., and Agosto, G. M. (1971). Studies of human chorionic gonadotrophin. *Recent Prog. Hormone Res.*, **27**, 121–156.

Cantor, H. and Boyse, E. A. (1977). Lymphocytes as models for the study of mammalian cellular differentiation. *Immunol. Rev.*, **33**, 105–124.

Catt, K. J., Dufau, M. L., and Vaitukaitis, J. L. (1975). Appearance of hCG in pregnancy plasma following the initiation of implantation of the blastocyst. *J. Clin. Endocrin. Metab.*, **40**, 537–540.

Chaffee, J. K. and Schacner, M. (1978a). NS-6 (nervous system antigen-6), a new cell surface antigen of mature brain, kidney and spermatozoa. *Develop. Biol.*, **62**, 173–184.

Chaffee, J. K. and Schacner, M. (1978b). NS-7 (nervous system antigen-7). A cell surface antigen of mature brain, kidney and spermatozoa shared by embryonal tissue and transformed cells. *Develop. Biol.*, **62**, 185–192.

Channing, C. P., Stone, S. L., Sakai, C. N., Haour, F., and Saxena, B. B. (1978). A stimulatory effect of the fluid from preimplantation rabbit blastocyst upon luteinization of monkey granulosa cell cultures. *J. Reprod. Fertil.*, **54**, 215–220.

Chapman, V. M., West, J. D., and Adler, D. A. (1977). Genetics of early mammalian embryogenesis. In M. I. Sherman (Ed.) *Concepts in Mammalian Embryogenesis* pp. 95–135. MIT, Cambridge.

Chatterjee-Hasrouni, S. and Lala, P. K. (1979). Localization of H-2 antigens on mouse trophoblast cells. *J. Exp. Med.*, **149**, 1238–1253.

Coggin, J. H., Ambrose, K. R., Bellomy, B. B., and Anderson, N. G. (1971). Tumour immunity in hamsters immunised with fetal tissues. *J. Immunol.*, **107**, 526–533.

Coggin, J. H. and Anderson, N. G. (1974). Cancer differentiation and embryonic antigens: some central problems. *Adv. Cancer Res.*, **19**, 105–165.

Coombs, R. R. A., Marks, J., and Bedford, D. (1956). Specific mixed agglutination: mixed erythrocyte–platelet antiglobulin reaction for the detection of platelet antibodies. *Brit. J. Haematol.*, **2**, 84–94.

Coombs, R. R. A., Wilson, A. B., Eremin, O., Gurner, B. W., Haegert, D. G., Lawson, Y. A., Bright, S., and Munro, A. J. (1977). Comparison of the direct antiglobulin rosetting reaction with the mixed antiglobulin rosetting reaction for the detection of immunoglobulin on lymphocytes. *J. Immunol. Methods*, **18**, 45–54.

Cullen, S. E. and Schwarz, B. D. (1976). An improved method for isolation of H-2 and Ia alloantigens with immune precipitation induced by protein A bearing staphylococci. *J. Immunol.*, **117**, 136–142.

Dalianus, T., Anderson, B., and Klein, G. (1977). Separation of cells with different H-2 antigens by passage through cellular immuno-absorbent columns. *Europ. J. Immunol.*, **7**, 154–158.

Delovitch, T. L. and McDevitt, H. O. (1975). Isolation and characterisation of murine Ia antigens. *Immunogenetics*, **2**, 39–00.

Delovitch, T. L., Press, J. L., and McDevitt, H. O. (1978). Expression of murine Ia antigens during embryonic development. *J. Immunol.*, **120**, 818–824.

Dickmann, Z., Dey, S. K., and Sen Gupta, J. (1976). A new concept: control of early pregnancy by steroid hormones originating in the preimplantation embryo. *Vit. Horm.*, **34**, 215–242.

Diwan, S. B. and Stevens, L. C. (1976). Development of teratomas from the ectoderm of mouse egg cylinders. *J. Natl. Cancer Inst.*, **57.**, 937–942.

Douglas, T. C. (1972). Occurrence of a theta-like antigen in rats. *J. Exp. Med.*, **136**, 1054–1062.

Dreskin, R., Spicer, S., and Greene, W. (1970). Ultrastructural localisation of chorionic gonadotrophin in human term placenta. *J. Histochem. Cytochem.*, **18**, 862–874.

Ducibella, T. (1977). Surface changes of the developing trophoblast cell. In M. H. Johnson (Ed.) *Development in Mammals*, volume 1, pp. 5–30, North Holland, Amsterdam.

Dziadek, M. (1978). Modulation of alpha-fetoprotein synthesis in the early post implantation mouse embryo. *J. Embryol. Exp. Morphol.*, **46**, 135–146.

Dziadek, M. and Adamson, E. (1978). Localisation and synthesis of alpha-fetoprotein in post-implantation mouse embryos. *J. Embryol. Exp. Morphol.*, **43**, 289–313.

Edidin, M,. (1964). Transplantation antigens in the early mouse embryo. *Transplantation*, **2**, 627–637.

Edidin, M. (1972). The tissue distribution and cellular location of transplantation antigens. In B. D. Kahan and R. A. Reisfeld (Eds) *Transplantation Antigens*, pp. 75–114. Academic Press, New York.

Edidin M,. (1976). The appearance of cell-surface antigens in the development of the mouse embryo: a study of cell-surface differentiation. In *Embryogenesis in Mammals,* CIBA Foundation Symposium 40 (new series), pp. 177–197. Elsevier, Amsterdam.

Edidin, M., Gooding, L. R., and Johnson, M. H. (1974). Surface antigens of normal early embryos and a tumour model system useful for their further study. In E. Diczfalusy (Ed.) *Immunological Approaches to Fertility Control. Karolinska Symposium No. 7,* pp. 336–356. Bogtrykkeriet Forum, Copenhagen.

Edwards, R. G. (1976). In R. G. Edwards and M. H. Johnson (Eds) *Physiological Effects of Immunity against Reproductive Hormones*, pp. 268, Cambridge University Press, Cambridge.

Edwards, R. G. and Johnson, M. H. (1976). *Physiological Effects of Immunity against Reproductive Hormones.* Cambridge University Press, Cambridge.

Eguchi, G. (1979). Transdifferentiation in pigmented epithelial cells of vertebrate eyes *in vitro*. In J. D. Ebert and T. S. Okada (Eds) *Mechanisms of Cell Change*, pp. 273–291. John Wiley, New York.

Elson, J.,Jenkinson, E. J., and Billington, W. D. (1975). Fc receptors on mouse placenta and yolk sac cells. *Nature*, **255**, 412–414.

Engvall, E. and Carlson, H. E. (1976). Enzyme-linked immunosorbent assay ELISA. In G. Feldman, P. Druet, J. Bignon, and S. Avrameas (Eds) *1st International Symposium on Immunoenzymatic Techniques* , pp. 135–147. North-Holland/American Elsvier, Amsterdam.

Erickson, R. P. (1972). Alternative modes of detection of H-2 antigens on mouse spermatozoa. In R. A. Beatty and S. Gluecksohn-Waelsch (Eds) *Genetics of the Spermatozoan* , pp. 191–200. Bogtrykkeriet Forum, Copenhagen.

Erickson, R. P. (1977). Differentiation and other alloantigens of spermatozoa. In M. Edidin and M. H. Johnson (Eds) *Immunobiology of Gametes*, pp. 85–114, Cambridge University Press, London.

Erickson, R. P., Gachelin, G., Fellous, M., and Jacob, F. (1977) Absorption analysis of H-2D and K antigens on spermatozoa. *J. Immunogenetics*, **4**, 47–51.

Fagraeus, A. and Espmark, J. A. (1961). Use of a mixed haemadsorption method in virus infected tissue cultures. *Nature*, **190**, 370–371.

Fagraeus, A., Espmark, J. A., and Jonsson, J. (1965). Mixed haemadsorption: a mixed antiglobulin reaction applied to antigens on a glass surface. Preparation and evaluation of indicator red cells; survey of present applications. *Immunology*, **9**, 161–175.

Faulk, W. P., Chonochie, L. D., Trenchev, P., and Dorling, J. (1974). An immunohistological study of the distribution of immunoglobulins, collagen and contractile proteins in human placentae. *Protides Biol. Fluids*, **22**, 303–307.

Faulk, W. P. and Jeannet, M. (1976). Immunological studies of immunoglobulins from human placentae. In W. A. Hemmings (Ed.) *Maternofoetal Transmission of Immunoglobulins*, pp.47–59. Cambridge University Press, London.

Faulk, W. P. and Johnson, P. M. (1977). Immunological studies of human placentae: identification and distribution of proteins in mature chorionic villi. *Clin. Exp. Immunol.*, **27**, 365–375.

Faulk, W. P., Sanderson, A. R., and Temple A. (1977). Distribution of MHC antigens in human placental chorionic villi. *Transpl. Proc.*, **IX**, 1379–1384.

Faulk, W. P., Temple, A., Lovins, R. E., and Smith, N. (1978). Antigens of human trophoblast: a working hypothesis for their role in normal and abnormal pregnancies. *Proc. Natl. Acad. Sci. USA.*, **75**, 1947–1951.

Fellous, M. and Dausset, J. (1973). Histocompatibility antigens of human spermatozoa. In K. Bratanov (Ed) *Immunology of Reproduction*, pp. 332–338, Bulgarian Academy of Science, Sofia.

Feteanu, A. (1978). *Labelled Antibodies in Biology and Medicine*, Abacus Press, England.

Fraser, H. M. (1976). Physiological effects of antibody to luteinising hormone releasing hormone. In R. G. Edwards and M. H. Johnson (Eds) *Physiological Effects of Immunity against Reproductive Hormones*, pp. 137–165. Cambridge University Press, London.

Gachelin, G. (1978). The cell surface antigens of mouse embryonal carcinoma cells. *Biochim. Biophys. Acta*, **516**, 27–60.

Gachelin, G., Fellous, M., Guenet, J. L., and Jacob, F. (1976). Developmental expression of an early embryonic antigen common to mouse spermatozoa and cleavage embryos, and to human spermatozoa: its expression during spermatogenesis. *Develop. Biol.*, **50**, 310–320.

Gachelin, G., Kemler, R., Kelly, F., and Jacob, F. (1977). PCC4, a new cell surface antigen common to multipotential embryonal carcinoma cells, spermatozoa and mouse early embryos. *Develop. Biol.*, **57**, 199–209.

Gardner, P. J. (1975). Immunocytochemical localisation of steroids in the testis: a preliminary study. *Anat. Rec.*, **181**, 359–360.

Gardner, R. L. and Johnson, M. H. (1973). Investigation of early mammalian development using interspecific chimaeras between rat and mouse. *Nature New Biol.*, **246**, 86–89.

Ghetie, V., Mota, G., and Sjoqvist, J. (1978). Separation of cells by affinity chromatography on SpA-sepharose 6MB. *J. Immunol. Methods*, **21**, 133–141.

Glass, L. E. and Hanson, J. E. (1976). Molecular specificity in serum antigen transfer to mouse embryos cleaving *in vivo*. In W. A. Hemmings (Ed.) *Maternofoetal Transmission of Immunoglobulin*, pp. 299–312, Cambridge University Press, London.

Goldberg, E. H., Aoki, T., Boyse, E., and Bennett, D. (1970). Detection of H-2 antigens on mouse spermatozoa by the cytotoxicity test. *Nature*, **228**, 570–572.

Goldberg , E. H., Boyse, E. A., Bennett, D., Scheid, M., and Carswell, E. A. (1971).

Serological demonstration of H-Y (male) antigen on mouse sperm. *Nature*, **232**, 478–480.

Goldschneider, I. and Moscona, A. A. (1972). Tissue specific cell surface antigens in embryonic cells. *J. Cell Biol.*, **53**, 435–449.

Goodfellow, P. N., Barnstaple, C. J., Bodmer, W. F., Snary, D., and Crumpton, M. J. (1976). Expression of HLA System Antigens on Placenta. *Transplantation*, **22**, 595–603.

Gooding, L. R. and Edidin, M. (1974). Cell surface antigens of a mouse testicular teratoma. Identification of an antigen physically associated with H-2 antigens on tumour cells. *J. Exp. Med.*, **140**, 61–78.

Gotze, D. and Ferrone, S. (1972). A rapid micromethod for direct H-2 typing of mouse cultured lymphoid cells. *J. Immunol. Methods*, **1**, 203–206.

Grant, J. (1978). Immunological methods in bacteriology. In D. M. Weir (Ed.) *Handbook of Experimental Immunology*, 3rd edn, pp. 39.1–39.15. Blackwell Scientific Publications, London.

Gustafson, T. and Wolpert, L. (1967). Cellular movement and contact in sea urchin morphogenesis. *Biol. Rev. Cambridge Phil. Soc.*, **42**, 442–448.

Håkansson, S., Heyner, S., Sundqvist, K. G., and Bergstrom, S. (1975). The presence of paternal H-2 antigens on hybrid mouse blastocysts during experimental delay of implantation and the disappearance of these antigens after onset of implantation. *Int. J. Fertil.*, **20**, 137–140.

Halim, A., Abbassi, K., and Festenstein, H. (1974). The expression of the HLA antigens on human spermatozoa. *Tissue Antigens*, **4**, 1–6.

Hammerling, G. J., Mauve, G., Goldberg, E., and McDevitt, H. O. (1974). Tissue distribution of Ia antigens. Ia on spermatozoa, macrophages and epidermal cells. *Immunogenetics*, **1**, 428–437.

Hammerling, U., Oaki, T., Harven de E., Boyse, E. A., and Old, L. J. (1968). Use of hybrid antibody with anti-γG and anti-ferritin specificities in locating cell surface antigens by electron microscopy. *J. Exp. Med.* **128**, 1461–1469.

Hammerling, U., Stackpole, C. W., and Koo, G. (1973). Hybrid antibodies for labelling cell surface antigens. In H. Busch (Ed.) *Methods in Cancer Research* , volume 9 pp. 225–282. Academic Press, New York.

Handyside, A. H. and Barton, S. C. (1977). Evaluation of the technique of immunosurgery for the isolation of inner cell masses from mouse blastocysts. *J. Embryol. Exp. Morphol.*, **37**, 217–226.

Hausman, S. J. and Palm, J. (1973).Variable expression of Ag-B and non-Ag-B histocompatibility antigens on cultured rat cells of different histological origin. *Transplantation*, **16**, 313–324.

Hearn, J. P. (1979). Long term suppression of fertility by immunisation with hCG-β subunit and its reversibility in female marmoset monkeys. In G. P. Talwar (Ed.) *Recent Advances in Reproduction and Regulation of Fertility*, pp. 427–438. Elsevier/North Holland, Amsterdam.

Hellstrom, K. E. and Hellstrom, I. (1974). Lymphocyte-mediated cytotoxicity and blocking serum activity to tumour antigens. *Adv. Immunol.*, **18**, 209–277.

Hemmings, W. A. (1976). *Maternofoetal Transmission of Immunoglobulins*, Cambridge University Press, London.

Herzenberg, L. A. and Herzenberg, L. A. (1978). Analysis and separation using the fluorescence activated cell sorter FACS. In D. M. Weir (Ed.) *Handbook of Experimental Immunology*, 3rd edn, volume 2, pp. 22.1–22.21. Blackwell Scientific Publications, Oxford.

Heyner, S. (1973). Detection of H-2 antigens on the cells of the early mouse embryo. *Transplantation*, **16** 675–678.

Heyner, S. and Hunziker, R. D. (1979). Differential expression of alloantigens of the major histocompatibility complex on unfertilized and fertilized mouse eggs. *Develop. Genet.*, **1** (in press).

Hillier, S. G. and Cameron, E. H. D. (1976). Physiological effects of immunity against steroids in the rat. In R. G. Edwards and M. H. Johnson (Eds) *Physiological Effects of Immunity against Reproductive Hormones* pp. 91–120, Cambridge University Press, London.

Hodges, J. K. and Hearn, J. P. (1979). Long term suppression of fertility by immunisation against LHRH and its reversibility in female and male marmoset monkeys. In G. P. Talwar (Ed.) *Recent Advances in Reproduction and Regulation of Fertility* pp. 87–96. Elsevier/North Holland, Amsterdam.

Hunter, W. M. (1978). Radioimmunossay . In D. M. Weir (Ed.) *Handbook of Experimental Immunology*, 3rd edn, pp. 14.1–14.40. Blackwell Scientific Publications, London.

Ibsen, K. I. and Fishman, W. H. (1979). Developmental gene expression in cancer. *Biochim. Biophys. Acta*, **560**, 243–280.

Ikonicoff, L. K. (1974). Ultrastructural localization of human chorionic somato-mammotrophic hormone (HCS) in the human placenta by the peroxidase immunocytoenzymological method. In E. Wisse, W. T. L. Daems, I. Molenaar, and P. Duijn (Eds) *Electron Microscopy and Cytochemistry*, pp. 151–153. North Holland Publishing Co., Amsterdam.

Ikonicoff, L. K. and Cedard, L. (1973). Localisation of human chorion gonadotropic and somato-mammotropic hormones by the peroxidase immunohistoenzymologic method in villi and amniotic epithelium of human placenta. *Amer. J. Obstet Gynec.*, **116**, 1124–1132.

Jacob, F. (1977). Mouse teratocarcinoma and embryonic antigens. *Immunol. Rev.*, **33**, 3–32.

Jeffcoate, S. L., Holland, D. T., and Fraser, H. M. (1976). Anti-LH-RH sera in the investigation of reproduction. In R. G. Edwards and M. H. Johnson (Eds) *Physiological Effects of Immunity against Reproductive Hormones*, pp. 121–136. Cambridge University Press, London.

Jenkinson, E. J. and Billington, W. D. (1977). Cell surface properties of early mammalian embryos. In M. I. Sherman (Ed.) *Concepts in Mammalian Embryogenesis* pp. 235–266. MIT Press, Cambridge, Mass.

Jenkinson, E. J., Billington, W. D., and Elson, J. (1976). Detection of receptors for immunoglobulin on human placenta by EA rosette formation. *Clin. Exp. Immunol.*, **23**, 456–461.

Johnson, G. D., Holborrow, E. J., and Dorling, J. (1978). Immunofluorescence and immunoenzyme techniques. In D. M. Weir (Ed.) *Handbook of Experimental Immunology*, 3rd edn, pp. 15.1–15.30. Blackwell Scientific Publications, London.

Johnson, M. H. (1974). Studies using antibodies to the macromolecular secretions of the early pregnant uterus. In A. Centaro and N. Carretti (Eds) *Immunology in Obstetrics and Gynaecology Proceedings of the First International Congress, Padua* pp. 123–133. Excerpta Medica, Amsterdam.

Johnson, M. H. (1975a). Antigens of peri-implantation trophoblast. In R. G. Edwards, C. W. S. Howe, and M. H. Johnson (Eds) *Immunobiology of Trophoblast* , pp. 87–100. Cambridge University Press, London.

Johnson, M. H. (1975b). The macromolecular organization of membranes and its bearing on events leading up to fertilization. *J. Reprod. Fertil.*, **44**, 167–184.

Johnson, M. H. (1976). Fertilization and implantation. In J. S. Scott and W. R. Jones (Eds) *Immunology of Human Reproduction*, pp. 33–60. Academic press, London.

Johnson, M. H. and Edidin, M. (1972). H-2 antigens on mouse spermatozoa. *Transplantation*, **14**, 781–786.

Johnson, M. H., Hekman, A., and Rumke, P. (1975). The male and female genital tracts in allergic diseases. In P. G. H. Gell, R. R. A. Coombs, and P. Lachman (Eds) *Clinical Aspects of Immunology*, pp. 1509–1544. Blackwell Scientific Publications, London.

Johnson, P. M. Faulk, W. P. and Wang, A. C. (1976). Immunological studies of human placentae: subclass and fragment specificity of binding of aggregated IgG by placental endothelial cells. *Immunology*, **31**, 659–664.

Joshi, M. S. and Murray, I. M. (1974). Immunological studies of rat uterine fluid peptidase. *J. Reprod. Fertil.*, **37**, 361–365.

Karkinen-Jaaskelainen, M. (1978). Permissive and directive interactions in lens induction. *J. Embryol. Exp. Morphol.*, **44**, 167–179.

Kawarai, Y. and Nakane, P. K. (1970). Localisation of tissue antigens on ultrathin sections with peroxidase labelled antibody method. *J. Histochem. Cytochem.*, **18.**, 161–166.

Kemler, R., Babinet, C., Condamine, H., Gachelin, G., Guenet, J. L., and Jacob, F. (1976). Embryonal carcinoma antigen and the T/t locus of the mouse. *Proc. Natl. Acad. Sci.*, **73**, 4080–4084.

Kemler, R., Babinet, C., Eisen, H., and Jacob, F. (1977). Surface antigens in early differentiation. *Proc. Natl. Acad. Sci. USA*, **74**, 4449–4452.

Kirchner, C. (1972). Immune histologic studies on the synthesis of a uterine specific protein in the rabbit and its passage through the blastocyst coverings. *Fertil. Steril.*, **23**, 131–136.

Klein, J. (1965). The ontogenetic development of H-2 antigens *in vivo* and *in vitro*. In J. Matousek (Ed.) *Blood Groups of Animals*, pp. 405–414, Jonk, The Hague.

Klein, J. (1975). *Biology of the Mouse Histocompatibility-2 Complex*. Springer-Verlag, New York.

Klein, J. (1979). The major histocompatibility complex of the mouse. *Science*, **203**, 516–521.

Koo, G. C., Boyse, E. A., and Wachtel, S. S. (1977). Immunogenetic techniques and approaches in the study of sperm and testicular cell surface. In M. Edidin and M. H. Johnson (Eds) *Immunobiology of Gametes*, pp. 73–84. Cambridge University Press, London.

Kosasa, T. S., Levesque, L. A., Taylor, M. L., and Goldstein, D. P. (1974). Measurement of early chorionic activity with radioimmunoassay specific for human chorionic gonadotropin following spontaneous and induced ovulation. *Fert. Steril.*, **25**, 211–216.

Krco, C. J. and Goldberg, E. H. (1976). H-Y(male) antigen detection on eight cell mouse embryos. *Science*, **193**, 1134–1135.

Krco, C. J. and Goldberg, E. H. (1977). Major histocompatibility antigens on pre-implantation mouse embryos. *Transpl. Proc.*, **IX** 1367–1370.

Lamm, M. E., Koo, G. C., Stackpole, C. W., and Hammerling, U. (1972). Hapten-conjugated antibodies and visual markers used to label cell surface antigens for electron microscopy; an approach to double labelling. *Proc. Natl. Acad. Sci. USA.*, **69**, 3732–3736.

Lee, C. Y. and Ryan, R. J. (1975). Radioreceptor assay for human chorionic gonadotrophin. *J. Clin. Endocrin. Metab.*, **40**, 228–233.

Mage, M. G., McHugh, L. L., and Rothstein, T. L. (1977). Mouse lymphocytes with and without surface immunoglobulins: preparative scale preparation in polystyrene culture dishes coated with specifically purified anti-immunoglobulin. *J. Immunol. Methods*, **15**, 47–56.

Marchesi, V. T., Ginsburg, V., Robbins, P. W., and Fox, C. F. (1978). Cell surface carbohydrates and biological recognition. In *Clinical and Biological Research*, volume 23. A. R. Liss Inc. New York.

Matre,, R. and Johnson, P. M. (1977). Multiple Fc receptors in the human placenta. *Acta Path. Microbiol. Scand. Sect. C*, **85**, 314–316.

Matre, R., Tonder, O., and Endresen, C. (1975). Fc receptors in human placenta. *Scand. J. Immunol.*, **5**, 741–745.

McAvoy, J. W. (1978). Cell division, cell elongation and distribution of α, β and γ crystallins in the rat lens. *J. Embryol. Exp. Morphol.*, **44**, 149–165.

McClay, D. R. and Chambers, A. F. (1978). Identification of four classes of cell surface antigens appearing at gastrulation in sea urchin embryos. *Devlop. Biol.*, **63**, 179–186.

McClay, D. R., Chambers, A. F., and Warren, R. H. (1977). Specificity of cell–cell interactions in sea urchins embryos. Appearance of new cell surface determinants at gastrulation. *Develop. Biol.*, **56**, 343–355.

McIntyre, J. A., and Faulk, W. P. (1978). Suppression of mixed lymphocyte cultures by antibodies against human trophoblast membrane antigens. *Transpl. Proc.*, **X**, 919–922.

McNatty, K. P., Bennie, J. G., Hunter, W. M., and McNeilly, A. S. (1976). The effects of antibodies to human gonadotrophins on the viability and rate of progesterone secretion by human granulosa cells in tissue culture. In R. G. Edwards and M. H. Johnson (Eds) *Physiological Effects of Immunity against Reproductive Hormones*, pp. 41–66. Cambridge University Press, London.

Miles, L. E. M. and Hales, C. N. (1968). Labelled antibodies and immunological assay systems. *Nature (Lond.)*, **219**, 186–189.

Mishell, D. R., Thorneycroft, I. H., Nagata, Y., Murata, J., and Nakamura, R. M. (1973). Serum gonadotrophin and steroid patterns in early human gestation. *Amer. J. Obstet. Gynaec.*, **117**, 631–645.

Moller, G. and Moller, E. (1962). Phenotypic expression of mouse isoantigens. *J. Cell. Comp. Physiol.*, **60** (Suppl), 107–128.

Morello, D., Gachelin, G., Dubois, PH., Tanigaki, N., Pressman, D., and Jacob, F. (1978). Absence of reaction of a xenogenic anti-H-2 serum with mouse embryonal carcinoma cells. *Transplantation*, **26**, 119–125.

Moriarty, G. C., Moriarty, C. M., and Sternberger, L. A. (1973). Ultrastructural immunocytochemistry with unlabelled antibodies and the peroxidase–anti–peroxidase complex. A technique more sensitive than radioimmunoassay. *J. Histochem. Cytochem.*, **21**, 825–833.

Moscona, A. A. (1965). Recombination of dissociated cells and the development of cell aggregates. In E. N. Willmer (Ed.) *Cells and Tissues in Culture* , pp. 489–529. Academic Press, New York.

Moscona, A. A. and Moscona, M. H. (1962). Specific inhibition of cell aggregation by antisera to suspensions of embryonic cells. *Anat. Rec.*, **142**, 319–320.

Moskalewski, S. and Koprowski, H. (1972). Presence of egg antigen in immature oocytes and pre-implantation embryos. *Nature*, **237**, 167.

Muller, K. and Gerisch, G. (1978). A specific glycoprotein as the target site of adhesion blocking Fab in aggregating *Dictyostelium* cells. *Nature*, **274**, 445–449.

Nieschlay, E. (1975). Immunisation with Hormones. In *Reproduction Research*. Elsevier/North Holland, Amsterdam.

Nowinski, R. C. and Klein, P. A. (1975). Anomalous reactions of mouse alloantisera with cultured tumour cells. II Cytotoxicity is caused by antibodies to leukaemia viruses. *J. Immunol.*, **115**, 1261–1268.

Ohno, S. (1977). The original function of MHC antigens as the general plasma membrane anchorage site of organogenesis directing proteins. *Immunol. Rev.*, **33**, 59–69.

Ohno, S., Nagai, Y., and Ciccarese, S. (1978). Testicular cells lyostripped of H-Y antigen organise ovarian follicle-like aggregates. *Cytogenet. Cell Genet.*, **20**, 351–364.

Owen, J. J. T. (1979). Developmental aspects of the lymphoid system. In E. S. Lennox (Ed.) *International Review of Biochemistry*, volume 22, pp. 1–27. University Park Press, Baltimore.

Parish, C. R. and Hayward J. A. (1974). The lymphocyte surface I Relation between Fc receptors, C3 receptors and surface immunoglobulin. *Proc. Roy. Soc. Lond. B*, **187**, 47–63.

Parish, C. R. and McKenzie, I. F. C. (1978). A sensitive rosetting method for detecting subpopulations of lymphocytes which react with alloantisera. *J. Immunol. Methods*, **20**, 173–183.

Pizzaro, O., Hoecker, G., Rubinstein, P., and Ramos, A (1961). The distribution in the tissues and development of H-2 antigens of the mouse, *Proc. Natl. Acad. Sci. USA.*, **47**, 1900–1906.

Raj, Madwa, H. G. (1976). Anti-gonadotrophins and the endocrine function of the ovary. In R. G. Edwards and M. H. Johnson (Eds) *Physiological Effects of Immunity against Reproductive Hormones*, pp. 187–204. Cambridge University Press, London.

Reddy, A. L., Hudes, M. I., Karp, R. D., and Mullen, Y. (1977). Micromixed hemadsorption assay—a sensitive method for detecting antibodies against tumour associated antigens. *J. Immunol. Methods.*, **17**, 293–307.

Reddy, S. and Watkins, W. B. (1978). Immunofluorescence localisation of ovine placental lactogen. *J. Reprod. Fertil.*, **52**, 173–174.

Revillard, J. P., Brochier, J., Robert, M., Bonneau, M., and Traeger, J. (1976). Immunologic properties of placental eluates. *Transplant. Proc.*, **8**, 275–279.

Rocklin, R. E., Kitzmiller, J. L., Carpenter, C. B., Garovoy, M. R., and David, J. R. (1976). Maternal–fetal relation. Absence of an immunologic blocking factor from the serum of women with chronic abortions. *N. Engl. J. Med.*, **295**, 1209–1213.

Rogan, E. G., Schafer, M. P., Anderson, N. G., and Coggin, J. H. (1973). Cyclic AMP levels in the developing hamster foetus: a correlation with the phasing of foetal antigen in membrane maturation, *Differentiation*, **1**, 199–204.

Romanovsky, A. (1964a). Studies on antigenic differentiation in the embryonic development of *Rana temporaria*: I Agar precipitation tests. *Folia Biol. (Prague)*, **10**, 1–11.

Romanovksy, A. (1964b). Studies of antigenic differentiation in the embryonic development of *Rana temporaria*: II Ring test. *Folia Biol. (Prague)*, **10**, 12–22.

Rosen, S. D., Chang, C.-M., and Barondes, S. H. (1977). Intercellular adhesion in the cellular slime-mold *Polysphondylium pallidum* inhibited by interaction of asialofetuin or specific univalent antibody with endogenous cell surface lectin. *Develop. Biol.*, **61**, 202–213.

Rosenberg, S. A., Schwarz, S., Anding, H., Hyatt, C., and Williams, M. G. (1977). Comparison of multiple assays for detecting human antibodies against surface antigens on normal and malignant human tissue culture cells. *J. Immunol. Methods*, **17**, 225–239.

Rossant, J. (1977). Cell commitment in early rodent development. In M. H. Johnson (Ed.) *Development in Mammals*, volume 2, pp. 119–150. North Holland, Amsterdam.

Roth, G. (1977). Literature search: labelling of living cells by means of ferritin and synthetic polymeric microspheres (January 1975–October 1976). *J. Immunol. Methods*, **18**, 1–15.

Rutishauser, U., Gall, W. E., and Edelman, G. M. (1978a). Adhesion among neural cells of the chick embryo: IV Role of the cell surface molecule CAM in formation of neurite bundles in cultures of spinal ganglion. *J. Cell Biol.*, **79**, 382–392.

Rutishauser, U., Thiery, J. P., Brackenbury, R., and Edelman, G. M. (1978b). Adhesion among neural cells of the chick embryo: III Relationship of the surface molecule CAM to cell adhesion and the development of histotypic patterns. *J. Cell Biol.*, **79**, 371–381.

Sandrin, M. S., Potter, T. A., Morgan, G. M., and McKenzie, I. F. C. (1978). Detection of mouse alloantibodies by rosetting with protein A coated sheep red blood cells. *Transplantation*, **26**, 126-130.

Saxena, B., Hasan, S., Haour, F., and Schmidt-Gollwitzer, M. (1974). Radioreceptor assay of 'human chorionic gonadotrophin. Detection of early pregnancy. *Science*, **184**, 793–795.

Scaramuzzi, R. J. (1976). Physiological effects of immunising sheep against oestradiol-17β. In R. G. Edwards and M. H. Johnson (Eds) *Physiological Effects of Immunity against reproductive Hormones*, pp. 67–90. Cambridge University Press, London.

Schacner, M. (1974). NS-1 (Nervous system antigen-1), a glial-cell-specific antigenic component of the surface membrane. *Proc. Natl. Acad. Sci. USA.*, **71**, 1795–1799.

Schlesinger, M. (1964). Serologic studies of embryonic and trophoblastic tissues of the mouse. *J. Immunol.*, **93**, 255–263.

Schultz, G. A. and Church, R. B. (1975). Transcriptional patterns in early mammalian development. In R. Weber (Ed.) *The Biochemistry of Animal Development*, volume 3, pp. 47–90. Academic Press, New York.

Searle, R. F. and Jenkinson, E. J. (1978). Localization of trophoblast defined surface antigens during early mouse embryogenesis. *J. Embryol. Exp. Morphol.*, **43**, 147–156.

Searle, R. F., Sellens, M. H., Elson, J., Jenkinson, E. J., and Billington, W. D. (1976). Detection of alloantigens during pre-implantation development and early trophoblast differentiation in the mouse by immunoperoxidase labelling. *J. Exp. Med.*, **143**, 348–359.

Seigler, H. F. and Metzgar, R. S. (1970). Embryonic development of human transplantation antigens. *Transplantation*, **9**, 478–486.

Sellens, M. H. (1977). Antigen expression on early mouse trophoblast. *Nature*, **269**, 60–61.

Sellens, M. H., Jenkinson, E. J., and Billington, W. D. (1978). Major histocompatibility and non-major histocompatibility antigens on mouse ectoplacental cone and placental trophoblastic cells. *Transplantation*, **25**, 173–179.

Sen Gupta, J., Gupta, P. D., Manchanda, S. K., and Talwar, G. P. (1978). Immunocytochemical localisation of binding sites for LH and hCG in preimplantation mouse embryos. *J. Reprod. Fertil.*, **52**, 163–165.

Setchell, B. P. and Edwards, R. G. (1976). The effect of immunisation against gonadotrophins on the testis and male reproductive tract. In R. G. Edwards and M. H. Johnson (Eds) *Physiological Effects of Immunity against Reproductive Hormones*, pp. 167–186. Cambridge University Press, London.

Sherman, M. I. and Wudl, L. R. (1977). T-complex mutations and their effects. In M. I. Sherman (Ed.) *Concepts in Mammalian Embryogenesis*, pp. 136–234. MIT Press, Cambridge, Mass.

Shivers, C. A. (1974). Immunological interference with implantation. In E. Diczfalusy (Ed.) *Immunological Approaches to Fertility Control. Karolinska Symposium no. 7*, pp. 223–244. Bogtrykkeriet Forum, Copenhagen.

Smith, G. (1978). Inhibition of cell-mediated microcytotoxicity and stimulation of mixed lymphocyte reactivity by mouse pregnancy serum. *Transplantation*, **26**, 278–283.

Solter, D. and Knowles, B. B. (1975). Immunosurgery of mouse blastocyst. *Proc. Natl. Acad. Sci. USA*, **72**, 5099–5102.

Solter, D. and Knowles, B. B. (1978). Monoclonal antibody defining a stage specific mouse embryonic antigen (SSEA-1), *Proc. Natl. Acad. Sci. USA*, **75**, 5565–5569.

Solter, D. and Schacner, M. (1976). Brain and sperm cell surface antigen (NS-4) on pre-implantation embryos. *Develop. Biol.,* **52**, 98–104.

Stenman, S. and Vaheri, A. (1978). Distribution of major connective tissue protein fibronectin in normal human tissues. *J. Exp. Med.,* **147**, 1054–1064.

Sternberger, L. A. (1972). The unlabelled-antibody-peroxidase and the quantitative-immunouranium methods in light and electron immunohistochemistry. In D. Glick and R. M. Rosenbaum (Eds) *Techniques of Biochemical and Biophysical Morphology,* pp. 67–88, Wiley-Interscience, New York.

Sternberger, L. A. and Petrale, J. P. (1976). The unlabelled antibody enzyme method immunocytochemistry of hormone receptors at target cells. In G. Feldman, P. Druet, J. Bignon, and S. Avrameas (Eds) *Proc. 1st International Symposium on Immunoenzymatic Techniques,* pp. 43–58. North Holland Publishing Co., Amsterdam.

Stevens, L. C. (1967). The biology of teratomas. *Adv. Morphogenesis,* **6**, 1–31.

Stevens, L. C. (1970). The development of transplantable teratocarcinomas from intra-testicular grafts of pre- and post-implantation mouse embryos. *Develop. Biol.,* **21**, 364–382.

Strickland, S., Reich, E., and Sherman, M. I. (1976). Plasminogen activator in early embryogenesis: enzyme production by trophoblast and parietal endoderm. *Cell,* **9**, 231–240.

Sundaram, K., Connell, K., and Passantino, T. (1975). Implication of absence of hCG-like gonadotrophin in the blastocyst for control of corpus luteum function in the pregnant rabbit. *Nature (Lond.),* **256**, 739–741.

Talwar, G. P. (1979). *Recent Advances in Reproduction and Regulation of Fertility.* Elsevier/North Holland, Amsterdam.

Talwar, G. P., Ramakrishnan, S., Das, C., Dubey, S. K., Salahuddin, M., Shastri, N., Tandon, A., and Singh, O. (1979). Anti-hCG immunization. In G. P. Talwar (Ed.) *Recent Advances in Reproduction and Regulation of Fertility,* pp. 453–466. Elsevier/North Holland, Amsterdam.

Tamerius, J., Hellstrom, I., and Hellstrom, K. E. (1975). Evidence that blocking factors in the sera of multiparous mice are associated with immunoglobulins. *Int. J. Cancer,* **16**, 456–464.

Taylor, R. B., Duffus, W. P., Raff, M. C., and de Petris, S. (1971). Redistribution and pinocytosis of lymphocyte surface immunoglobulin molecules induced by anti-immunoglobulin antibody. *Nature New Biol.,* **233**, 225–229.

Ten Have-Opbroek, A. A. W. (1979). Immunological studies of lung development in the mouse embryo. II. First appearance of the great alveolar cells as shown by immunofluorescence. *Develop. Biol.,* **69**, 408–423.

Terry, W. D., Henkart, P. A., Coligan, J. E., and Todd, C. W. (1974). Carcinoembryonic antigen: characteristics and clinical application. *Transpl. Rev.,* **20**, 100–129.

Thesleff, I., Stenman, S., Vaheri, A., and Timpl, R. (1979). Changes in the matrix proteins fibronectin and collagen during differentiation of the tooth germ. *Develop. Biol.,* **70**, 116–126.

Ting, C.-C., Sandford, K. K., and Price, F. M. (1978). Expression of foetal antigens in foetal and adult cells in long term culture. *In vitro,* **14**, 207–211.

Trenker, E. (1979). Post-natal cerebellar cells of staggerer mutant mice express immature components on their surface. *Nature,* **277**. 566–567.

Trenker, E. and Sarkar, S. (1978). Microbial carbohydrate specific antibodies distinguish between different stages of differentiating mouse cerebellum. *Prog. in Clinical and Biological Res..,* **23**, 67–74.

Van Blerkom, J. and Manes, C. (1977). The molecular biology of the peri-implantation embryo. In M. I. Sherman (Ed) *Concepts in Mammalian Embryogenesis,* pp. 37–94. MIT Press, Cambridge, Mass.

Vitetta, E. S., Artzt, K., Bennett, D., Boyse, E. A., and Jacob, F. (1975). Structural similarities between a product of the T/t locus isolated from sperm and teratoma cells, and H-2 antigens isolated from splenocytes. *Proc. Natl. Acad. Sci. USA, 72*, 3215–3219.

Voisin, G. A. and Chaouat, G. (1974). Demonstration, nature and properties of maternal antibodies fixed on placenta and directed against paternal antigens. *J. Reprod. Fertil (Suppl.)*, **21**, 87–103.

Vojtiskova, M. and Pokorna, Z. (1972). Developmental expression of H-2 antigens in the spermatogenic cell series: possible bearing on haploid gene action. *Folio Biol. (Prague)*, **18**, 1–9.

Vojtiskova, M., Pokorna, Z., Viklicky, V., Boubelik, M., and Hattikudur, N. S. (1974). The expression of H-2 and differentiation antigens on mouse spermatozoa. *Folia Biol. (Prague)*, **20**, 321–324.

Wachtel, S. S., Koo, G. C., Breg, W. R., Elias, S., Boyse, E. A. and Miller, J. O. (1975). Expression of H-Y antigen in human males with two Y chromosomes. *New Engl. J. Med.*, **293**, 1070–1072.

Wagner, M. (1973). Methods of labelling antibodies for electron microscopic localisation of antigens. In J. B. G. Kwapinski (Ed.) *Research in Immunochemistry and Immunobiology*, pp. 182–252. University Park Press, Baltimore.

Wartiovaara, J., Leino, I., and Vaheri, A. (1979). Expression of the cell surface associated glycoprotein, fibronectin, in the early mouse embryo. *Develop. Biol.*, **69**, 247–267.

Webb, C. G., Gall, W. E., and Edelman, G. M. (1977). Synthesis and distribution of H-2 antigens in pre–implantation mouse embryos. *J. Exp. Med.*, **146**, 923–932.

Weemen, B. K., and Schuurs, A. H. W. M. (1976). Sensitivity and specificity of hapten enzyme-immunoassays. In G. Feldman, P. Druet, J. Bignon, and S. Avrameas (Eds) Proc. 1st. International Symposium on *Immunoenzymatic Techniques*, pp. 125–133. North Holland Publishing Company, Amsterdam.

Wegmann, T. G., Singh, B., and Carlson, G. A. (1979). Allogeneic placenta is a paternal strain immunoabsorbent. *J. Immunol.*, **122**, 271–274.

Welsh, K. I. and Batchelor, J. R. (1978). Assays for antibodies against histocompatibility antigens. In D. M. Weir (Ed.) *Handbook of Experimental Immunology*, 3rd edn, volume 2, pp. 35.1–35.20. Blackwell Scientific Publications, Oxford.

West, J. D. (1978). Analysis of clonal growth using chimaeras and mosaics. In M. H. Johnson (Ed.) *Development in Mammals*, volume 3, pp. 413–460. North Holland, Amsterdam.

Wild, A. E. and Dawson, P. (1977). Evidence for Fc receptors on rabbit yolk sac endoderm. *Nature*, **268**, 443–445.

Wiley, L. D. (1974). Presence of gonadotrophin on the surface of preimplanted mouse embryos. *Nature*, **252**, 715–716.

Wiley, L. D. and Calarco, P. G. (1975). The effects of anti-embryo sera and their localization on the cell surface during mouse pre-implantation development. *Develop. Biol.*, **47**, 407–418.

Willison, K. R. and Stern, P. L. (1978). Expression of a Forssman antigenic specificity on the preimplantation mouse embryo. *Cell*, **14**, 785–793.

Winzler, R. (1970). Carbohydrates in cell surfaces. *Int. Rev. Cytol.*, **29**, 77–125.

Wolk, M. and Eyat-Giladi, H. (1977). The dynamics of antigenic changes in the epiblast and hypoblast of the chick during the processes of hypoblast, primitive streak and head process formation, as revealed by immunofluorescence. *Develop. Biol.*, **55**, 33–45.

Wood, G. W. and Barth, R. F. (1975). Detection of cell bound immunoglobulins by a radioisotopic micro-mixed hemadsorption reaction with technetium-99m-labelled erythrocytes. *J. Immunol.*, **114**, 944–949.

Yanagisawa, K., Bennett, D., Boyse, E. A., Dunn, L. C., and Dimeo, A. (1974). Serological identification of sperm antigens specified by lethal t-alleles in the mouse. *Immunogenetics*, **1**, 57–67.

Youtananukorn, V. and Matangkasombut, P. (1973). Specific plasma factors blocking human maternal cell mediated immune reaction to placental antigens. *Nature New Biol.*, **242**, 110–111.

Zenges, M. T., Wolf, U., Gunther, E., and Engel, W. (1978). Studies on the function of H-Y antigen: dissociation and re-organisation experiments on rat gonadal tissue. *Cytogenet. Cell Genet.*, **20**, 365–372.,

Zetter, B. R. and Martin, G. R. (1978). Expression of a high molecular weight cell surface glycoprotein (LETS protein) by preimplantation mouse embryos and teratocarcinoma stem cells. *Proc. Natl. Acad. Sci. USA*, **75**, 2324–2328.

Zwaan, J. (1968). Lens specific antigens and cytodifferentiation in the developing lens. *J. Cell Physiol.*, **72** (Suppl 1), 47–72.

Antibody as a Tool
Edited by J. J. Marchalonis and G. W. Warr
© 1982 John Wiley & Sons Ltd.

Chapter 13

Antibodies as Pharmacologic and Medicinal Tools

SAUL B. KADIN

Department of Medicinal Chemistry, Pfizer Central Research, Groton, CT 06340, USA

and

IVAN OTTERNESS

Department of Pharmacology, Pfizer Central Research, Groton, CT 06340, USA

I. INTRODUCTION

The breadth of application of antibodies in the areas of pharmacology and therapeutics has been immense. Passively administered antibodies have been used both prophylactically and therapeutically in infectious diseases, to prevent erythroblastosis foetalis, to prolong allograft survival and in the treatment of neoplastic diseases. As pharmacomimetic agents, antibodies can mimic the action of certain drugs or natural hormones by binding to specific receptors. Anti-drug antibodies can also behave as specific drug antagonists by binding drug and thereby preventing association with specific pharmacologic receptors. Finally, antibodies may be used to carry drugs to specific target tissues. These uses of antibodies have not been limited to laboratory studies since γ-globulins, specific immune sera, anti-Rh globulin, anti-venom antibodies, anti-lymphocyte sera, and anti-drug antibodies have all been employed successfully in the clinic.

Equally important, antibodies have become primary tools in the elucidation of drug mechanisms of action. As the key reagent of radioimmunoassay procedures, antibodies have been used to quantify drug absorption, distribution, and excretion pathways. Radioimmunoassay procedures are outlined in Chapter 6 and a comprehensive list of drugs that have been assayed by this technique has been given by Butler (1977). Antibodies may also be used for histologic localization of drug at specific tissue binding sites. This use is in its infancy and has thus far been applied principally to endogeneous substances

447

such as cyclic GMP (Chan-Palay and Palay, 1979), the enkephalins (Hökfelt *et al.*, 1977; Simantov *et al.*, 1977), and other hormones. Antibodies are of paramount importance in the study of the mechanism of certain disease processes where anti-receptor antibodies appear to play an important role. Examples include acanthosis nigricans and anti-insulin receptor antibody (Flier *et al.*, 1975; Kahn *et al.*, 1976), myasthenia gravis and anti-acetylcholine receptor antibody (Lennon and Carnegie, 1971; Toyka *et al.*, 1975), and Graves disease and anti-thyrotropin receptor antibody (Dorrington and Munro, 1966; Smith *et al.*, 1969). Finally, specific antibodies may be used to elucidate normal physiological mechanisms through the study of their effects upon endogenous hormones such as oestradiol (Ferin *et al.*, 1968, 1969, 1974), gastrin (Lipshutz *et al.*, 1972), renin (Romero *et al.*, 1973), chorionic gonadotrophin (Thanavala *et al.*, 1978; Talwar *et al.*, 1976), and testosterone (Nieschlag and Wickings, 1977).

This chapter will focus on the uses of passively administered antibodies that may favourably affect the course of non-infectious diseases and will concentrate particularly on describing those instances where drugs are directly involved. These include situations where the exquisite specificity of antibodies is used to direct drugs precisely to target tissues and where antibodies are used to reverse the toxic effects of specific drugs. Circumstances where antibodies are used, for example, as immunoregulants are omitted since such topics have been reviewed elsewhere: anti-lymphocyte sera (ALS) (Lance *et al.*, 1973; Russell, 1977), anti-Ia sera (Davies and Staines, 1976), anti-Rh sera (Gorman, 1975; Woodrow, 1974), and anti-idiotypic sera (Geczy *et al.*, 1978).

II. ANTIBODIES AS CARRIERS OF BIOLOGICAL ACTIVITY

A substantial body of information now exists which shows that many autologous tumours are immunogenic and so may be recognized and subsequently destroyed by the host's immune system (Cerottini and Brunner, 1974; Hellström and Hellström, 1974; Herberman, 1974). Evidence for a correlation between prognosis and immune competence in clinical disease has been presented (Hersh *et al.*, 1976). The continued growth of tumours, therefore, often in the presence of cells that are capable of destroying such tumours *in vitro*, remains a perplexing problem. Several possible explanations for such anomalous behaviour include: (a) the existence of serum 'blocking factors' that inhibit cell-mediated tumour cytotoxicity (Currier and Basham, 1972; Sjögren *et al.*, 1971); (b) the demonstration that some oncogenic agents display immunosuppressive qualities which may subvert immunologic responsiveness (Stutman, 1975); (c) the phenomenon of 'sneaking through' by which tumour cells develop beyond some critical stage before detection by the immune system (Klein, 1973); (d) the elaboration by tumour tissue of factors that depress the activity of tumoricidal macrophages (Mahoney and Leighton,

1962; Fauve *et al.*, 1974; Boetcher and Leonard, 1974; Snyderman and Pike, 1977); (e) the active participation by elements of the immune system in promoting tumour growth (Prehn, 1977).

Despite the frequently observed clinical failure of the host to mount an immune response commensurate with the requirements for tumour elimination or to respond predictably to the passive administration of anti-tumour antibodies (Rosenberg and Terry, 1977), tumour tissues are sufficiently immunogenic to have been employed to elicit xenogeneic antibodies, and such antibodies have been used as carriers to localize therapeutic agents specifically at tumour sites. Since the use of most anti-cancer agents is governed by severe constraints that arise from their generally cytotoxic nature, the preparation and utilization of complexes derived from tumour-specific antibodies plus a therapeutic agent can constitute more effective treatment than either of the component parts of the complex in terms of both efficacy and toleration. The mechanisms by which such complexes display synergistic effects have not been fully elucidated, but may be related to the following:

(i) 'homing' effects where the antibody molecule causes the therapeutic agent to localize at a target tissue (Ghose and Nigam, 1972);
(ii) augmentation of the anti-tumour activity of one component of the complex by the other (Davies, 1974; Davies *et al.*, 1974; Segerling *et al.*, 1975; Rubens *et al.*, 1975);
(iii) antibody-facilitated cell penetration for those agents that act intracellularly (Guclu *et al.*, 1975);
(iv) prolongation of drug activity ('depot' effect) due to slow release from or slow degradation of the complex (Szekerke *et al.*, 1972);
(v) increased numbers of cells passing through a drug-sensitive part of the cell cycle as a result of interaction with antibodies (Macpherson, 1974).

Ideally, an immunotherapeutic complex should retain the antigenic specificity of the antibody as well as the intrinsic therapeutic activity of the second component of the complex. Additionally, the physical and chemical forces that bind the complex should be sufficiently firm as to allow dissociation or the expression of biological activity only after the target site is reached. Finally, antibodies with specificities against tissues other than those for which the therapeutic agent is intended should not be present. Adverse reactions such as anaphylaxis and serum sickness may be encountered because of the use of xenogeneic antibodies. Rapid elimination of the complex from the host also may occur if an immune response is elicited against the heterologous antibody.

Drugs that have been used to form immunochemotherapeutic complexes include chlorambucil, *p*-phenylenediamine mustard, triaziquone, daunomycin, adriamycin, and methotrexate (Figure 1). Antibodies also have been used as carriers of toxins, enzymes, radioactivity, and boron.

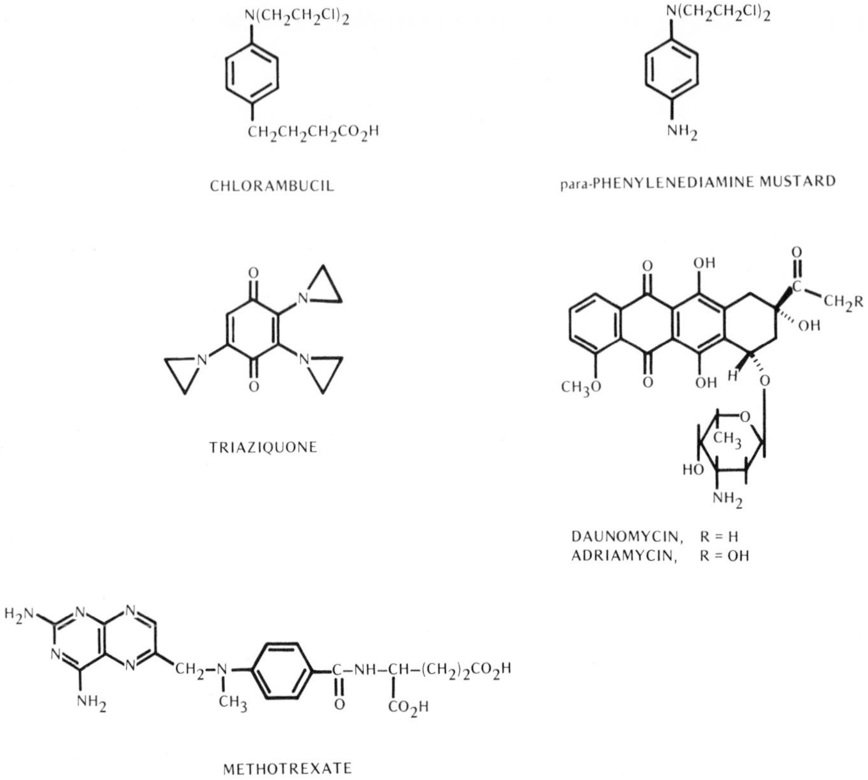

Figure 1. Structures of drugs used in the preparation of drug–antibody complexes

A. Chlorambucil

The drug–antibody complex that has been the subject of the most intense scrutiny is that derived from chlorambucil (Figure 1), a cytotoxic, alkylating agent that reacts with biologically important nucleophiles such as phosphate, amine, sulphydryl, hydroxyl, imidazole, and carboxyl groups. Ghose and Nigam (1972) reported that a non-covalent chlorambucil–goat anti-Ehrlich ascites tumour antibody complex, which was prepared by mixing the immunoglobulin and drug in a ratio of greater than 10 : 1 by weight and which retained both antibody specificity and alkylating activity, was a more effective inhibitor of tumour growth, both *in vitro* and in mice, than either drug or antibody alone. Chlorambucil bound to normal goat γ-globulin was no more effective than drug alone. In a complementary study, Ghose *et al.* (1972) found that a complex consisting of chlorambucil and rabbit anti-EL4 antibodies exhibited greater activity in EL4-challenged mice than did chlorambucil alone, antibody alone, or chlormabucil complexed to normal rabbit globulins. Similar results using chlorambucil and rabbit anti-Ehrlich ascites tumour antibodies were reported shortly thereafter by Flechner (1973). A study in the Novikoff ascites tumour system with chlorambucil and rabbit antibodies demonstrated that this non-covalent complex was far superior to drug or antibody alone or to a complex derived from drug and normal γ-globulin in inhibiting tumour formation and lowering mortality in tumour-challenged rats (Smith *et al.*, 1975).

The exact chemical nature of the non-covalently linked chlorambucil–antibody complexes has not been elucidated. However, chlorambucil is protected from rapid hydrolysis and resultant loss of alkylating activity in the presence of serum of various species, and this is presumably a consequence of the ability of the drug to bind non-specifically to serum proteins (Israels and Linford, 1963). That a reduced rate of degradation can not, however, account entirely for the favourable effects observed using chlorambucil–antibody complexes is evident by the failure of complexes prepared from chlorambucil and normal immunoglobulins to demonstrate enhanced activities.

Davies and O'Neill (1973), following a protocol similar to that described by the Ghose group, also found that a chlorambucil–rabbit anti-EL4 antibody complex afforded protection against EL4-challenged mice that was greater than that provided by either drug or antibody alone. However, these authors could not attribute the heightened effects of the non-covalent complex to a homing mechanism because similarly beneficial effects were obtained when the drug and antibody were administered separately. Their dosing procedure required, moreover, that the drug be administered approximately 1 hour prior to antibody (Davies, 1974; Davies *et al.*, 1974). Data substantiating this thesis were obtained by Rubens and Dulbecco (1974) who studied a complex derived from chlorambucil and immune rabbit serum containing antibodies to polyoma-transformed cells. While the chlorambucil–antibody complex was more effective in inhibiting the cloning efficiency of these cells than was either serum or drug alone, the separate addition of drug and immune serum to the tissue culture afforded growth inhibition equal to that observed for the complex. Further support for the concept that the cytotoxic activity of chlorambucil and antibodies used in tandem was equivalent at least to that of a drug–antibody complex was found in a system using cultured human melanoma cells (Vennegoor *et al.*, 1975).

The apparent discrepancies between these sets of results, one requiring the use of pre-formed complexes for the expression of optimal anti-tumour activity and the other requiring the administration merely of the constituents of the complexes, have not been resolved. Using an AKR mouse lymphoma model, Ghose *et al.* (1975a) reported that the use of a chlorambucil–anti-tumour immunoglobulin complex was associated with significantly greater survival rates than those observed following the separate administration of equivalent amounts of chlorambucil and antibody. The Davies group compared the *in vitro* cytotoxic activity displayed by chlorambucil-antibody complexes pre-pared at pH 3.5 and pH 8 with that obtained using the components of the complex (O'Neill *et al.*, 1975). They found that the successive addition of drug and antibody afforded cytotoxic effects greater than that provided by either of the complexes. Moreover, the complex prepared at acidic pH, for which a preparative method similar to one subsequently described by Guclu *et al.* (1976) was utlized, lacked immunologic specificity, suggesting that this drug–antibody complex had dissociated under the experimental conditions. The complex prepared at alkaline pH exhibited diminished cytotoxicity, probably as a result of loss of alkylating activity of chlorambucil at the pH used for complex formation, but retained immunologic specificity, indicating that the pH 8 complex was stable.

Several other groups of investigators have studied the nature of chlorambu-cil–protein interactions, but none appears to have examined complexes prepared under strongly acidic conditions (Guclu *et al.*, 1976). Hopwood and Stock (1971) reported that the rate of hydrolysis of chlorambucil is retarded in the presence of bovine γ-globulin. Ross (1974) obtained similar results using human γ-globulin and showed, furthermore, that most of the protein-bound chlorambucil arose from alkylation. In contrast, substantial non-covalent binding of chlorambucil to rabbit immunoglobulin G was reported by Blakeslee and Kennedy (1974). They later showed that chlorambucil forms a high molecular weight aggregate under the experimental conditions used for complex formation. The aggregate has a molecular weight greater than 200,000, retains alkylating activity and is much more resistant to hydrolysis than non-aggregated chlorambucil (Blakeslee *et al.*, 1975). Consequently, the presence of aggregated, non-dialysable chlorambucil may have led to divergent estimates concerning the degree to which chlorambucil is non-covalently bound to antibodies.

Several clinical studies have been conducted using chlorambucil–antibody complexes. A single patient with malignant melanoma was treated with chlorambucil bound to goat anti-melanoma antibodies (Ghose *et al.*, 1972). The complex was injected both intravenously and directly into metastatic nodules and, after 2 weeks of treatment, regression of metastatic nodules was noted. No adverse reactions or complications were observed. Another study in a single patient was associated with beneficial effects, but had to be discontinued because of the appearance of an anaphylactic reaction (Ghose *et al.*, 1975c). Suggestions of anti-tumour activity in the treatment of melanoma and neuroblastoma were found using chlorambucil bound to human γ-globu-lin, but no control values were reported (Oon *et al.*, 1974). Four patients with widespread metastatic melanoma were treated for several weeks to several months with separate injections of chlorambucil and goat anti-melanoma antibodies (Everall *et al.*, 1977). Side effects, other than those associated with the cytotoxic drug, were not observed. Although the trial did not include controls the patients were reported to survive beyond the expected median survival time based on historical results. A more extensive and detailed study of the effects of a chlorambucil–antibody complex in the treatment of malignant melanoma was described by Ghose *et al.* (1977) who found that 7 of 13 patients had objective responses or stabilized disease following treatment with this immunochemotherapeutic regimen whereas none of 11 patients treated with DTIC, 5-(3,3-dimethyl-1-triazenyl)-imidazole-4-carboxamide, showed objective tumour regression. Significantly prolonged survival times were also observed for the drug–antibody complex treated group compared to the DTIC group. Two patients receiving the drug-antibody complex developed anaphylactic reactions.

In related experiments, the use of a complex prepared from chlorambucil and anti-lymphocyte globulin led to marked delays in rejection times of skin and heart allografts in rats (Papachristou *et al.*, 1977). The drug–antibody complex afforded results superior to those obtained by the separate administration of the components of the complex although the latter protocol proved superior to those in which only drug or antibody was utilized.

The meaningful accomplishments associated with the use of chlorambucil–tumour specific antibody complexes, both in the laboratory and clinic, have been clouded by the lack of adequate chemical characterization of the complexes and by conflicting reports concerning the demonstration of equivalent biological activities following administration of the individual components of the complexes. Continued efforts to explore the nature of the physicochemical forces that maintain the complexes, particuarly as they are affected by various experimental procedures, will be necessary to reconcile the discordant observations. Likewise, the methodologies used for preparing the complexes and the protocols by which they are subsequently evaluated will need to be standardized so that results emanating from different laboratories can be equitably compared.

B. *p*-Phenylenediamine Mustard

p-Phenylenediamine mustard or *N,N-bis*-(2-chloroethyl)-*p*-phenylenediamine (Figure 1) is, like chlorambucil, an alkylating agent. However, in contrast to the latter substance, *p*-phenylenediamine mustard has been linked covalently, through the interposition of spacer molecules, to rabbit anti-EL4 lymphoma antibodies (Rowland *et al.*, 1975; Rowland, 1977). This approach was utilized in order to synthesize complexes that contained relatively high drug to antibody ratios while avoiding the problems of reduced antibody specificity and diminished aqueous solubility which often accompany efforts to prepare heavily substituted antibodies.

Employing 1-dimethylaminopropyl-3-ethylcarbodiimide (Table 1) as the coupling agent, *p*-phenylenediamine mustard was first linked, via an amide bond, to polyglutamic acid in a 45 to 1 molar ratio. Subsequent covalent

Table 1. Some reagents used to link antibodies to drugs, toxins, and enzymes, and types of chemical functionalities formed

Reagent	Formula	New functionality formed
1-Dimethylamino-propyl-3-ethyl-carbodiimide	$(CH_3)_2N(CH_2)_3N=C=NC_2H_5$	Amide
Dithiothreitol	$HSCH_2CHOHCHOHCH_2SH$	Thioether
Glutaraldehyde	$OHC(CH_2)_3CHO$	Imine
Nitrous acid	HNO_2	Azo
Toluene diisocyanate	$H_3C-\langle\quad\rangle-NCO$ NCO	Ureide
Diethyl malonimidate	$C_2H_5O-C-CH_2-C-OC_2H_5$ $\quad\ \ \|\|\qquad\quad\|\|$ $\quad\ \ NH\qquad\ \ NH$	Amidine

attachment of the drug–polyglutamic acid intermediate to the anti-EL4 immunoglobulin also was achieved using the water-soluble diimide reagent. Thus, the carboxylic acid groups of polyglutamic acid served as points of attachment for both drug and antibody. Administration of the covalently linked, three-component complex to mice challenged with approximately 10,000 times the LD_{50} of EL4 cells led to a median survival time of greater than 100 days. In contrast, mice given antibody alone or the drug–polyglutamic acid intermediate complex alone exhibited median survival times only slightly greater than those observed following saline treatment (13 days). The use of the intermediate complex plus specific antibody afforded results that were not as good as those obtained with the covalently linked tripartite complex (38 days versus more than 100 days median survival times), suggesting that the latter may be functioning through a true homing mechanism (Rowland *et al.*, 1975).

A similar study, in which the survival times of mice challenged with EL4 cells were compared following treatment either with *p*-phenylenediamine mustard covalently linked to antibody through dextran, a water-soluble glucose polymer, or with the drug–dextran complex plus antibody, showed that the fully covalently linked complex displayed significantly superior effects, again suggesting that a homing mechanism was operative (Rowland, 1977).

C. Triaziquone

Triaziquone, 2,3,5-tris(aziridino)-1,4-benzoquinone (Figure 1), is a cytotoxic agent containing aziridine groups that are capable of alkylating tissue nucleophiles. The quinone moiety can also interact with cysteine and other thiols to afford thioether derivatives of aziridine-substituted hydroquinones which retain alkylating activity (Linford, 1973). When triaziquone was linked covalently to dithiothreitol (Table 1) -treated rabbit antibodies that had been elicited against a methylcholanthrene-induced guinea pig sarcoma, the resulting complex, which was estimated to contain 5 moles of triaziquone per mole of antibody, displayed greater activity against monolayers of sarcoma cells than did drug alone, antibody alone or the same complex that had first been absorbed with sarcoma cells (Linford *et al.*, 1974). Although triaziquone formed cytotoxic conjugates with non-immune γ-globulin, such covalent complexes were much less active than conjugates prepared using immunospecific globulins (Linford and Froese, 1978).

Skin allograft survival times in mice were prolonged significantly following treatment with mixtures of triaziquone and rabbit anti-mouse thymocyte globulin. A covalently linked complex of drug and anti-thymocyte globulin, while yielding results superior to those obtained using saline, was not as effective as the drug–antibody mixture (Beatty *et al.*, 1978). The reasons for the failure of the covalently linked conjugate to demonstrate results superior to those of the drug–antibody mixture are not clear, but may be related to the small number of triaziquone molecules incorporated into the complex or to the restricted access of the complex to only those cells carrying thymocyte antigens.

D. Daunomycin and Adriamycin

Daunomycin (daunorubicin) and adriamycin (doxorubicin) are chemically related natural products (Figure 1) that are clinically effective anti-tumour agents (Tan *et al.*, 1967; O'Bryan *et al.*, 1973). Each consists of a substituted anthraquinone moiety in glycosidic linkage to the amino sugar, daunosamine. Following incorporation into drug–antibody conjugates, both drugs showed retention of pharmacologic activity (Hurwitz *et al.*, 1975).

Covalent attachment of daunomycin to rabbit anti-mouse B-cell leukaemia antibodies was carried out in three different ways in order to study the effects on biologic activity of various types of drug–antibody combinations (Hurwitz *et al.*, 1975). In the first example, periodate oxidation of daunomycin, which cleaves the bond between the amino- and hydroxyl-bearing carbon atoms of the sugar moiety, generated a carbonyl function containing intermediate that was allowed to react with the amino substituents of the antibody, and the imine groups thus formed were reduced by sodium borohydride. A second method used for covalently joining the drug and antibody utilized glutaraldehyde (Table 1) to link the amino groups of the respective components of the complex. Finally, 1-dimethylaminopropyl-3-ethylcarbodiimide was used to forge an amide functionality between the amino substituent of the drug and a carboxylic acid group of the antibody.

The most cytotoxic complex, as measured by inhibition of cellular RNA synthesis, was that prepared using glutaraldehyde, but this may have been due to the liberation of free daunomycin as a consequence of the aqueous lability of this conjugate. The antibody activity of the complex made with glutaraldehyde was, however, markedly diminished. In evaluating the capacity of the different complexes to retain both drug and antibody effects, that complex prepared using the periodate–sodium borohydride method demonstrated optimal activity (Hurwitz *et al.*, 1975).

Additional studies with complexes prepared from daunomycin and antibodies directed against either mouse B-cell leukaemia or PC5 plasmacytoma showed that each conjugate displayed preferential cytotoxicity against those target cells which the antibodies were capable of recognizing. Daunomycin linked to rabbit anti-bovine serum albumin antibodies exhibited little or no activity against either tumour type (Levy *et al.*, 1975).

The importance of the Fc fragment of the antibody molecule to the manifestation of *in vitro* cytotoxic activity by the complex was examined by preparing covalent conjugates of daunomycin and (Fab')$_2$ fragments derived from antibodies elicited against bovine serum albumin and YAC lymphoma cells (Hurwitz *et al.*, 1976). The drug–anti-YAC (Fab')$_2$ complex displayed greater anti-YAC cytotoxicity than did free daunomycin or the complex prepared from the (Fab')$_2$ fragments of anti-bovine serum albumin antibodies. The use of (Fab')$_2$ fragments may have important *in vivo* consequences since the functional activity of the antibody component of the complex will more nearly resemble that of a pure carrier in the absence of the complement activating Fc fragment. In addition, a complex lacking the Fc fragment, which contains the major species-specific determinants, should elicit fewer anaphylactic reactions following multiple courses of therapy.

A comparison of the beneficial effects afforded by daunomycin alone and by daunomycin covalently linked to specific as well as non-specific antibodies was carried out by measuring increased lifespan and survival rates in mice challenged with PC5 plasmacytoma tumour cells (Hurwitz *et al.*, 1978). While the drug–anti-PC5 plasmacytoma antibody complex furnished results better than those obtained with control animals or animals treated with daunomycin linked to irrelevant antibodies, it was not superior to daunomycin alone and was less effective than a mixture of daunomycin and specific antibodies. Augmented therapeutic effects obtained with mixtures of drugs and specific antibodies have been described previously (Davies, 1974; Davies *et al.*, 1974; Rubens *et al.*, 1975; Segerling *et al.*, 1975), but it is not known whether a further improvement in benefits could be obtained if daunomycin were administered prior to antibody (Davies and O'Neill, 1973; Davies, 1974; Davies *et al.*, 1974).

The concentration of daunomycin within the drug–antibody complex was increased by using dextran as an intermolecular bridge (Hurwitz *et al.*, 1978). Periodate-mediated oxidation of dextran afforded a polyaldehyde derivative that was allowed to interact first with daunomycin and then with anti-YAC lymphoma antibodies, and the resulting imine linkages were reduced with sodium borohydride. The daunomycin–dextran–anti-YAC antibody complex was superior to daunomycin alone in increasing survival rates of YAC-challenged mice, but was no better, at high doses, than a drug–dextran complex or a drug–dextran–normal immunoglobulin conjugate. At low doses, however, the daunomycin–dextran–specific antibody complex displayed more favourable effects than did the conjugate prepared using normal immunoglobulins, suggesting selective concentration of drug at tumour sites.

E. Methotrexate

Methotrexate (Figure 1), an inhibitor of dihydrofolate reductase, was covalently coupled, through the use of nitrous acid (Table 1), to hamster antibodies raised against mouse L1210 cells (Mathe *et al.*, 1958). The drug–antibody complex, when compared to methotrexate alone, specific antibodies alone, methotrexate plus specific antibodies or methotrexate coupled to normal immunoglobulins, demonstrated significant advantages in increasing survival rates in L1210-challenged mice. An analogous study, in which methotrexate was linked, also via a diazotization reaction, to rabbit anti-human reticulum cell sarcoma antibodies, showed that the drug–antibody complex retained immunologic specificity *in vitro* (Calendi *et al.*, 1969). Closer inspection of the chemistry involved in the diazotization of methotrexate revealed, however, the occurrence of several competing reaction sequences that yield, depending upon reaction conditions, up to 14 products (Robinson *et al.*, 1973). Therefore, without further substantial chemical characterization of the methotrexate–antibody complexes used in earlier studies (Mathe *et al.*, 1958; Calendi *et al.*, 1969), it would appear difficult to assess with certainty the importance of the results obtained.

When methotrexate was conjugated to rabbit anti-L1210 antibodies through the carbodiimide-promoted formation of an amide link, the resulting complex displayed substantially greater activity than mixtures of methotrexate and antibodies in increasing the survival times of L1210-challenged mice (Robinson *et al.*, 1973).

F. Toxins and Enzymes

Diphtheria toxin is an extraordinarily toxic protein of molecular weight *c.* 62,000 which acts by inhibiting protein synthesis through the inactivation of a polypeptide chain elongation factor (Collier, 1967; Honjo *et al.*, 1968; Baseman *et al.*, 1970). It has been estimated that fewer than ten molecules of the enzymatically active Fragment A of the toxin may be all that is required to kill a cell (Gill *et al.*, 1973).

These properties of diphtheria toxin were exploited by showing that conjugates of toxin and guinea pig anti-mumps virus antibodies, covalently linked by means of toluene diisocyanate (Table 1) which forms ureido linkages with the amino substituents of each reactant, exhibited much greater activity in lysing mumps-infected rhesus monkey kidney cells than did antibodies alone (Moolten and Cooperband, 1970). The selectivity of the conjugate for mumps infected, in contrast to uninfected, cells was demonstrated by the low level of activity expressed by the conjugate against the latter. Unfortunately, this series of experiments did not measure the cytotoxic effects of simple mixtures of toxin and antibodies. In an analogous manner, the use of diethyl malonimidate (Table 1), which reacts readily with amino groups to form amidine functions, afforded a covalently-linked complex consisting of diphtheria toxin and rabbit anti-trinitrophenyl (TNP) antibodies. This complex displayed significantly greater cytotoxicity against TNP-substituted HeLa cells than it did against unmodified HeLa cells (Philpott *et al.*, 1973a). Additional evidence for the selective cytotoxicity of the toxin–antibody complex was obtained by showing that the presence of a hapten, ε-dinitrophenyl (DNP)-lysine, inhibited the activity of the conjugate. Diphtheria toxin alone was non-selective, being equally toxic to both TNP-HeLa cells and HeLa cells.

When the effects of a diphtheria–toxin anti-DNP antibody conjugate, which was prepared using glutaraldehyde as the linking agent, were examined in hamsters challenged with DNP-modified hamster sarcoma cells it was found that the complex was effective in delaying the appearance of tumours and prolonging the lifespan of the animals (Moolten *et al.*, 1972). Moreover, the covalently bound conjugate was found to be more effective than a simple mixture consisting of toxin and anti-DNP antibodies. Hamsters challenged with simian virus-40-transformed sarcoma cells showed a reduction in tumour incidence and prolongation of lifespan following administration of single doses of diphtheria toxin–anti-sarcoma antibody conjugates that had been linked covalently using glutaraldehyde (Moolten *et al.*, 1975). Despite the administration of repeated doses, however, established sarcomas continued to progress. In contrast, established lymphomas in hamsters did regress following weekly treatment with toxin–antibody conjugate, suggesting that differences in susceptibility to the complex may exist among various tumours. The separate administration of toxin and specific antibodies at different subcutaneous sites in hamsters bearing established lymphomas afforded results similar to those seen in untreated control animals.

The possibility that diphtheria toxin–antibody conjugates that had been prepared using glutaraldehyde demonstrated less than optimal cytotoxic activity as a result of intramolecular cross-linking of the chains of the toxin molecule led to the use of a novel method for the synthesis of such complexes (Thorpe *et al.*, 1978). The reaction of chlorambucil with triethylamine and butyl chloroformate generated a mixed anhydride which, following nucleophi-

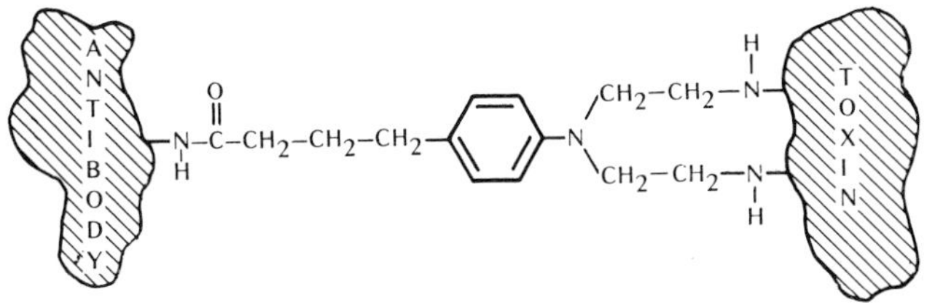

Figure 2. Schematic representation of a toxin–antibody complex prepared using chlorambucil as the linking agent

lic attack by the amino substituents of horse anti-human lymphocyte globulin, provided a chlorambucil–antibody covalent complex connected via an amide group. Subsequent interaction of this complex with diphtheria toxin resulted in alkylation of the toxin. Thus, the reactive sites of chlorambucil served to bridge the toxin and antibody molecules (Figure 2). When tested against a human lymphoblastoid line the conjugate exhibited activity 1000-fold that of equivalent concentrations of diphtheria toxin alone. Mixtures of toxin and specific antibody displayed activity that was no greater than that of the toxin alone, suggesting that a homing mechanism rather than an augmentation effect was responsible for the activity of the conjugate.

The report that enzymes coupled to antibodies afforded conjugates that retained both immunologic and enzymatic activities was instrumental in the later development of enzyme–antibody conjugates designed to demonstrate anti-tumour cytotoxic activities (Avrameas, 1969). Diethyl malonimidate was used to furnish a covalently linked conjugate composed of glucose oxidase and anti-TNP antibodies which, in the presence of lactoperoxidase and potassium iodide, destroyed TNP-substituted HeLa and Hep-2 tumour cells (Philpott *et al.*, 1973b; Philpott *et al.*, 1973c). The biochemical rationale of this cytotoxic reaction is based on the generation of hydrogen peroxide as a result of the oxidation of cellular glucose by the tissue-targeted glucose oxidase. Lactoperoxidase, in the presence of iodide ion and the newly formed hydrogen peroxide, catalyses the iodination of cellular constituents, thereby causing cell death. The presence of each component of the toxic triad, the enzyme–antibody conjugate, lactoperoxidase and potassium iodide, was necessary for the manifestation of cytotoxic activity. Selectivity was demonstrated by showing the ability of a hapten, ε-DNP-lysine, to block the reaction and by the failure to observe cytotoxicity against non-hapten-substituted HeLa and Hep-2 cells at concentrations where TNP-substituted cells were readily killed. Similar results were obtained when a combination of a glucose oxidase–anti-TNP antibody conjugate, horseradish peroxidase and arsphenamine, in which cytotoxicity is probably ultimately effected by an oxidized derivative of arsphenamine, was used to kill TNP-substituted HeLa and Hep-2 cells (Philpott *et al.*, 1974). A study in which glucose oxidase was coupled to antibodies elicited against a human colonic cancer line and against carcinoembryonic antigen, a specific marker for entodermally-derived digestive tract tumours (Gold and Freedman, 1966), showed that such enzyme–antibody conjugates, in the presence of lactoperoxidase and iodide ion, were significantly more cytotoxic to colonic tumour cells than were similar complexes prepared from normal immunoglobulins (Shearer *et al.*, 1974).

A unique approach to the design of enzyme–antibody conjugates exhibiting anti-tumour activity involved the covalent linkage of alcohol dehydrogenase and anti-TNP antibodies (Philpott *et al.*, 1979). Following incubation with a mixture of this conjugate, nicotinamide adenine dinucleotide and allyl alcohol, which together constitute a system designed to generate acrolein, the highly toxic oxidation product of allyl alcohol, a greater degree of killing was observed with TNP-substituted than with unsubstituted Hep-2 tumour cells. As with previously described model systems, the presence of a hapten suppressed the expression of cytotoxicity. Treatment of TNP-Hep-2 cells with a non-covalently linked mixture of alcohol dehydrogenase and anti-TNP antibodies, together with the other factors required for the formation of acrolein, failed to demonstrate significant cytotoxicity, indicating the probable importance of the antibody in directing the enzyme to specific target sites.

A covalent complex prepared from glutaraldehyde, phospholipase C, and antibodies raised against Friend leukaemia was significantly more cytotoxic to leukaemic spleen cells than to normal spleen cells derived from the same strain of mice (Flickinger and Trost, 1976).

G. Radioactivity

The use of antibodies as carriers of anti-tumour activity began with the work of Pressman's group who found that specific antibodies labelled with ^{131}I retained immunologic specificity (Pressman and Keighley, 1948), although later work showed that antibodies heavily substituted with iodine lost activity (Johnson *et al.*, 1960). Following administration to tumour-bearing animals of radioactive iodine that had first been allowed to react with specific anti-tumour antibodies, localization of radiolabel was found to occur largely, but not exclusively, in tumour tissue (Pressman and Korngold, 1953; Bale *et al.*, 1955). However, extensive absorption of the radiolabelled complex with normal tissues led to improved selectivity (Day *et al.*, 1956).

As a result of the finding that antibodies raised against some tumour antigens cross-reacted with fibrinogen (Day *et al.*, 1959), efforts were initiated to treat experimental tumours with ^{131}I-labelled anti-fibrin antibodies (Day *et al.*, 1959; Spar *et al.*, 1959; Bale *et al.*, 1960), the principle for this mode of treatment being the increase in fibrin deposition often observed at tumour sites, possibly as a consequence of an inflammatory reaction. Unfortunately, this type of therapeutic regimen was found to have limited effectiveness (Spar *et al.*, 1960; Day *et al.*, 1960), and a clinical trial using ^{131}I-labelled rabbit anti-human fibrinogen antibodies in the treatment of 172 cancer patients was not successful (Spar *et al.*, 1967).

Radioiodinated rabbit antibodies elicited against a human glioma were found to bind preferentially to the glioma following intravenous administration (Day *et al.*, 1965; Mahaley *et al.*, 1965). Mice inoculated with Ehrlich ascites cells that had been incubated with ^{131}I-labelled rabbit anti-Ehrlich ascites cell antibodies failed to develop tumours in contrast to mice that were inoculated with cells that had been treated with non-iodinated antibodies or with ^{131}I-labelled normal immunoglobulins (Ghose *et al.*, 1967). A comparison of radiolabelled specific and non-specific immunoglobulins showed that only the former localized at homologous tumour sites (Izzo *et al.*, 1972). Preferential localization of radioiodinated specific antibodies was also observed using rabbit antibodies that had been elicited against rat mammary tumours (Kellen and Lo, 1973), and with antibodies raised against a microsome fraction of a hamster malignant melanoma (Smith and Gökcen, 1974). An example of the failure of radioiodinated antibodies to localize extensively at a specific tumour site *in vivo* occurred using rabbit anti-mouse myeloma protein antibodies, injection of which resulted in significant interactions with normal γ-globulin and with circulating myeloma proteins (Reif, 1971).

When heterologous antibodies elicited against mouse EL4 lymphoma were iodinated with ^{131}I and then administered to EL4-challenged mice partial or complete tumour suppression was obtained, depending upon the quantity of labelled antibody utilized (Ghose and Guclu, 1974; Ghose *et al.*, 1975b). Neither antibody alone nor radioiodinated normal immunoglobulins produced beneficial effects. Two of four tumour-bearing individuals, following treatment with ^{131}I-labelled specific antibodies, appeared to concentrate the radioactive complex in metastatic tissues (Ghose *et al.*, 1975b). After goat antibodies against carcinoembryonic antigen (CEA) were labelled with ^{125}I and injected into hamsters bearing CEA-producing tumours preferential uptake of iodinated antibodies was found to occur in tumour tissue (Goldenberg *et al.*, 1974). In a comparable clinical situation, however, no evidence was found for localization of ^{131}I-labelled anti-CEA antibodies, possibly because a high level of circulating CEA prevented the antibodies from reaching metastatic sites (Reif *et al.*, 1974).

H. Boron

Bombardment of boron with slow neutrons leads to the following reaction:

$$^{10}_{5}B + ^{1}_{0}n \rightarrow ^{7}_{3}Li + ^{4}_{2}He$$

The nuclear fragments liberated during the fission process are of considerably higher energy than the incident neutrons and, furthermore, dissipate their

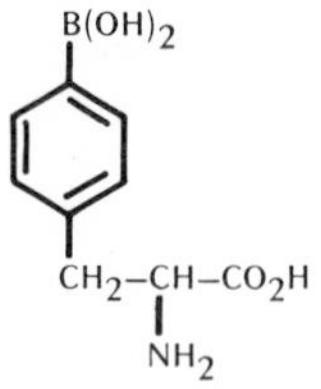

D,L-4-BORONOPHENYLALANINE 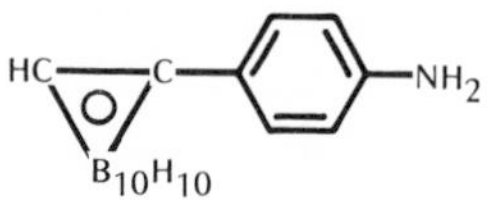   1-(4-AMINOPHENYL)-1,2-DICARBA-*closo*-
                                        DODECABORANE

Figure 3. Structures of boron-containing compounds that have been covalently linked
to antibodies

energy over short distances, making boron fission an attractive procedure for destroying tumours while minimizing toxicity to normal tissues (Kruger, 1940). In fact, early studies indicated the potential utility of this therapeutic approach by showing that irradiation of boron-containing tumours in mice could lead to tumour regression (Kruger, 1940; Zahl *et al.*, 1940). The challenge of preferentially localizing boron in tumour tissue appeared, therefore, to be particularly well suited to the use of antibodies as carriers or homing agents.

The feasibility of employing boron containing amino acid derivatives to prepare boron–antibody conjugates was demonstrated by the successful coupling of D,L-4-boronophenylalanine (Figure 3) to bovine γ-globulin (Mallinger *et al.*, 1972). Incorporation of boron into antibodies raised against two different antigens was also accomplished by the diazotization process using 1-(4-aminophenyl)-1,2-dicarba-*closo*-dodecaborane (Figure 3) as the boron-containing species (Hawthorne *et al.*, 1972). When coupled to rabbit anti-bovine serum albumin antibodies, the boron-containing conjugate retained most of the precipitating activity of the unmodified antibody. Following covalent attachment to antibodies directed against human histocompatibility antigens, the resulting boron–antibody conjugate, after neutron radiation, displayed significant cytotoxicity against human lymphocytes.

Attempts to enhance biological activity by incorporating greater amounts of boron per antibody molecule without diminishing the aqueous solubility of the newly formed conjugate led to the preparation of numerous boron derivatives exhibiting polar functional groups (Wong *et al.*, 1974; Tolpin *et al.*, 1974). Although increased levels of boron binding were achieved the extent of such conjugation was not considered sufficient to mediate tumour cell distruction *in vivo* (Sneath *et al.*, 1974). Recently, boron-containing reactive intermediates that also display gluconamide groups were found to react with human γ-globulin to provide conjugates that not only incorporated high levels of boron but also exhibited good aqueous solubility (Sneath *et al.*, 1976).

III. ANTIBODY REVERSAL OF DRUG EFFECTS

The principles by which the elicitation of antibodies to low molecular weight organic substances such as drugs is accomplished were established by Landsteiner (1945). He demonstrated that an antibody response to small molecules could be successfully elicited if such molecules were first coupled to carrier proteins. The development of the radioimmunoassay procedure by Yalow and Berson (1959, 1960) has led to the routine elicitation of antibodies to drugs in order to measure their concentration and tissue localization (Butler, 1977). The systematic utilization of antibodies to reverse the effects of drugs is of more recent occurrence but its development was foreshadowed by work on the neutralization of the activity of endogenous hormones by either active immunization or passively administered antibodies (Clutton *et al.*, 1938; Lieberman *et al.*, 1959).

Ideally, the development of antibodies capable of reversing drug action *in vivo* should proceed through several well defined steps. First, anti–drug antibody of suitable affinity and specificity must be elicited. This can usually be accomplished by utilizing immunization techniques like those developed for radioimmunoassay. It is a relatively simple matter to determine the affinity constant of drug and antibody (Chapter 4). The greater the affinity constant of drug and antibody compared with that of drug and receptor, the more effectively will antibody compete for drug with the pharmacologically active receptor. Specificity is not ordinarily a problem unless there exists a natural pharmacophor displaying structural similarity to the drug. Second, having shown that antibody will strongly bind drug, it is also important to show that antibody will antagonize the biological activity of drug both *in vitro* and *in vivo*. The former, of course, depends upon the presence of suitable tissue preparations whereas the latter requires whole animal studies. Antibody must be administered after the development of an adequate pharmacologic or toxic response to prove that a true reversal has occurred; it is insufficient to demonstrate that the administration of admixed antibody and drug has less effect than drug alone. Reversal is, therefore, the important laboratory demonstration of potential clinical utility. The relationship between antibody dose and efficacy can subsequently be established in animals, and a clinical sample prepared using purified, unaggregated and pyrogen free antibody. After suitable safety studies the preparation may be considered ready for human trials. Obviously, frequent administration of xenogeneic antibodies may lead to serum sickness and anaphylaxis. Thus, the clinical applications of anti-drug antibody have focused on the treatment of drug toxicity since reversal usually requires but a single administration of antibody. Only in the case of the

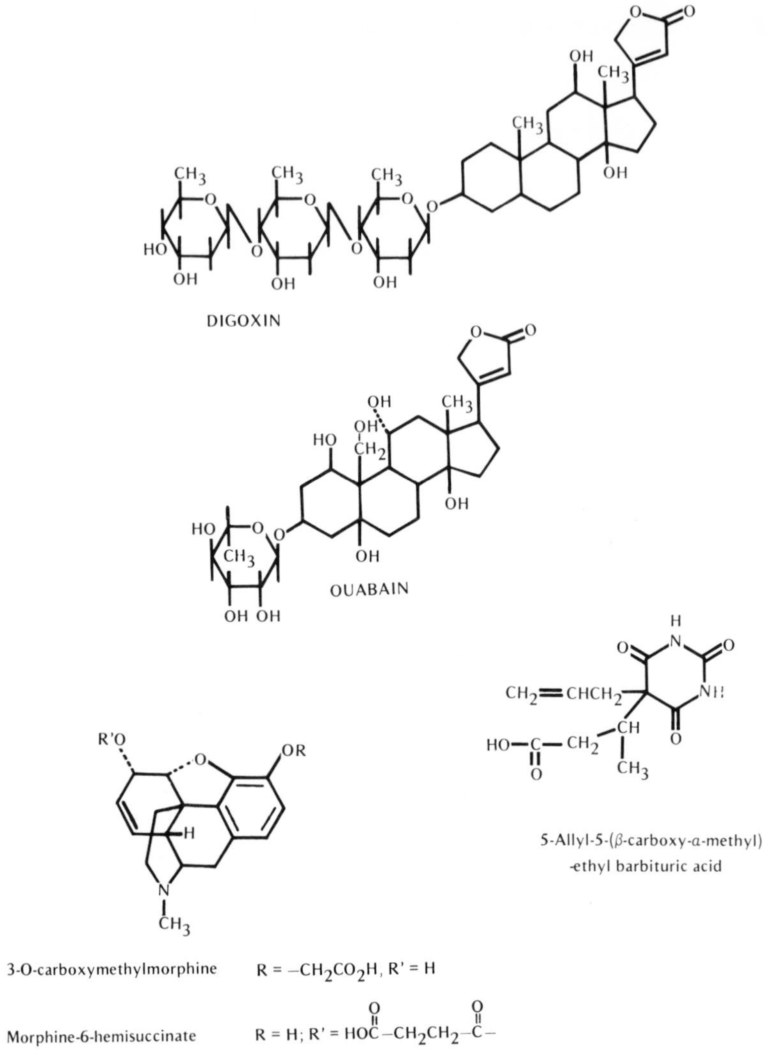

DIGOXIN

OUABAIN

5-Allyl-5-(β-carboxy-α-methyl)
-ethyl barbituric acid

3-O-carboxymethylmorphine   R = $-CH_2CO_2H$, R' = H

Morphine-6-hemisuccinate   R = H; R' = $HOC-CH_2CH_2-C-$

Figure 4. Structures of drugs and haptens that have been used in toxicity reversal studies

cardiac glycosides have both *in vitro* and *in vivo* studies of antibody reversal of drug effects been carried out fully and clinical efficacy established in man.

A. Digoxin

Antibody reversal of the effects of digoxin has been reviewed by Butler *et al.* (1973, 1977a) and by Smith *et al.* (1977). Digoxin (Figure 4), which is a cardiac stimulant consisting of the digoxigenin aglycone linked to three digitoxose sugar moieties, is not sufficiently immunogenic to elicit antibodies by direct immunization. Therefore, Butler and Chen (1967) coupled digoxin to bovine serum albumin (BSA) to prepare a suitable immunogen. The terminal sugar of digoxin was cleaved to the corresponding dialdehyde by sodium metaperiodate, and the excess metaperiodate consumed using ethylene glycol. The dialdehyde functions were allowed to react with the lysyl ε-amino groups of the carrier molecule to form an imine which was reduced by sodium borohydride. Immunization with the conjugate led, after several months, to the production of antibodies with affinity constants of the order of $10^{10} M^{-1}$ (Smith *et al.*, 1970). Although the aglycone of digoxin may be considered a steroid-like structure, the antibody exhibited no significant cross-reactivity in ligand displacement reactions with a number of naturally occurring steroids (Smith *et al.*, 1969, 1970). This is not unexpected since digitoxin, which like the steroids lacks a hydroxyl group at position 12 of the cardenolide structure, shows a 40–50-fold lower affinity for anti-digoxin antibodies than digoxin.

The effects of antibodies on digoxin binding to erythrocytes is particularly informative and appears to have general applicability to the mechanism of antibody reversal of drug effects. Gardner *et al.* (1973) considered the erythrocyte-associated digoxin to be in two compartments: intracellular (unbound) and bound to specific membrane receptor. Addition of antibody to the digoxin-laden erythrocytes led to rapid (within minutes) clearance of intracellular digoxin. Removal of membrane-bound digoxin, however, was much slower and remained incomplete after 5 hours. Since a similarly slow rate of loss of specifically bound digoxin occurred in the presence of a large excess of ouabain, a competitive cardiac glycoside, it was concluded that the rate limiting step in this process was the dissociation of bound digoxin from specific receptor. Kuschinsky *et al.* (1968) obtained similar results using cardiac tissue. This indicates that antibodies can serve as a 'sink' to bind free drug and so prevent the reassociation of drug with its specific receptor. The rate at which a drug effect is reversed, however, cannot be faster than the rate of dissociation of drug from receptor and *in vivo* it may be even slower. For example, if a drug is highly lipophilic and partitions only poorly into plasma where it can interact with antibody, the rate of reversal of the drug effect could be much slower than that of receptor dissociation.

Specific antibodies raised against digoxin were shown to reverse a number of digoxin effects *in vitro*. Antibodies antagonized the digoxin-induced increases in tension development of guinea pig atrial strips (Curd *et al.*, 1971). Antibodies reversed a number of toxic electrophysiological effects of digoxin on isolated Purkinje fibres (Mandel *et al.*, 1972). Finally, antibodies counteracted the digoxin-mediated decrease in potassium transport in erythrocytes at a rate equivalent to the loss of membrane-bound, but not intracellular, digoxin (Gardner *et al.*, 1973).

Specific antibodies were shown to reverse the effects of digoxin in digoxin-intoxicated dogs (Schmidt and Butler, 1971). Seventeen dogs were administered 0.09 mg/kg of digoxin daily for 3 days, and all developed toxic arrhythmias within 3 hours of the last dose. While all control animals died within 48 hours, each of 8 dogs treated with digoxin-specific antibodies survived with the majority reverting to normal sinus rhythm within 3 hours of antibody administration (Schmidt and Butler, 1971).

The fate of antibody-bound drug is important in the *sequela* of the reversal phenomenon. The work of Schmidt *et al.* (1974) in actively immunized animals showed that the half-life of digoxin increased from a mean 3.4 days (controls) to 9.4 days (immunized with BSA only) to a mean of 72 days in digoxin-immunized dogs. Moreover, plasma levels were almost 100-fold higher in the specifically immunized animals. Digoxin was readily detectable in the sera of immunized animals 1 year later. Since autologous γ-globulin (Spiegelberg and Weigle, 1965; Waldman and Strober, 1969; Schmidt *et al.*, 1974) is eliminated from rabbits with a half-life of 4–8 days, these results suggest that as antibody which has bound digoxin is metabolized, digoxin is released into the plasma where it is available for reassociation with other digoxin antibodies or the digoxin receptor. Confirming these findings, Schmidt *et al.* (1974) found no significant differences in the half-life of autologous anti-digoxin antibody and control γ-globulin. Butler (1970) suggested, therefore, that Fab fragments of antibodies should be used in place of whole antibody molecules since Fab is excreted directly in the urine (Wochner *et al.*, 1967), and, consequently, a significant portion of the Fab-bound digoxin would be rapidly eliminated. Compared to the intact antibody molecule, Fab fragments possess a number of potential advantages that include: (a) their lack of species specific determinants which would render them less immunogenic and, therefore, less prone to induce anaphylactoid side effects (Butler *et al.*, 1973); (b) their shorter half-life (4 to 12 hours) which leads to more rapid clearance (Spiegelberg and Weigle, 1965; Wochner *et al.*, 1967; Janeway *et al.*, 1968; Lloyd and Smith 1978); (c) their lack of aggregating properties which may result in greater safety margins following intravenous administration (Janeway *et al.*, 1968); and (d) their smaller molecular size which leads to a faster distribution phase and perhaps a larger volume of distribution culminating in a more rapid and efficient reversal of drug effects. Curd *et al.* (1971) proposed that a further increase in the safety of the antibody preparation might be achieved by eliminating non-specific γ-globulins through the use of affinity columns, and succeeded in showing that specifically purified Fab fragments could reverse digoxin-induced ventricular tachycardia in dogs. Their work on *in vivo* reversal of digoxin-induced toxicity by specifically purified antibodies or their Fab fragments has been confirmed and extended by Lloyd Smith (1978), Ochs *et al.* (1978), and Hougen *et al.* (1979).

Butler *et al*. (1977b) compared the serum levels and urinary excretion patterns of [^{3}H]digoxin in dogs receiving either sheep anti-digoxin serum, specifically purified sheep anti-digoxin Fab fragments, or control serum. Following a dose of 0.02 mg/kg i.v., control dogs had peak blood levels of *c*. 10 ng/ml which decreased to below 1 ng/ml within 1 day. Antiserum-treated dogs had peak blood levels of over 100 ng/ml after the first day which persisted for several days before declining slowly to a concentration of 10 ng/ml on day 10. Dogs treated with the specific Fab fragments achieved peak blood levels during the first day of 30–40 ng/ml which decreased to below 1 ng/ml after 6 days. As might be expected, most of the digoxin was protein bound after treatment with either anti-digoxin antisera or Fab, and thus pharmacologically inactive. Urinary excretion was measured and found to be similar in control dogs and Fab-treated dogs, although, particularly at early times, a large proportion of the digoxin eliminated by the urinary pathway was protein bound (presumably to Fab) in the Fab-treated dogs. Urinary excretion of digoxin in the antisera-treated dogs was not significant during the first 96 hours following dosing. It was presumed that urinary excretion became measurable only after significant catabolism of specific antibody occurred. These results demonstrate the ability of Fab to enhance the *in vivo* elimination of drugs compared to the intact antibody molecule.

The kinetics of toxicity reversal were studied by Lloyd and Smith (1978) who examined the hypothesis that the small size of the Fab fragment would permit more rapid distribution in interstitial spaces and thereby affect a more rapid reversal of digoxin-induced toxicity than the whole antibody molecule. In dogs, the distribution phase for sheep antibody was found to be much faster for Fab ($t_{1/2} = 0.54$ hours) than for unchanged γ-globulin ($t_{1/2} = 2.28$ hours). The elimination rates were also faster for Fab ($t_{1/2} = 17$ hours) compared to whole antibody ($t_{1/2} = 51$ hours). When the ability of the two preparations to reverse a lethal dose of digoxin was compared, the Fab fragment restored normal sinus rhythm in 36 minutes while whole antibody required 85 minutes, thus substantiating part of the rationale for the preferential use of Fab. Hess *et al*. (1978) found a similar reversal time (43 minutes) using specifically purified (Fab')$_2$ fragments in cats. Excess amounts of Fab were reported to be no faster in reversing toxicity than stoichiometric quantities, a result that would appear to confirm the *in vitro* finding that the rate limiting step in toxicity reversal is drug dissociation from specific receptor.

Smith *et al*. (1976) reversed advanced digoxin intoxication in the clinic by using specifically purified sheep anti-digoxin Fab fragments. Precautionary skin tests were carried out with intradermal injections of 5, 50, and 100 μg of the specific Fab fragments at 5 minute intervals prior to intravenous administration of Fab. When no skin reactions were observed, a test infusion of 2 mg of Fab in 1 ml of saline was administered. After 5 minutes of uneventful observation, the calculated dose of Fab (1100 mg) was infused in 600 ml of physiological saline over 2 hours. Within 10 minutes of completing the infusion a stable sinus rhythm was restored in the patient. The digoxin serum concentration rose rapidly from *c*. 18 to 120 ng/ml, but the free digoxin concentration fell below measurable levels (less than 1 ng/ml). Renal excretion of digoxin was shown initially to be almost totally Fab bound. Free digoxin levels remained low and the patient recovered. No evidence for either adverse immune reactions or an immune response to the Fab fragment was observed during the post-recovery period.

B. Digitoxin

Ochs and Smith (1977) did not elicit specific anti-digitoxin antibodies, but selected digoxin antibodies which cross-reacted with and bound digitoxin with an intrinsic asociation constant of 10^{10}M^{-1}. Studies were carried out in dogs where digitoxin and digoxin have comparable pharmacokinetics. Digitoxin toxicity was reversed with specific Fab fragments prepared from anti-digoxin antibodies, but not with non-specific Fab. The reappearance of conducted sinus beats occurred with a mean time of 18 minutes following Fab administration and a stable sinus rhythm was obtained in 54 minutes.

Digitoxin has an extremely long half-life in man (Lukas, 1972). Its very slow elimination rate is attributed to extensive albumin binding which prevents excretion by the kidney (Lukas and DeMartino, 1969) and allows continued recirculation. In addition, the apolar nature of the molecule lowers the ratio of free drug to tissue-bound drug (Kuschinsky *et al.*, 1968; Runge, 1977). The long half-life of digitoxin compounds the problems of drug intoxication.

In the rhesus monkey, digitoxin has a half-life for elimination of 136 hours. Administration of non-specific Fab or IgG had no effect on the rate of elimination, but intravenous injection of specific anti-digitoxin Fab fragments led to a rapid fourfold increase in plasma digitoxin levels which subsequently declined with a half-life of *c*. 4 hours. After 12 to 16 hours, the half-life reverted to that of normal controls, *c*. 136 hours. When specific IgG antibody was administered, the plasma concentration rose rapidly to thirteen times that of control animals. Only after 2 weeks did the digitoxin plasma levels begin to approach those of the controls. More importantly, while cumulative urinary excretion was greatly augmented by specific Fab compared to that of control, it was diminished by specific IgG. No data on reversal of toxicity were reported in the monkey.

C. Ouabain and Acetyl Strophanthidin

Ciofalo and Ash (1971) showed that the toxic effects of ouabain (Figure 4) were inhibited *in vivo* in rabbits following active immunization, but no toxicity reversal studies were carried out. Gold and Smith (1974) examined the effects of antibodies on the reversal of the inotropic effects of ouabain and acetyl strophanthidin on cardiac muscle *in vitro*. The differences in reversal times, 124 ± 6 minutes for anti-ouabain antibody versus 37 ± 3 minutes for anti-acetyl strophanthidin antibody, were attributed to the differences in the rates of dissociation from the respective drug receptors.

D. Morphine

The elicitation of antibodies to morphine has been reported by a number of investigators as part of the development of radioimmunoassay procedures (Spector and Parker, 1970; Spector, 1971; van Vunakis *et al.*, 1972; Wainer *et al.*, 1972, 1973a) and haemagglutination assays (Adler *et al.*, 1971, 1972). Synthetic modification of the morphine molecule has been required to prepare a morphine–carrier protein conjugate for immunization (Figure 4). Spector and Parker (1970) prepared 3-O-carboxymethyl morphine and conjugated this derivative to carrier protein via 1-dimethylaminopropyl-3-ethylcarbodiimide. Wainer *et al.* (1972) prepared morphine-6-hemisuccinate and linked it to the carrier protein via formation of a mixed anhydride with isobutyl chloroformate.

Morphine depresses the contractions of isolated electrically stimulated guinea pig ileum and this effect can be inhibited by addition of specific antibody to the tissue bath prior to addition of morphine (Wainer *et al.*, 1973b; DeCato and Adler, 1973). However, Bleiberg *et al.* (1973), using a slightly different ileal preparation that contained no antihistamine, reported that anti-morphine antibodies in the presence of morphine give Schultz–Dale contractions. The excellent correlation between the morphine binding capacity and the pharmacologic blocking capacity of the antisera strongly supports the concept that morphine is neutralized by antibody and the activity remaining in the antibody–morphine mixture is attributable to free morphine (DeCato and Adler, 1973).

Wainer *et al.* (1973b) demonstrated that the morphine-induced inhibition of ileal contractions could be reversed by subsequent addition of anti-morphine antibody. When only a stoichiometric amount of antibody was added, the morphine effect was reduced by *c.* 80%; a twofold excess of antibody was required to neutralize all morphine activities. Antibody reversed the depression of ileal contraction after a few minutes. Thus, unlike the cardiac glycosides, the reversal of morphine effects is rapid and apparently not limited by the rate of drug dissociation from receptor.

The passive administration of anti-morphine antibodies has a pronounced effect on the pattern of tissue distribution observed for morphine. After mice were treated with either 0.2 ml of anti-morphine antisera or with control sera and subsequently injected with morphine, plasma levels of morphine were 90-fold higher in mice receiving the specific antisera compared to those receiving control sera. Total morphine concentration was higher in the brains of the passively immunized mice, but, after subtraction of the amount of morphine in the vascular compartment, the tissue levels of morphine in the brains were in fact calculated to be far lower (Berkowitz *et al.*, 1975). It appears that antibody preferentially binds morphine and the resultant complex circulates in the plasma, greatly diminishing the amount of drug available for tissue binding. To confirm this, the brains of morphine-treated rats were perfused with saline to remove the antibody-bound morphine in plasma and, under these circumstances, it was determined that the concentration of morphine in brain tissue of antibody-treated rats was less than 25% that of rats that were treated with control sera. This further substantiates the conclusion that the primary effect of specific antibody is to sequester drug in the plasma, elevating plasma concentrations of drug and making less available for binding to specific tissue receptors.

Numerous studies have shown that active immunization against morphine inhibits the effects of subsequently administered drug (Berkowitz and Spector, 1972; Bonese *et al.*, 1974; Berkowitz *et al.*, 1975; Meisheri and Isom, 1978). It also has been suggested that opiate tolerance may partially depend upon antibody production to the opiate (Ringle and Herndon, 1972; Ryan *et al.*, 1972; Miller *et al.*, 1977). Miller *et al.* (1975) examined the effect of passively administered antibody on subsequently administered morphine in the rat, and demonstrated the ability of antibody to attenuate the electroencephalographic changes normally induced by drug. Reversal studies have not been done although they could be carried out readily using the reversal of opiate-induced myopia as an end point.

E. Barbiturates

Antibodies to the barbiturates were elicited (Spector and Flynn, 1971; Flynn and Spector, 1972) by using a barbiturate hapten, 5-allyl-5-(β-carboxy-α-methyl)ethyl barbituric acid (Figure 4), coupled to bovine γ-globulin. In actively immunized mice, the pharmacologic response (measured as depression of rotarod activity) to an active dose of pentobarbital was decreased (Flynn *et al.*, 1977) and serum levels following phenobarbital administration were increased (Flynn and Cerreta, 1978). Moreover, the absolute increase in the serum levels of pentobarbital were related directly to the antibody binding capacity of the pentobarbital antisera.

Cerreta *et al.* (1979) examined the effect of passively administered rabbit antibodies on the pharmacokinetic response to phenobarbital. Barbiturate binding capacity in mice that received 0.1 ml of rabbit anti-barbiturate antisera exhibited a half-life of about 6 days reflecting the half-life of the specific barbiturate antibody. Serum levels of [^{3}H]phenobarbital were about four times higher in mice pre-treated with the specific antibody than in controls. The additional serum phenobarbital appeared to be bound to antibody but a surprising amount, about 25%, was unbound, reflecting presumably either a low affinity constant for the antibody or administration of less than stoichiometric quantities of specific antibodies. Assuming a blood volume of 2 ml per mouse, 45 pmol of phenobarbital were bound compared to a total binding capacity of 90 pmol for the 0.1 ml antisera added. The possibility that low affinity antibody was utilized in these experiments seems likely since the rate of phenobarbital clearance was only marginally slower than that of free phenobarbital (8 hours versus 6 hours). This may be contrasted with the case of high affinity antibody against the cardiac glycosides where the kinetics of drug clearance were dictated by the half-life of the specific antibody rather than that of free drug. Finally, it is not clear whether the differences between normal and immune sera in the antagonism of the pentobarbital effects on rotarod ataxia are due to antibody since at the lowest dose, 15 mg/kg i.v., each mouse received slightly over 1 μmol pentobarbital, while the authors determined the binding capacity of the passively administered antisera to be only 990 pmol per ml. Therefore it remains to be documented whether antibody can reverse the pharmacologic effects of barbiturates *in vivo*. Based on the *in vitro* work, specific antibodies offer a potential therapeutic approach to barbiturate poisoning. Studies on long-acting barbiturates such as phenobarbital should provide ample opportunity to study reversal of drug toxicity in comatose animals and provide a test of the feasibility for human application.

A more serious problem may inhibit the development of clinical applications of anti-barbiturate antibodies. A typical poisoning dose of barbiturate is 5–15 times the usual hypnotic dose of 100–200 mg in man. Assuming at least 1 g of drug (molecular weight 250) has been ingested then 4 mmol of drug need to be neutralized by specific Fab fragments (molecular weight of 50,000 per binding site), *i.e.* 200 g of Fab anti-barbiturate would have to be administered. If Fab could be infused at a concentration approximating that of high normal values for total plasma protein, *i.e.* 8 g per 100 ml, at least 2.5 litres of fluid would be required. Smith *et al.* (1976), however, used only 0.2 g/100 ml Fab in man. Not only may there be problems in administering 2.5 litres by infusion to normal individuals but there may be severe logistic problems in obtaining such large quantities of antibody. Assuming that hyperimmune sera contain 10 mg of specific antibody per ml or about 6 mg specific Fab/ml (assuming a near 100% yield), then 33 litres of starting antisera would be required to produce the necessary Fab. It can be concluded at this time that antibody reversal of drug intoxication appears to be practical only in the case where milligrams (cardiac glycosides) rather than grams (barbiturates) of drug need to be neutralized.

IV. SUMMARY AND CONCLUSIONS

The pharmacologic and medicinal applications of antibody have been examined in detail in two selected areas: (1) the use of antibodies as carriers that transport specific therapeutic agents to precise target sites and (2) the use of antibodies to reverse the activity of drugs. These two areas have been chosen as prototypical in that they illustrate many of the newer aspects of the clinical applications of antibody.

Antibodies have been used to carry drugs, toxins, enzymes, radioactivity, and boron to specific tissue sites, and evidence that chemical complexes prepared from specific antibodies and therapeutic agents display augmented levels of activity has been presented. In efforts to maximize the therapeutic ratios of drugs, particularly those that have previously demonstrated promising anti-tumour activities as single agents, drug–antibody complexes have received the major share of attention. Immunochemotherapeutic complexes that utilize (a) toxins and enzymes, which offer the opportunities of designing potential therapeutic regimens around highly specific biochemical mechanisms of action, (b) radioiodinated antibodies, which deliver tumour-destroying radioactivity to precise tumour sites, and (c) boron derivatives of antibodies, which sensitize tumours to the subsequent effects of neutron radiation, have been less well studied as novel approaches to cancer chemotherapy.

The synthetic immunochemotherapeutic complexes have been shown to retain the biologic spectrum of activities of their component parts. The mechanisms by which the complexes display enhanced activities appear to result from the ability of the antibody to 'home' to a specific tissue site and thereby intensify the effect of the therapeutic agent to which it is linked, although several reports have appeared describing the attainment of equally beneficial effects following the separate administration of drugs and antibodies *in vivo* or the use of non-complexed drug–antibody mixtures *in vitro*.

No systematic attempts have been made to define which drugs or classes of drugs, if any, are best suited to the preparation of drug–antibody complexes. Likewise, the comparative attributes of covalently and non-covalently linked drug–antibody complexes have not been established. This issue is particularly important in view of the questions that have been raised concerning the immunologically specific anti-tumour activities of non-covalently bonded conjugates of chlorambucil and anti-tumour antibodies.

The requirement for the development of greater potency and selectivity suggests that other issues in need of resolution include (a) the identification of those chemical methodologies and functionalities that may be optimal in producing biologically active complexes, (b) the relative value of linking drugs and antibodies directly or through spacer molecules, (c) the preparation of complexes having relatively high drug to antibody ratios which, nevertheless, retain both drug activity and antibody specificity, and (d) the investigation of the potential value of using monoclonal antibodies in the preparation of various conjugates. The study of immunotherapeutic complexes in mixed populations of normal and target cells should allow *in vitro* competitive evaluation of the selectivity and killing efficiency of the complexes and greatly expedite the identification of those complexes having the greatest therapeutic potential.

The use of antibodies to reverse the pharmacologic activities of drugs is a natural outgrowth of the use of antibodies to neutralize bacterial toxins. However, a series of important changes have taken place. First, antibody has been specifically purified using affinity columns, thereby eliminating many of the problems associated with administration of large amounts of heterologous sera or γ-globulin. Second, it was found that if the class-specific region of the antibody molecule (Fc) was removed by proteolytic cleavage so that only the combining site fragment (Fab) was used, drug toxicity could be reversed more rapidly and drug eliminated more efficiently via renal excretion. The results of these studies have documented the clinical advantages of the use of specific Fab fragments.

Antibody-mediated reversal of drug intoxication has found clinical utility in the case of cardiac glycosides. Smith *et al.* (1977) suggested the extension of this procedure to red tide paralytic shell fish (Johnson *et al.*, 1964) and DDT poisoning (Centeno *et al.*, 1970). Butler suggested its application to thyrotoxic crisis (Burman *et al.*, 1976), and potential applications to other abused drugs are limited only by knowledge of the identity of the toxic substance. The studies with barbiturates suggest that antibodies are not currently applicable to all forms of poisoning. The logistics involved in obtaining and administering the quantities of antibody or Fab that would be necessary to reverse a typical case of barbiturate poisoning are currently prohibitive. This may be true of most toxic agents that are administered in close to gram quantities.

The development of the methodology for producing monoclonal antibody-producing hybridomas (Chapter 9) will have a great impact on future work done in these areas. The findings of Koprowski *et al.* (1978) and Steplewski *et al.* (1979), for example, suggest that, at least in the case of melanoma, production of tumour-specific monoclonal antibody can be accomplished by the hybridoma technique. This may obviate the problems that have been associated with the production of antibodies that cross-react with normal tissue. Moreover, their initial work suggests that some anti-melanoma hybridoma antibodies cross-react with melanomas of other patients. A further demonstration of a cross-reactive tumour antigen detected by monoclonal hybridoma antibody has been reported by Herlyn *et al.* (1979) in colorectal carcinoma. The finding of common tumour antigens could greatly expand the opportunities for the use of immunochemotherapeutic agents in man.

The use of hybridomas also will allow the solution of several unanswered questions concerning the optimal utilization of antibodies as carriers. It may be possible to identify whether the class of antibody used to prepare the immunotherapeutic complex is important. The Fc fragment could be useful for internalizing the complex by promoting phagocytosis or pinocytosis. Conversely, it may prove more useful, as in the case of drug toxicity reversal, to use the Fab fragment to obtain a complex with 'pure' transport function. The employment of the hybridoma technique will allow the use of antibody that is highly specific, pure, and of a particular class. Finally, with the advent of anti-idiotypic antisera and the demonstration of idiotypic determinants on the surfaces of helper and suppressor T cells, immunotherapeutic complexes derived from antibody with anti-idiotypic specificities may offer a method of selectively suppressing the response to a specific antigen without affecting the overall status of the immune system.

REFERENCES

Adler, F. L. and Liu, C. -T. (1971). Detection of morphine by hemagglutination inhibition. *J. Immunol.*, **106**, 1684–1685.

Adler, F.L., Liu, C. -T., and Catlin, D. H. (1972). Immunological studies on heroin addiction. I. Methodology and application of a hemagglutination inhibition test for the detection of morphine. *Clin. Immunol. Immunopath.*, **1**, 53–68.

Avrameas, S. (1969). Coupling of enzymes to proteins with glutaraldehyde. *Immunochemistry*, **6**, 43–52.

Bale, W. F., Spar, I. L., and Goodland, R. L. (1960). Experimental radiation therapy of tumors with ^{131}I-carrying antibodies to fibrin. *Cancer Res.*, **20**, 1488–1494.

Bale, W. F., Spar, I. L., Goodland, R. L., and Wolfe, D. E. (1955). *In vivo* and *in vitro* studies of labeled antibodies against rat kidney and Walker carcinoma. *Proc. Soc. Exp. Biol. Med.*, **89**, 564–568.

Baseman, J. B., Pappenheimer, A. M., Jr., Gill, D. M., and Harper, A. A. (1970). Action of diphtheria toxin in the guinea pig. *J. Exp. Med.*, **132**, 1138–1152.

Beatty, J. D., Friesen, E., Linford, J. H., and Israels, L. G. (1978). Effects of conjugated and nonconjugated antithymocyte globulin and Trenimon on T lymphocytes and skin graft refection. *Transplantation*, **25**, 197–203.

Berkowitz, B., Cerreta, K., and Spector, S. (1975). Influence of active and passive immunity on the disposition of dihydromorphine-^{3}H. *Life Sci.*, **15**, 1017–1029.

Berkowitz, B. and Spector, S. (1972). Evidence for active immunity to morphine in mice. *Science*, **178**, 1290–1292.

Blakeslee, D., Chen, M., and Kennedy, J. C. (1975). Aggregation of chlorambucil *in vitro* may cause misinterpretation of protein binding data. *Brit. J. Cancer*, **31**, 689–692.

Blakeslee, D. and Kennedy, J. C. (1974). Factors affecting the non-covalent binding of chlorambucil to rabbit immunoglobulin G. *Cancer Res.*, **34**, 882–885.

Bleiberg, M. J., Janicki, B. N., and Leahy, W. (1973). Effects of a morphine-rabbit anti-morphine antibody mixture on guinea pig isolated ileum. *Brit. J. Pharmacol.*, **49**, 721–723.

Boetcher, D. A. and Leonard, E. J. (1974). Abnormal monocyte chemotactic response in cancer patients. *J. Natl. Cancer Inst.*, **52**, 1091–1099.

Bonese, K. F., Wainer, B. H., Fitch, F. W., Rothberg, R. M., and Schuster, C. R. (1974). Changes in heroin self-administration by a rhesus monkey after morphine immunization. *Nature (Lond.)*, **252**, 708–710.

Burman, K. D., Yeager, H. C., Briggs, W. A., Earll, J. M., and Wartofsky, L. (1976). Resin hemoperfusion: A method of removing circulating thyroid hormones. *J. Clin. Endocrinol.*, **42**, 70–78.

Butler, V. P., Jr. (1970). Digoxin: Immunologic approaches to measurement and reversal of toxicity. *New Engl. J. Med.*, **283**, 1150–1156.

Butler, V. P., Jr. (1977). Immunological assay of drugs. *Pharm. Rev.*, **29**, 103–184.

Butler, V. P., Jr. and Chen, J. P. (1967). Digoxin specific antibodies. *Proc. Natl. Acad. Sci., USA*, **57**, 71–78.

Butler, V. P., Jr., Schmidt, D. H., Smith, T. W., Haber, E., Raynor, B. D., and DeMartini, P. (1977b). Effects of sheep digoxin-specific antibodies and their Fab fragments on digoxin pharmacokinetics in dogs. *J. Clin. Invest.*, **59**, 345–359.

Butler, V. P., Jr., Smith, T. W., Schmidt, D. H., and Haber, E. (1977a). Immunologic reversal of the effects of digoxin. *Fed. Proc.*, **36**, 2235–2241.

Butler, V. P., Jr., Watson, J. F., Schmidt, D. H., Gardner, J. D., Mandel, W. J., and Skelton, C. L. (1973). Reversal of the pharmacological and toxic effects of cardiac glycosides by specific antibodies. *Pharm. Rev.*, **25**, 239–248.

Calendi, E., Costanzi, G., Indiveri, F., Lotti, G., and Zini, C. (1969). Histoimmunologic specificity of an anti-lymphoid tissue sarcoma γ-globulin bound to methotrexate. *Boll. Chim. Farm.*, **108**, 25–28.

Centeno, E. R., Johnson, W. J., and Sehon, A. H. (1970). Antibodies to two common pesticides, DDT and malathion. *Int. Arch. Allergy Appl. Immunol.*, **37**, 1–13.

Cerottini, J. C. and Brunner, K. T. (1974). Cell-mediated cytotoxicity, allograft rejection, and tumor immunity. *Adv. Immunol.*, **18**, 67–132.

Cerreta, K. V., Flynn, E. J., and Spector, S. (1977). Immunization of mice against barbiturates and effect on disposition of phenobarbital-H-3. *Clin. Immunol. Immunopath.*, **7**, 203–218.

Cerreta, K. V., Flynn, E. J., and Spector, S. (1979). Pharmacologic response to pentobarbital in passively immunized mice. *Eur. J. Pharm.*, **54**, 365–371.

Chan-Palay, V. and Palay, S. L. (1979). Immunochemical localization of cyclic GMP: Light and electron microscopic evidence for involvement of neuroglia. *Proc. Natl. Acad. Sci., USA*, **76**, 1485–1488.

Ciofalo, F. and Ashe, H. (1971). Ouabain-induced ventricular arrhythmia in rabbit: influence of antibodies. *Life Sci.*, **10**, 341–345.

Clutton, R. F., Harington, C. R., and Yuill, M. E. (1938). CXLVII Studies in synthetic immunochemistry. III. Preparation and antigenic properties of thyroxyl derivatives of proteins, and physiological effects of their antisera. *Biochem. J.*, **32**, 1119–1132.

Collier, R. J. (1967). Effect of diphtheria toxin on protein synthesis: inactivation of one of the transfer factors. *J. Mol. Biol.*, **25**, 83–98.

Curd, J., Smith, T. W., Jaton, J. -C., and Haber, E. (1971). The isolation of digoxin-specific antibody and its use in reversing the effects of digoxin. *Proc. Natl. Acad. Sci. USA*, **68**, 2401–2406.

Currie, G. A. and Basham, C. (1972). Serum mediated inhibition of the immunological reactions of the patient to his own tumor: a possible role for circulating antigen. *Brit. J. Cancer*, **26**, 427–438.

Davies, D. A. L. (1974). The combined effect of drugs and tumor-specific antibodies in protection against a mouse lymphoma. *Cancer Res.*, **34**, 3040–3043.

Davies, D. A. L., Buckham, S., and Manstone, A. J. (1974). Protection of mice against syngeneic lymphomata. *Brit. J. Cancer*, **30**, 305–311.

Davies, D. A. L. and O'Neill, G. J. (1973). *In vivo* and *in vitro* effects of tumor specific antibodies with chlorambucil. *Brit. J. Cancer (Suppl. 1)*, **28**, 285–298.

Davies, D. A. L. and Staines, N. A. (1976). A cardinal role for I-region antigens (Ia) in immunological enhancement and the clinical implications. *Transplant. Rev.*, **30**, 18–39.

Day, E. D., Lassiter, S., Woodhall, B., Mahaley, J. L., and Mahaley, M. S., Jr. (1965). The localization of radioantibodies in human brain tumors. I. Preliminary exploration. *Cancer Res.*, **25**, 773–778.

Day, E. D., Planinsek, J., Korngold, L., and Pressman, D. (1956). Tumor-localizing antibodies purified from antisera against Murphy rat lymphosarcoma. *J. Natl. Cancer Inst.*, **17**, 517–532.

Day, E. D., Planinsek, J. A., and Pressman, D. (1959). Localization *in vivo* of radioiodinated anti-rat-fibrin antibodies and radioiodinated rat fibrinogen in the Murphy rat lymphosarcoma and in other transplantable rat tumors. *J. Natl. Cancer Inst.*, **22**, 413–426.

Day, E. D., Planinsek, J. A., and Pressman, D. (1960). Localization of radioiodinated antibodies in rats bearing tumors induced by *N*-2-fluorenylacetamide. *J. Natl. Cancer Inst.*, **25**, 787–802.

DeCato, L., Jr. and Adler, F. L. (1973). Neutralization of morphine activity by antibody. *Res. Commun. Chem. Pathol. Pharmacol.*, **5**, 775–788.

Dorrington, K. J. and Munro, D. S. (1966). The long acting thyroid stimulator. *Clin. Pharm. Therap.*, **7**, 788–806.

Everall, J. D., Dowd, P., Davies, D. A. L., O'Neill, G. J., and Rowland, G. F. (1977). Treatment of melanoma by passive humoral immunotherapy using antibody drug synergism. *Lancet*, **i**, 1105–1106.

Fauve, R. M., Hevin, B., Jacob, H., Gaillard, J. A., and Jacob, F. (1974). Antiinflammatory effects of murine malignant cells. *Proc. Natl. Acad. Sci. USA*, **71**, 4052–4056.

Ferin, M., Dyrenforth, I., Cowchock, S., Warren, M., and Vande Wiele, R. L. (1974). Active immunization to 17β-estradiol and its effects upon the reproductive cycle of the rhesus monkey. *Endocrinology*, **94**, 765–776.

Ferin, M., Tempone, A., Zimmering, P. E., and Vande Wiele, R. L. (1969). Effects of antibodies to 17β-estradiol and progesterone on the estrous cycle of the rat. *Endocrinology*, **85**, 1070–1078.

Ferin, M., Zimmering, P. E., Lieberman, S., and Vande Wiele, R. L. (1968). Inactivation of the biological effects of exogenous and endogenous estrogens by antibodies to 17β-estradiol. *Endocrinology*, **83**, 565–571.

Flechner, I. (1973). The cure and concomitant immunization of mice bearing Ehrlich ascites tumors by treatment with an antibody-alkylating agent complex. *Eur. J. Cancer*, **9**, 741–745.

Flickinger, R. A. and Trost, S. R. (1976). Cytotoxicity of antibody–phospholipase C conjugates on cultured Friend leukemia cells. *Eur. J. Cancer*, **12**, 159–160.

Flier, J. S., Kahn, C. R., Roth, J., and Bar, R. S. (1975). Antibodies that impair insulin receptor binding in an unusual diabetic syndrome with severe insulin resistance. *Science*, **190**, 63–65.

Flynn, E. J. and Cerreta, K. V. (1978). Contribution of phenobarbital antibody-binding capacity to increased serum levels of [^{3}H]-phenobarbital. *Clin. Immunol. Immunopath.*, **9**, 80–86.

Flynn, E. J., Cerreta, K. V., and Spector, S. (1977). Pharmacologic response to pentobarbital in actively immunized mice. *Eur. J. Pharmacol.*, **42**, 21–29.

Flynn, E. J. and Spector, S. (1972). Determination of babiturate derivatives by radioimmunoassay. *J. Pharm. Exp. Therap.*, **181**, 547–554.

Gardner, J. D., Kiino, D. R., Swartz, T. J., and Butler, V. P., Jr. (1973). Effects of digoxin-specific antibodies on accumulation and binding of digoxin by human erythrocytes. *J. Clin. Ivest.*, **52**, 1820–1833.

Geczy, A. F., deWeck, A. L., Geczy, C. L., and Toffler, O. (1978). Suppression of reaginic antibody formation in guinea pigs by anti-idiotypic antibodies. *J. Allergy Clin. Immunol.*, **62**, 261–270.

Ghose, T., Cerini, M., Carter, M., and Nairn, R. C. (1967). Immunoradioactive agent against cancer. *Brit. Med. J.*, **1**, 90–93.

Ghose, T. and Guclu, A. (1974). Cure of a mouse lymphoma with radioiodinated antibody. *Eur. J. Cancer*, **10**, 787–792.

Ghose, T., Guclu, A., and Tai, J. (1975a). Suppression of an AKR lymphoma by antibody and chlorambucil. *J. Natl. Cancer Inst.*, **55**, 1353–1357.

Ghose, T., Guclu, A., Tai, J., MacDonald, A. S., Norvell, S. T., and Aquino, J. (1975b). Antibody as a carrier of ^{131}I in cancer diagnosis and treatment. *Cancer (Philadelphia)*, **36**, 1646–1657.

Ghose, T. and Nigam, S. P. (1972). Antibody as carrier of chlorambucil. *Cancer (Philadelphia)*, **29**, 1398–1400.

Ghose, T., Norvell, S. T., Guclu, A., Bodurtha, A., Tai, J., and MacDonald, A. S. (1977). Immunochemotherapy of malignant melanoma with chlorambucil-bound antimelanoma globulins: preliminary results in patients with disseminated disease. *J. Natl. Cancer Inst.*, **58**, 845–852.

Ghose, T., Norvell, S. T., Guclu, A., Cameron, D., Bodurtha, A., and MacDonald, A. S. (1972). Immunochemotherapy of cancer with chlorambucil-carrying antibody. *Brit. Med. J.*, **3**, 495–499.

Ghose, T., Norvell, S. T., Guclu, A., and MacDonald, A. S. (1975c). Immunotherapy of human malignant melanoma with chlorambucil-carrying antibody. *Eur. J. Cancer*, **11**, 321–326.

Gill, D. M., Pappenheimer, A. M., Jr., and Uchida, T. (1973). Diphtheria toxin, protein synthesis, and the cell. *Fed. Proc.*, **32**, 1508–1515.

Gold, H. K. and Smith, T. W. (1974). Reversal of ouabain and acetyl strophanthidin effects in normal and failing cardiac muscle by specific antibody. *J. Clin. Invest.*, **53**, 1655–1661.

Gold, P. and Freedman, S. O. (1966). Specific carcinoembryonic antigens of the human digestive system. *J. Exp. Med.*, **122**, 467–481.

Goldenberg, D. M., Preston, D. F., Primus, F. J., and Hansen, H. J. (1974). Photoscan localization of GW-39 tumors in hamsters using radiolabeled anticarcinoembryonic antigen immunoglobulin G. *Cancer Res.*, **34**, 1–9.

Gorman, J. G. (1975). *The Role of the Laboratory in Hemolytic Disease of the Newborn.* Lea & Febiger, Philadelphia, PA.

Guclu, A., Ghose, T., Tai, J., and Mammen, M. (1976). Binding of chlorambucil with antitumor globulins and its effect on drug and antibody activities. *Eur. J. Cancer*, **12**, 95–100.

Guclu, A., Tai, J., and Ghose, T. (1975). Endocytosis of chlorambucil-bound anti-tumor globulin following 'capping' in EL4 lymphoma cells. *Immunol. Commun.*, **4**, 229–242.

Hawthorne, M. F., Wiersema, R. J., and Takasugi, M. (1972). Preparation of tumor-specific boron compounds. 1. *In vitro* studies using boron-labeled antibodies and elemental boron as neutron targets. *J. Med. Chem.*, **15**, 449–452.

Hellström, K. E. and Hellström, I. (1974). Lymphocyte-mediated cytotoxicity and blocking serum activity to tumor antigens. *Adv. Immunol.*, **18**, 209–277.

Herberman, R. B. (1974). Cell-mediated immunity to tumor cells. *Adv. Cancer Res.*, **19**, 207–263.

Herlyn, M., Steplewski, Z., Herlyn, D., and Koprowski, H. (1979). Colorectal carcinoma-specific antigen: Detection by means of monoclonal antibodies. *Proc. Natl. Acad Sci. USA*, **76**, 1438–1442.

Hersh, E. M., Mavligit, G. M., and Gutterman, J. U. (1976). Immunodeficiency in cancer and the importance of immune evaluation of the cancer patient. *Med. Clin. North Am.*, **60**, 623–639.

Hess, T., Scholtysik, G., and Riesen, W. (1978). The prevention and reversal of digoxin intoxication with specific antibodies. *Am. Heart J.*, **96**, 486–495.

Hökfelt, T., Ljungdahl, A., Terenius, L., Elde, R., and Nilsson, G. (1977). Immunohistochemical analysis of peptide pathways possibly related to pain and analgesia: Enkephalin and substance P. *Proc. Natl. Acad Sci. USA*, **74**, 3081–3085.

Honjo, T., Nishizuka, Y., Hayaishi, O., and Kato, I. (1968). Diphtheria toxin-dependent adenosine diphosphate ribosylation of aminoacyl transferase II and inhibition of protein synthesis. *J. Biol. Chem.*, **243**, 3553–3555.

Hopwood, W. J. and Stock, J. A. (1971). The effect of macromolecules upon the rates of hydrolysis of aromatic nitrogen mustard derivatives. *Chem. Biol. Interact.*, **4**, 31–39.

Hougen, T. J., Lloyd, B. L., and Smith, T. W. (1979). Effects of inotropic and arrhythmogenic digoxin doses and of digoxin-specific antibody on myocardial monovalent cation transport in the dog. *Circulation Res.*, **44**, 23–31.

Hurwitz, E., Levy, R., Maron, R., Wilchek, M., Arnon, R., and Sela, M. (1975). The covalent binding of daunomycin and adriamycin to antibodies, with retention of both drug and antibody activities. *Cancer Res.*, **35**, 1175–1181.

Hurwitz, E., Maron, R., Arnon, R., and Sela, M. (1976). Fab dimers of antitumor immunoglobulins as covalent carriers of daunomycin. *Cancer Biochem. Biophys.*, **1**, 197–202.

Hurwitz, W., Maron, R., Bernstein, A., Wilchek, M., Sela, M., and Arnon, R. (1978). The effect *in vivo* of chemotherapeutic drug–antibody conjugates in two murine experimental tumor systems. *Int. J. Cancer*, **21**, 747–755.

Israels, L. G. and Linford, J. H. (1963). Some observations on the reactions of chlorambucil, azo-mustard (CB 1414), and cyclophosphamide. *Proc. Fifth Can. Cancer Conf.*, 399–415.

Izzo, M. J., Buchsbaum, D. J., and Bale, W. F. (1972). Localization of a ^{125}I-labeled rat transplantation antibody in tumors carrying the corresponding antigen. *Proc. Soc. Exp. Biol. Med.*, **139**, 1185–1188.

Janeway, C. A., Merler, E., Rosen, F. S., Salmon, S., and Crain, J. D. (1968). Intravenous gamma globulin. Metabolism of gamma globulin fragments in normal and agammaglobulinemic persons. *New Engl. J. Med.*, **278**, 919–923.

Johnson, A., Day, E. D., and Pressman, D. (1960). The effect of iodination on antibody activity. *J. Immunol.*, **84**, 213–220.

Johnson, H. M., Frey, P. A., Angelotti, R., Campbell, J. E., and Lewis, K. H. (1964). Haptenic properties of paralytic shellfish poison conjugated to proteins by formaldehyde treatment. *Proc. Soc. Exp. Biol. Med.*, **117**, 425–430.

Kahn, C. R., Flier, J. S., Bar, R. S., Archer, J. A., Gorden, P., Martin, M. M., and Roth, J. (1976). The syndromes of insulin resistance and acanthosis nigricans. *New Engl. J. Med.*, **294**, 739–745.

Kellen, J. A. and Lo, J. S. (1973). Localization of ^{125}I labeled antibodies against tumor-associated proteins from experimental rat mammary neoplasms. *Res. Commun. Chem. Pathol. Pharmacol.*, **5**, 411–420.

Klein, G. (1973). Immunological surveillance against neoplasia. *Harvey Lect.*, **69**, 71–102.

Koprowski, H., Steplewski, Z., Herlyn, D., and Herlyn, M. (1978). Study of antibodies against human melanoma produced by somatic cell hybrids. *Proc. Natl. Acad Sci. USA*, **75**, 3405–3409.

Kruger, P. G. (1940). Some biological effects of nuclear disintegration products on neoplastic tissue. *Proc. Natl. Acad. Sci. USA*, **26**, 181–192.

Kuschinsky, K., Lullmann, H., and Van Zwieten, P. A. (1968). A comparison of the accumulation and release of ^{3}H-ouabain and ^{3}H-digitoxin by guinea pig heart muscle. *Br, J. Pharm. Chemother.*, **30**, 317–328.

Lance, E. M., Medawar, P. B., and Taub, R. N. (1973). Antilymphocyte serum. *Adv. Immunol.*, **17**, 1–92.

Landsteiner, K. (1945). *The Specificity of Serological Reactions*. Harvard Univ. Press, Boston, Massachusetts.

Lennon, V. A. and Carnegie, P. R. (1971). Immunological disease: A break in tolerance to receptor sites. *Lancet*, **i**, 630–633.

Levy, R., Hurwitz, E., Maron, R., Arnon, R., and Sela, M. (1975). The specific cytotoxic effects of daunomycin conjugated to antitumor antibodies. *Cancer Res.*, **35**, 1182–1186.

Lieberman, S., Erlanger, B. F., Beiser, S. M., and Agate, F. J., Jr. (1959). Steroid–protein conjugates: their chemical, immunochemical and endocrinological properties. *Rec. Prog. Horm. Res.*, **15**, 165–200.

Linford, J. H. (1973). 2,3,5-Tris-ethyleneimino-1,4-benzoquinone (Trenimon): some chemical and biological properties. *Chem. Biol. Interact.*, **6**, 149–168.

Linford, J. H. and Froese, G. (1978). Comparisons of the chemical and biological properties of triaziquone and triaziquone–protein conjugates. *J. Natl. Cancer Inst.*, **60**, 307–316.

Linford, J. H., Froese, G., Berczi, I., and Israels, L. G. (1974). An alkylating agent–globulin conjugate with both alkylating and antibody activity. *J. Natl. Cancer Inst.*, **52.**, 1665–1667.

Lipshutz, W., Hughes, W., and Cohen, S. (1972). The genesis of lower esophageal sphincter pressure: its identification through the use of gastrin antiserum. *J. Clin. Invest.*, **51**, 522–529.

Lloyd, B. L. and Smith, T. W. (1978). Contrasting rates of reversal of digoxin toxicity by digoxin specific Ig and Fab fragments. *Circulation*, **58**, 280–283.

Lukas, D. S. (1972). Of toads and flowers. *Circulation*, **46**, 1–4.

Lukas, D. S. and DeMartino, A. G. (1969). Binding of digitoxin and some related cardenolides to human plasma proteins. *J. Clin. Invest.*, **48**, 1041–1053.

Macpherson, I. (1974). Cancer immunotherapy: the role of immunostimulation. *Lancet*, **i**, 1058.

Mahaley, M. S., Jr., Mahaley, J. L., and Day, E. D. (1965). The localization of radioantibodies in human brain tumors. II. Radioautography. *Cancer Res.*, **25**, 779–793.

Mahoney, M. J. and Leighton, J. (1962). The inflammatory response to a foreign body within transplantable tumors. *Cancer Res.*, **22**, 334–338.

Mallinger, A. G., Jozwiak, E. L., Jr., and Carter, J. C. (1972). Preparation of boron-containing bovine γ-globulin as a model compound for a new approach to slow neutron therapy of tumors. *Cancer Res.*, **32**, 1947–1950.

Mandel, W. J., Bigger, J. T., Jr., and Butler, V. P., Jr. (1972). The electrophysiological effects of low and high digoxin concentration on isolated mammalian cardiac tissue: reversal by digoxin specific antibody. *J. Clin. Invest.*, **51**, 1378–1387.

Mathe, G., Loc, T. B., and Bernard, J. (1958). Effet sur la leucemie 1210 de la Souris d'une combinasion par diazotization d'A-methopterine et de γ-globulines de hamsters porteurs de cette leucemie par heterogreffe. *C. R. Acad. Sci.*, **246**, 1626–1628.

Meisheri, K. D. and Isom, G. E. (1978). Influence of immune stimulation and suppression on morphine physical dependence and tolerance. *Res. Commun. Chem. Pathol. Pharmacol.*, **19**, 85–99.

Miller, C., Nakamura, J., Leung, C. Y., Winters, W. D., and Benjamini, E. (1975). Immunological specificity of antibodies to morphine and their effect on the electroencephalographic activity of morphine. *Neuropharmacology*, **14**, 385–396.

Miller, C. H., Winters, W. D., and Benjamini, E. (1971). Opiate tolerance: independence from immunological mechanisms. *J. Pharm. Exp. Therap.*, **203**, 213–221.

Moolten, F. L., Capparell, N. J., and Cooperband, S. R. (1972). Antitumor effects of antibody–diphtheria toxin conjugates: use of hapten-coated tumor cells as an antigenic target. *J. Natl. Cancer Inst.*, **49**, 1057–1062.

Moolten, F. L., Capparell, N. J., Zajdel, S. H., and Cooperband, S. R. (1975). Antitumor effects of antibody–diphtheria toxin conjugates. II. Immunotherapy with conjugates directed against tumor antigens induced by simian virus 40. *J. Natl. Cancer Inst.*, **55**, 473–477.

Moolten, F. L. and Cooperband, S. R. (1970). Selective destruction of target cells by diphtheria toxin conjugated to antibody directed against antigens on the cells. *Science*, **169**, 68–70.

Nieschlag, E. and Wickings, E. J. (1977). Neutralization of testosterone by antibodies. In L. Martini and M. Molta (Eds.) *Androgens and Antiandrogens*, pp. 115–125. Raven press, New York.

O'Bryan, R. M., Luce, J. K., Talley, R. W., Gottlieb, J. A., Baker, L. H., and Bonadonna, G. (1973). Phase II evaluation of adriamycin in human neoplasia. *Cancer (Philadelphia)*, **32**, 1–8.

Ochs, H. R. and Smith, T. W. (1977). Reversal of advanced digitoxin toxicity and modification of pharmacokinetics by specific antibodies and Fab fragments. *J. Clin. Invest.*, **60**, 1303–1313.

Ochs, H. R., Vatner, S. F., and Smith, T. W. (1978). Reversal of inotropic effects of digoxin by specific antibodies and their Fab fragments in the conscious dog. *J. Pharm. Exp. Therap.*, **207**, 64–71.

O'Neill, G. J., Pearson, B. A., and Davies, D. A. L. (1975). *In vitro* cytotoxicity of anti-θ (thy-1) antibodies combined with chlorambucil. *Immunology*, **28**, 323–329.

Oon, C. J., Apsey, M., Buckleton, H., Cooke, K. B., Hanham, I., Hazarika, P., Hobbs, J. R., and McLeod, B. (1974). Human immune γ-globulin treated with chlorambucil for cancer therapy. *Behring Inst. Mitt.*, **56**, 228–235.

Papachristou, D., Zaki, A. F., and Fortner, J. G. (1977). Chlorambucil-carrying ALG as an immunosuppressive agent in the rat. *Transplant. Proc.*, **9**, 1059–1062.

Philpott, G. W., Bower, R. J., and Parker, C. W. (1973a). Improved selective cytotoxicity with an antibody–diphtheria toxin conjugate. *Surgery*, **73**, 928–935.

Philpott, G. W., Bower, R. J., and Parker, C. W. (1973b). Selective iodination and cytotoxicity of tumor cells with an antibody–enzyme conjugate. *Surgery*, **74**, 51–58.

Philpott, G. W., Bower, R. J., Parker, K. L., Shearer, W. T., and Parker, C. W. (1974). Affinity cytotoxicity of tumor cells with antibody–glucose oxidase conjugates, peroxidase, and arsphenamine. *Cancer Res.*, **34**, 2159–2164.

Philpott, G. W., Grass, E. H., and Parker, C. W. (1979). Affinity cytotoxicity with an alcohol dehydrogenase–antibody conjugate and allyl alcohol. *Cancer Res.*, **39**, 2084–2089.

Philpott, G. W., Shearer, W. T., Bower, R. J., and Parker, C. W. (1973c). Selective cytotoxicity of hapten-substituted cells with an antibody–enzyme conjugate. *J. Immunol.*, **111**, 921–929.

Prehn, R. T. (1977). Immunostimulation of the lymphodependent phase of neoplastic growth. *J. Natl. Cancer Inst.*, **59**, 1043–1049.

Pressman, D. and Keighley, G. (1948). The zone of activity of antibodies as determined by the use of radioactive tracers; the zone of activity of nephritoxic antikidney serum. *J. Immunol.*, **59**, 141–146.

Pressman, D. and Korngold, L. (1953). The *in vivo* localization of anti-Wagner-osteogenic-sarcoma antibodies. *Cancer (Philadelphia)*, **6**, 619–623.

Reif, A. E. (1971). Studies on the localization of radiolabeled antibodies to a mouse myeloma protein. *Cancer (Philadelphia)*, **27**, 1433–1439.

Reif, A. E., Curtis, L. E., Duffield, R., and Shauffer, I. A. (1974). Trial of radiolabeled antibody localization in metastases of a patient with a tumor containing carcinoembryonic antigen. *J. Surg. Oncol.*, **6**, 133–150.

Ringle, D. A. and Herndon, B. L. (1972). *In vitro* morphine binding by sera from morphine treated rabbits. *J. Immunol.*, **109**, 174–175.

Robinson, D. A., Whiteley, J. M., and Harding, N. G. L. (1973). Cell-directed antimetabolites: alternative syntheses of cytotoxic methotrexate-containing macromolecules. *Biochem. Soc. Trans.*, **1**, 722–726.

Romero, J. C., Hubler, S. W., Cosak, T. J., and Warzynski, T. J. (1973). Effect of anti-renin on blood pressure of rabbits with experimental renin hypertension. *Am. J. Physiol.*, **225**, 810–817.

Rosenberg, S. A. and Terry, W. D. (1977). Passive immunotherapy of cancer in animals and man. *Adv. Cancer Res.*, **25**, 323–388.

Ross, W. C. J. (1974). The interaction of chlorambucil with human γ-globulin. *Chem. Biol. Interact.*, **8**, 261–267.

Rowland, G. F. (1977). Effective antitumor conjugates of alkylating drug and antibody using dextran as the intermediate carrier. *Eur. J. Cancer*, **13**, 593–596.

Rowland, G. F., O'Neill, G. J., and Davies, D. A. L. (1975). Suppression of tumor growth in mice by drug–antibody conjugate using a novel approach to linkage. *Nature (Lond.)*, **255**, 487–488.

Rubens, R. D. and Dulbecco, R. (1974). Augmentation of cytotoxic drug action by antibodies directed at cell surface. *Nature (Lond.)*, **248**, 81–82.

Rubens, R. D., Vaughan-Smith, S., and Dulbecco, R. (1975). Augmentation of cytotoxic drug action and X-irradiation by antibodies. *Brit. J. Cancer*, **32**, 352–354.

Runge, T. M. (1977). Clinical implications of differences in pharmacodynamic action of polar and nonpolar cardiac glycosides. *Amer. Heart. J.*, **93**, 248–255.

Russel, P.S. (1977). Antilymphocyte sera for immunosuppression: a powerful class of agents awaiting full application to patient care. In E. Haber and R. M. Krause (Eds.) *Antibodies in Human Diagnosis and Therapy*, pp. 303–357. Raven Press, New York.

Ryan, J. J., Parker, C. W., and Williams, R. C., Jr. (1972). Gamma-globulin binding of morphine in heroin addicts. *J. Lab. Clin. Med.*, **80**, 155–164.

Schmidt, D. H. and Butler, V. P., Jr. (1971). Immunological protection against digoxin toxicity. *J. Clin. Invest.*, **50**, 866–871.

Schmidt, D. H., Kaufman, B. M., and Butler, V. P., Jr. (1974). Persistence of hapten–antibody complexes in the circulation of immunized animals after a single intravenous injection of hapten. *J. Exp. Med.*, **139**, 278–294.

Segerling, M., Ohanian, S. H., and Borsos, T. (1975). Chemotherapeutic drugs increase killing of tumor cells by antibody and complement. *Science*, **188**, 55–57.

Shearer, W. T., Turnbaugh, T. R., Coleman, W. E., Aach, R. D., Philpott, G. W., and Parker, C. W. (1974). Cytotoxicity with antibody–glucose oxidase conjugates specific for a human colonic cancer and carcinoembryonic antigen. *Int. J. Cancer*, **14**, 539–547.

Simantov, R., Kuhar, M. J., Uhl, G., and Snyder, S. H. (1977). Opioid peptide enkephalin: Immunohistochemical mapping in rat central nervous system. *Proc. Natl. Acad. Sci. USA*, **74**, 2167–2171.

Sjögren, H. O., Hellström, I., Bansal, S. C., and Hellström, K. E. (1971). Suggestive evidence that the 'blocking antibodies' of tumor-bearing individuals may be antigen–antibody complexes. *Proc. Nat. Acad. Sci. USA*, **68**, 1372–1375.

Smith, B. R., Dorrington, K. J., and Munro, D. S. (1969). The thyroid-stimulating properties of long-acting, thyroid stimulator γG-globulin subunits. *Biochim. Biophys. Acta*, **192**, 277–285.

Smith, G. V., Grogan, J. B., Stribling, J., and Lockard, J. (1975). Immunochemotherapy of hepatoma in rats. *Amer. J. Surg.*, **129**, 146–155.

Smith, H. J. and Gökcen, M. (1974). Tumor localizing antibodies directed against the malignant melanoma of hamsters. *Res.Commun. Chem Pathol. Pharmacol.*, **7**, 725–743.

Smith, T. W., Butler, V. P., Jr., and Haber, E. (1969). Determination of therapeutic and toxic serum digoxin concentrations by radioimmunoassay. *New Engl. J. Med.*, **281**, 1212–1216.

Smith, T. W., Butler, V. P., Jr., and Haber, E. (1970). Characterization of antibodies of high affinity and specificity for the digitalis glycoside digoxin. *Biochemistry*, **9**, 331–337.

Smith, T. W., Butler, V. P., Jr., and Haber, E. (1977). Cardiac glycoside-specific antibodies in the treatment of digitalis intoxication. In E. Haber and R. M. Krause (Eds.) *Antibodies in Human Diagnosis and Therapy*, pp. 365–389. Raven Press, New York.

Smith, T. W., Haber, E., Yeatman, L., and Butler, V. P., Jr. (1976). Reversal of advanced digoxin intoxication with Fab fragments of digoxin-specific antibodies. *New Engl. J. Med.*, **294**, 797–800.

Sneath, R. L., Jr., Soloway, A. H., and Dey, A. S. (1974). Protein-binding polyhedral boranes. 1. *J. Med. Chem.*, **17**, 796–799.

Sneath, R. L, Jr., Wright, J. E., Soloway, A. H., O'Keefe, S. M. and Smolnycki, W. D. (1976). Protein-binding polyhedral boranes. 3. *J. Med. Chem.*, **19**, 1290–1294.

Snyderman, R. and Pike, M. C. (1977). Macrophage migratory dysfunction in cancer. *Amer. J. Pathol.*, **88**, 727–739.

Spar, I. L., Bale, W. F., Goodland, R. L., Casarett, G. W., and Michaelson, S. M. (1960). Distribution of injected ^{131}I-labeled antibody to dog fibrin in tumor-bearing dogs. *Cancer Res.*, **20**, 1501–1504.

Spar, I. L., Bale, W. F., Marrack, D., Dewey, W. C., McCardle, R. J., and Harper, P. V. (1967). ^{131}I-labeled antibodies to human fibrinogen. *Cancer (Philadelphia)*, **20**, 865–870.

Spar, I. L., Goodland, R. L., and Bale, W. F. (1959). Localization of ^{131}I labeled antibody to rat fibrin in transplantable rat lymphosarcoma. *Proc. Soc. Exp. Biol. Med.*, **100**, 259–262.

Spector, S. (1971). Quantitative determination of morphine in serum by radioimmunoasay. *J. Pharm. Exp. Therap.*, **178**, 253–258.

Spector, S. and Flynn, E. J. (1971). Barbiturates: Radioimmunoassay. *Science*, **174**, 1036–1038.

Spector, S. and Parker, C. W. (1970). Morphine: Radioimmunoassay. *Science*, **168**, 1347–1348.

Speigelberg, H. L. and Weigle, W. O. (1965). The catabolism of homologous and heterologous 7S gamma globulin fragments. *J. Exp. Med.*, **121**, 323–338.

Steplewski, Z., Herlyn, M., Herlyn, D., Clark, W. H., and Koprowski, H. (1979). Reactivity of monoclonal anti-melanoma antibodies with melanoma cells freshly isolated from primary and metastatic melanoma. *Eur. J. Immunol.*, **9**, 94–96.

Stutman, O. (1975). Immunodepression and malignancy. *Adv. Cancer Res.*, **22**, 261–422.

Szekerke, M., Wade, R., and Whisson, M. E. (1972). The use of macromolecules as carriers of cytotoxic groups (Part I). Conjugates of nitrogen mustards with proteins, polypeptidyl proteins and polypeptides. *Neoplasma*, **19**, 199–209.

Talwar, G. P., Sharma, N. C., Dubey, S. K., Salahuddin, M., Das, C., Ramakrishnan, S., Kumar, S., and Hingorani, V. (1976). Isoimmunization against human chorionic gonadotropin with conjugates of processed β-subunit of the hormone and tetanus toxoid. *Proc. Natl. Acad. Sci., USA*, **73**, 218–222.

Tan, C., Tasaka, H., Yu, K. P., Murphy, M. L., and Karnofsky, D. A. (1967).

Daunomycin, an antitumor antibiotic, in the treatment of neoplastic disease. *Cancer (Philadelphia)*, **20**, 333–353.

Thanavala, Y. M., Hay, F. C., and Stevens, V. C. (1978). Immunological control of fertility: measurement of affinity of antibodies to human chorionic gonadotrophin. *Clin. Exp. Immunol.*, **33**, 403–409.

Thorpe, P. E., Ross, W. C. J., Cumber, A. J., Hinson, C. A., Edwards, D. C., and Davies, A. J. S. (1978). Toxicity of diphtheria toxin for lymphoblastoid cells is increased by conjugation to antilymphocytic globulin. *Nature (Lond.)*, **271**, 752–755.

Tolpin, E. I., Wong, H. S., and Lipscomb, W. N. (1974). Binding studies of boron hydride derivatives to proteins for neutron capture therapy. *J. Med. Chem.*, **17**, 792–796.

Toyka, K. V., Drachman, D. B., Pestronk, A., and Kao, I. (1975). Myasthenia gravis: passive transfer from man to mouse. *Science*, **190**, 397–399.

van Vunakis, H., Wasserman, E., and Levine, L. (1972). Specificities of antibodies to morphine. *J. Pharm. Exp. Therap.*, **180**, 514–521.

Vennegoor, C., Van Smeerdÿk, D., and Rumke, Ph. (1975). Effects of mixtures and complexes of chlorambucil and antibody on a human melanoma cell line. *Eur. J. Cancer*, **11**, 725–732.

Wainer, B. H., Fitch, F. W., Fried, J., and Rothberg, R. M. (1973a). A measurement of the specificities of antibodies to morphine-6-succinyl-BSA by competitive inhibition of ^{14}C-morphine binding. *J. Immunol.*, **110**, 667–673.

Wainer, B. H., Fitch, F. W., Rothberg, R. M., and Fried, J. (1972). Morphine-3-succinyl-bovine serum albumin: an immunogenic hapten–protein conjugate. *Science*, **176**, 1143–1144.

Wainer, B. H., Fitch, F. W., Rothberg, R. M., and Schuster, C. R. (1973b). *In vitro* morphine antagonism by antibodies. *Nature (Lond.)*, **241**, 537-538.

Waldman, T. A. and Strober, W. (1969). Metabolism of immunoglobulins. *Prog. Allergy*, **13**, 1–110.

Wochner, R. D., Strober, W., and Waldman, T. A. (1967). The role of the kidney in the metabolism of Bence Jones proteins and immunoglobulin fragments. *J. Exp. Med.*, **126**, 207–221.

Wong, H. S., Tolpin, E. I., and Lipscomb, W. N. (1974). Boron hydride derivatives for neutron capture therapy. Antibody approach. *J. Med. Chem.*, **17**, 785–791.

Woodrow, J. C. (1974). Rh immunization and its prevention. *Pathobiol. Annual*, pp. 65–86, Appleton-Century-Crofts, New York.

Yalow, R. S. and Berson, S. A. (1959). Assay of plasma insulin by immunological methods. *Nature (Lond.)*, **184**, 1648–1649.

Yalow, R. S. and Berson, S. A. (1960). Immunoassay of endogenous plasma insulin in man. *J. Clin. Invest.*, **39**, 1157–1175.

Zahl, P. A., Cooper, F. S., and Dunning, J. R. (1940). Some *in vivo* effects of localized nuclear disintegration products on a transplantable mouse sarcoma. *Proc. Natl. Acad. Sci. USA*, **26**, 589–598.

RECENT PAPERS

After completion of this manuscript the following relevant papers appeared in the literature:

(a) Dullens *et al.* (*Cancer Treatment Reports*, **63**, 99 (1979)) reported the comparative effects of a non-covalently bonded chlorambucil–antibody complex in two different mouse tumour systems.

(b) Dullens *et al.* (*Eur. J. Cancer*, **15**, 69 (1979)) found that a non-covalently linked chlorambucil-antibody complex was more effective in a mouse tumour system than was a mixture of the unlinked components.

(c) Latif *et al.* (*Cancer*, **45**, 1326 (1980)) evaluated the cytotoxicity of three covalently linked drug–antibody complexes against human tumour cells growing in nude mice. Whereas a conjugate derived from chlorambucil demonstrated anti-tumour activity, neither a methotrexate–antibody conjugate nor a daunomycin–antibody conjugate was effective.

(d) Chu and Whiteley (*Molec. Pharmacol.*, **17**, 382 (1980)) suggested that methotrexate–protein complexes may be transported into cells by mechanisms different from those for the parent drug.

(e) Shearer and Mettes (*J. Immunol.*, **123**, 2763 (1979)) showed that a mixture of cytosine arabinoside and goat anti-L cell antiserum acted synergistically to produce inhibition of L cell growth *in vitro*. The antibody caused stimulation of uptake of drug by the cells and subsequent incorporation into nuclear DNA.

(f) Gilliland *et al.* (*Proc. Nat. Acad. Sci., USA*, **77**, 4539 (1980)) synthesized covalently linked toxin–antibody complexes using the A chain of diphtheria toxin or of ricin and a monoclonal antibody directed against colorectal carcinoma antigens. The conjugates showed toxicity for the colorectal cells in culture but not for a variety of other cell lines.

(g) Gilliland and Collier (*Cancer Res.*, **40**, 3564 (1980)) reported that when the A chain of diphtheria toxin was covalently bonded to anti-Concanavalin A antibodies the resulting conjugate was selectively toxic for cells bearing Concanavalin A on their surfaces.

(h) Philpott *et al.* (*J. Immunol.*, **125**, 1201 (1980)) used IgE as a cytotoxic carrier to destroy rat basophilic leukaemia cells which have surface receptors for IgE.

(i) Hess *et al.* (*Eur. J. Clin. Inv.*, **10**, 93 (1980)) found that digoxin-specific sheep $F(ab')_2$-antibody fragments were sufficiently effective in reversing digitoxin-induced tachycardia in cats to warrant their clinical use.

Chapter 14

Immunological Studies on Parasites

Leslie Hudson

*Department of Immunology, St George's Hospital Medical School,
London, UK*

and

David Snary

*Department of Immunochemistry,
Wellcome Research Laboratories, Beckenham, Kent, UK*

I. INTRODUCTION

The incidence of parasitic disease and of scientists studying parasites is increasing. Fortunately, the latter seems to be growing at a faster rate. In this review we have not even attempted to do justice to what is now an immense field: the immunology of host–parasite relations. Instead, we have considered the limited past successes, the current major problems, and some of the approaches by which these problems might be overcome.

The role of immunology in the study of infection and control of disease is both ancient and modern.

The basic principles by which infection is resisted, becomes established or is overcome have been known for many years. Although spectacular success has been achieved in the immunological control of infectious diseases of viral and bacterial origin, the obvious lack of success in parasitic diseases has endowed them with almost magical and sinister qualities. At present the balance is entirely in the parasites' favour; they have evolved complex and fascinating mechanisms that allow them to survive and multiply in an immunologically hostile environment.

Much of the research over the last two decades has concentrated on the demonstration of acquired immunity without attempting to investigate its basis, control, and potential exploitation for immunoprophylaxis. It is clear that progress towards effective immunoprophylaxis will only come with a more detailed understanding of the molecular basis of the host–parasite relationship.

It is not necessary to justify the search for effective immunoprophylactic methods purely in terms of the limited success achieved with drugs or vector control; parasites do provoke a vigorous immune response, although immunity (protection) is rarely complete and is often only achieved after long-term repeated exposure.

A. Scope

Although the state of parasitism is found throughout the animal kingdom, parasites rarely produce overt disease and only few parasites, those of man and his domestic animals, are considered to be economically important.

This review is intended to reflect the current trends of research and so is limited to those parasites that are at present the subject of intense interest. Even so, the remit is immense, such that it has been necessary to concentrate on specific approaches from particular systems that might have wider implications in future studies.

The main parasites of man and his domestic animals are listed in Table 1.

II. PARASITE MECHANISMS OF SURVIVAL

The quality of the immune response provoked by parasites is not special, on the contrary, parasites are excellent immunogens that can stimulate both the specific and non-specific elements of the immune response. It is surprising, therefore, that parasitic infection is almost invariably chronic and often associated with lingering, debilitating disease which can completely obscure the existence of immunity. It is probable that parasites owe their undoubted success to the complex series of mechanisms described below by which they evade or compromise the immune system.

A. Antigenic Variation

The plasma membrane of African trypanosomes is covered by a surface coat composed of a virtually single molecular species of glycoprotein. In a susceptible host, a population of trypanosomes develops which express one predominant antigen type of coat protein. Under immune pressure, probably an antibody response against this coat protein (Vickerman, 1974), the trypanosomes are eliminated, only to be replaced by many subsequent populations each displaying entirely different coat proteins (Mansfield, 1978). There is tentative evidence that *Plasmodium* (Brown, 1977), *Babesia* (Doyle, 1977), and *Schistoma* (Smith and Clegg, 1979) might also change their antigenic properties during the course of infection.

The molecular basis of antigenic variation is discussed later in this chapter (Section IV. E).

B. Acquisition of Host Characteristics

Upon entry into an unsensitized host, invasive forms of *Schistosoma* are able to adsorb host antigens to their surface in advance of the developing immune response (Clegg *et al.*, 1971; Sell and Dean, 1972). It is probable that this mechanism facilitates the survival of adult schistosomes in an immune host capable of resisting a second challenge of invasive forms (Smithers, 1976).

Athough there is evidence that blood-stream forms of *Trypanosoma vivax* (Ketteridge, 1972), *T. gambiense* (Seed, 1974), and *T. lewisi* (Dwyer, 1976) also adsorb host plasma proteins, it has not been established whether this phenomenon is essential for their survival.

An equally effective way of attaining host characteristics and evading the immune response is to seek an immunologically privileged intracellular site. Parasites have exploited virtually every available host cell type in this way, even to the extent of invading the very doyens of the immune system, the macrophages (*Trypansoma cruzi, Toxoplasma*) or the lymphocytes themselves (*Theileria*).

C. Interference with the Host's Immune Response

Several mechanisms for specific and non-specific interference with the induction and expression of the host's immune response have been suggested, but, as yet, not all have been systematically investigated. Their overall importance may be inferred from their diverse nature:

(i) Many animal species have been shown to have a generally depressed response to specific immunization when infected with various protozoa and worms. Suppression tends to involve humoral rather than cell-mediated immunity (e.g. in *Babesia* infections of mice; see Purvis, 1977) and might be mediated by an increased number of suppressor T lymphocytes or antigenic competition in the common macropohage pathway of 'antigen processing'.

(ii) The basic malevolence of parasitic infection may be appreciated by the massive, but ineffective, humoral immune response induced by malarial or trypanosome infections where a reversal of the immunoglobulin/albumin concentrations in the serum can occur. It has been suggested (Greenwood, 1974), with some evidence, that these parasites secrete 'polyclonal activators' which stimulate a large proportion of lymphocytes without regard to antigen specifity. This would explain why anti-parasite antibody is such a small fraction of the total immunoglobulin elicited during infection with these parasites.

(iii) The secretion or excretion of soluble exoantigens is a feature of virtually all parasitic infections. Clearly, these antigens might be capable of blocking immune induction or effector mechanisms, for example, by

Table 1. Major parasites of man and domestic animals*

Organism	Disease	Vertebrate host of clinical or economic importance	Invertebrate host	Laboratory maintenance
PROTOZOA				
Plasmodium Several spp. *P. falciparum* most serious	Malaria	Man	Mosquito	Primates; but some rodent-specific species as laboratory models *In vitro* culture in human erythrocytes
Trypanosoma Several spp. (a) *T. brucei*, and subspecies	African trypanosomiasis or 'sleeping sickness'	Man and cattle	Tsetse-fly	Rodents. *In vitro* culture in liquid media or mammalian continuous cell lines
(b) *T. cruzi*	American trypanosomiasis or Chagas's disease	Man	Reduvid or 'kissing bug'	Rodent, but rabbit and dog models for pathological studies liquid media or mammalian cell lines

Parasite	Disease	Host	Vector	Laboratory maintenance
Leishmania Several spp.	Several names related to the nature of the disease	Man	Sand-fly	Mice. *In vitro* culture in liquid media or cell lines
Piroplasms (a) *Babesia*	Babesiasis or 'cattle tick fever'	Cattle	Tick	Cattle, or splenectomized calves for attenuation. Rodent-specific species as laboratory models
(b) *Theileria*	Theileriosis or 'East Coast fever'	Cattle	Tick	Cattle. *In vitro* culture in bovine lymphoblastoid cell lines
RIKETTSIA *Anaplasma*	Anaplasmosis	Cattle	Tick	Cattle. Sheep or deer for attenuation
METAZOA *Schistosoma* Several spp.	Schistosomiasis or bilharziasis	Man	Snail	Mouse or hamster. Snail for production infective cercarial forms

*Severally clinical important helminth parasites have not yet been adapted to routine laboratory maintenance, for example *Onchocera*.

complexing with circulating antibodies at a site remote from the parasite or by the formation of 'blocking' immune complexes in a manner similar to that described (but equally, not understood) in tumour systems (Bansal *et al.*, 1972).

Although the precise origin of these exoantigens has not been determined, they do show serological cross-reactions with intact parasites. They are probably produced by at least two mechanisms:(a) active—shedding or secretion; and (b) passive—accelerated membrane turnover, induced by antibody, or immune lysis of parasites.

(iv) Parasites that normally reside in macrophages have evolved mechanisms by which they gain entry via a phagocytic vesicle and then either escape into the cell's cytoplasm (e.g. *Trypanosoma cruzi* ; see Nogueira *et al.*, 1977) or prevent their own digestion by stopping lysosome–phagosome fusion (e.g. *Toxoplasma*; see Hirsch et al., 1974).

(v) Fabulation is a mechanism that has thus far only been described for free-living ciliates (Eisen and Tallan, 1977) but it is such an elegant mechanism that we feel that some parasite must be using it somewhere. Briefly, if *Tetrahymena* organisms are immobilized by antibodies attached to their cilia, they rapidly regain motility using membrane-bound proteolytic enzymes to cleave each divalent IgG molecule into monovalent Fab fragments. The Fab fragments remain attached to the cilia and so prevent further hindrance by more antibody of the same type.

III. STUDIES ON IMMUNOPROPHYLAXIS

The apparent contradiction in the observation that parasites provoke an efficient immune response and yet still produce infection, and often disease, is a function of the complexity of the parasite's mechanisms of survival. In the majority of the parasite systems studied it is clear that significant, or complete, clinical protection can be achieved under well-defined laboratory conditions. Although well-defined conditions do not prevail in Nature, it is only through the simplicity provided by a defined system that a valid approach can be made to the production of candidate vaccines.

A. Laboratory Models

Ethical considerations do not allow the immediate testing of vaccines on human subjects and so great reliance must be placed on laboratory models, often modelling both the host and the parasite, for example, the use of *Babesia rodhaini* in mice as a model of *Babesia argentina* in cattle.

1. Experimental Host

For obvious reasons, the mouse or rat is usually the host of choice for studies of the immune response against parasites, particularly where the rodent is susceptible to infection with the human pathogen. Because it has been found that regimes giving good rodent protection are often ineffective in other species, the initial rodent screen is almost invariably followed by tests on primate species before proceeding to clinical trials.

Inter-host variation can also be a problem within the same species, for example, the difference in *Leishmania* infection between two genetically inbred strains of mice has been found to be as great as that between two different host species (Blackwell *et al.*, 1980).

2. Parasite

In the extreme case (e.g. *Trypanosoma brucei*), protection has only been found when the same species, strain, and even clone of parasite is used for immunization and challenge (Cross, 1975). Fortunately, this is not the finding in the majority of systems studied, for example, there is evidence for good inter-species protection in *Plasmodium* (Nussenzweig, 1977) and *Schistosoma* (Smithers, 1976).

In cases where protection is related to the parasite strain and where the number of strains in a natural challenge is limited (for example, vaccination against bovine babesiosis; see Callow, 1977) it has been possible to immunize with several strains, either consecutively or as a mixture.

3. Immunization Schedule

Although the ideal anti-parasite vaccine would require a single inoculation of a low concentration of parasite antigen, available evidence suggests that the anti-parasite immune response is highly dose dependent and develops only after long-term immunization at frequent intervals (for example, immune response to malarial sporozoites in rodents and primates; (Nussenzweig 1977).

4. Nature of Challenge

The challenge infection is the only valid method currently available for assessing the degree of host protection. For reliability, the challenging infection should parallel natural conditions as far as possible, for example using the life cycle stage transmitted by the invertebrate host in a graded series representing multiples of the natural challenge dose. Although sometimes inconvenient, it is often highly advantageous to assess protection using parasites derived from the invertebrate host. For example, mice immunized with killed *T. cruzi* organisms can control challenge with bug-derived parasites and yet still be susceptible to an artificial syringe-passaged blood infection (Hudson, L. Unpublished observations).

5. Adjuvant Requirements

In studies on malaria, it has been found that attenuated (γ-irradiated) live sporozoite vaccines do not require an adjuvant (Nussenzweig, 1977), whereas killed merozoite vaccines are effective only when administered in complete Freund's adjuvant (Cohen *et al.*, 1977). The need for an effective and clinically acceptable adjuvant is a problem central to virtually every anti-parasite vaccine system intended for human use.

B. Animal Versus Human Vaccines

Because vaccines intended for animal use have to meet less exacting criteria of acceptability and need only provide a measurable economic benefit, rather than complete protection, the application of immunoprohylaxis in animal parasitic diseases is far in advance of its application in humans. Several factors favour the development of vaccines for animal use:

(i) Clinical protection without sterile immunity is acceptable in animal, and perhaps some human, parasitic diseases. However, this would not be acceptable in Chagas' disease, for example, where there is evidence suggesting that any remaining low level chronic infection might still produce overt disease (see Section VI. B).

(ii) Candidate vaccines can often be tested in the host species for which they are intended. The associated time saving is further enhanced by a diminished need to eliminate potential side effects of vaccination, for example, when cattle were immunized against babesiosis, a low incidence of haemolytic anaemia was observed in newborn calves (Langford *et al.*, 1971). This resulted from sensitization of pregnant females with blood group substances contaminating the vaccine preparation. Haemolytic anaemia resulted when the offspring had inherited the same blood group as that contaminating the vaccine.

(iii) As with other infectious organisms, for example, viruses or bacteria, a vaccine based upon live attenuated parasites would be expected to give better long-term protection than a vaccine based upon killed organisms. The relatively short life expectancy of farm animals would lessen the chance of reversion back to full virulence and would limit the problem of infection arising from parasites avoiding the attenuation process. An associated advantage is that adjuvants of high irritancy (granuloma formation) or carcinogenicity (oil-based adjuvants) are not precluded from animal use.

IV. TARGET ANTIGENS FOR VACCINATION

Parasites have complex life cycles with morphologically and biochemically distinct stages. Although an ideal vaccine would protect against all life cycle stages, in practice the choice is usually between the prevention of invasion or the prevention of dissemination of a minimally established infection. This situation is well illustrated by the current studies in malaria immunoprophylaxis using immunization with (a) live, γ-irradiated sporozoites (the mosquito stage which can infect man) (Nussenzweig *et al.*, 1972, Clyde *et al.*, 1975) and (b) killed merozoites (the stage responsible for erythrocyte invasion and reinvasion) plus adjuvant (Cohen *et al.*, 1977).

The use of sporozoite-based vaccines is conceptually attractive in that, if effective, it would afford complete resistance to natural infection. However, as immunity is entirely stage specific (Nussenzweig *et al.*, 1969) it would be necessary to maintain a continuous immune response in those individuals at risk. The time scale required for parasite invasion and stage transformation is much less than that required to reactivate a quiescent immune response. In addition, this regime would be protective only if all invading sporozoites were eliminated immediately upon entry into the immunized host.

Merozoite-based vaccines have the advantage that protection is not stage specific (reviewed Cohen *et al.*, 1977) and in simian models have allowed virtually complete survival, with a transient reduced parasitaemia, against homologous and heterologous variant challenge. Unfortunately, as mentioned previously, they have the gross disadvantage of a total reliance on complete Freund's adjuvant for their effect.

Although whole-organism vaccines might, on present evidence, be acceptable for use against human malaria it is known that this would be unacceptable in other systems, for example, *T. cruzi* infection and Chagas' disease. *Trypanosoma cruzi* organisms possess antigens that show serological cross-reactivity with host tissues (Reviewed in Teixeira, 1979). The possibility that vaccination with whole organisms might lead to human disease by an autoimmune mechanism indicates that in this disease a potential vaccine would have to be based upon purified protective antigens, free of potentially cross-reactive components (Hudson and Ribeiro dos Santos, 1980).

A. Protective Antigens

The identification of parasite antigens which are capable of inducing protective immunity is important. This statement is especially true when vaccines using the whole organism cannot be used either because, for reasons such as antigenic competition, they do not protect or because the presence of cross-reacting antigens means the vaccines themselves may be harmful (Teixeira *et al.*, 1975).

Attempts have been made to identify protective antigens in *T. cruzi* using sera from infected patients (Afchain *et al.*, 1970). However, even a single-celled organism such as *T. cruzi* is antigenically complex and gives rise to an even more complex spectrum of antibodies. In addition, it may be argued that this approach might define the very antigens one wishes to avoid, that is, those which elicit a vigorous but ineffective immune response.

An alternative approach is to define certain characteristics which a protective antigen should possess and use these criteria to select antigens for further study. In studying *T. cruzi* we have selected antigens according to the following criteria:

(i) They should be common to all stages of the life cycle.
(ii) They should be major antigens, this is essential if preparative techniques are to yield enough material for characterization.
(iii) They should be derived from the cell surface, thus ensuring that the antigens are readily available to immune effector mechanisms.

It is possible to apply the constraints listed above to studies on *T. cruzi*, but they may not be as applicable to other systems, for example, it may not be possible to identify protective antigens in *Plasmodium* species which are common throughout the life cycle (Miller, 1977).

Studies of the type to be discussed have one essential prerequisite; a reliable supply of defined parasite material in sufficient quantities. Fortunately, the major blood protozoan parasites can now be produced by *in vitro* culture (*Plasmodium*—Trager and Jensen, 1976; *T. brucei*—Hirumi *et al.*, 1977 *T. cruzi*—Pan, 1978). However, multicellular parasites such as *Schistosoma* cannot yet be grown continuously *in vitro*, and shortage of material for antigen characterization studies is a serious limitation.

Evidence is available for protozoa to support the notion that important protective antigens will be cell surface in origin. Cell surface antigens (Snary and Scott, 1979) and cell surface membrane (Segura *et al.*, 1977) of *T. cruzi* are capable of inducing protective immunity. The origins of protective antigens in multicellular parasites is less clear, it is possible that protection might be achieved by neutralization of important secretory products (Sadun and Lin, 1959), although there is evidence to suggest that cell surface structures still might be the most likely origin of protective antigens (Hayunga *et al.*, 1979).

B. Antigen Identification

Two alternative approaches have been used: (a) isolated surface membranes have been prepared by subcellular fractionation techniques; or (b) biochemical and immunological probes have been used to label the membrane of the intact cell before breakage. Both approaches have been applied to *T. cruzi* and the results of these studies will be reviewed in detail below.

C. Plasma Membrane Preparation from *Trypanosoma cruzi*

Purified plasma (surface) membrane fractions are known to be capable of inducing protective immunity, but little work has yet been reported on the detailed characterization of these preparations.

It is possible that cell breakage is the most critical stage in the preparation of plasma membranes. The type and intensity of disruptive sheer forces used determines the nature of the membrane vesicles formed. There are also important biochemical considerations, for example, *T. cruzi* organisms contain high concentrations of membrane-bounded proteases that are released by cell breakage (Itow and Camargo, 1977). If these proteases are not inactivated or removed they rapidly degrade the disrupted membranes.

Flagellar and surface membrane fractions have been prepared from epimastigotes using either a Ribi cell disintegrator (Segura *et al.*, 1977) or by Dounce homogenization after hypotonic shock treatment (Pereira *et al.*, 1978). Highly purified plasma membrane has also been recovered by inducing epimastigotes to release membrane vesicles by treatment with acetate buffer at pH 4 (da Silveira *et al.*, 1979).

The membrane preparations recovered from *T. cruzi* all appear to have been isolated free of their subcellular microtubule array. A method has been described for the isolation of membranes from *T. brucei* using hypotonic shock and Dounce homogenization which produces membranes which still have associated microtubules (Voorheis *et al.*, 1979). It is possible that membranes prepared in this manner approximate more closely to the intact cell surface and so may be more suitable for studies which require the preservation of functional properties.

D. Immunological Probes

The approaches included in this section have relied on the specificity of antibodies in the detection of potentially important antigens.

1. Immunochemical Techniques

Immunoelectrophoretic techniques have been applied to trypanosome species with some success (Afchain *et al.*, 1979), although it is probable that the analytically more powerful technique of crossed immune electrophoresis will now supersede the original methods. In this new procedure antigen is separated by electrophoresis in one dimension in agarose and then electrophoresed in the second dimension into an agarose gel containing immune sera.

Precipitin arcs are produced which are readily detected and enumerated. This technique has been applied to a study of *Plasmodium knowlesi* (Deans *et al.*, 1978).

The separation given by immunoelectrophoresis can be exploited to generate antisera specific for individual parasite components. It is possible to recover single precipitin arcs from a complex immune electrophoresis pattern and, by immunizing animals with the immune complex, produce antisera specific for the parasite antigen in the precipitin arc (Afchain *et al.*, 1978). In studies on *T. cruzi* the precipitin arc against a protein designated 'component 5' was used to produce an antiserum which allowed 'component 5' to be identified at the cell surface (Fruit *et al.*, 1978). As these studies were performed primarily with acqueous extracts of *T. cruzi*, 'component 5' is either not an integral membrane component or is the hydrophilic part of an integral membrane component released by proteolysis during extraction. No information is available on the ability of 'component 5' to confer protection by immunization.

2. Somatic Cell Hybridization

The recent production, by somatic cell fusion, of hybrid cells secreting monoclonal antibodies should significantly increase the use of immunological probes for the identification of antigens. (Monoclonal antibodies are discussed in detail in Chapter 9.) Briefly, spleen cells from immune mice or rats are fused with non-secreting plasmocytoma cell lines to produce hybrid cells, secreting specific antibodies, which are then selected and cloned. In this way complex mixtures of antigens can be analysed and the antibodies generated used for immune affinity chromatography for the purification of antigens. Because this approach has been used very successfully in the study of rat thymocyte membrane antigens (McMaster and Williams, 1979), its application to parasites is obvious and will be, without doubt, equally successful. Monoclonal antibodies capable of conferring passive protection against *Plasmodium yoelii* have already been prepared (Freeman *et al.*, 1980) and have specificity for the merozoite stage of the life cycle.

Monoclonal antibodies have been used to identify a sporozoite-specific protein with a molecular weight of 44,000 daltons on the surface of *Plasmodium berghei* sporozoites. Pretreatment of sporozoites with the monoclonal antibody before infection of mice protected the mice from the lethal effects of the malaria (Yoshid *et al.*, 1980). The protection mediated by this antibody should be stage specific and any sporozoite which escapes to develop into a merozoite could produce clinical malaria.

3. Serodiagnosis

It is perhaps in the area of serodiagnosis that the real advantages of monoclonal antibodies will be seen. The high degree of specificity that can be achieved with these antibodies has been exploited in the serodiagnosis of infection by the cestode *Mesocestoides corti* (Mitchell *et al.*, 1979). The current techniques for the serodiagnosis of *T. cruzi* infection can give positive reactions when individuals are infected with other trypanosomes (Kagan *et al.*, 1978). Development of methods which utilize specific monoclonal antibodies should alleviate this problem.

E. Cell Surface Specific Labels

Reagents capable of labelling proteins or carbohydrates which cannot transverse lipid bilayers have been extremely useful in the study of cell surface antigens. Studies which have involved labelling cell surface proteins with ^{125}I using lactoperoxidase have been carried out on trypanosomes (Snary and Hudson, 1979; Rovis *et al.*, 1978) and schistosomes (Ramasamy, 1979). In addition, the *N*-acylating reagent, [35S]formylmethionine sulphone, has been used to label specifically the cell surface variant antigen of *T. brucei* (Cross, 1975). Specific labelling of cell surface carbohydrates/glycoproteins using NaB^3H_4 and galactose oxidase has also been applied to studies on trypanosomes, (Alves *et al.*, 1979, Rovis *et al.*, 1978).

Studies on *T. cruzi* using cell surface labelling techniques have demonstrated the presence of many cell surface antigens, the majority of which are present throughout the life cycle (Snary and Hudson, 1979). This result is in contrast to that achieved with African trypanosomes where the blood-stream trypomastigotes express only one antigen (Cross, 1975; Rovis *et al.*, 1978). Application of lectin affinity chromatography (for example, with the lectin from *Lens culinaris* which has affinity for glucose and mannose) to the fractionation of ^{125}I]lactoperoxidase-labelled cell surface antigens of *T. cruzi* demonstrated that only one of the many iodinated surface components was a glycoprotein. Furthermore, this glycoprotein was antigenically constant, not only throughout the life cycle, but also among a series of different strains (Snary, 1980). Indeed, this glycoprotein fraction of *T. cruzi* fulfils many of the requirements listed above, for a candidate vaccine:

(i) It elicits a protective immune response in mice when injected with complete Freund's adjuvant or saponin (Scott and Snary, 1979).

(ii) It does not contain determinants which cross-react with human heart and nerve tissue (Scott and Snary, 1979).

(iii) It is a major cell surface component which does not vary antigenically throughout the parasite's life cycle (Snary, 1980).

(iv) It can be readily isolated from *in vitro* culture-derived organisms (Snary and Hudson, 1979).

It must be stressed, however, that although immunization with this antigen reduced parasitaemia and mortality during the acute infection: protection was

Table 2. Composition of lipopolysaccharide from *Trypanosoma cruzi*

		Per cent by weight*	
Carbohydrate	galactose	23 ⎫	
	mannose	36 ⎪	
	glucose	1.0 ⎬	63.3
	glucosamine	0.8 ⎪	
	inositol	2.5 ⎭	
Protein			9.5
Phosphate			2.0
Fatty acids	palmitic	6.9 ⎫	
	lignoceric	4.6 ⎪	
	stearic	0.6 ⎬	12.5
	oleic	0.2 ⎭	
	myristic	0.2	
Bases	17-methyl sphingamine	4.8 ⎫	
	sphingamine	1.5 ⎬	6.3

*Data compiled from de Lederkremer *et al.*, 1977, 1978.

not complete. The few parasites surviving in the immunized host might still produce pathology, albeit reduced, in the chronic phase (Teixeira, 1979).

Specific labelling of cell surface carbohydrate of *T. cruzi* by galactose oxidase and NaB^{3}H$_4$ gives a rather different result from that described above when lectin affinity chromatography and lactoperoxidase were used. The galactose oxidase method labelled a lipopolysaccharide and three glycoproteins on the surface of *T. cruzi*. The three glycoproteins have molecular weights much lower (in the region of 30,000 daltons) than the 90,000 dalton glycoprotein identified by [^{125}I]lactoperoxidase label and lectin affinity chromatography. Phenol extraction has been used to isolate these three low molecular weight glycoproteins and the lipopolysaccharide, and the lipopolysaccharide further purified (de Lederkremer *et al.*, 1977). This lipopolysaccharide, which the authors have described very aptly as a lipopeptidophosphoglycan, has an unusual composition (Table 2) for a eukaryoptic cell constituent, although a similar lipopolysaccharide has been found in *Acanthamoeba castellanii* (Korn *et al.*, 1974). The structure isolated from *T. cruzi* is unusual in that it contains high levels of neutral sugars, phospholipid components, and amino acids. The similarity of these components to bacterial lipopolysaccharides suggests that they, or similar compounds, may be responsible for endotoxin-type properties associated with some protozoa, (Seneca *et al.*, 1966; Clark, 1978). (See polyclonal activation Section II. C). The phenol extracted glycoproteins and lipopolysaccharides are cell surface in origin (Alves *et al.*, 1979) and, although they are immunogenic, they do not induce protective immunity. As they are found in the serum of infected animals during the acute phase of the disease (Gottlieb, 1977) it is possible that the detection of this antigen could be used as the basis of a diagnostic test.

F. Variant Antigens of *Trypanosoma brucei*

Variant specific antigens of African trypanosomes are a special class of cell surface glycoproteins. The ability of *T. brucei* to avoid the immune response of a host is mediated by the ability of the trypanosome to change its cell surface coat. (The coat is almost entirely composed of variant specific glycoprotein; Cross, 1978.) Amino acid sequence data suggest that the antigenic variants do not arise by point mutations (Bridgen *et al.*, 1976) and, although common determinants have been detected on different variant antigens (Barbet and McGuire, 1978), inhibition studies with isolated glycopeptides suggest that these antigenically common determinants are in the carbohydrate side chains rather than the polypeptide chain (A. A. Holder and G. A. M. Cross, personal communication). The recent reports of the cloning of genes specific for a variant antigen (Williams *et al.*, 1979; Hoeijmakers *et al.*, 1980a,b) is probably the first step in answering many of the outstanding questions concerning antigenic variations, these include : the structural relationships between different variants: the total repertoire of variants capable of being expressed by a single organism; and the exact mechanism involved in the antigenic change. Even though variant-specific antigens are associated with the cell membrane in intact trypanosomes they can be isolated into aqueous solution. The way in which the antigen associates with the membrane through the C-terminal portion of the molecule is still not understood (Cross and Johnson, 1976).

G. Host Cell Modification

Protozoa which invade cells in an attempt to avoid the host's immune response often modify the cell membrane of the invaded cell. In some instances this modification can be passive, for example, in *T. cruzi* both infected and uninfected cells can adsorb parasite antigen to their surface (Ribeiro dos Santos and Hudson, 1980a). The importance of this finding in relation to immunopathology will be discussed at the end of the chapter (Section VI. B).

In malaria the host cell modification appears to be more active. Strain-specific modification of *Plasmodium knowlesi* infected erythrocytes has been detected serologically and shows evidence of antigenic variation (Brown, 1977). Biochemical changes have also been detected (Wallach and Conley, 1977), involving the appearance of a new glycoprotein and the loss of other components. The new antigens which appear on red cells infected by *Plasmodium falciparum* are associated with knob-like protrusions which appear only on infected erythrocytes (Langreath and Reese, 1979). It is believed that the knobs on infected erythrocytes are involved in the adherence of older parasitized erythrocytes to the endothelial cells of vascular tissue (Miller, 1972). Any role the parasite-induced changes of the erythrocyte surface may have in the host's resistance, or potential resistance, to malaria is not yet known.

V. HOST IMMUNE RESPONSE

The immune response of the host to parasite antigens in natural infection and deliberate immunization has been the subject of several recent books and reviews that are strongly recommended to the reader requiring a more detailed treatment of this field (Cohen and Sadun, 1976; Miller *et al.*, 1977; Clegg and Smith, 1978; Dick, 1979).

The parasite genus *Leishmania* deserves a special mention in this section, not because it has been studied in the manner reviewed here for similar parasites, but because it is the only human parasitic infection that is naturally terminated by the host's immune response. After transmission via the sand fly host, the invasive forms of the parasite divide intracellularly to produce a superficial sore which, provided that the host's immune response is normal, is infiltrated by lymphoid cells and usually heals within a few months. Parasite elimination is usually complete and is accompanied by lifelong cell-mediated immunity which is parasite species specific. Only a low concentration of antibody can be detected in the serum of recovered, solidly immune patients.

The central role of the immune response is evidenced by the disseminated infection and serious disease produced by the same parasite in those patients who fail to develop cell-mediated immunity, but instead produce high levels of serum antibody (Turk and Bryceson, 1971).

Further understanding of the precise nature and control of the immune response against parasite antigens is likely to be required before the 'natural' success of the immune system against *Leishmania* infection can be imitated in other parasite infections. Thus, although antibody is thought to play a major role in the control of acute infection of *Plasmodium, T. cruzi* and *T. brucei*, it is possible that sterile immune response might only be achieved with a strong cell-mediated immune response in the absence of high levels of circulating antibody.

A. Successes in Immunoprophylaxis

For reasons mentioned earlier (Section III. B), control of the cattle diseases babesiosis (Callow, 1977) and anaplasmosis (Ristic and Carson, 1977) by immunoprophylaxis is far in advance of similar human studies. *Babesia* organisms are attenuated by passage in young splenectomized calves and the parasitized blood is used to induce low grade infections in susceptible adult cattle. Although vaccinated animals become parasitaemic with a mild fever, they are otherwise clinically protected and fail to develop an acute infection after challenge with virulent organisms (Callow, 1977).

Intriguingly, when *Babesia* is attenuated in the calf host, concomitant with the loss of virulence is a loss of infectivity for the tick invertebrate host. This brings a twofold benefit, firstly, the disease is not transmitted from vaccinated to unvaccinated animals and secondly, if a sufficiently large number of animals can be vaccinated (infected with attenuated organisms) then natural transmission cycles could be broken.

VI. IMMUNOPATHOLOGY

Yet another aspect of the failure of the immune system in parasitic disease is the occurrence of secondary, host induced pathology. Not only is the immune response unable to eliminate those infections which cause disease but also some human parasites are not directly pathogenic, the lesions associated with the disease are often caused by the host's own immune response against parasite antigens. In schistomiasis, for example, the adult worms do not multiply and the eggs do not secrete cytotoxic substances; the 'pipestem' lesions formed in the liver of infected patients are entirely due to the host's immune response.

A. Immune Complexes

Immune complexes are probably a feature of all chronic infections and although they are usually without pathological consequence, they can produce vascular and glomerular lesions. For example, in *P. falciparum* infections immune complexes become deposited in the kidney and produce an acute glomerulonephritis which resolves after curative anti-parasite chemotherapy. By contrast, *P. malariae* infections can result in a chronic, immune complex mediated glomerulonephritis which persists after parasite cure (Reviewed in Casali *et al.*, 1979).

B. Autoimmunity

Although autoimmune phenomena have been recognized in a wide variety of infectious diseases (Glynn, 1979; Boreham, 1979), it has been proposed that in Chagas' disease the autoimmune response is one of the primary pathogenic mechanisms (Texeira *et al.*, 1975; Texeira, 1979). Initial studies showed that *T. cruzi* has antigens in common with human muscle and nervous tissue, and so infection was thought to give rise to cytotoxic humoral and cell-mediated responses that destroyed self tissue (Hudson and Ribeiro dos Santos, 1980).

More recent experimental evidence (Ribeiro dos Santos and Hudson, 1980a,b) indicates that parasite antigens can become associated with the surface membrane of both infected and uninfected host cells. Such parasite-modified cells become susceptible to elements of the host's anti-parasite immune response. If parasite antigen production and subsequent host cell death are sustained over a sufficiently long period then the chronic release of self components might elicit an anti-self immune response (Khoury *et al.*, 1979) which, in genetically predisposed individuals, might become self-sustaining after parasite cure.

Both these sets of observations are of great relevance to the immunop-rophylaxis of *T. cruzi* infection, host sensitizing and cross-reactive antigens would have to be eliminated from a candidate vaccine either by biochemical isolation (Section IV) or, by analogy to the bacterial toxin–toxoid vaccines, by destruction of their membrane binding activity without loss of their immunogenicity.

VII. CONCLUDING REMARKS

Research into the molecular basis of the immune response to parasites still has tremendous scope for development. It is clear, however, that research momentum is building up to the level where the control of malaria and Chagas' disease by immunoprophylaxis seems a real possibility. In leish-maniasis and schistosomiasis more basic work is required on the existing laboratory models, whereas in filariasis valid laboratory models have yet to be developed.

African trypanosomiasis stands alone in that it is the only important parasitic disease where the development of a vaccine is considered as 'perhaps the last practical possibility which would occur to most people whose daily business is concerned with the control of trypanosomiasis in the field' (Murray and Urquhart, 1977). One wonders, therefore, whether the novel approach required to overcome the problem of antigenic variation will have to come from the laboratory?

Much of this review has been devoted, of necessity, to experimental studies of the immune response to parasites rather than to its practical applications. Although it is beyond the scope of this review to deal with practical vaccination, there are several trans-disease problems that need to be solved before the present analytical techniques can be used on a preparative scale:

1. Supply of Antigen

If a candidate vaccine is based upon killed or attenuated whole organisms then it would be necessary to grow the parasite itself on a large scale. However, if protective antigens can be characterized and isolated it is possible to envisage other more biologically convenient techniques for the production of antigens. With *Schistosoma*, for example, it might be possible to establish cell lines, either directly or by fusion with existing eukaryotic cell lines. More compelling, of course, is the use of bacterial or yeast cloning vehicles for the propagation of genes coding for protective antigens, as has already been done for *T. brucei* variant antigens (Williams *et al.*, 1979; Hoeijmakers *et al.*, 1980a,b). The large-scale production of protective antigens by fermentation techniques not only would be cheaper but also, in the case of *T. cruzi*, for example, might simplify the whole problem of removing harmful from protective antigens.

2. Adjuvants

Vaccination studies using killed parasites (Mitchell *et al.*, 1975) or fractions thereof (Scott and Snary, 1979) have relied upon clinically unacceptable adjuvants for their effects. Reports of successful vaccination using clinically acceptable adjuvants are rare.

Selection of cell surface membrane proteins as protective antigens might have distinct advantages when their adjuvant requirements are considered. Vaccination studies using *P. falciparum* merozoite antigens mixed with muramyl dipeptide (MDP) with hydrophobic side chains in liposomes (Siddiqui *et al.*, 1978) suggests that MDP-liposomes act both as carrier and adjuvant for these antigens. Alternatively, work with Semliki forest viral antigens suggests that a liposome might not even be required. When these viral antigens were prepared in the absence of detergent, their hydrophobic tails self-associate to form protein micelles which produced good protective immunity in the absence of adjuvants (Morein *et al.*, 1978).

Although there is still room to doubt the feasibility of parasite control by immunoprophylaxis, there is no doubt that much basic immunological information will be generated by the present intense research interest in host–parasite relations.

ACKNOWLEDGEMENTS

We wish to thank Dr G. A. M. Cross for help and advice, and Margaret Williams for the preparation of the manuscript.

REFERENCES

Afchain, D., Capron, A., and Prata, A. (1970). Les anticorps precipitants dans la trypanosomiase americaine humaine. *Aaz. Med. Bahia*, **70**, 141–147.

Afchain, D., Fruit, J., Yarazabel, L., and Capron, A. (1978). Purification of a specific antigen of *Trypanosoma cruzi* from culture forms. *Am. J. Trop. Med. Hyg.*, **27**, 478–482.

Afchain, D., Le Ray, D., Fruit, J., and Capron, A. (1979). Antigenic make-up of *Trypanosoma cruzi* culture forms: identification of a specific component. *J. Parasitol.*, **65**, 507–514.

Aikawa, M. (1977). Variations in structure and function during the life cycle of malarial parasites. *Bull. WHO*, **55**, 139–156.

Alves, M. J. M., de Silveria, J. F., de Paiva, C. H. R., Tanaka, C. T., and Colli, W. (1979). Evidence for the plasma membrane localization of carbohydrate-containing macromolecules from epimastigote forms of *Trypanosoma cruzi*. *FEBS Lett.*, **99**, 81–85.

Bansal, S. C., Hargreaves, R., and Sjogren, O. (1972). Facilitation of polyoma tumour growth in rats by blocking sera and tumour eluate. *Int. J. Cancer*, **9**, 97–108.

Barbet, A. F. and McGuire, T. C. (1978). Cross-reacting determinants in variant-specific surface antigens of African trypanosomes. *Proc. Natl. Acad. Sci.*, **75**, 1989–1993.

Blackwell, J., Freeman, J., and Bradley, D. (1980). Influence of H-2 complex on acquired resistance to *Leishmania donovani* infection in mice. *Nature*, **283**, 72–74.

Boreham, P. F. L. (1979). The pathogenesis of African and American trypanosomiasis. *Biochim. Physiol. Protozoa*, **2**, 429–457.

Bridgen, P. J., Cross, G. A. M., and Bridgen, J. (1976). *N*-terminal amino acid sequences of variant-specific surface antigens from *Trypanosoma brucei*. *Nature*, **263**, 613–614.

Brown, K. N. (1977). Antigenic variation in malaria. *Adv. Exp. Med. Biol.*, **93**, 5–29.

Callow, L. L. (1977). Vaccination against bovine babesiosis. *Adv. Exp. Med. Biol.*, **93**, 121–149.

Casali, P., Perrin, L. H., and Lambert, P. H. (1979). Immune complexes and tissue injury. In G. Dick (Ed.) *Immunological Aspects of Infectious Diseases*, pp. 295–342. MTP Press.

Clark, I. A. (1978). Does endotoxin cause both disease and parasite death in acute malaria and babesiosis? *Lancet*, **2**, 75–77.

Clegg, J. A. and Smith M. A. (1978). Prospects for the development of dead vaccines against helminths. *Adv. Parasit.*, **16**, 165–218.

Clegg, J. A., Smithers, S. R., and Terry, R. J. (1971). Concomitant immunity and host antigens associated with schistosomiasis. *Int. J. Parasit.*, **1**, 43–49.

Clyde, D. F., McCarthy, V. C., Miller, R. M., and Woodward, W. E. (1975). Immunisation of man against *falciparum* and *vivax* malaria by use of attenuated sporozoites. *Am. J. Trop. Med. Hyg.*, **24**, 397–401.

Cohen, S., Butcher, G. A., and Mitchell, G. H. (1977). Immunisation against erythrocytic forms of malaria parasites. *Adv. Exp. Med. Biol.*, **93**, 89–112.

Cohen, S. and Sadun, E. (Eds.) (1976). Immunology of parasitic infections. Blackwell Scientific Publications, Oxford.

Cross, G. A. M. (1975). Identification, purification and properties of clone-specific glycoprotein antigens constituting the surface coat of *Trypanosoma brucei*. *Parasitology*, **71**, 393–417.

Cross, G. A. M. (1978). Antigenic variation in trypanosomes. *Proc. R. Soc. Lond. B*, **202**, 55–72.

Cross, G. A. M. and Johnson, J. G. (1976). Structure and organisation of the variant-specific antigens of *Trypanosoma brucei*. In van den Bossche (Ed.) *Biochemistry of Parasites and Host–Parasite Relationships*, pp. 413–420. Elsevier, Amsterdam.

Deans, J. A., Dennis, E. D., and Cohen, S. (1978). Antigenic analysis of sequential erythrocytic stages of *Plasmodium knowlesi*. *Parasitology*, **77**, 333–344.

Dick, G. (Ed.) (1978). *Immunological Aspects of Infectious Diseases*. MTP Press.

Doyle, J. J. (1977). Antigenic variation in *Babesia*. *Adv. Exp. Med. Biol.*, **93**, 27–29.

Dwyer, D. M. (1976). Immunological and fine structure evidence of avidly bound host serum proteins in the surface coat of a bloodstream trypanosome. *Proc. Natl. Acad. Sci.*, **73** (4), 1222–1226.

Eisen, H. and Tallan, I. (1977). *Tetrahymena pyriformis* recovers from antibody immobilisation by producing univalent antibody fragments. *Nature*, **270**, 514–515.

Freeman, R. R., Trejdosiewiez, A. J., and Cross, G. A. M. (1980). Protective antibodies recognizing stage-specific merozoite antigens of a rodent malaria parasite. *Nature*, **284**, 366–368.

Fruit, J., Afchain, D., Petitprez, A., and Capron, A. (1978). *Trypanosoma cruzi*: location of a specific antigen on the surface of bloodstream trypomastigote and culture epimastigote forms. *Exp. Parasitol.*, **45**, 183–189.

Glynn, L, E. (1979). In G. Dick (Ed.) *Autoimmunity in Infectious Diseases*, pp. 389–420. MTP Press.

Gottlieb, M. (1977). A carbohydrate containing antigen from *Trypanosoma cruzi* and its detection in the circulation of infected mice. *J. Immunol.*, **119**, 465–470.

Greenwood, B. N. (1974). Possible role of B-cell mitogen in hypergammaglobulinaemia in malaria and trypanosomiasis. *Lancet*, **1**, 435.

Hayunga, E. G., Murrell, K. D., Taylor, D. W., and Vannier, W. E. (1979). Isolation and characterisation of surface antigens from *Schistosoma mansoni*. *J. Parasitol.*, **65**, 497–506.

Hirsch, J. G., Jones, T. C., and Len, L. (1974). Interaction *in vitro* between Toxoplasma gondii and mouse cells. In Porter and Knight (Eds.) *Parasites in the Immunised Host: mechanisms of survival*, p. 205. Associated Science Publishers, Amsterdam.

Hirumi, H., Doyle, J. J., and Hirumi, K. (1977). African trypanosomes: cultivation of animal-infective *Trypanosoma brucei in vitro*. *Science*, **196**, 992–994.

Hoeijmakers, J. H. J., Borst, P., van den Burg, J., Weissmann, C., and Cass, G. A. M. (1980a).Isolation of plasmids containing DNA complementary to messenger RNA for variant surface glycoproteins of *Trypanosoma brucei*. *Gene*, **8**, 391–497.

Hoeijmakers, J. H. J., Frasch, A. C. C., Bernards, A., Borst, P., and Cross, G. A. M. (1980b). Expression of variant surface antigen in trypanosomes is associated with the appearance of an altered copy of the gene coding for the antigen. *Nature*, **284**, 78–80.

Hudson, L. and Ribeiro dos Santos, R. (1981). Immunological aspects of chagasic cardiopathy. In H. Lessof (Ed.) *Immunological Aspects of Cardiovascular Disease*. Marcel Dekker pp 141–155.

Itow, S. and Camargo, E. P. (1977). Proteolytic activities in cell extracts of *Trypanosoma cruzi*. *J. Protozool.*, **24**, 591–595.

Kagan, I. G., Goldsmith, R. S., Zarate-Castaneda, R., and Allain, D. S. (1978). Evaluation of serologic tests for studies on Chagas' disease. *Bull. Pan. Am. Hlth. Org.*, **12**, 341–348.

Ketteridge, D. S. (1972). *Trypanosoma vivax*: surface interrelationships between host and parasite. *Trans. R. Soc. Trop. Med. Hyg.*, **66**, 324.

Khoury, E. L. *et al.* (1979). Circulating antibodies to peripheral nerve in American trypanosomiasis. (Chagas' disease). *Clin. Exp. Immunol.*, **36** (1), 8–15.

Korn, E. D., Dearborn, D. G., and Wright, P. L. (1974). Lipophosphoglycan of the plasma membrane of *Acanthamoeba castellanii*. *J. Biol. Chem.*, **249**, 3335–3341.

Langford, G., Knot, S. G., Dimmock, C. K., and Derrington, P. (1971). Haemolytic disease of newborn calves in a dairy herd in Queensland. *Aust. Vet. J.*, **47**, 1–4.

Langreth, S. G. and Reese, R. T. (1979). Antigenicity of the infected-erythrocyte and merozoite surfaces in *falciparum* malaria. *J. Exp. Med.*, **150**, 1241–1254.

de Lederkremer, R. M., Casal, O. L., Tanaka, C. T., and Colli, W. (1978). Ceramide and inositol content of the lipopeptidophosphoglycan from *Trypanosoma cruzi*. *Biochem. Biophys. Res. Comm.*, **85**, 1268–1274.

de Lederkremer, R. M., Tanaka, C. T., Alves, M. J. M., and Colli, W. (1977). Lipopeptidophosphoglycan from *Trypanosoma cruzi*. *Eur. J. Biochem.*, **74**, 263–267.

McMaster, W. R. and Williams, A. F. (1979). Identification of Ia glycoproteins in rat thymus and purification from rat spleen. *Eur. J. Immunol.*, **9**, 426–433.

Mansfield, J. M. (1978). Immunobiology of African Trypanosomiasis. *Cell. Immunol.*, **39**, 204–210.

Miller, L. H. (1972). The ultrastructure of red cells infected by *Plasmodium falciparum* in Man. *Trans. R. Soc. Trop. Med. Hyg.*, **66**, 459–462.

Miller, L. M. (1977). A critique of merozoite and sporozoite vaccines in malaria. In L. H. Miller, J. A. Pine, and J. J. McKelvey (Eds.) *Immunity to Blood Parasites*, pp. 113–120. Plenum Press, New York.

Miller, L. H., Pino, J. A., and McKelvey, J. J. (Eds.) (1977). Immunity to blood parasites of animals and man. In *Advances in Experimental Medical Biology*, volume 93, Plenum Publ. Corp., New York.

Mitchell, G. F., Cruise, K. M., Chapman, C. B., Anders, R. F., and Howard, M. C. (1979). Hybridoma antibody immunoassays for the detection of parasitic infection: development of a model system using a larval cestode infection in mice. *Aust. J. Exp Biol. Med. Sci.*, **57**, 287–302.

Mitchell, G. H., Butcher, G. A., and Cohen, S. (1975). Merozoite vaccination against *Plasmodium knowlesi* malaria. *Immunology*, **29**, 397–407.

Morein, B., Helenius, A., Simons, H., Pettersson, R., Kaariarnen, L., and Schirrmacher, V. (1978). Effective subunit vaccines against enveloped animal virus. *Nature*, **276**, 715–718.

Murray, M. and Urquhart, G. M. (1977). Immunoprophylaxis against African trypanosmiasis. *Adv. Exp. Med. Biol.*, **93**, 209–241.

Nogueira, N., Gordon, S. and Cohen, Z. (1979). *Trypanosoma cruzi*: modification of macrophage function during infection. *J. Exp. Med.*, **146** (1), 157–171.

Nussenzweig, R. S. (1977). Immunoprophylaxis of malaria: sporozoite-induced immunity. *Adv. Exp. Med. Biol.*, **93**, 75–87.

Nussenzweig, R. S., Vanderberg, J. P., Most, H., and Orton, C. (1969). Specificity of protective immunity produced by X-irradiated *Plasmodium berghei* sporozoites. *Nature*, **222**, 488–489.

Nussenzweig, R. S., Vanderberg, J., Spitalny, G. L., Rivera, CIO, Orton, C., and Most, H. (1972). Sporozoite-induced immunity in mammalian malaria. A review. *Am. J. Trop. Med. Hyg.*, **21**, 722–728.

Pan, S. C. (1978). *Trypanosoma cruzi*: Cultivation in a macromolecule-free semisynthetic and synthetic media. *Exp. Parasitol.*, **46**, 108–112.

Pereira, N. M.,Timm, S. L., da Costa, S. C. G., Rabello, M. A., and de Souza, W. (1978). *Trypanosoma cruzi*: isolation and characterisation of membrane and flagellar fractions. *Exp. Parasitol.*, **46**, 225–234.

Purvis, A. C. (1977). Immunodepression to *Babesia microti* infection. *Parasitology*, **75**, 197.

Ramasmy, R. (1979). Surface proteins of schistosomula and cercaria of *Schistosoma mansoni*. *Internat. J. Parasitol.*, **9**, 491–493.

Ribeiro dos Santos, R. and Hudson, L. (1980a). *Trypanosoma cruzi*: adsorption of parasite antigens to mammalian cell surfaces. *Parasite Immunol.*, 2 1–10.

Ribeiro dos Santos, R. and Hudson, L. (1980b). *Trypanosoma cruzi*: immunological consequences of parasite modification of host cells. *Clin. Exp. Immunol.*, **40**, 36–41.

Ristic, M. and Carson, C. A. (1977). Methods of immunoprophylaxis against bovine anaplasmosis with emphasis on use of the attenuated *Anaplasma marginale* vaccine. *Adv. Exp. Med. Biol.*, **93**, 158–188.

Rovis, L., Barbet, A. F., and Williams, R. O. (1978). Characterisation of the surface coat of *Trypanosoma congolense*. *Nature*, **271**, 654–656.

Sadun, E. H. and Lin, S. S. (1959). Studies on the host–parasite relationhsip of *Schistosoma japonicum*. IV. Resistance acquired by infection, by vaccination, and by injection of immune serum, in monkeys, rabbits and mice. *J. Parasitol.*, **45**, 543–547.

Scott, M. T. and Snary, D. (1979). Protective immunisation of mice using cell surface glycoprotein from *Trypanosoma cruzi*. *Nature*, **282**, 73–74.

Seed, J. R. (1974). Antigens and antigenic variability of the African trypanosomes. *J. Protozool.*, **21**, 639–646.

Sell, K. W. and Dean, D. A. (1972). Demonstration of host antigens on schistosomula and adult worms using the mixed antiglobulin test. *Clin. Exp. Immunol.*, **12**, 315.

Segura, E. L., Vazquez, C., Bronzina, A., Campas, J. M., Cerisola, J. A., and Gonzalez-Cappa, S. M. (1977). Antigens of the subcellular fractions of *Trypanosoma cruzi*. II. Flagellar and membrane fraction. *J. Protozool.*, **24**, 540–543.

Seneca, H., Per, P., and Hampar, B. (1966). Active immunisation of mice with chagastoxin. *Nature*, **209**, 309–310.

Siddiqui, W. A., Taylor, D. W., Kan, S. C., Kramer, K., Richmond-Crum, S. M., Kotani, S., Shiba, T., and Kusumoto, S. (1978). Vaccination of experimental monkeys against *Plasmodium falciparum*: a possible safe adjuvant. *Science*, **201**, 1237–1239.

da Silveiaa, J. F., Abrahamsohn, P. A., and Colli, W. (1979). Plasma membrane vesicles isolated from epimastigote forms of *Trypanosoma cruzi*. *Biochem. Biophys. Acta*, **550**, 222–232.

Smith, M. A. and Clegg, J. A. (1979). Different levels of immunity to *Schistosoma mansoni* in the mouse: the role of variant cercariae. *Parasitology*, **78** (3), 311–321.

Smithers, S. R. (1976). Immunity to trematode infections. In Cohen and Sadun (Eds.) *Immunology of Parasitic Infections*, p. 296. Blackwell Scientific Publications.

Snary, D. (1980). *Trypanosoma cruzi*: Antigenic invariance of the cell surface glycoprotein. *Exp. Parasitol.*, **49**, 68–77.

Snary, D. and Hudson, L. (1979). *Trypanosoma cruzi* cell surface proteins: identification of one major glycoprotein. *FEBS Lett.*, **100**, 166–170.

Teixeira, A. R. L. (1979). Chagas' disease; trends in immunological research and prospects for immunoprophylaxis. *Bull. WHO*, **57** (5), 697–710.

Teixeira, A. R. L., Teixeira, M. L., and Santos-Buch, C. A. (1975). The immunology of experimental Chagas' disease IV. Production of lesions in rabbits similar to those of chronic Chagas' disease in man. *Amer. J. Path.*, **80** (1), 163–178.

Trager, W. and Jensen, J. B. (1976). Human malaria parasites in continuous culture. *Science*, **193**, 673–675.

Turk, J. L. and Bryceson, A. D. M. (1971). Immunological phenomena in leprosy and related diseases. *Adv. Immunol.*, **13**, 209.

Vickerman, K. (1974). Antigenic variation in African trypanosomes. In Porter and Knight (Eds.) *Parasites in the Immunised Host: mechanisms of survival*, p. 53. Associated Science Publishers, Amsterdam.

Voorheis, H. P., Gale, J. S., Owen, M. J., and Edwards, W. (1979). The isolation and partial characterisation of the plasma membrane from *Trypanosoma brucei*. *Biochem. J.*, **180**, 11–24.

Wallach, D. F. H. and Conley, M. (1977). Altered membrane proteins of monkey erythrocytes infected with simian malaria. *J. Mol. Med.*, **2**, 119–136.

Williams, R. O., Young, J. R., and Majiwa, P. O. (1979). Genomic rearrangements correlated with antigenic variation in *Trypanosoma brucei*. *Nature*, **282**, 847–849.

Yoshida, N., Nussenzweig, R. S., Potoanjak, P., Nussenzweig, V., and Aikawa, M. (1980).Hybridoma produces protective antibodies directed against the sporozoite stage of malaria parasite. *Science*, **207**, 71–73.

Antibody as a Tool
Edited by J. J. Marchalonis and G. W. Warr
© 1982 John Wiley & Sons Ltd

Chapter 15

Isolation and Characterization of Plasma Membranes

KERMIT L. CARRAWAY

and

CORALIE A. CAROTHERS CARRAWAY
*Department of Anatomy and Cell Biology and Oncology,
University of Miami School of Medicine, Miami,
Florida 33101, USA*

I. INTRODUCTION

The plasma membrane, which is the external cell surface of most animals cells, is involved in many critical cell phenomena, including recognition processes which are important in immunology. Such phenomena are dependent upon the nature of the components present in the plasma membrane, their specific functions (e.g. enzyme or transport activities), their organization in the membrane and the ability to undergo changes in that organization after receiving specific stimuli. Although many of these studies can be performed on intact cells or tissues, others require the more traditional biochemical approach, isolation, and characterization of the plasma membrane. Because of the great specificity of antibodies, immunochemistry can potentially make outstanding contributions to the understanding of plasma membrane structure function relationships. Examples of such studies can be cited from work on spectrin, the cytoskeletal protein associated with the cytoplasmic surface of the erythrocyte membrane. By use of antibody against spectrin, it can be identified as a ubiquitous component of erythrocyte membranes which is absent from more complex cells (Hiller and Weber, 1977), and is distinguishable from myosin (Sheetz *et al.*, 1975), with which it has been compared (Guidotti, 1972). Its localization at the membrane cytoplasmic surface was established by immune electron microscopy (Nicolson *et al.*, 1971). In addition divalent antibodies against spectrin, which bound to the cytoplasmic cell surface, could alter the distribution of cell surface components (Nicolson and Painter, 1973) and intramembrane particles (Elgsaeter and Branton, 1974) and accelerate shape changes of ghosts induced by Mg-ATP (Sheetz and Singer, 1977). These observations provide evidence for transmembrane linkages (Nicolson, 1976) which may be important in transmitting information from the exterior surface to the interior of the cell. Fewer successes have been obtained in attempting to extend these types of studies to more complex cells. The requisite criteria are obvious: specific antibody against the plasma membrane component in question and plasma membranes which are relatively unperturbed from their native state, representative of the portion of the cell surface to be investigated and free of contaminating membranes which could lead to erroneous interpretations. Preparation of plasma membranes from complex cells has proven to be a major stumbling block. Therefore in this review we shall concentrate on methods for obtaining and analysing plasma membranes to assure that they meet the criteria necessary for further studies, whether they be immunochemical investigations or other types of studies.

The major difficulty in isolating plasma membranes from nucleated cells is that the membrane barrier must be disrupted during the isolation procedure. Thus it is impossible to isolate a plasma membrane which has not been perturbed. A critical question is the degree of perturbation involved. Even if the perturbation can be minimized, it is important to remember that the plasma membrane is a dynamic, functional part of the cell (Nicolson and Poste, 1976a) and that its isolation from the cell necessarily removes some cellular factors and alters some interactions which may be important in membrane integrity and function. This point becomes particularly significant in view of recent observations of cytoskeleton–membrane interactions which can alter cell surface organization and behaviour (Nicolson, 1976; Berlin *et al.*, 1974; Schreiner and Unanue, 1977; Nicolson and Poste, 1976a,b; Edelman, 1976; Pastan and Willingham, 1978).

These considerations alone lead to a simple but necessary philosophy for choosing a particular plasma membrane isolation scheme. The procedure should be designed to fit the purpose for which the membranes are being isolated. For example, isolation of a plasma membrane antigen would not require very stringent control of the degree of purification of the plasma membrane, since further purification of the antigen would be performed. In contrast a compositional study of plasma membranes would have stricter requirements. Biochemical localization of an antigen or other molecule to the plasma membrane requires a careful assessment of purity which would not be necessary for many functional (e.g. plasma membrane enzyme behaviour) studies. Isolation of plasma membranes for the purpose of studying organization of membrane components requires special attention to membrane integrity, i.e., consideration of the perturbations of membrane structure involved in membrane preparation. Both yield and purity are also important if average properties of the membrane population are to be measured, since an unrepresentative population or contaminants will lend a bias to the results. Finally, some studies have requirements which supersede all other considerations. For example, transport measurements require a closed system, which must be attained regardless of whether there can be optimization of other factors. In this review we will concentrate on the most recent and best characterized methods for plasma membrane isolation. We will try to provide, whenever possible, some understanding of the bases for the methods to aid the investigator in adjusting the method to the particular problem under investigation. It should always be remembered that every cell or tissue type will behave differently in any particular membrane preparation procedure. We have concentrated almost exclusively on animal cells. Since prokaryotes do not have substantial internal organelles, the procedures for isolating plasma membranes from them are generally less complex. Work on plasma membranes from plant cells has been scant and has not deviated to a substantial degreee from similar studies on animal cells.

Membrane isolation procedures require three basic steps: disruption, fractionation, and identification. The key step is the disruption procedure, since it will dictate the strategies which can be employed in subsequent steps. For the purposes of this article the cell disruption techniques have been divided into three categories according to the nature of the cells: cells in suspension, cells attached to a substratum, and cells in tissues. For a number of reasons which will be discussed below cells in the first category are usually the easiest to handle. Therefore in many membrane isolations from substrate-attached cells the cells are suspended before begining the procedure. Tissue cells may also be isolated before membrane preparation. Details of many of the specific procedures used in several of the more common membrane isolation methods are provided in an excellent recent monograph by Evans (1978). Neville (1975) and Glick (1976) have presented compendia of membrane isolation procedures. An earlier article by DePierre and Karnovsky (1973) provides an excellent review of methods for identifying plasma membranes and for assessing disruption procedures.

II. CELL DISRUPTION

A. Cells in Suspension

1. Preparation of Cells

A number of advantages accrue from the use of cells in suspension. One is the relative uniformity of the mixture, which reduces variations in the forces applied to the different cells in the population during disruption. If desired, the cell population can be fractionated so that there is also homogeneity with respect to cell types present. A second advantage is that suspended cells generally have fewer cell surface specializations (e.g. junctions, in the case of tissues or substratum attachments, in the case of monolayer cultured cells). The specializations in suspended cells (e.g. microvilli, blebs, ruffles) appear to be dynamic and transient structures in most cases and are often lost or modified in membrane isolation procedures. If cells are to be isolated or suspended before membrane preparation, it is important that no critical membrane components or functions be altered. The definition of critical components or functions is the prerogative of the investigator. If specific membrane functions are to be investigated in the course of the study, these should be monitored for changes which may occur during cell suspension or isolation of a cell population. Otherwise, more general techniques for assessing membrane integrity will have to be used: cell viability, cell surface labelling, metabolic labelling or enzyme, transport or binding activities.

The most commonly used techniques for isolation of cells from tissues involve digestion of the tissue with enzymes which degrade connnective tissue, exemplified by the isolation of adipocytes by brief collagenase digestion of adipose tissue (Rodbell, 1964). Since procedures for isolating cells (for examples see Table 1) often involve the use of degradative enzymes (including possible contaminants, such as proteases in commercial preparations of collagenase) which can alter membrane components, it is necessary to be able to evaluate degradation. One potentially useful method is to label the cells by techniques which incorporate radioactivity into cell surface components. For example, enzymatic labelling with lactoperoxidase and ^{125}I or metabolic pulse labelling with glucosamine or fucose can be used on tissue samples (Barchi *et al.*, 1977). The samples can be subjected to SDS–polyacrylamide gel electrophoresis before and after the enzymatic digestion to determine whether there are significant losses of components due to degradation. If such losses occur, the degraded components will often be resynthesized and incorporated into the cell membrane if the isolated cells are incubated in an appropriate medium. This 'repair process can also be monitored by metabolic pulse labelling if electrophoretic patterns of surface components can be established.

Dissociation of cells from tissues by mechanical means, a technique which minimizes the problem of degradative enzymes, is usually not a reasonable alternative, because the forces necessary to achieve tissue dissociation can also cause substantial membrane damage and loss of cell viability. Viable cells can, however, be obtained mechanically in some cases. Tumour tissues are often more readily dissociable than normal. Kawai and Spiro (1977) have reported a sieving procedure which yields fat cells from adipose tissue for which plasma membranes were subsequently prepared.

Another significant problem with the preparation of isolated cells from tissue is that the functional polarity which the cells have in the tissue may be lost during the dissociation and cell isolation. Little work has been done on this

Table 1. Selected procedures for cell dissociation from tissues*

Tissue type	Procedure used for dissociation	Reference
Epididymal fat pad	Digestion with collagenase in albumin/bicarbonate/glucose	Rodbell (1964)
Perirenal fat tissue (rabbits)	Disruption by forcing through sieves	Kawai and Spiro (1977)
Liver (rat)	Perfusion with modified Hanks/EGTA/BSA followed by perfusion with modified Hanks/collagenase/BSA	Moldeus et al. (1978)
Liver (rat)	Perfusion with Hanks followed by perfusion with (a) Hanks/collagenase/hyaluronidase, (b) Hanks/collagenase or (c) Hanks/collagenase/STI	Wisher and Evans (1977)
Liver (rat)	Incubation of liver slices in Ca^{2+}/Mg^{2+}-free PBS, then incubation in EGTA/PBS, followed by incubation in Hanks/Ca^{2+}/collagenase/hyaluronidase	Fry et al. (1976)
Virgin mammary gland (mouse)	Chopped tissue incubated in Ca^{2+}/Mg^{2+}-free BSS, digested in collagenase/hyaluronidase/BSA, then in Pronase/medium 199	Wiepjes and Prop (1970)
Lactating mammary gland (rat)	Minced, incubated in collagenase/BSA with stirring	Schroeder et al. (1977)
Mid-pregnant mammary gland (rabbit)	Injection of collagenase/elastase/chymotrypsin/KRB into interstitial space of gland and digestion followed by treatment with KRB/EDTA, then additional enzyme digestion and gentle pipetting	Kraehenbuhl (1977)
Intestinal tissue (chicken)	Intestinal segments incubated with hyaluronidase/BSA and stirred gently	Kimmich (1975)

*Abbreviations used: BSA, bovine serum albumin; PBS, phosphate-buffered saline; STI, soybean trypsin inhibitor; BSS, balanced salts solution; KRB, Krebs–Ringer buffer.

problem. However, Wisher and Evans (1977) have determined that the plasma membrane fractions obtained from hepatocytes isolated by a standard collagenase perfusion procedure are quite similar to those obtained from disruption of the tissue. Since the fractionation scheme is based upon separation of the various morphological units (membrane faces) of the cells, these results indicate that the hepatocytes still maintain significant functional polarity. Whether this observation will hold for other tissue types and dissociation procedures is unknown. Obviously, the rate of dissociation of cells from the tissues, the extent of cell disruption, and the speed with which the cells are isolated could be significant factors in determining maintenance of cell polarity.

2. Preparation of Envelopes

The goal in disrupting cells for membrane preparation is to obtain a uniform population of plasma membranes which can be separated from nuclei, internal organelles, and other cytoplasmic constituents. There are two basic strategies for achieving this goal. One is to stabilize the cell surface such that the plasma membrane can be isolated as a relatively intact cell surface 'envelope' or 'ghost' after internal constituents have been extruded through a tear in the surface by homogenization (Warren and Glick, 1969). The second is to disrupt the cell surface completely, reducing it to a relatively uniform population of plasma membrane vesicles, which can then be separated from other cellular constituents (Wallach and Schmidt-Ullrich, 1977).

The objective in stabilizing the membrane is to permit it to be identified by microscopy, thus simplifying the control of conditions of homogenization and the assessment of fractionation. A number of protocols for stabilization and homogenization of suspended cultured cells have been developed (Warren *et al.*, 1966; Warren and Glick, 1969). In applying these procedures to ascites cells we found considerable variability in the response of different cell types. Thus the procedure must be optimized for each cell type. Figure 1 shows the protocol used for Sarcoma 180 cells (Shin and Carraway, 1973a; Huggins, 1975; Moore *et al.*, 1978). When investigating a new cell type, we begin with this procedure and vary the parameters of homogenization shown in Table 2. The objectives are to optimize cell breakage, minimize nuclear disruption, and maximize the number of intact cell envelopes. Whether these criteria are fulfilled can be monitored simply by phase contrast microscopy of the homogenates.

Polyacrylamide gel electrophoresis in SDS of Zn^{2+}-stabilized envelope preparations compared to unstabilized membrane vesicles from Sarcoma 180 cells showed that the envelopes contained three high molecular weight polypeptides which were greatly reduced in amount in the vesicles (Shin and Carraway, 1973a). Two of these polypeptides (Figure 2) were later identified as myosin and actin binding protein (Moore *et al.*, 1976; Moore *et al.*,1978),

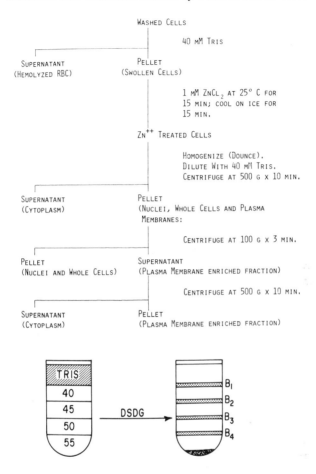

Figure 1. Scheme for isolation of cell surface envelopes of Sarcoma 180 ascites tumour cells using stabilization with $ZnCl_2$

components associated with the cellular cytoskeleton which is believed to be involved in maintaining cell shape and controlling the membrane organization (Nicolson, 1976). We have postulated that the envelope stabilization results from stabilization of the association of these cytoskeletal elements with the membrane (Moore *et al.*, 1978). Release of cytoskeletal proteins and fragmentation of the envelopes occur concomitantly upon extraction with hypotonic alkaline buffers. Extraction with nonionic detergent removes the bilayer of the envelope, leaving an envelope-shaped cytoskeletal residue. Myosin has been localized at the cytoplasmic surface of plasma membranes by immune electron microscopy (Painter *et al.*, 1975; Rikihisa and Mizuno, 1977). Previous immunochemical results indicating the presence of myosin at the cell

Table 2. Conditions for disruption in the preparation of cell surface envelopes by Zn^{2+} or Mg^{2+} stabilization*

Operation	Range	Effects
Swelling at 4 °C		
Salt concentration	40 mM Tris, 0–0.1 M NaCl	Cell diameter should increase 50–100%.
Time	3–10 min	Bleb formation should be avoided by increasing salt concentration or decreasing time
Stablization		
Agent	$ZnCl_2$ (0.1–5 mM), or $MgCl_2$ (2–20 mM)	Phase image of plasma membrane darkens. If divalent cation concentration too high, homogenization becomes difficult and cyto- plasmic organelle contamination increases.
Time	5–30 min	Increased cation, time or temperature will
Temperature	4–25 °C	increase 'hardening' of membrane
Homogenization		
Cell concentration	Dilute loose cell pellet × 8–15	Monitor number of envelopes and nuclei by phase contrast microscopy. Optimal per- formance will give > 80% broken cells and
Homogenizer	Tight pestle optimum	nearly equal numbers of nuclei and envelopes.
Disruption	5–20 slow, strong strokes with 3–5 min interval after each 5 strokes	Too much homogenization or inadequate stabilization results in vesiculation, which can be determined from envelope counts
Post-homogenization	Return to isotonic conditions with salt or sucrose	Membranes and nuclei are stabilized before fractionation

*Data provided by Dr John Huggins (Huggins, 1975, and unpublished results).

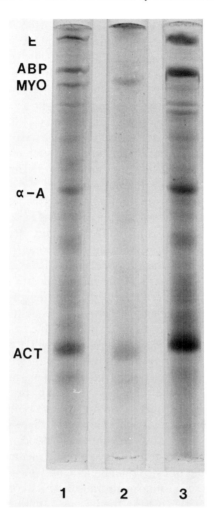

Figure 2. Polypeptides of isolated cell surface envelopes of Sarcoma 180 ascites cell surface envelopes (gel 1). The pattern is dominated by cytoskeletal polypeptides. Gel 2 shows purified gizzard actomyosin. Gel 3 shows the proteins extracted by glycine–EDTA–mercaptoethanol. Bands have been identified as actin (ACT), α-actinin (α-A), myosin (MYO), and actin binding protein (ABP). (Figure is revised from Moore, 1978)

surface (Kemp *et al.*, 1971; Willingham *et al.*, 1974) have been questioned (Gröschel-Stewart *et al.*, 1976).

We suspect that the hypotonic medium used for swelling the cells and the shear forces present during homogenization disrupt the membrane–cytoskeleton organization or association. By changing the medium and/or reducing the shear force applied, we have been able to isolate envelopes from some ascites cells without the use of external stabilizing agents. However, the disruption is less easily controlled in these cases, and the variability among different cell types is more pronounced. Atkinson (1973) has provided a detailed description of the isolation of HeLa cell ghosts which apparently does not involve the use of stabilizing agents.

For some other cell types, notably adipocytes, 'ghosts' can also be obtained by brief homogenization without prior stabilization (Rodbell, 1967). The large size and high fat content of the cells probably contribute to the ease of disruption of these cells. Further investigations of such procedures are needed with other cell types to provide methods for envelope isolations which eliminate deleterious effects which occur with some of the stabilizing agents.

The isolation of envelopes from stabilized cells provides not only the ease of identification but also a decreased likelihood of loss of portions of the plasma membrane. Since the surface is probably a mosaic, such losses could yield membrane preparations with significantly different properties from the original. However, it should be recognized that there is little experimental evidence to show that some parts of the membrane are not lost in stabilized preparations. Microvilli are particularly sparse in envelope preparations. In most cells they disappear during the cell swelling; engulfed into the expanding cell body, their membrane becomes indistinguishable from the rest of the cell surface. In cell types with particularly stable microvilli they may remain intact and be 'shed' from the cell during membrane disruption procedures. Obviously such losses can alter the composition of the isolated plasma membrane.

Another advantage of the envelope isolation procedure is that the membranes are not sealed, thus obviating the possibility that cytoplasmic material is trapped during isolation. However, there is concern that the stabilization methods can cause adventitious association of cytoplasmic components with the membrane. We have already mentioned the association and possible contribution of cytoskeletal elements. Such considerations raise the question of how the plasma membrane and its constituents should be defined. It is clear that the plasma membrane cannot be considered as an isolated entity in the intact cell and that some cytoskeletal structural elements and cytoplasmic and extracellular components can be associated with the plasma membrane in its native state. As yet we have no good operational criteria for assessing such associations. The problem is illustrated by considering glyceraldehyde-3-phosphate dehydrogenase in erythrocytes. It is specifically associated with erythrocyte membranes isolated by standard hypotonic lysis (Shin and Carraway, 1973b; Kant and Steck, 1973; McDaniel *et al.*, 1974). However, it is removed from the membranes in isotonic salt solutions and from cells treated with digitonin in isotonic salt solutions, ionic conditions which one supposes are present in the intact erythrocyte. The nature and function of the enzyme-membrane association and whether it exists in the intact cell are still matters for debate.

Other isolation procedures have been reported to yield plasma membrane 'ghosts' or envelopes. McCollester (1970) used borate buffers in hypotonic solutions for lysing Meth A ascites tumour cells and recovered the surface membranes by centrifugation. The borate was reported to destabilize endoplasmic reticulum without causing vesiculation of the plasma membrane. Since borate can interact strongly with carbohydrates, some cell surface stabilization may also be involved.

Stabilization of plasma membranes can also be achieved by the use of chemical cross-linking agents such as glutaraldehyde (Dods *et al.*, 1972; Warley and Cook, 1976). However, the effects of the chemical modifications on membrane functions, membrane composition, membrane component isolation, and membrane polypeptide analysis reduce the usefulness of such procedures for many purposes. Cross-linking conditions must be carefully chosen for these preparations to minimize artefacts. Stabilization of plasma membrane by Concanavalin A (Con A) has been used in membrane isolations from *Dictyostelium discoideum* (Parrish and Müller, 1976) and a wall-less mutant of *Neurospora crassa* (Scarborough, 1975). Triton X-100 was used for cell disruption of the *Dictyostelium*. More recently, Condeelis (1978) has reported isolation of both ghosts and Con A 'caps' from *Dictyostelium*. Cap formation occurs when the cells are incubated at 22 °C for a period of time before lysis.

Table 3 provides a compilation of selected preparations of ghosts, envelopes, or membrane sheets from cells in suspension. Erythrocyte membrane preparation techniques are not included.

Phagocytosis of beads by cells prior to disruption has been used to isolate plasma membrane material (Wetzel and Korn, 1969; Heine and Schnaitman, 1971; Charalampous *et al.*, 1973). Obviously, this procedure simplifies separation and identification problems. A significant difficulty is that many phagocytic vesicles rapidly fuse with lysosomes (Rikihisa and Mizuno, 1978), leading to contamination with lysosomal membranes and possibility of degradation. In addition the phagocytic activity of different cell types is highly variable. Since the cytoplasmic face is presumably external in the membranes isolated as phagocytic particles, they have been used to try to identify transmembrane proteins by dual labelling procedures, labelling the intact cells with impermeant reagents (Hunt and Brown, 1975; Evans and Fink, 1977), isolating phagocytic particles and labelling with a second reagent. It is critical in such procedures to perform appropriate controls to demonstrate the impermeability of the phagocytic particle membrane to the reagent. In addition the orientation of 'phagolysosomes' obtained by some methods seems to be inverted (Rikihisa and Mizuno, 1978). Obviously, such preparations need to be characterized carefully before they are used for investigating transmembrane proteins.

Another procedure for isolating cell surface membranes from suspended cells involves adsorption of the cell onto positively charged beads, which can be prepared by covalently coupling polylysine to glass or polyacrylamide beads

Table 3. Selected preparations of cell surface ghosts, envelopes, or large fragments*

Cell type	Medium for disruption	Agent for disruption	Method of fractionation	Morphological evaluation	Plasma membrane markers	Contamination markers
L cells[a]	2.2. mM FMA, 20 mM Tris, pH 8.0	Dounce	DC, DSDG	PCM, TEM	—	—
L cells[a]	1 mM ZnCl$_2$, 0.05% Tween-20	Dounce	Glass bead column and CSDG or DC/CSDG	PCM, TEM	—	—
L cells[a]	0.075 M acetic acid	Dounce	Linear glycerol gradient	PCM, TEM	—	—
L cells[a]	50 mM Tris, 2.5 mM MgCl$_2$ pH 7.4	Dounce	DC, DSDG	PCM, TEM	—	—
L cells[b]	1 mM ZnCl$_2$	Dounce	2 phase	PCM, TEM	S-ATPase, cell surface antigens	NADH diaphorase, [3H]DNA, cyt oxidase
HeLa[c]	10 mM Tris, 15 mM IAA	Dounce	Zonal	PCM, TEM	[3H]fucose	—
Meth A ascites[d]	2.5 mM borate 0.2 mM EDTA, pH 9.2	Magnetic stirring	DC	PCM, TEM	—	DNA, RNA
Sarcoma 180[e]	1–2 mM ZnCl$_2$	Dounce	DC/DSDG or 2 phase	PCM, TEM	Chol, SA, S-ATPase	NADH diaphorase
L 1210[f] CHO[g]	1 mM ZnCl$_2$ 1 mM ZnCl$_2$ or 2 mM MgCl$_2$	Dounce Dounce	DC/DSDG 2 phase	PCM PCM, TEM	5N 5N, S-ATPase, SA	SDH, G6Pase SDH, cyt c reductase, DNA, RNA
Normal lymphoidal or ALL[h]	20 mM borate, 0.2 mM EDTA, pH 9.2	Magnetic stirring	Glass bead column	PCM, TEM	5N	NADH oxidoreductase, SDH

Cell type	Homogenization medium	Disruption	Gradient / centrifugation	Microscopy	Plasma-membrane markers	Contamination markers
Neuroblastoma[i]	1 mM ZnCl$_2$	Dounce	Ficoll gradient	PCM, TEM	AcCholase, Chol, SA	—
L 5178 Y leukemia[j]	10 mM Tris, 20 mM KCl	Syringe	DC	PCM	5N, S-ATPase	RNA
L 5178 Y leukemia[k]	0.25 M sucrose, 1 mM EDTA, glutaraldehyde after homogenization	Syringe	DSDG	PCM		G6Pase, SDH, AcPase
Fat cells[l]	2.5 mM ATP, 2.5 mM MgCl$_2$, 0.1 mM CaCl$_2$, 0.1 mM NAD, 0.05 mM NADP, 1 mM KHCO$_3$	Inversion	DC	PCM	Adenylate cyclase	LDH
Sperm (acrosomal membrane)[m]	0.15 M NaCl, 5 mM HEPES	Dounce	DSDG	PCM, TEM	Glycosidases	APase
Dictyostelium[n]	0.1 M Tris, pH 8.5, after incubation in 100 µg/ml Con A	0.2% Triton X-100	DC	PCM, TEM	APase, cAMP-PDE	
Neurospora[o]	10 mM Tris, 5 mM MgSO$_4$ after incubation with 0.5 mg/ml Con A in isotonic medium	Dounce	DC	PCM, TEM	5N, S-ATPase	DNA, RNA, SDH

* Abbreviations used: FMA, fluoresceine mercuric acetate; IAA, iodoacetic acid; DC, differential centrifugation; DSDG and CSDG, discontinuous and continuous sucrose density gradient centrifugation; PCM, phase contrast microscopy; TEM, transmission electron microscopy; S-ATPase, Na$^+$, K$^+$-ATPase; Chol, cholesterol; SA, sialic acid; 5N, 5′-nucleotidase; G6Pase, glucose 6-phosphatase; AcCholase, acetylcholinesterase; APase, alkaline phosphatase; cAMP-PDE, cyclic AMP phosphodiesterase; cyt, cytochrome; SDH, succinic dehydrogenase; LDH, lactic dehydrogenase; AcPase, acid phosphatase. ALL, acute lymphocytic leukaemia.
[a]Warren et al. (1966); [b]Brunette and Till (1971); [c]Atkinson and Summers (1971); [d]McCollester (1970); [e]Shin and Carraway (1973a); [f]Huggins (1975); [g]Juliano and Gagalang (1975); [h]Warley and Cook (1973); [i]Truding et al. (1974); [j]Dods et al. (1972); [k]Rodbell (1967); [m]Zahler and Doak (1975); [n]Scarborough (1975); [o]

(Jacobson, 1977; Jacobson and Branton, 1977; Cohen *et al.*, 1977; Kalish *et al.*, 1978; Jacobson *et al.*, 1978). Since most cells have negatively charged surfaces, they adhere strongly to the beads. Vortexing shears away cells, leaving attached surface membrane and some intracellular debris, which is removed by brief low power sonication (Cohen *et al.*, 1977). The vortexing procedure is performed in sucrose/acetate at pH 5, a condition similar to one previously used for 'stabilizing' plasma membranes (Warren *et al.*, 1966). The subsequent sonication and washing steps are performed in 10 mM Tris at pH 7.4. The fate of surface specializations such as microvilli and blebs during the isolation procedure and the possibility of selectivity in binding of different regions of the cell surface to the beads are still uncertain. One might envision that a highly villous cell would be bound to the beads only by the microvilli, if these survive the pH 5 acetate treatment. Shearing might then remove only the microvilli from the cells.

In at least one cell type which we have investigated, microvilli can be removed from the cell rather easily. The 13762 MAT-C1 rat mammary adenocarcinoma has numerous branched microvilli extending from the cell body (Figure 3). We found that these microvilli, which are relatively stable, are released from the cells during hypotonic swelling in the presence of fluoresent Con A, which provides a means of visualization (Figure 4) (Huggins *et al.*, 1980). Later experiments showed that the microvilli are spontaneously shed by the cells *in vitro* and *in vivo*. Isolation of these microvilli (Carraway *et al.*, 1980) then provides a source of plasma membrane from this specialized region of the cell.

3. Membrane Vesiculation

The opposite extreme of isolation of envelopes or ghosts is to reduce the plasma membrane to vesicles. Vesiculation is required for some types of cells for which disruption to envelopes is not feasible. The goal is to obtain plasma membrane vesicles without disrupting nuclei, lysosomes, or mitochondria, whose contents and membranes complicate fractionation procedures. Because plasma membranes, endoplasmic reticulum and Golgi are all disrupted to different extents in different types of cells, it is important to control disruption conditions carefully. Evans (1978) has discussed conditions and procedures used for disruption, including homogenization, sonication, shearing, and gas cavitation. The last technique has been discussed extensively by Wallach and Schmidt-Ullrich (1977).The integrity of cellular organelles is strongly influenced by the medium used for disruption, including type of buffer, salt concentration, osmolality, and divalent cation concentration. A selection of procedures and conditions used for disruption to vesicles is given in Table 4. Often the selection of the disruption medium involves a series of compromises. Low ionic strength facilitates plasma membrane disruption but may also result

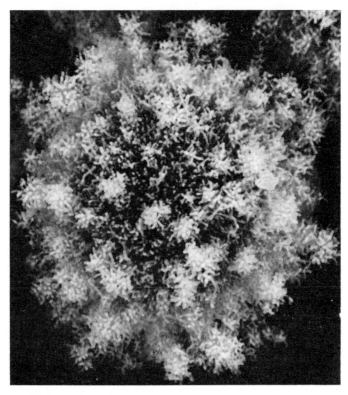

Figure 3. Scanning electron micrograph of 13762 MAT-Cl mammary adenocarcinoma
cell showing branched microvilli

in fragmentation of lysosomes, nuclear membranes, and the outer mitochondrial membrane. Raising the osmotic strength, but not the ionic strength, by
including sucrose may reduce organelle disruption but also tends to stabilize
the plasma membrane against vesiculation. Addition of divalent cations
Mg^{2+} or Ca^{2+} also stabilizes organelles but may cause aggregation of
vesicles and complicate fractionation. Some buffers are toxic to certain cells
and may induce morphological changes, such as blebbing, which interfere with
uniform cell disruption. This may also occur due to the increased dissociation of
cytoskeletal elements at higher pH values (Moore *et al.*, 1978).

An obvious disadvantage of vesiculation procedures is the loss of an
identifiable morphology. This greatly complicates fractionation methods, since
alternate means of identification of the plasma membrane are required. The
stringent disruption conditions often lead to sealed vesicles, which provide
both an advantage and a disadvantage. Sealed vesicles, required if any type of
translocation or permeability measurements are to be performed on the
membranes, can be manipulated osmotically to aid in fractionation. However,

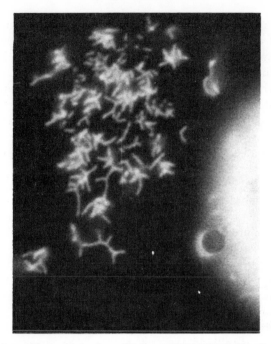

Figure 4. Shedding of branched microvilli from 13762 MAT-Cl induced by hypotonic
swelling in the presence of fluorescent Con A

the sealed vesicles can also trap soluble cellular components. Although the
amount of trapped materials can be reduced by osmotic lysis of the vesicles, this
procedure may also release some loosely bound membrane constituents. The
problem of loss of membrane components is also a disadvantage of vesiculation
procedures in general because of the severity of the disruption forces
employed. In this sense these methods face exactly the opposite criticisms of
the stabilization procedures. The two strategies should probably be considered
complementary in systems where both can be applied. Unfortunately, there
have been too few comparisons of membranes isolated by the different
procedures from the same cell system.

As noted in Table 4 lymphocytes are predominant among the cells for which
vesiculation procedures have been used. Due to the small cell size and large
nucleus : cell volume ratio, disruption to yield envelopes has proven difficult or
impossible. Since the nucleus dominates the cell, the major problem in the
lymphocyte is to break the membrane without disrupting the nucleus. The use
of hypertonic sucrose solutions as a disruption medium may prove a solution to
this problem (Monneron and d'Alayer, 1978).

It should be clear from the previous discussions that the two ideal situations,
cell breakage to give intact envelopes or fragmentation into a uniform
population of vesicles, will not be possible with many cell types and may not be

achievable in the most rigorous sense with any cell, because of the inherent heterogeneity of the cell surface, regardless of the source of the cell. In fact most plasma membrane preparations fall into a broad category between these two ideals, yielding a mixed population of plasma membranes as vesicles and fragments of various sizes. It is quite common to find multiple fractions possessing the characteristics of plasma membranes, as delineated in later sections. For example, Perdue *et al.* (1971) found two plasma membrane fractions from chick embryo fibroblasts which were separated on continuous sucrose density gradients. The lower fraction contained vesicles, while the upper was predominantly large sheets or fragments and vesicles, depending on the mode of homogenization. Although these results suggest a fragmentation of the plasma membrane into functional or morphological domains, it has rarely been possible to assign the isolated fractions to their subcellular origins in suspended or cultured cells.

Most of the disruption techniques discussed above are based upon mechanical disruption or on pressure changes (cavitation) which cause disruption by bubble formation. Another frequently used pressure change technique is osmotic lysis, which is the most common basis for erythrocyte membrane preparations (e.g. Dodge *et al.*, 1963). Lysis of more complex cells in hypotonic media tends to cause disruption of intracellular organelles. An alternative method is to 'load' the cells with an osmotically active substance such as glycerol. Barber and Jamieson (1970) have used such a procedure for isolation of platelet plasma membrane fractions with no apparent damage to intracellular organelles. In addition Jett *et al.* (1977) have used a similar procedure for preparing plasma membranes from RAJI lymphoid cells.

B. Plasma Membranes from Attached Cells in Culture

Cells such as fibroblasts attached to a substratum in culture exhibit a definite polarity, both parallel and perpendicular to the substratum. In addition to a leading and trailing edge, these cells also have a top (dorsal) surface which is not equivalent to the bottom (attached) surface. When the cells are removed from the substratum, this polarity is lost. If the cells are removed by scraping, the polarity loss occurs in a time-dependent fashion after the cell is removed. One can potentially fix or stabilize the cells in these intermediate states. Such considerations complicate the isolation of membranes from attached cells. Clearly the cell and its plasma membrane are no longer the same after the cells have been removed from the substratum. Thus there is a need for procedures which can be used to isolate plasma membranes without prior detachment of the cells from the substratum.

Since fibroblasts have upper and lower surfaces relative to the substratum, it is potentially possible to isolate different membrane fractions representative of these. In a procedure based on prior experiments of Barland and Schroeder

Table 4. Selected methods for preparation of plasma membrane vesicles from cells in suspension*

Cell type	Medium for disruption	Agent for disruption	Method of fractionation	Morphological evaluation	Plasma membrane markers	Contamination markers
Ehrlich ascites[a]	0.25 M sucrose, 0.2 mM MgSO$_4$,	N$_2$ cavitation	DC, Ficoll gradient	—	S-ATPase, 'surface antigen'	NADH diaphorase
3T3, SV-3T3, BHK-21 or BHK-Py, L cells[b]	0.25 M sucrose	N$_2$ cavitation	DC Dextran gradient	—	5N transport systems	NADH dehydrogenase, SDH
Fat cells[c]	0.25 M sucrose, 5 mM Tris, pH 7.4	Sieve	SDG, Dextran gradient	—	5N, S-ATPase	NADH oxidase, succinate-cyt c reductase
HEp and HSV-HEp cells[d]	0.25 M sucrose 0.02 mM MgSO$_4$, 0.5 g/l BSA, 1 mM HEPES, pH 7.4	N$_2$ cavitation	DC, DSDG	TEM	5N, [^{3}H]fucose	NADH diaphorase
Lymph node lymphocytes[e]	0.15 M NaCl, 10 mM Tris, pH 7.4	Tissue press	DC, CSDG	PCM, TEM	5N, cell surface antigens	AcPase, G6Pase, SDH
Br18 lymphoblasts[f]	Eagle's MEM	Cell rupturing pump	DC, DSDG	—	5N, histocompatibility antigen	—
Calf thymocytes[g]	Hanks	N$_2$ cavitation	DC, Ficoll gradient	TEM	5N, M-ATPase, pNPase, SA, chol	NADH reductase, succinate-cyt c reductase, G6Pase DNA, RNA

Cell type	Medium	Homogenization	Centrifugation	Microscopy	Plasma membrane markers	Other markers
Calf thymocytes[h]	0.25 M sucrose, 50 mM Tris, 1 mM EDTA	Frozen cells in Waring Blendor	DC, DSDG	TEM	5N, SA	SDH, glucosaminidase, DNA
RAJ1 lymphoid cells[i]	10 mM Tris, 1 mM MgCl₂, 1 mM CaCl₂	Hypotonic lysis of glycerol-loaded cells	DC, DSDG	TEM	PDE	glucosaminidase, G6Pase, SDH, LDH, esterase
Calf thymocytes	50 mM Tris, 25 mM KCl, 5 mM MgCl₂, 60% sucrose	Potter homogenizer	DC, DSDG	TEM, freeze-fracture EM	5N, 3N, S-ATPase, γ-GT, APase	SDH, Cyt oxidase, NADH-cyt c reductase, gal transferase, TPPase, AcPase, esterase, glucosaminidase
CEF[k]	0.25 M sucrose, 50 mM Tris, 1 mM Mg(OAC)₂	Dounce	DC, Dextran T-40 gradient	—	5N, S-ATPase	NADPH-cyt c reductase, SDH
Neurospora membrane ghosts[l]	10 mM Tris	glass–Teflon homogenizer	DC	TEM	5N, S-ATPase	SDH, RNA, DNA
HeLa ghosts[m]	10 mM Tris, 1 mM MgCl₂, 0.25 M sucrose	sonication	DC, CSDG	TEM	S-Atpase, [125I]antibody	NADH-cyt c reductase, RNA
Fat cells[n]	0.25 M sucrose, 10 mM Tris, 1 mM EDTA	Potter–Elvehjehm homogenizer	DC, CSDG or Ficoll gradient	TEM	Adenylate cyclase, ATPase	SDH, RNA, NADH-cyt c reductase
Dictyostelium[o]	8.6% sucrose, 5 mM Tris, PMSF (saturated)	Stirred with glass beads	DC, DSDG	TEM	APase, 5N	SDH, NADPH-cyt c reductase, RNA

*Abbreviations used: see lists in Tables 2 and 3; M-ATPase, Mg²⁺ ATPase; PDE, phosphodiesterase; 5N, 5′-nucleotidase; γ-GT, γ-glutamyl transferase, gal transferase, galactosyl transferase; TPPase, thiamine pyrophosphatase.
[a] Wallach and Kamat (1964, 1966); [b] Hochstadt et al. (1975); [c] Avruch and Wallach (1971); [d] Heine et al. (1972); [e] Allan and Crumpton (1970); [f] Snary et al (1974); [g] van Blitterswijk et al. (1973); [h] Kornfeld and Siemers (1974); [i] Jett et al., (1977); [j] Monneron and d'Alayer (1978); [k] Bingham and Burke (1972); [l] Scarborough (1975); [m] Boone et al. (1969); [n] McKeel and Jarrett (1970); [o] Gilkes and Weeks (1977).

(1970), Noonan *et al.* (1976) have used stabilization methods to obtain such fractions. Fibroblasts were incubated for 15 minutes with 1 mM ZnCl$_2$, in dimethylsulphoxide at 37°C, then for 10 minutes on ice in 2.2 mM fluorescein mercuric acetate in 20 mM Tris (pH 8.1). The fixed cells were fragmented by shaking and the dislodged membrane fragments decanted and collected by low speed centrifugation. The membranes in this fraction were considered the upper plasma membrane. The material remaining attached to the substratum was removed by scraping and homogenizing in 1 mM ZnCl$_2$ to remove the nuclei. Material isolated by density gradient centrifugation from this fraction was considered to be the lower plasma membrane. More recent experiments suggest that the results are not so straightforward (McClure *et al.*, 1979). Scanning electron microscopy indicates that membranes are released only from the population of cells with an 'epitheloid' morphology. In addition only the membrane from the area of the cell surface circumscribing the nucleus is released. That which is directly apposed to the nucleus or at the edge of the cell is maintained. Thus the basis for the pronounced compositional differences between 'upper plasma membrane' and membrane isolated by other techniques is unclear, although it does appear that the isolation technique for 'upper membrane' involves selection of a particular cell fraction.

An alternative, almost obverse, procedure involves vesiculation of the plasma membrane of attached cells by chemical treatment of the cell with formaldehyde, other low molecular weight aldehydes, or sulphhydryl blocking agents (Scott, 1976). The released vesicles are heterogeneous in size, ranging from 0.5 to 1.5 μm in diameter. An obvious disadvantage of this procedure is that the chemical modifications may alter membrane functions. Since glycerol does not react covalently, a potentially less damaging procedure involves glycerol 'blistering' of myoblasts and fibroblasts (Vandenburgh, 1977). It seems likely that other cellular perturbants will be found which can cause similar effects. The mechanism of vesicle or blister formation and release is unclear. Temperature, divalent cations, and an energy source appear to be important (Scott and Maercklein, 1979). Blebbing of erythrocyte membranes apparently involves a disruption of the cytoskeleton (spectrin–actin) or cytoskeleton–membrane association (Lutz *et al.*, 1977). Such an effect may also be important in the vesiculation of fibroblast plasma membranes, but the vesiculation is not inhibited by cytoskeletal perturbants such as colchicine or cytochalasin (Scott and Maercklein, 1979). It seems likely that these vesiculation procedures are releasing a selected fraction of the membrane from the cell which will be representative of only a portion of the cell surface. In addition the vesicles will almost certainly contain trapped soluble cytoplasmic components. Further characterization is needed to evaluate the nature of these processes and components, but the sinplicity of the procedures suggest that they may be useful in many kinds of studies.

C. Plasma Membranes from Tissues

Membrane isolation from tissues is complicated by the presence of multiple cell types and membrane specializations of the different cell types. Thus there is no 'plasma membrane' which can be isolated as a uniform, homogeneous unit representing all of the cellular surfaces. The problem of surface specializations can be transformed into an advantage if one is seeking a specialized cell function or morphological unit. In that case the best disruption procedure is the minimal perturbation which gives the particular unit in an isolable, identifiable form in sufficient quantity. As an example, one can cite procedures for isolating intestinal brush borders (Miller and Crane, 1961) as a morphological unit. Unfortunately, although most tissues and their cells are very complex, they do not have such well-defined units. The most thoroughly studied tissue has been liver. Many of the plasma membrane preparations from this tissue are based on the original method of Neville (1960), which employs homogenization in 1 mM $NaHCO_3$. Others have criticized this procedure (Takeuchi and Terayama, 1965; Coleman *et al.*, 1967), arguing that the hypotonic conditions result in extensive plasma membrane and organelle fragmentation and yield predominantly the bile canalicular fronts (Steck and Wallach, 1970), which are stabilized by junctional complexes. Ray (1970) includes Ca^{2+} in the medium to provide stabilization of membrane regions other than the bile canalicular fronts. However, calcium does not act as a stabilizing agent for membranes in all tissues. More frequently homogenization is performed in an isotonic sucrose medium. Using both isotonic and hypotonic disruption media, Evans (1978) has reported isolation of six plasma membrane subfractions, which have been assigned to the three primary faces in liver cells, blood sinusoidal, lateral, and bile canalicular, based on morphological and enzymic criteria. The bile canalicular fronts and lateral surfaces were isolated by rate-zonal centrifugation from the nuclear pellets of the first differential centrifugation after homogenization in 1 mM $NaHCO_3$. The blood sinusoidal faces were obtained from a microsomal fraction after homogenization in isotonic medium.

Attempting to transfer protocols of membrane isolation from one tissue type to another, even from normal to malignant tissues from the same organ, can be fraught with difficulties. Thus it is desirable to work out the optimal conditions for isolation of the desired fractions for each individual tissue type. This necessarily involves heavy reliance upon fractionation and membrane identification methods. Liver is a relatively soft tissue which is easily homogenized. Other tissues require harsher conditions for disruption and greater care to assure that nuclear disruption and release of nucleic acids is minimized. For example, muscle contains myofibrils and extensive connective tissue which make homogenization difficult. Extensive shearing followed by extraction of myofibrillar protein is usually performed before additional fractionation to obtain sarcolemma is attempted (Smith and Appel, 1977). Likewise the extensive connective tissue of mammary gland necessitates a vigorous disruption procedure (Keenan *et al.*, 1970; Shin *et al.*, 1975), which complicates subsequent fractionation and identification schemes by destroying morphological units such as Golgi and reducing both internal and external membranes to vesicles and fragments of variable sizes.

Because of its complexity brain tissue provides a particular challenge. Most of the work on isolation of plasma membranes of this tissue has been done on synaptosomes, sealed fragments of nerve endings which are released when cerebral cortex is subjected to a mild shearing procedure in isotonic medium. Plasma membranes from synaptosomes can be released by hypotonic shock and purified further. Because of the complexity of this organ further work on brain plasma membranes will almost certainly require isolation of individual cell types. Although cell isolation presents its own challenges and pitfalls, as indicated previously, these appear far less demanding than attempting to sort out the membrane fractions produced on disrupting brain tissue. In addition many of the problems of cell isolation can be overcome with appropriate controls and ancillary experiments to evaluate degradation. Some progress has been made in isolating plasma membranes from cells dissociated from neural tissues, notably with neural retina and cerebellum (Merrell and Glaser, 1973), glial cells (Levitan *et al.*, 1972; Blomstrand and Hamberger, 1969), neuronal cell bodies (Henn *et al.*, 1972), and cells dissociated from immature brain (Hemminki and Suovaniemi, 1973).

Plasma membranes representative of two cell faces in kidney tissue, brush border and basolateral, have been prepared after mild shearing. Microvilli are obtained from brush border by more vigorous disruption using Mg^{2+} as a stabilizing agent (Booth and Kenny, 1974). However, fragmentation to vesicles from the microvillar plasma membrane can also occur, depending on the conditions (Booth and Kenny, 1976). Isolation of plasma membranes from intestinal brush borders is achieved after vesiculation in 1 M Tris (Eichholz and Crane, 1974).

Table 5 provides a list of plasma membrane isolation procedures which have been used with various types of tissue.

III. FRACTIONATION

A. Centrifugation

Virtually every plasma membrane purification scheme developed uses centrifugation at some stage. Centrifugal fractionations are based on two principles, separation by weight and separation by density. Sedimentation coefficients, upon which differential centrifugation (separation by weight) is based, are actually complex functions of size, shape, medium, and other

Table 5. Selected preparations of plasma membranes from tissues*

Cell type	Medium for disruption	Agent for disruption	Method of fractionation	Morphological evaluation	Plasma membrane markers	Contamination markers
Liver or hepatomas[a]	1 mM bicarbonate	Potter–Elvehjem homogenizer	DC, DSDG	PCM, TEM	S-ATPase, 5N, APase, PNPase, adenylate cyclase, others	G6Pase, esterase, NADPH-cyt c reductase, G3PDH, others
Liver[b]	0.25 M sucrose, 5 mM Tris, ph 8	Potter–Elvehjem	DC, DSDG	PCM, TEM	5N, PDE-I	G6Pase, NADPH-cyt c reductase, cyt c oxidase, glucosaminidase, others
Liver[c]	1 mM bicarbonate, 0.5 mM CaCl₂ pH 7.6	Dounce	DC, zonal DSDG	TEM	5N, LAP, APase, adenylate cyclase, PDE	SDH, AcPase, monoamine oxidase, G6Pase, NADPH-cyt c reductase
Liver[c]	0.25 M sucrose, 5 mM Tris, pH 8	Dounce	DC, DSDG	TEM	Same as previous	Same as previous
Kidney cortex[d]	0.25 M sucrose, 20 mM bicarbonate	Dounce	DC, DSDG	TEM, brush border	APase	AcPase, G6Pase, succinate-cyt c reductase
Kidney cortex[e]	10 mM mannitol, 2 mM Tris, pH 7.1	Blender	Mg²⁺ treatment, DC	TEM, microvilli	APase, endopeptidase, amino peptidase, γ-GTase	S-ATPase, Cathepsin C' SDH, NADPH-cyt c reductase
Kidney cortex[f]	0.25 M sucrose, 10 mM TEA, pH 7.6	Dounce	DC (brush border), free flow electrophoresis (vesicles, microvilli)	TEM, microvilli *and* basolateral vesicles	S-ATPase (vesicles), APase (microvilli)	G6Pase, SDH, AcPase
Kidney cortex[g]	0.25 M sucrose, 1 mM EDTA, 4 mM Tris, pH 7.6	Potter–Elvehjem	DC, DSDG	TEM, (basolateral membranes)	S-ATPase, aminopeptidase	APase, LDH, G6Pase, SDH

Table 5. *Cont.* Selected preparations of plasma membranes from tissues*

Cell type	Medium for disruption	Agent for disruption	Method of fractionation	Morphological evaluation	Plasma membrane markers	Contamination markers
Muscle (skeletal, smooth, or heart)[h]	0.25 M sucrose, 0.2 mM EDTA, 0.2 mM Tris, pH 7.6	Polytron	LiBr extraction, DC, CSDG	TEM	S-ATPase, SA, ^{125}I incorp. by LPO	C-ATPase
Muscle (skeletal)[i]	0.25 M sucrose, 0.5 mM EDTA, pH 7.4	Waring Blendor	DC, CSDG	TEM	[^{3}H]ouabain	—
Heavy microsomal fraction of previous prep.[j]	0.25 M sucrose	French press	CSDG	TEM, transverse tubules	[^{3}H]ouabain	—
Muscle skeletal[k]	0.25 M sucrose, 0.5 mM EDTA, 0.1 M Tris, pH 7.4	Polytron	LiBr extraction, DC, DSDG	TEM	S-ATPase, 5 N, chol	LDH, SDH, IDPase, NADP-cyt c reductase, NADPH-cyt c reductase, AcPase, DNA
Brain (cerebral cortex)[l,m]	0.32 M sucrose, 1 mM phosphate, 0.1 mM EDTA pH 7.4	Teflon glass homogenizers	D-Ficoll grad.	TEM (synaptosomes)	S-Atpase	NADH-cyt c reductase, monoamine oxidase, SDH, RNA, NADPH-cyt c reductase
Cerebral cortex synaptosomes[m]	1 mM phosphate, 0.1 mM EDTA	14 gauge cannula, alkaline lysis	DSDG	TEM (synaptosomal membranes)	As above	As above
Spinal cord[n]	0.3 M Tricine, 0.5 mM MnCl$_2$, pH 5	Teflon-glass homogenizer	DC, DSDG	TEM	5N, cAMP PDE, Accholase	NADH-cyt c reductase NADPH-cyt c reductase, AcPase
Intestine mucosal scrape	5 mM EDTA, pH 7.4	Waring Blendor	DC	PCM, TEM (brush border)	Apase, ATPase, sucrose, others	—
Brush border (see above)[o]	1 M Tris	Incubation	DSDG	TEM (hollow tubes)	As above	As above
Brush border[p]	17 mM EDTA	Stirring	DC, DSDG	TEM	Apase, LAP, M-Anase	G6Pase

				(vesicles, hollow sacs)	ATPase, invertase, others	
Bladder[q]	FMA (sat'd), 20 mM Tris	Epithelium scraped after FMA treatment, homogenized in 20 mM Tris in Ten Broeck homogenizer	DC, DSDG	TEM	—	—
Intestine (mucosal scrape)[r]	0.25 mM sucrose, 5 mM H/I, 0.5 mM EDTA	Dounce	DC, DSDG	TEM (brush border and basolateral vesicles)	Apase, S-ATPase, sucrose, peptide hydrolase	G6Pase, NADH oxidase, NADH-cyt c reductase, succinate-cyt c reductase
Thyroid[s]	1 mM NaHCO$_3$	Dounce	DC, DSDG	TEM	5N, S-ATPase, APase, M-ATPase, adenylate cyclase	NADH-cyt c reductase, cyt c oxidase
Pancreas[t]	0.25 M sucrose, 40 mM Tris, 5 mM BME, 3 mM MgCl$_2$, 1 mM EDTA, 200 μg/ml SBT1	Teflon-glass homogenizer	DC. DSDG	TEM	5N, adenylate cyclase, M-ATPase	SDH. amylase, RNA
Pancreas (Islets of Langerhans)[u]	10 mM borate, 0.2 mM MgCl$_2$, pH 8.0	Beckman micromixer	CSDG	TEM	5N, APase, S-ATPase, M-ATPase, adenylate cyclase, [^{125}I]WGA	AcPase, cyt c oxidase, insulin, RNA
Mammary[v]	1 mM NaHCO$_3$	Polytron	DC, DSDG	TEM	Electrophoresis comparisons with MFGM	—
Mammary[w]	0.25 M sucrose, 20 mM Tris, pH 7.4	Sorvall Omni-Mixer	DC, DSDG, digitonin shift	TEM	5N, S-ATPase	SDH, NADPH-cyt c reductase, gal trans

*Abbreviations used: See lists for previous tables; PDE-I, phosphodiesterase I; LAP, leucine aminopeptidase; TEA, triethanolamine; G3PDH, glyceraldehyde 3-phosphate dehydrogenase; LPO, lactoperoxidase; C-ATPase, Ca^{2+}-ATPase; WGA, wheat germ agglutinin. [a]Emmelot et al. (1974); [b]Aronson and Touster (1974); [c]Wisher and Evans (1975); [d]Neville (1974), Wilfong and Neville (1970); [e]Booth and Kenny (1974); [f]Heidrich et al. (1972); Bode et al (1976); [g]Ebel et al. (1976); [h]Andrew and Appel (1973); Smith and Appel (1977); [i]Caswell et al. (1976); [j]Lau et al. (1977); [k]Schapira et al. (1974); [l]Gurd et al. (1974), Wang and Mahler (1977); [m]Babitch et al (1976); [n]Ghosh and Koenig (1977); [o]Eicholz and Crane (1974); [p]Forstner et al. (1968); [q]Hicks and Ketterer (1970); [r]Fujita et al (1972); [s]Yamishita and Field (1974); Suzuki et al. (1977); [t]Poirier et al. (1977); [u]Lernmark et al. (1976); [v]Keenan et al. (1970); [w]Shin et al. (1975), Huggins and Carraway (1976).

parameters, but the other factors are generally ignored in fractionation of cellular organelles. Thus intact cells, nuclei, ghosts, mitochondria, lysosomes, membrane fragments, and membrane vesicles can be separated into rough classes by pelleting with increasing centrifugal forces. Since pelleting is dependent upon the rate of sedimentation and the distance the particle must travel, there will be cross-contamination of fractions due to the original distribution of particles in the centrifuge tube. Multiple washing and centrifugation steps are required to overcome this difficulty. A more serious problem is the variation and overlap in weights among the various morphological units, particularly membrane fragments, depending on the extent of disruption. In cases where the plasma membranes are fractured into pieces of varying size but uniform density, differential centrifugation can possibly complicate membrane isolation.

Separation by density can be achieved on gradients of appropriate compositions and densities. A number of factors must be considered in choosing the type and range of gradient to be used (Evans, 1978). Foremost among these are the nature of the membranes to be isolated and the nature of the contaminating materials. Obviously, sealed vesicles and open fragments will respond differently on gradients depending on the gradient material and its osmotic activity. Since the density of the vesicle is the sum of its membrane density (with associated materials, such as water of hydration) and the density of the intravesicular contents, its position on a gradient will depend on its permeability to the gradient material. A permeant solute, such as glycerol, will 'load' the vesicle and the density of the vesicle will reflect only the contributions of the membrane and its associated components, since internal and external densities are equalized. A non-permeant, small solute such as sucrose, presents the vesicle with a large osmotic gradient as well as a density gradient. Sedimentation thus will cause shrinkage of the vesicle and concentration of the non-permeant intravesicular contents as water is removed. Density gradients of a large uncharged, non-permeant molecules such as Ficoll or dextran, do not produce such large osmotic effects. It should be clear that the densities obtained for vesicles can be influenced by a number of factors (Wallach and Schmidt-Ullrich, 1977).

Open membrane fragments are not subject to these influences. Since osmotic forces are not considered important, separations are usually performed on sucrose gradients. For analytical separations continuous gradients are preferred, but discontinuous gradients are often used for preparative work, since they facilitate collection of the membrane fractions. It is always advisable to analyse by continuous gradient centrifugation any preparation that is to be separated on a discontinuous gradient. This permits a more judicious choice of the densities to be used for the discontinuous gradient. It should also be recognized that the bands collected at the interfaces of the discontinuous gradient result from artificial narrowing of the gradient which destroys its resolving power over that range.

In either continuous or discontinuous gradients the sample can be sedimented (loaded at the top) or floated (loaded from below). Since plasma membranes band at low densities (Evans, 1978), flotation has the advantage of eliminating contamination due to trapping of other constituents at the centrifuge tube wall or gradient interfaces. It also decreases contamination from incomplete sedimentation, i.e., failure to achieve isopycnic conditions. However, these factors will tend to decrease plasma membrane yields in flotation experiments. When the densities of the desired membranes and their major contaminants are known, a sandwich gradient technique (Louvard *et al.*, 1973; Evans, 1978) can be useful. The sample is loaded at a density intermediate between the two, so that they are moved in opposite directions on the gradient during centrifugation.

Because of the configuration and ability to be loaded and unloaded while revolving, zonal rotors offer advantages in resolving power. Both rate-zonal and density separations can be performed, and the large capacity of the commercial rotors is a boon for preparative work. However, the large capacity also tends to limit the analytical and developmental studies on membrane preparative procedures, so the zonal rotors have not been widely utilized. In addition the capital investment tends to discourage those not extensively involved in membrane preparation.

Materials which form their own gradient during centrifugation offer obvious technical advantages. Use of the alkali metal salts (e.g. CsCl) has been limited because the high concentrations necessary tend to disrupt membranous elements. It is clearly important that no interaction occur between membranes and the gradient material. Percoll, a silica sol coated with polyvinylpyrrolidone to reduce its interaction with cellular components, will form a density gradient upon centrifugation. We have recently been able to separate microvilli shed from 13762 mammary adenocarcinoma cells from intact cells and membrane vesicles using a Percoll gradient (Carraway *et al.*, 1980). Attempts to achieve this separation with sucrose gradients were unsuccessful.

Further purification of membrane fractions can sometimes be achieved by density perturbation, i.e., treatment of the membranes to alter their densities. Upon recentrifugation the perturbed membranes migrate to a new position on the gradient and are separated from contaminating membranes which were not perturbed by the treatment and which migrate to the original position. An example of this procedure is the use of digitonin to perturb the densities of cholesterol-enriched plasma membrane (Amar-Costesec *et al.*, 1974; Lewis *et al.*, 1975). Figure 5 and Table 6 show the use of this method to facilitate the separation of plasma membranes (enriched in 5'-nucleotidase) and Golgi (enriched in galactosyltransferase) from rat mammary tissue (Huggins and Carraway, 1976). An interesting facet of these results is that one shifted fraction is enriched in both nucleotidase and galactosyltransferase (Huggins *et al.*, 1980). Membrane isolation using phagocytosis of or adsorption to beads also depends on the density difference between the beads and cellular constituents for separation of the membranes.

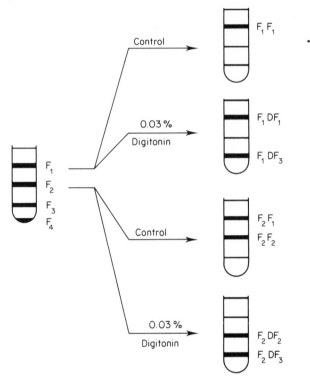

Figure 5. Scheme for isolating plasma membranes from lactating rat mammary gland using the digitonin shift procedure. Fractions F_1 and F_2 were obtained as described previously. (Shin *et al.*, 1975)

Wallach *et al.* (1972) introduced the term affinity density perturbation to describe the technique in which reagents (e.g. lectins) which bind to the cell surface are covalently coupled to beads, which can then bind to membranes and alter their densities. Plasma membranes which bind specifically to the beads can be separated from the other cellular constituents by density gradient centrifugation. The critical factor is the specificity of the reagent for the cell surface. Specific antibodies against cell surface components would be an obvious reagent of choice (Lim *et al.*, 1975). However, it should be remembered that according to the membrane flow hypothesis endomembranes will also contain cell surface constituents which are destined for the plasma membrane. Thus it is not so simple to differentiate operationally between the cell surface and endomembranes, even when fractionation procedures are available. Another difficulty with the affinity techniques is removing the membranes from the beads without perturbing the membrane. Hapten elution techniques are sometimes not successful because of multiple attachments of the membranes to the beads. Methods for disrupting antibody–antigen interac-

Table 6. Effect of digitonin shift fractionation on distribution
of mammary membrane enzyme markers[*]

Fraction	5'-Nucleotidase μmol/hour/mg protein	Galactosyl transferase
Homo	4.7	0.09
F_1	136	2.4
F_1DF_1	56	4.9
F_1DF_3	340	0
F_2	125	3.2
F_2DF_1	96	4.6
F_2DF_3	170	4.14

[*]Designation of fractions as in Figure 5.

tions may also perturb membrane structures of interest. Clearly the usefulness
of the method will depend strongly on the ultimate purpose of the membrane
preparation.

B. Chromatographic Separation

The same principles can be applied to separation by affinity chromatography.
Membranes from homogenates or partially purified fractions can be passed
through columns derivatized with appropriate binding reagents. Lectins have
been most often used to obtain the binding specificity. However, it should be
recognized that endomembranes as well as plasma membranes contain lectin
binding sites. It has been suggested that 'plasma membrane vesicles' which do
not bind to Con A columns are inside-out vesicles (Zachowski and Paraf, 1974;
Walsh *et al.*, 1976). Other possibilities are that these non-binding membranes
are from compositionally distinct regions of the plasma membrane (Resch *et
al.*, 1978) or from rightside-out endomembranes, whose carbohydrate
components would be inside the vesicle.

An interesting application of affinity chromatography was used to purify
hormonally sensitive plasma membranes from rat fat cells (Luzio *et al.*, 1976).
Taking advantage of the ability of antisera against rat erythrocytes to
cross-react with isolated rat fat cells, the fat cells were coated with rabbit
anti-erythrocyte serum before homogenization. The homogenate was then
passed over an immunoabsorbent column of donkey anti-(rat globulin).
Binding of plasma membranes was detected by assaying adenylate cyclase and
5'-nucleotidase. Removal of the membranes from the adsorbent was not
reported, illustrating one of the difficulties with this type of technique.

Chromatography on glass beads has also been used for the isolation of the
plasma membranes (Warley and Cook, 1973). The basis for this method is not
clear, but it probably involves some type of adsorption phenomenon.

C. Partition Techniques

Partition methods (Albertsson, 1971) have been used for separation of cells and proteins using a simple two-phase separation or a more elaborate countercurrent distribution (Walter, 1975). Brunette and Till (1971) used a dextran–polyethylene glycol aqueous two-phase system to purify L-cell surface membranes afer homogenization of Zn^{2+}-treated cells. The method is rapid and can be performed without high speed centrifugation. Plasma membranes are found in the interface between the phases. Multiple partitions can be performed to remove nuclei and other contaminants which become trapped at the interface. Depending on the purpose for which the membranes are intended, a significant problem with the method might be the adsorption of the polymeric phase components to the membranes.

D. Electrophoresis and Isoelectric Focusing

Because of differences in charge between plasma membranes and other organelles electrophoretic separation is potentially very useful. The technique of free flow electrophoresis, pioneered and developed by Hannig (1972), has been used for a number of separations (Evans, 1978). Unfortunately, the technique is experimentally very demanding and the commercial equipment for performing the operation is expensive. The use of the technique is illustrated by fractionation of kidney brush border preparations into microvilli and basolateral surfaces (Heidrich *et al.*, 1972; Bode *et al.*, 1976). It has also been used for fractionation of gastric mucosal membranes (Saccomani *et al.*, 1977). Isoelectric focusing has been used for separation of membranes from erythrocytes, lymphocytes, and platelets (Jamieson and Groh, 1971), but the method has not seen extensive use.

IV. PLASMA MEMBRANE IDENTIFICATION

A. Morphology

In cases where intact envelopes or ghosts can be isolated the simplest means of identification is microscopy. Envelopes or large fragments are usually observed by phase contrast or dark field microscopy, which also permits assessment of nuclear contamination. These techniques can be used for a semi-quantitative evaluation of the yield of the isolation in terms of ghosts per number of cells homogenized. The light microscope does not have sufficient resolution to assess contamination by smaller organelles, such as lysosomes, mitochondria, and fragments of Golgi or endoplasmic reticulum. Usually transmission electron microscopy of thin sections of membrane pellets is used to assess contamination with other organelles, since the organellar structures show characteristic patterns by this method. Negative staining is less frequently used because the differentiating characteristics are less clearly delineated.

Vigorous disruption of cells not only breaks down the plasma membrane into fragments and vesicles, but also will fragment Golgi, endoplasmic reticulum, the nuclear envelope, and outer mitochondrial membrane, depending on the conditions and the stability of these elements in the individual system. Thus the identifying morphology of these organelle membranes may be lost. For this reason morphological identification of plasma membranes and assessment of yields from vigorously disrupted cells are difficult, if not impossible.

As mentioned earlier, certain morphological features associated with surfaces of tissue cells can be used as an aid in identifying plasma membranes, if they have not been too severely disrupted. The presence of junctional complexes has been useful in identifying and assigning cell surface regions from liver membrane preparations. Microvilli, when they survive homogenizing conditions, are also a useful morphological marker for the cell surface. Recently it has become apparent that microfilaments are attached to the inner surface of the plasma membrane (Korn, 1978) and could potentially be used for identification. However, these structures are rather readily disrupted by conditions used for membrane preparation, and one must be concerned about adventitious association of actin microfilaments with other cellular elements. A major difficulty in using morphological markers is their quantitation. Morphometric techniques (Weibel, 1969) have not been used routinely in plasma membrane isolation.

B. Enzyme Markers

1. Plasma Membrane Enzymes

For preparations which have lost morphological integrity, the most common method for identifying plasma membranes is through the use of enzyme markers. The degree of purification of these markers provides an estimate of the purification of the plasma membranes, providing that certain conditions are met. DePierre and Karnovsky (1973) have discussed critically factors which are important in the use of marker enzymes for identification and evaluation of plasma membrane preparations. The most important criteria are that the enzyme be localized predominantly, if not exclusively, at the cell surface and that any changes in its specific activity be accountable. The former can be assessed by histochemical or biochemical techniques. Our own bias is to use ectoenzymes as markers whenever possible, because there are more and better procedures for evaluating the localization of these enzymes. DePierre and Karnovsky (1974) have used substrate permeability, product localization, and inactivation by a non-permeant reagent to assess the localization of 5'-nucleotidase, Mg^{2+}-ATPase, and *p*-nitrophenylphosphatase of lymphoid cells.

We have used similar procedures for evaluating the localizations of 5'-nucleotidase (Carraway *et al.*, 1976) and a Ca^{2+}- and Mg^{2+}-dependent ATPase of mammary tumour cells (C. A. C. Carraway *et al.*, 1980). When beginning work on any new system for which markers have not been defined, it is always advisable to perform such localization studies. The activities of various plasma membrane enzymes can vary widely with cell type, as can the fraction of the total cellular activity of a particular enzyme localized in the plasma membrane.

The problem of activation or inactivation of the marker enzyme during the preparation procedure can be circumvented by careful book-keeping. Inactivation usually results from perturbation of the enzyme structure during disruption or separation procedures. Activation is less frequent but can be observed if an inhibitor of the enzyme is removed during fractionation, as has been postulated for galactosyltransferase (Mitranic *et al.*, 1974), or if enzyme perturbation enhances enzyme activity.

Another problem in using enzyme markers is the overlapping specificities of some of the enzymes. Thus the assays used will often measure the activities of more than one enzyme, which may have different localizations. For example, phosphate release assays for 5'-nucleotidase often also measure a contribution from alkaline phosphatase. The spectrophotometric and radiochemical assays usually include phosphate compounds such as β-glycerophosphate as alkaline phosphatase inhibitors. For 5'-nucleotidase the plant lectin Concanavalin A can be used as an inhibitor (Riordan and Slavik, 1974; Carraway and Carraway, 1976; Riemer and Widnell, 1975) to estimate the contribution of other enzymes. Sensitivity to levamisole is used to assess the specificity of alkaline phosphatase (Beaufay, 1974).

The problem of overlapping specificities is particularly acute for the ATPases, which are differentiated primarily by their cation specificities. There are possibly five different ATPases which can be associated with plasma membranes: Na^+, K^+-ATPase, the alkali metal pump enzyme which is inhibited by ouabain; Ca^{2+}, Mg^{2+}-ATPase, the Ca^{2+} pump enzyme; Mg^{2+}-ATPase, which is usually expressed as the residual activity; Ca^{2+}- or Mg^{2+}-ATPase, which is an ectoenzyme showing approximately equivalent activation by either divalent cation; and myosin. Few efforts have been made to differentiate among the last four of these. In fact there is no consistent scheme for doing so, even though such a scheme would enhance their usefulness as plasma membrane markers. It is possible that the reported ecto Mg^{2+}-ATPase (Trams and Lauter, 1974; DePierre and Karnovsky, 1974; Smolen and Weissman, 1978) is the same enzyme as the Ca^{2+}- or Mg^{2+}-ATPase (Stefanovic *et al.*, 1976; Ronquist and Agren, 1975; C. A. C. Carraway *et al.*, 1980). Obviously, the discovery of specific inhibitors for these various enzymes would be of great benefit to the use of these enzymes as markers.

From the above considerations it should be discerned that the use of enzyme markers to calculate the degree of plasma membrane purification is fraught with difficulties. First, one must know the fraction of the total amount of a given enzyme which is present in the plasma membrane. Second, one must be able to ascertain how much of the enzyme fraction is obtained in the final product. Third, one must contend with the probability that the enzyme marker is not uniformly distributed over the entire plasma membrane of the cells, even for homogeneous cell populations. It is possible to attain a purification of the enzyme marker which is higher than the theoretical purification of total plasma membrane if one isolates a membrane region enriched in the enzyme. Thus purification factors should be reported for the species assayed, not for the membranes, since the relationship between the two is not always straightforward.

The localization of certain enzymes to discrete regions of the plasma membrane can be used to advantage in identifying membrane fractions from complex tissues. Evans (1978) has shown that leucine aminopeptidase, 5'-nucleotidase, alkaline phosphatase, and nucleotide pyrophosphatase are more highly concentrated in bile canalicular membranes than in contiguous or blood sinusoidal membranes. In contrast adenylyl cyclase activity is highest in blood sinusoidal membranes. Membrane fractions from kidney separated by free flow electrophoresis showed a high alkaline phosphatase and low Na^+, K^+-ATPase for microvilli-containing fractions from the apical (brush border) region of the cell and a high Na^+, K^+-ATPase and low alkaline phosphatase for vesicles from the basal region (Heidrich *et al.*, 1972).

Immunochemical procedures can be used in some instances as an aid in characterizing enzymes present in membrane fractions. By combining histochemical staining procedures for the enzymes with immunoelectrophoresis of detergent-soluble membrane components, one can identify different enzymes possessing the same specificity (Blomberg and Raftell, 1973; Raftell and Blomberg, 1973) and determine how they distribute among various membrane fractions.

Table 7 provides a listing of some of the enzymes which have been used as plasma membrane markers. It should be recognized that the localization of these enzymes to the plasma membrane has not necessarily been validated in all cases.

2. Enzyme Markers for Contaminating Membranes

In the absence of morphological criteria contaminating organelles are best determined from enzyme markers. As with the plasma membrane markers the localization criteria used are usually not absolute and are often undefined for any particular system. Nevertheless, such enzyme data are a useful adjunct in

Table 7. Commonly used plasma membrane marker enzymes

Enzyme	Comments	References
5'-Nucleotidase	Ectoenzyme. Most widely used marker. Localization to plasma membrane not exclusive in most cell types	De Pierre and Karnovsky (1973); Solyom and Trams (1972)
Na^+, K^+-ATPase	Ion pump enzyme. Localized to basal surface of cells in some tissues	Solyom and Trams (1972)
Mg^{2+}-ATPase	Function and localization ill-defined. Has been reported to be ectoenzyme in some cells. Confusion with Ca^{2+}- or Mg^{2+}-ATPase possible	Solyom and Trams (1972)
Ca^{2+}- or Mg^{2+}-ATPase	Ectoenzyme in some cells. Activation by Ca^{2+} or Mg^{2+} approximately equivalent	Stefanovic *et al.* (1976); C. A. C. Carraway *et al.* (1980)
γ-Glutamyltrasnferase	Implicated in amino acid transport. Abundant in kidney brush border, but present in many cell types	Tate and Meister (1975); Monneron and d'Alayer (1978); Resch *et al.* (1978)
Adenylate cyclase	Ubiquitous, but variable activity. Hormones and F^- stimulate. Assay complex	Solyom and Trams (1972)
Alkaline phosphatase	Term encompasses several enzymes with different substrate specificities and localizations	Solyom and Trams (1972)
Phosphodiesterase I, nucleotide pyrophosphatase	Possibly the same enzyme	Touster *et al.* (1970)
Leucine aminopeptidase	Usually assayed as naphthylamidase	Solyom and Trams (1972)

Table 8. Commonly used marker enzymes for contaminating subcellular fractions in plasma membrane preparations

Organelle	Enzyme	References
Mitochondria		
Outer membrane	Monamine oxidase	Amar-Costesec *et al.* (1974)
Inner membrane	Succinic dehydrogenase	Allan and Crumpton (1972)
	Cytochrome oxidase	Allan and Crumpton (1972)
Endoplasmic reticulum	NADH-cytochrome c	Beufay *et al.* (1974)
	reductase, Glucose-6-	Amar-Costesec *et al.* (1974)
	phosphatase, Esterase,	Allan and Crumpton (1972)
	NADH diaphorase	Dallner *et al* (1966)
Golgi	Galactosyltransferase	Bergeron *et al.* (1973)
	Thiamine pyrophosphatase	Cheetham *et al.* (1971)
Lysosomes	*N*-Acetylglucosaminidase	Gianetto and de Duve (1955)
	Acid phosphatase	Gianetto and de Duve (1955)
Peroxisomes	Catalase	Baudhuin *et al.* (1964)
Cytoplasm	Lactic dehydrogenase	Neilands (1955)

assessing plasma membrane purity. Again there is a problem of variability of enzyme activity with source. For example, glucose-6-phosphatase is often used as a marker for endoplasmic reticulum, but its activity is greatly reduced in some cells. Succinic dehydrogenase is the most commonly used marker for mitochondria. However, it should be remembered that vigorous disruption can fragment the outer mitochondrial membrane, releasing it as fragments or vesicles which do not contain succinic dehydrogenase. Monoamine oxidase can be used then as an outer membrane marker. Golgi contamination is often not evaluated in plasma membrane preparations. The most frequently used Golgi marker enzyme is galactosyltransferase, but there is a question whether it may also occur in some plasma membranes. We have found substantial amounts of galactosyltransferase in mammary membrane fractions that are high in 5'-nucleotidase, sialic acid, and cholesterol, nominally plasma membrane components.

Table 8 lists commonly used markers for contaminating organelles.

C. Chemical Markers

Analysis of chemical compositions of plasma membrane preparations can be used in assessing purification or contamination, although there are few absolute markers. Since sialic acid and cholesterol are enriched in plasma membranes, their contents are reported for many preparations. As expected, there is considerable variability among different systems. The cholesterol/phospholipid ratio is another parameter which has been considered diagnostic for plasma membranes, but there is no universal agreement on what the ratio is (a value near 1 is often cited as appropriate), probably due to both variations in the purity of the preparations reported and in the systems examined. Glycolipids, particularly sialic acid containing gangliosides (Morgan *et al.*, 1971), should be useful plasma membrane markers, but they have not been routinely used. Of the phospholipids sphingomyelin appears to be generally more concentrated in plasma membranes than other organelles (Evans, 1978), but results for different species of red cells indicate that its specific content can be highly variable (Nelson, 1967).

Chemical markers are probably more useful for assessment of contaminants. The presence of nucleic acids suggests contamination by nuclei, rough endoplasmic reticulum or adsorbed ribosomes, although the presence of RNA at the cell surface has been reported. Cardiolipin appears to be present exclusively in mitochondria. Since membrane preparations can easily be analysed for their constituent polypeptides, it would be useful to have specific diagnostic polypeptides for identification of membrane components. Unfortunately, no useful scheme for such an approach is available. Plasma membranes generally contain larger amounts of higher molecular weight polypeptides, possibly cytoskeletal components, but these are often dissociable from the membrane, and there is a question concerning native association. Actin appears to be a ubiquitous component of plasma membrane preparations, but its occurrence in other insoluble non-membranous structural elements and its tendency to associate with many different proteins render it useless as a marker.

D. Antigens and Other Binding Proteins

Relatively little use has been made of plasma membrane antigens (see refs. in Tables 3 and 4) as markers for evaluating membrane isolations, primarily for two reasons. First, the localization criteria are the same as for enzyme markers, and antigen localization is often even less well defined. Second, quantitative assays for the antigens, described elsewhere in this volume, are usually more complex than those for enzymes. Somewhat more utility has been made of other binding proteins (e.g. hormones, toxins) which associate with plasma membranes (Andrew *et al.*, 1974; Suzuki *et al.*, 1977; Matlib *et al.*, 1979). Purification can be assessed by measuring the binding activity of membrane fractions. The complexity of the binding functions and techniques for measuring binding tend to reduce the attractiveness of this approach, although it has been used in a number of systems. For example, binding of [^{125}I]luteinizing hormone was found to parallel 5′-nucleotidase activity in membrane fractions from bovine corpus luteum (Gospadarowicz, 1973). Similarly, [^{14}C]fructose binding activity was greater in membrane fractions enriched in nucleotidase and Na$^+$, K$^+$-ATPase from bovine circumvallate papillae, presumably reflecting the presence of 'taste receptors' in the plasma membranes from this tissue (Lo, 1973).

Table 9. Isolation of plasma membranes labelled with membrane-specific or surface-associated ligands*

Cell or tissue type	Ligand	Specificity	References
Fat cells	[^{125}I]Insulin	Insulin receptor	Chang *et al*. (1975)
	[^{125}I]WGA	NAG-containing oligosaccharides	
	[^{125}I]Cholera toxin	G_1-ganglioside	
Muscle cells (cultured)	[^{125}I α-]Bungarotoxin	Acetylcholine receptor	Schimmel *et al*. (1973)
Human skin fibroblasts	[^{125}I]WGA	NAG of oligosaccharides	Kartner *et al*. (1977)
HeLa	[^{125}I]Antiserum (horse)	Unspecified cell surface antigens	Boone *et al*. (1969)
Skeletal muscle	[^{3}H]Ouabain	Na$^+$, K$^+$-ATPase of transverse tubules	Caswell *et al*. (1976) Lau *et al*. (1977)
Pancreas islets of Langerhans	[^{125}I]WGA	NAG of oligosaccharides	Lernmark *et al*. (1976)
Platelets	[^{125}I]Lentil lectin		Rittenhouse-Simmons and Deykin (1976)

*Abbreviations used: WGA, wheat germ agglutinin; NAG, *N*-acetyl glucosamine.

An alternative is to bind the ligand to the cells before disruption of the plasma membrane (Chang *et al*., 1975). If radioactive ligand is used, the radioactivity can be assayed to localize its binding sites among the fractions produced during the preparation. Such an approach obviously is favoured by a high association constant for the ligand. If the plasma membrane is impermeable to the ligand, this technique eliminates contributions from intracellular binding components, assuming that no exchange occurs during preparation. Controls for exchange reactions can be performed with appropriate mixing experiments. A number of different ligands have been used for such preparations, including lectins, antibodies, hormones, toxins, and ouabain (Table 9). To correct for non-specific binding Boone *et al*. (1969) used [^{125}I]immune and [^{131}I]non-immune antisera and monitored the ratio of the two during fractionation of HeLa cells after reaction of the intact cells with the labelled antisera.

E. Labelling of the Cell Surface

The ideal situation in identifying plasma membranes would be to label uniformly every plasma membrane molecule and no other molecules in the cell. Obviously there are no labelling procedures which can approach such a standard. However, specific covalent labelling of the cell surface by imper-

Table 10. Use of cell surface labelling for identification of plasma membranes

Cell or tissue	Labelling reagent	References
Lymphocytes	^{125}I and lactoperoxidase	Marchalonis *et al* (1971)
L cells	^{125}I and lactoperoxidase	Hubbard and Cohn (1975)
Cardiac cells (cultured)	^{125}I and lactoperoxidase	Heller and Harary (1977)
Rat muscle	^{125}I and lactoperoxidase	Barchi *et al*. (1977)
L-1210	^{125}I and lactoperoxidase	Tsai *et al*. (1975)
Rat dermal fibroblasts	Periodate and [^{3}H]borohydride	Thom *et al*. (1977)
Placental micro-villus membrane	[^{32}P]phosphate incorporation into alkaline phosphatase	Carlson *et al*. (1976)
Human neutrophil	Galactose oxidase and [^{3}H] borohydride	Klempner *et al*. (1980)

meant probes is a useful technique for monitoring membrane isolations. Either chemical or enzymatic incorporation of label can be used (Carraway, 1975). The former employs non-penetrating molecules containing reactive functional groups. As with any other marker group it is necessary to assess the localization. For this purpose controls should be run on broken cells and comparisons made of specific activities of labelled isolated membranes and membranes isolated from labelled cells. Broken cells should incorporate much more label into more different components (e.g. polypeptides separated by SDS–poyacrylamide gel electrophoresis). Labelled isolated membranes should have a higher specific activity than membranes isolated from labelled cells. Another useful technique is to compare in intact and broken cells incorporation into a known major intracellular component, e.g. actin or histones. Autoradiography can also be informative. Because of the heterogeneity of plasma membranes it is advantageous to have a relatively non-specific reactive functional group so that it is not specifically incorporated into particular domains of the cell surface. The major problem in labelling with chemical reagents is the permeation of the reagent (Carraway, 1975), which will be variable with different cell types. For that reason enzymatic labelling has been more frequently used.

Lactoperoxidase and galactose oxidase are most often used for labelling cells before membrane isolation. In our hands transglutaminase, another enzyme which has been used for labelling membranes (Brewer and Singer, 1974), is not efficient enough in labelling cell surfaces to be very useful. Criteria for determining the localization of the label have been discussed previously and should include those controls discussed for chemical reagents. For the iodination reaction with lactoperoxidase controls without peroxide (or a peroxide generating system) and without lactoperoxidase are important.

Likewise the incorporation of radioactive borohydride in the absence of galactose oxidase treatment should be determined. Pretreatment of cells with neuraminidase often enhances galactose oxidase–borohydride labelling. Proteolytic cleavage, monitored by label released or electrophoresis, can be used to determine whether the incorporated label is surface located, assuming that the cells are not also leaky to protease. The major difficulty with enzymatic labelling is labelling of leaky or dead cells (Juliano and Behar-Bannelier, 1975). A significant proportion of dead cells in a preparation will exhibit by electrophoresis heavily labelled histone bands, providing a simple assessment procedure for intactness of cells.

A possible problem with galactose oxidase–borohydride labelling is that the aldehyde produced by oxidation can react with an amino group on another protein before the reductive labelling (Carraway, 1975). This would alter the properties of the proteins in question but would not necessarily affect the use of the procedure for monitoring membrane isolations. In addition such cross-linking reactions appear less frequent in labelling whole cells than isolated membranes, and they can be reduced by running the borohydride reduction simultaneously with the oxidation.

The lactoperoxidase and galactose oxidase procedures are complementary in a sense. The former is less specific, since it will label any accessible tyrosine residues in protein at the cell surface. The latter is directed only towards glycoproteins with accessible galactose or galactosamine. Heavily glycosylated proteins are often deficient in accessible tyrosine. A significant criticism of these methods is that they necessarily involve oxidative perturbations of the cells. Metabolic labelling with radioactive substrates does not cause such perturbations, but it requires that the substrate be incorporated specifically into the plasma membrane. Fucose labelling has been used to a limited extent for such studies because it is incorporated specifically into the cell surface in some cells (Atkinson and Summers, 1971). The use of this procedure for new cell types would require substantiation of unique or preferential plasma membrane localization.

Surface labelling procedures can be particularly helpful in evaluating the heterogeneity of the cell surface and the distribution of the cell surface elements during fractionation procedures. For example collagenase-dissociated guinea pig intestine showed two ^{125}I-labelled peaks after lactoperoxidase labelling, homogenization, and density gradient centrifugation. Enzyme markers and morphological studies indicated that these came from brush border and basolateral faces of the intestinal cells (Lewis *et al.*, 1975). In a similar study Graham *et al.* (1975) found that [25]I-labelled fibronectin, a major surface glycoprotein of normal fibroblasts, did not fractionate with plasma membrane markers after disruption of the labelled cells by nitrogen cavitation. Apparently fibronectin is an extracellular matrix component which is only loosely associated with the plasma membrane. This study emphasizes a hazard in using cell surface labelling as the sole plasma membrane marker. Extracellular components, including serum proteins, can be labelled and then lost from the membrane during fractionation.

V. CONCLUSIONS

Our objective in this review has been to provide an understanding of the basic methodologies currently used in the isolation of plasma membranes from animal cells. We have attempted to provide considerations involved in the choice of the membrane preparation method(s) best suited to the needs of the investigator. Included in these considerations are discussions of the pitfalls which may be encountered in using the various methods and a sufficient bibliography to give the uninitated investigator some starting point(s) from which to begin his attempt at plasma membrane isolation. It should be clear that there is no simple method for plasma membrane isolation which will work for most cell types. However, there are certain criteria which are important enough to membrane preparation to bear reiteration in summarizing this area.

(i) The isolation procedure should be designed to fulfill the need of the investigation.

(ii) Thorough understanding of the tissue or cell from which the membranes are to be isolated is invaluable. Investigations of the cell surface components by chemical, enzymatic or metabolic labelling, localization of antigens or enzymes by histochemical or chemical methods and characterization of enzyme or transport functions by kinetic or chemical analyses provide information which can be used in evaluating degradation, purification, and recoveries of membranes during disruption and fractionation procedures.

(iii) Disruption should be carefully monitored to obtain the desired fragmentation of the plasma membrane without destruction of other organelles or membrane components. Microscopy and sedimentation can be used to evaluate organelle destruction, while labelling studies are useful in assessing degradation of membrane components.

(iv) Fractionation procedures should minimize membrane aggregation and carefully control perturbation.

(v) A balance sheet of 'markers' should be prepared for all fractionation procedures to permit evaluation of purification and recoveries.

Adherence to these criteria will not guarantee successful plasma membrane preparations, but it will enhance the probability of obtaining membranes with the properties sought for the investigation to be performed.

The use of antibodies in the preparation and characterization of plasma membranes is still in its infancy, but this approach has outstanding potential. A major difficulty has been the acquisition of purified antibodies against components localized in the plasma membrane. The use of monoclonal antibodies from hybridomas (Kohler and Milstein, 1975) may aid in overcoming this difficulty. However, it must be recognized that no technology will override the fact that most proteins are not uniquely localized in the cell. Thus methods for detection and quantitation continue to be a concern. For membranes the insolubility of the constituents has complicated most immunological analyses. For many systems this problem can be overcome by using the solubilizing power of dodecyl sulphate and the resolving power of polyacrylamide gel electrophoresis. After removal of the detergent the antigen can be detected on the gels by an indirect staining procedure, applying antibody and ^{125}I-labelled Staph A protein (Adair *et al.*, 1978). If the procedures described previously can provide specific antibodies and relatively unperturbed plasma membranes, it should be possible to perform immunochemical localization studies and antibody perturbations similar to those described earlier for anti-spectrin antibody and erythrocyte membranes. This type of study should enormously enhance our knowledge of membrane structure/function relationships.

ACKNOWLEDGMENTS

We thank Drs Ulrich Melcher, John Huggins, and Anne Sherblom for reading the manuscript, Dr Robert E. Scott for preprints of his work and Eileen Huggins for assistance with the preparation of the manuscript. Original investigations described in this chapter were conducted in cooperation with the USDA, Agricultural Research Service, Southern Region, supported by NIH, the American Cancer Society, and the Oklahoma Agricultural Experiment Station and performed in the Dept. of Biochemistry, Oklahoma State Univ., Stillwater, OK.

REFERENCES

Adair, W. S., Jurivich, D., and Goodenough, U. W. (1978). Localization of cellular antigens in sodium dodecyl sulfate-polyacrylamide gels. *J. Cell Biol.*, **79**, 281–285.
Albertsson, P. -Å. (1972). *Partition of Cell Particles and Macromolecules*, 2nd edn. Wiley-Interscience, New York.
Allan, D. and Crumpton, M. J. (1970). Preparation and characterization of the plasma membrane of pig lymphocytes. *Biochem. J.*, **120**, 133–143.
Allan, D. and Crumpton, M. J. (1972). Isolation and composition of human thymocyte plasma membrane. *Biochim Biophys. Acta*, **274**, 22–27.
Amar-Costesec, A., Wibo, M., Thinès-Sempoux, D., Beaufay, H., and Berthet, J. (1974). Analytical study of microsomes and isolated subcellular membranes from rat liver IV. Biochemical, physical, and morphological modifications of microsomal components induced by digitonin, EDTA, and pyrophosphate. *J. Cell Biol.*, **62**, 717–745.
Andrew, C. G. and Appel, S. H. (1973). Macromolecular characterization of muscle membranes. I. Proteins and sialic acid of normal and denervated muscle. *J. Biol. Chem.*, **248**, 5156–5163.

Aronson, N. N., Jr. and Touster, O. (1974). Isolation of rat liver plasma membrane fragments in isotonic sucrose. *Methods Enzymol.*, **31**, 90–102.

Atkinson, P. H. (1973). HeLa cell plasma membranes. *Methods Cell Biol.*, **1**, 157–188.

Atkinson, P. H. and Summers, D. F. (1971). Purification and properties of HeLa cell plasma membranes. *J. Biol. Chem.*, **246**, 5162–5175.

Avruch, J. and Wallach, D. F. H. (1971). Preparation and properties of plasma membrane and endoplasmic reticulum fragments from isolated rat fat cells. *Biochim. Biophys. Acta.*, **233**, 334–347.

Babitch, J. A., Breithaupt, T. B., Chiu, T. -C., Garadi, R., and Helseth, D. L. (1976). Preparation of chick brain synaptosomes and synaptosomal membranes. *Biochim. Biophys. Acta*, **433**, 75–89.

Barber, A. J. and Jamieson, G. A. (1970). Isolation and characterization of plasma membranes from human blood platelets. *J. Biol. Chem.*, **245**, 6357–6365.

Barchi, R. L., Bonilla, E., and Wong, M. (1977). Isolation and characterization of muscle membranes using surface-specific labels. *Proc. Natl. Acad. Sci. USA*, **74**, 34–38.

Barland, P. and Schroeder, E. A. (1970). A new rapid method for the isolation of surface membranes from tissue culture cells. *J. Cell Biol.*, **45**, 662–668.

Baudhuin, P., Evrard, P., and Berthet, J. (1967). Electron microscopic examination of subcellular fractions. I. The preparation of representative samples from suspensions of particles. *J. Cell. Biol.*, **32**, 181–191.

Beaufay, H., Amar-Costesec, A., Feytmans, E., Thines-Sempoux, D., Wibo, M., Robbi, M., and Berthet, J. (1974). Analytical study of microsomes and isolated subcellular membranes from rat liver. I. Biochemical methods. *J. Cell Biol.*, **61**, 188–200.

Bergeron, J. J. M., Ehrenreich, J. H., Siekevitz, P., and Palade, G. E. (1973). Golgi fractions prepared from rat liver homogenates. II. Biochemical characterization. *J. Cell Biol.*, **59**, 73–88.

Berlin, R. D., Oliver, J. M., Ukena, T. E., and Yin, H. H. (1974). Control of cell surface topography. *Nature*, **247**, 45–46.

Bingham, R. W. and Burke, D. C. (1972). Isolation of plasma membrane and endoplasmic reticulum fragments from chick embryo fibroblasts. *Biochim. Biophys. Acta*, **274**, 348–352.

Blomberg, F. and Raftell, M. (1973). Membrane fractions from rat hepatoma. II. Immunochemical characterization of detergent-soluble membrane esterases, glycosidases, and leucyl-β-napthylamidase. *Biochim. Biophys. Acta*, **291**, 431–441.

Blomstrand, C. and Hamberger, A. (1969). Protein turnover in cell-enriched fractions from rabbit brain. *J. Neurochem.*, **16**, 1401–1407.

Bode, F., Baumann, K., and Kinne, R. (1976). Analysis of the pinocytic process in rat kidney. II. Biochemical composition of pinocytic vesicles compared to brush border microvilli, lysosomes and basolateral plasma membranes. *Biochim. Biophys. Acta*, **433**, 294–310.

Boone, C. W., Ford, L. E., Bond, H. E., Stuart, D. C., and Lorenz, D. (1969). Isolation of plasma membrane fragments from HeLa cells. *J. Cell Biol.*, **41**, 378–392.

Booth, A. G. and Kenney, A. J. (1974). A rapid method for the preparation of microvilli from rabbit kidney. *Biochem. J.*, **142**, 575–581.

Booth, A. G. and Kenney, A. J. (1976). A morphometric and biochemical investigation of the vesiculation of kidney microvilli. *J. Cell Sci.*, **21**, 449–463.

Brewer, G. J. and Singer, S. J. (1974). On the disposition of the proteins of the membrane-containing bacteriophage PM2. *Biochemistry*, **13**, 3580–3588.

Brunette, D. M. and Till, J. E. (1971). A rapid method for the isolation of L-cell surface membranes using an aqueous two-phase polymer system. *J. Memb. Biol.*, **5**, 215–224.

Carlson, R. W., Wada, H. G., and Sussman, H. H. (1976). The plasma membrane of human placenta. *J. Biol. Chem.*, **251**, 4139–4146.

Carraway, C. A. and Carraway, K. L. (1976). Concanavalin A perturbation of membrane enzymes of mammary gland. *J. Supramol. Struc.*, **4**, 121–126.

Carraway, C. A. C., Corrado, F. J., Fogle, D. D., and Carraway, K. L. (1980a). Ecto-enzymes of mammary gland and its tumors. Ca^{2+}- or Mg^{2+}-stimulated adenosine triphosphatase and its perturbation by concanavalin A. *Biochem. J.*, **191**, 45–51.

Carraway, K. L. (1975). Covalent labeling of membranes. *Biochim. Biophys. Acta*, **415**, 379–410.

Carraway, K. L., Fogle, D. D., Chesnut, R. W., Huggins, J. W., and Carraway, C. A. C. (1976). Ecto-enzymes of mammary gland and its tumors. *J. Biol. Chem.*, **251**, 6173–6178.

Carraway, K. L., Huggins, J. W., Cerra, R. F., Yeltman, D. R., and Carraway, C. A. C. (1980b). α-Actinin-containing branched microvilli from an ascites adenocarcinoma. *Nature*, **285**, 508–510.

Caswell, A. H., Lau, Y. H., and Brunschwig, J. -P. (1976). Ouabain-binding vesicles from skeletal muscle. *Arch. Biochem. Biophys.*, **176**, 417–430.

Chang, K. -J., Bennett, V., and Cuatrecasas, P. (1975). Membrane receptors as general markers for plasma membrane isolation procedures. *J. Biol. Chem.*, **250**, 488–500.

Charalampous, F. C., Gonatas, N. K., and Melbourne, A. D. (1973). Isolation and properties of the plasma membrane of KB cells. *J. Cell Biol.*, **59**, 421–435.

Cheetham, R. D., Morre, D. J., Pannek, C., and Friend, D. S. (1971). Isolation of a Golgi apparatus-rich fraction from rat liver. IV. Thiamine pyrophosphatase. *J. Cell Biol.*, **49**, 899–905.

Cohen, C. M., Kalish, D. I., Jacobson, B. S., and Branton, D. (1977). Membrane isolation on polylysine-coated beads. *J. Cell Biol.*, **75**, 119–134.

Coleman, R., Michell, R. H., Finean, J. B., and Hawthorne, J. N. (1967). A purified plasma membrane fraction isolated from rat liver under isotonic conditions. *Biochim. Biophys. Acta*, **135**, 573–579.

Condeelis, J. (1978). A direct role for the actin cytoskeleton in the mobility of cell surface receptors. *J. Cell. Biol.*, **79**, 263a.

Dallner, G., Siekevitz, P., and Palade, G. E. (1966). Biogenesis of endoplasmic reticulum membranes. II. Synthesis of constitutive microsomal enzymes in developing rat hepatocyte. *J. Cell. Biol.*, **30**, 97–117.

DePierre, J. W. and Karnovsky, M. L. (1973). Plasma membranes of mammalian cells. *J. Cell Biol.*, **56**, 275–303.

DePierre, J. W. and Karnovsky, M. L. (1974). Ecto-enzymes of the guinea pig polymorphonuclear leukocyte. I. Evidence for an ecto-adenosine monophosphatase, adenosine triphosphatase, and *p*-nitrophenyl phosphatase. *J. Biol. Chem.*, **249**, 7111–7120.

Dodge, J. T., Mitchell, C., and Hanahan, D. J. (1963). The preparation and chemical characteristics of hemoglobin-free ghosts of human erythrocytes. *Arch. Biochem. Biophys.*, **100**, 119–130.

Dods, R. F., Essner, E., and Barclay, M. (1972). Isolation and characterization of plasma membranes from an L-asparaginase-sensitive strain of leukemia cells. *Biochem. Biophys. Res. Commun.*, **46**, 1074–1081.

Ebel, H., Aulbert, E., and Merker, H. J. (1976). Isolation of the basal and lateral plasma membranes of rat kidney tubule cells. *Biochim. Biophys. Acta*, **433**, 531–546.

Edelman, G. M. (1976). Surface modulation in cell recognition and cell growth. *Science*, **192**, 218–226.

Eichholz, A. and Crane, R. K. (1974). Isolation of plasma membranes from intestinal brush borders. *Methods Enzymol.*, **31**, 123–134.

Elgsaeter, A. and Branton, D. (1974). Intramembrane particle aggregation in erythrocyte ghosts. I. The effects of protein removal. *J. Cell Biol.*, **63**, 1018–1036.

Emmelot, P., Bos, C. J., van Hoeven, R. P., and van Blitterswijk, W. J. (1974). Isolation of plasma membranes from rat and mouse livers and hepatoma. *Methods Enzymol.*, **31**, 75–90.

Evans, R. M. and Fink, L. M. (1977). Identification of transmembrane bridging proteins in the plasma membrane of cultured mouse L-cells. *Proc. Natl. Acad. Sci. USA*, **74**, 5341–5344.

Evans, W. H. (1978). In T. S. Work and E. Work (Eds) *Preparation and Characterization of Mammalian Plasma Membranes*. North Holland, Amsterdam.

Forstner, G. G., Sabesin, S. M., and Isselbacher, K. J. (1968). Rat intestinal microvillus membranes. *Biochem. J.*, **106**, 381–390.

Fry, J. R., Jones, C. A., Wiebkin, P., Bellemann, P., and Bridges, J. W. (1976). The enzymic isolation of adult rat hepatocytes in a functional and viable state. *Anal. Biochem.*, **71**, 341–350.

Fujita, M., Ohta, H., Kawai, K., Matsui, H., and Nakao, M. (1972). Differential isolation of microvillous and basolateral plasma membranes from intestinal mucosa: mutually exclusive distribution of digestive enzymes and ouabain-sensitive ATPase. *Biochim. Biophys. Acta*, **274**, 336–347.

Ghosh, S. K. and Koenig, E. (1977). Isolation of non-myelin plasma membranes unique to white matter. *Biochim. Biophys. Acta*, **470**, 104–112.

Gianetto, R. and de Duve, C. (1955). Tissue fractionation studies. IV. Comparative study of the binding of acid phosphatase, β-glucuronidase and cathepsin by rat-liver particles. *Biochem. J.*, **59**, 433–438.

Gilkes, N. R. and Weeks, G. (1977). The purification and characterization of *Dictyostelium discoideum* plasma membranes. *Biochim. Biophys. Acta*, **464**, 142–156.

Glick, M. C. (1976). In P. L. Altman and D. D. Katz (Eds.) *Cell Biology, Biological Handbooks* volume I, pp. 92–95. Federation of American Societies for Experimental Biology, Bethesda, Maryland.

Gospodarowicz, D. (1973). Preparation and characterization of plasma membranes from bovine corpus luteum. *J. Biol. Chem.*, **248**, 5050–5056.

Graham, J. M., Hynes, R. O., Davidson, E. A., and Bainton, D. F. (1975). The location of proteins labeled by the ^{125}I-lactoperoxidase sytstem in the NIL 8 hamster fibroblast. *Cell*, **4**, 353–365.

Groeschel-Stewart, U., Chamley, J. H., McConnell, J. D., and Burnstock, G. (1976). Membrane alteration of trypsin-treated smooth muscle cells and penetration by antibodies to myosin. *Histochemistry*, **47**, 285–289.

Guidotti, G. (1972). Membrane proteins. *Ann. Rev. Biochem.*, **41**, 731–752.

Gurd, J. W., Jones, L. R., Mahler, H. R., and Moore, W. J. (1974). Isolation and partial characterization of rat brain synaptic plasma membranes. *J. Neurochem.*, **22**, 281–290.

Hannig, K. (1972). Separation of cells and particles by continuous free-flow electrophoresis. *Techniques Biochem. Biophys. Morphol.*, **1**, 191–232.

Heidrich, H. -G., Kinne, R., Kinne-Saffran, E., and Hannig, K. (1972). The polarity of the proximal tubule cell in rat kidney. *J. Cell Biol.*, **54**, 232–245.

Heine, J. W. and Schnaitman, C. A. (1971). A method for the isolation of plasma membrane of animal cells. *J. Cell Biol.*, **48**, 703–707.

Heine, J. W., Spear, P. G., and Roizman, B. (1972). Proteins specified by Herpes simplex virus. VI. Viral proteins in the plasma membrane. *J. Virol.*, **9**, 431–439.

Heller, M. and Harary, I. (1977). Plasma membranes from cardiac cells in culture.

Enzymatic radio-iodination, evaluation of preparation and properties of the sarcolemma. *Biochim. Biophys. Acta*, **467**, 29–43.

Hemminki, K. and Suovaniemi, O. (1973). Preparation of plasma membranes from isolated cells of newborn rat brain. *Biochim. Biophys. Acta*, **298**, 75–83.

Henn, F. A., Hansson, H. -A., and Hamberger, A. (1972). Preparation of plasma membrane from isolated neurons. *J. Cell Biol.*, **53**, 654–661.

Hicks, R. M. and Ketterer, B. (1970). Isolation of the plasma membrane of the luminal surface of rat bladder epithelium and the occurrence of a hexagonal lattice of subunits both in negatively whole mounts and in sectioned membranes. *J. Cell Biol.*, **45**, 542–553.

Hiller, G. and Weber, K. (1977). Spectrin is absent in various tissue culture cells. *Nature*, **266**, 181–183.

Hochstadt, J., Quinlan, D. C., Rader, R. L., Li, C. -C., and Dowd, D. (1975). Use of isolated membrane vesicles in transport studies. *Methods Membrane Biol.*, **5**, 117–162.

Hubbard, A. L. and Cohn, Z. A. (1975). Externally disposed plasma membrane proteins. I. Enzymatic iodination of mouse L-cells. *J. Cell Biol.*, **64**, 438–460.

Huggins, J. W. (1975). The isolation, characterization, and utilization of plasma membranes from tumor cells. *Ph.D. Thesis*, Oklahoma State University.

Huggins, J. W. and Carraway, K. L. (1976). Purification of plasma membranes from rat mammary gland by a density perturbation procedure. *J. Supramol. Struct.*, **5**, 59–63.

Huggins, J. W., Trenbeath, T. P., Chesnut, R. W., Carraway, C. A. C., and Carraway, K. L. (1980a). Purification of plasma membranes of rat mammary gland. Comparisons of subfractions with rat milk fat globule membrane. *Exp. Cell Res.*, **126**, 279–288.

Huggins, J. W., Trenbeath, T. P., Yeltman, D. R., and Carraway, K. L. (1980b). Restricted concanavalin A redistribution on the branched microvilli of an ascites tumor subline. *Exp. Cell Res.*, **127**, 31–46.

Hut, R. C. and Brown, J. C. (1975). Identification of a high molecular weight transmembrane protein in mouse L-cells. *J. Mol. Biol.*, **97**, 413–422.

Jacobson, B. S. (1977). Isolation of plasma membrane from eukaryotic cells on polylysine-coated polyacrylamide beads. *Biochim. Biophys. Acta*, **471**, 331–335.

Jacobson, B. S. and Branton, D. (1977). Plasma membrane: rapid isolation and exposure of the cytoplasmic surface by use of positively charged beads. *Science*, **195**, 302–304.

Jacobson, B. S., Cronin, J., and Branton, D. (1978). Coupling polylysine to glass beads for plasma membrane isolation. *Biochim. Biophys. Acta*, **506**, 81–96.

Jamieson, G. A. and Groh, N. (1971). Isoelectric focusing of human blood cell membranes. *Anal. Biochem.*, **43**, 259–268.

Jett, M., Seed, T. M., and Jamieson, G. A. (1977). Isolation and characterization of plasma membranes and intact nuclei from lymphoid cells. *J. Biol. Chem.*, **252**, 2134–2142.

Juliano, R. L. and Behar-Bannelier, M. (1975). An evaluation of techniques for labelling the surface proteins of cultured mammalian cells. *Biochim. Biophys. Acta*, **375**, 249–267.

Kalish, D. I., Cohen, C. M., Jacobson, B. S., and Branton, D. (1978). Membrane isolation on polylysine-coated glass beads. Asymmetry of bound membrane. *Biochim. Biophys. Acta*, **506**, 97–110.

Kant, J. A. and Steck, T. L. (1973). Specificity in the association of glyceraldehyde-3-phosphate dehydrogenase with isolated human erythrocyte membranes. *J. Biol. Chem.*, **248**, 8457–8464.

Kartner, N., Alon, M., Swift, M., Buchwald, M., and Riordan, J. R. (1977). Isolation of plasma membranes from human skin fibroblasts. *J. Membrane Biol.*, **36**, 191–211.

Kawai, Y. and Spiro, R. G. (1977). Fat cell plasma membranes. I. Preparation, characterization, and chemical composition. *J. Biol. Chem.*, **252**, 6229–6235.

Keenan, T. W., Morre', D. J., Olson, D. E., Yunghans, W. N., and Patton, S. (1970). Biochemical and morphological comparison of plasma membrane and milk fat globule membrane from bovine mammary gland. *J. Cell Biol.*, **44**, 80–93.

Kemp, R. B., Jones, B. M., and Groeschel-Stewart, U. (1971). Aggregative behaviour of embryonic chick cells in the presence of antibodies directed against actomyosins. *J. Cell Sci.*, **9**, 103–122.

Kimmich, G. A. (1975). Preparation and characterization of isolated intestinal epithelial cells and their use in studying intestinal transport. *Methods Membrane Biol.*, **5**, 51–115.

Klempner, M. S., Mikkelsen, R. B., Cortman, D. H., and Andre-Schwartz, J. (1980). Neutrophil plasma membranes. I. High-yield purification of human neutrophil plasma membrane vesicles by nitrogen cavitation and differential centrifugation. *J. Cell Biol.*, **86**, 21–28.

Kohler, G. and Milstein, C. (1975). Continuous cultures of fused cells secreting antibody of predefined specificity. *Nature*, **256**, 495–497.

Korn, E. D. (1978). Biochemistry of actomyosin-dependent cell motility (a review). *Proc. Nat. Acad, Sci. USA*, **75**, 588–599.

Kornfeld, R. and Siemers, C. (1974). Large scale isolation and characterization of calf thymocyte plasma membranes. *J. Biol. Chem.*, **249**, 1295–1301.

Kraehenbuhl, J. P. (1977). Dispersed mammary gland epithelial cells. I. Isolation and separation procedures. *J. Cell. Biol.*, **72**, 390–405.

Lau, Y. H., Caswell, A. H., and Brunschwig, J. -P. (1977). Isolation of transverse tubules by fractionation of triad junctions of skeletal muscle. *J. Biol. Chem.*, **252**, 5565–5574.

Lernmark, A., Nathans, A., and Steiner, D. F. (1976). Preparation and characterization of plasma membrane-enriched fractions from rat pancreatic islets. *J. Cell Biol.*, **71**, 606–623.

Levitan, I. B., Mushynski, W. E., and Ramirez, G. (1972). Highly purified synaptosomal membranes from rat brain. *J. Biol. Chem.*, **247**, 5376–5381.

Lewis, B. A., Elkin, A., Michell, R. H., and Coleman, R. (1975). Basolateral plasma membranes of intestinal epithelial cells. *Biochem J.*, **152**, 71–84.

Lim, R. W., Molday, R. S., Huang, H. V., and Yen, S. -P. S. (1975). Application of latex microspheres in the isolation of plasma membranes by affinity density perturbation of erythrocyte membranes. *Biochim. Biophys. Acta*, **394**, 377–387.

Lo, C. -H. (1973). The plasma membranes of bovine circumvallate papillae. Isolation and partial characterization. *Biochim. Biophys. Acta*, **291**, 650–661.

Louvard, D., Maroux, S., Baratti, J., Desnuelle, P., and Mutaftschiev, S. (1973). On the preparation and some properties of closed membrane vesicles from hog duodenal and jejunal brush border. *Biochim. Biophys. Acta*, **291**, 747–763.

Lutz, H. U., Lin, S. C., and Palek, J. (1977). Release of spectrin-free vesicles from human erythrocytes during ATP depletion. I. Characterization of spectrin-free vesicles. *J. Cell Biol.*, **73**, 548–560.

Luzio, J. P., Newby, A. C., and Hales, C. N. (1976). A rapid immunological procedure for the isolation of hormonally sensitive rat fat-cell plasma membrane. *Biochem. J.*, **154**, 11–21.

Marchalonis, J. J., Cone, R. E. and Santer, V. (1971). Enzymatic iodination: a probe for accessible surface proteins of normal and neoplastic lymphocytes. *Biochem J.* 124, 921–927.

Matlib, M. A., Crankshaw, J., Garfield, R. E., Crankshaw, D. J., Kwan, C. -Y., and Daniel, E. E. (1979). Characterization of membrane fractions and isolation of purified plasma membranes from rat myometrium. *J. Biol. Chem.*, **254**, 1834–1840.

McClure, J. A., Fischlschweiger, W., and Noonan, K. D. (1979). Characterization of the membrane fraction isolated by the fluorescein mercuric acetate technique of Barland and Schroeder. *Biochim. Biophys. Acta*, **550**, 16–37.

McCollester, D. L. (1970). Isolation of meth A cell surface membranes possessing tumor-specific transplantation antigen activity. *Cancer Res.*, **30**, 2832–2840.

McDaniel, C. F., Kirtley, M. E., and Tanner, M. J. A. (1974). The interaction of glyceraldehyde 3-phosphate dehydrogenase with human erythrocyte membranes. *J. Biol. Chem.*, **249**, 6478–6485.

McKeel, D. W. and Jarett, L. (1970). Preparation and characterization of a plasma membrane fraction from isolated fat cells. *J. Cell Biol.*, **44**, 417–432.

Merrell, R. and Glaser, L. (1973). Specific recognition of plasma membranes by embryonic cells. *Proc. Natl. Acad. Sci. USA*, **70**, 2794–2798.

Miller, D. and Crane, R. K. (1961). The digestive function of the epithelium of the small intestine. I. An intracellular locus of disaccharide and sugar phosphate ester hydrolysis. *Biochim. Biophys. Acta*, **52**, 281–293.

Mitranic, M. M., Sturgess, J. M., and Moscarello, M. A. (1974). Recovery of galactosyltransferase activity from sucrose gradients during isolation of Golgi membranes. *J. Membrane Biol.*, **19**, 397–408.

Moldeus, P., Högberg, J., and Orrenius, S. (1978). Isolation and use of liver cells. *Methods Enzymol.*, **52**, 60–71.

Monneron, A. and d'Alayer, J. (1978). Isolation of plasma and nuclear membranes of thymocytes. I. Enzymatic composition and ultrastructure. *J. Cell Biol.*, **77**, 211–231.

Moore, P. B. (1978). Cytoskeletal–membrane interactions in ascites tumor cells. *Ph.D. Thesis*, Oklahoma State University.

Moore, P. B., Anderson, D. R., Huggins, J. W., and Carraway, K. L. (1976). Cytoskeletal proteins associated with cell surface envelopes from sarcoma 180 ascites tumor cells. *Biochem. Biophys. Res. Commun.*, **72**, 288–294.

Moore, P. B., Ownby, C. L., and Carraway, K. L. (1978). Interactions of cytoskeletal elements with the plasma membrane of sarcoma 180 ascites tumor cells. *Exp. Cell Res.*, **115**, 331–342.

Morgan, I. G., Wolfe, L. S., Mandel, P., and Gombos, G. (1971). Isolation of plasma membranes from rat brain. *Biochim. Biophys. Acta*, **241**, 737–751.

Neilands, J. (1955). Lactic dehydrogenase of heart muscle. *Methods Enzymol.*, **1**, 449–454.

Nelson, G. J. (1967). Lipid composition of erythrocytes in various mammalian species. *Biochim. Biophys. Acta*, **144**, 221–232.

Neville, D. M., Jr. (1960). Isolation of cell surface membrane fractions from mammalian cells and organs. *J. Biophys. Biochem. Cytol.*, **8**, 413–422.

Neville, D. M., Jr. (1974). The isolation of kidney brush border. *Methods Enzymol.*, **31**, 115–123.

Neville, D. M., Jr. (1975). Isolation of cell surface membrane fractions from mammalian cells and organs. *Methods Membrane Biol.*, **3**, 1–49.

Nicolson, G. L. (1976). Transmembrane control of the receptors on normal and tumor cells. I. Cytoplasmic influence over cell surface components. *Biochim. Biophys. Acta*, **457**, 57–108.

Nicolson, G. L., Marchesi, V. T., and Singer, S. J. (1971). The localization of spectrin on the inner-surface of human red blood cell membranes by ferritin-conjugated antibodies. *J. Cell Biol.*, **51**, 265–272.

Nicolson, G. L. and Painter, R. G. (1973). Anionic sites of human erythrocyte membranes. II. Antispectrin-induced transmembrane aggregation of the binding sites for positively charged colloidal particles. *J. Cell Biol.*, **59**, 395–406.

Nicolson, G. L. and Poste, G. (1976a). The cancer cell: dynamic aspects and modifications in cell-surface organization. (Part 1). *New Engl. J. Med.*, **295**, 197–203.

Nicolson, G. L. and Poste, G. (1976b). The cancer cell: dynamic aspects and modifications in cell surface organization (Part 2). *New Engl. J. Med.*, **295**, 253–258.

Noonan, K. D., Lindberg, D. S., and McClure, J. A. (1976). Isolation and preliminary characterization of that part of the plasma membrane which is apposed to the substratum. *Prog. Clin. Biol. Res.*, **9**, 245–259.

Painter, R. G., Sheetz, M., and Singer, S. J. (1975). Detection and ultrastructural localization of human smooth muscle myosin-like molecules in human non-muscle cells by specific antibodies. *Proc. Natl. Acad. Sci. USA*, **72**, 1359–1363.

Parish, R. W. and Müller, U. (1976). The isolation of plasma membranes from the cellular slime mold *Dictyostelium discoideum* using Concanavalin A and Triton X-100. *FEBS Letts.*, **63**, 40–44.

Pastan, I. and Willingham, M. (1978). Cellular transformation and the 'morphologic phenotype' of transformed cells. *Nature*, **274**, 645–650.

Perdue, J. F., Kletzien, R., and Miller, K. (1971). The isolation and characterization of plasma membrane from cultured cells. I. The chemical composition of membrane isolated from uninfected and oncogenic RNA virus-converted chick embryo fibroblasts. *Biochim. Biophys. Acta*, **249**, 419–434.

Poirier, G. G., Lambert, M. P., Lebel, D., Sakr, F., Morrisset, J., and Beaudoin, A. R. (1977). Purification of plasma membranes from rat pancreas: a rapid method. *Proc. Soc. Exp. Biol. Med.*, **155**, 324–329.

Raftell, M. and Blomberg, F. (1973). Membrane fractions from rat hepatoma. III. Immunochemical characterization of detergent-soluble membrane phosphatases, electron transport chains and catalase. *Biochim. Biophys. Acta*, **291**, 442–453.

Ray, T. K. (1970). A modified method for the isolation of the plasma membrane from rat liver. *Biochim. Biophys. Acta*, **196**, 1–9.

Resch, K., Loracher, A., Mähler, B., Stoeck, M., and Rode, H. N. (1978). Functional mosaicism of the lymphocyte plasma membrane. Characterization of membrane subfractions obtained by affinity chromatography on Concanavalin A–Sepharose. *Biochim. Biophys. Acta*, **511**, 176–193.

Riemer, B. L. and Widnell, C. C. (1975). The demonstration of a specific 5'-nucleotidase activity in rat tissues. *Arch. Biochem. Biophys.*, **171**, 343–347.

Rikihisa, Y. and Mizuno, D. (1977). Demonstration of myosin on the cytoplasmic side of plasma membranes of guinea pig polymorphonuclear leukocytes with immunoferritin. *Exp. Cell Res.*, **110**, 87–92.

Rikihisa, Y. and Mizuno, D. (1978). Different arrangements of phagolysosome membranes which depend upon the particles phagocytized. *Exp. Cell Res.*, **111**, 437–449.

Riordan, J. R. and Slavik, M. (1974). Interactions of lectins with membrane glycoproteins. Effects of concanavalin A on 5'-nucleotidase. *Biochim. Biophys. Acta*, **373**, 356–360.

Rittenhouse-Simmons, S. and Deykin, D. (1976). Isolation of membranes from normal and thrombin-treated gel-filtered platelets using a lectin marker. *Biochim. Biophys. Acta*, **426**, 688–696.

Rodbell, M. (1964). Metabolism of isolated fat cells. I. Effects of hormones on glucose metabolism and lipolysis. *J. Biol. Chem.*, **239**, 375–380.

Rodbell, M. (1967). Metabolism of isolated fat cells. V. Preparation of 'ghosts' and their properties: adenyl cyclase and other enzymes. *J. Biol. Chem.*, **242**, 5744–5750.

Ronquist, G. and Agren, G. K. (1975). A Mg^{2+}- and Ca^{2+}-stimulated adenosine triphosphatase at the outer surface of Ehrlich ascites tumor cells. *Cancer Res.*, **35**, 1402–1406.

Saccomani, G., Stewart, H. B., Shaw, D., Lewin, M., and Sachs, G. (1977). Characterization of gastric mucosal membranes. IV. Fractionation and purification of K$^+$-ATPase-containing vesicles by zonal centrifugation and free-flow electrophoresis technique. *Biochim. Biophys. Acta*, **465**, 311–330.

Scarborough, G. A. (1975). Isolation and characterization of *Neurospora crassa* plasma membranes. *J. Biol. Chem.*, **250**, 1106–1111.

Schapira, G., Dobocz, I., Piau, J. P., and Delain, E. (1974). An improved technique for preparation of skeletal muscle cell plasma membrane. *Biochim. Biophys. Acta*, **345**, 348–358.

Schimmel, S. D., Kent, C., Bischoff, R., and Vagelos, P. R. (1973). Plasma membranes from cultured muscle cells: isolation procedure and separation of putative plasma-membrane marker enzymes. *Proc. Natl. Acad. Sci. USA*, **70**, 3195–3199.

Schreiner, G. F. and Unanue, E. R. (1976). Membrane and cytoplasmic changes in B lymphocytes induced by ligand–surface immunoglobulin interaction. *Adv. Immunol.*, **24**, 37–165.

Schroeder, B. T., Chakraborty, J., and Soloff, M. S. (1977). Binding of ^{3}H-oxytocin to cells isolated from the mammary gland of the lactating rat. *J. Cell Biol.*, **74**, 428–440.

Scott, R. E. (1976). Plasma membrane vesiculation: A new technique for isolation of plasma membranes. *Science*, **194**, 743–745.

Scott, R. E. and Maercklein, P. B. (1979). Plasma membrane vesiculation in 3T3 and SV3T3 cells. II. Factors affecting the process of vesiculation. *J. Cell Sci.*, **35**, 245–252.

Sheetz, M. P., Painter, R. G., and Singer, S. J. (1976). Relationships of the spectrin complex of human erythrocyte membranes to the actomyosins of muscle cells. *Biochemistry*, **15**, 4486–4492.

Sheetz, M. P. and Singer, S. J. (1977). On the mechanism of ATP-induced shape changes in human erythrocyte membranes. I. The role of the spectrin complex. *J. Cell Biol.*, **73**, 638–646.

Shin, B. C. and Carraway, K. L. (1973a). Cell surface constituents of sarcoma 180 ascites tumor cells. *Biochim. Biophys. Acta*, **330**, 254–268.

Shin, B. C. and Carraway, K. L. (1973b). Association of glyceraldehyde 3-phosphate dehydrogenase with the human erythrocyte membrane. *J. Biol. Chem.*, **248**, 1436–1444.

Shin, B. C., Ebner, K. E., Hudson, B. G., and Carraway, K. L. (1975). Membrane glycoprotein differences between normal lactating mammary tissue and the R3230 AC mammary tumor. *Cancer Res.*, **35**, 1135–1140.

Smith, P. B. and Appel, S. H. (1977). Isolation and characterization of the surface membranes of fast and slow mammalian skeletal muscle. *Biochim. Biophys. Acta*, **466**, 109–122.

Smolen, J. E. and Weissman, G. (1978). Mg^{2+}-ATPase as a membrane ectoenzyme of human granulocytes. Inhibitors, activators, and response to phagocytosis. *Biochim. Biophys. Acta*, **512**, 525–538.

Snary, D., Goodfellow, P., Hayman, M. J., Bodmer, W. F., and Crumpton, M. J. (1974). Subcellular separation and molecular nature of human histocompatibility antigens (HL-A). *Nature*, **247**, 457–461.

Solyom, A. and Trams, E. G. (1972). Enzyme markers in characterization of isolated plasma membranes. *Enzyme*, **13**, 329–372.

Steck, T. L. and Wallach, D. F. H. (1970). The isolation of plasma membranes. *Methods Cancer Res.*, **5**, 93–153.

Stefanovic, V., Ciesielski-Treska, J., Ebel, A., and Mandel, P. (1976). Neuroblast-glia interaction. The effect of co-cultivation upon ecto-ATPase activity of neuroblastoma and glioma cells. *Exp. Cell Res.*, **98**, 191–203.

Suzuki, S., Widnell, C. C., and Field, J. B. (1977). Preparation and characterization of subfractions of bovine thyroid plasma membranes. *J. Biol. Chem.*, **252**, 3074–3081.

Takeuchi, M. and Terayama, H. (1975). Preparation and chemical composition of rat liver cell membranes. *Exp. Cell Res.*, **40**, 32–44.

Tate, S. S. and Meister, A. (1974). Interaction of γ-glutamyl transpeptidase with amino acids, dipeptides, and derivatives and analogs of glutathione. *J. Biol. Chem.*, **249**, 7593–7602.

Thom, D., Powell, A. J., Lloyd, C. W., and Rees, D. A. (1977). Rapid isolation of plasma membranes in high yield from cultured fibroblasts. *Biochem. J.*, **168**, 187–194.

Touster, O., Aronson, N. N., Jr., Dulaney, J. T., and Hendrickson, H. (1970). Isolation of rat liver plasma membranes. Use of nucleotide pyrophosphatase and phosphodiesterase I as marker enzymes. *J. Cell Biol.*, **47**, 604–618.

Trams, E. G. and Lauter, C. J. (1974). On the sidedness of plasma membrane enzymes. *Biochim. Biophys. Acta*, **345**, 180–197.

Truding, R., Shelansky, M. L., Daniels, M. P., and Morell, P. (1974). Comparison of surface membranes isolated from cultured murine neuroblastoma cells in the differentiated or undifferentiated state. *J. Biol. Chem.*, **249**, 3973–3982.

Tsai, C. -M., Chen, K. -Y., and Canellakis, E. S. (1975). Isolation and characterization of the plasma membrane of L-1210 cells. Iodination as a marker for the plasma membrane. *Biochim. Biophys. Acta*, **401**, 196–212.

van Blitterswijk, W. J., Emmelot, P., and Feltkamp, C. A. (1973). Studies on plasma membranes. XIX. Isolation and characterization of a plasma membrane fraction from calf thymocytes. *Biochim. Biophys. Acta*, **298**, 577–592.

Vandenburgh, H. H. (1977). Separation of plasma membrane markers by glycerol-induced blistering of muscle cells. *Biochim. Biophys. Acta*, **466**, 302–314.

Wallach, D. F. H. and Kamat, V. B. (1964). Plasma and cytoplasmic membrane fragments from Ehrlich ascites carcinoma. *Proc. Natl. Acad. Sci. USA*, **52**, 721–728.

Wallach, D. F. H. and Kamat, V. B. (1966). Preparation of plasma–membrane fragments from mouse ascites tumor cells. *Methods Enzymol.*, **8**, 164–172.

Wallach, D. F. H., Kranz, B., Ferber, W., and Fischer, H. (1972). Affinity density perturbation: A new fractionation principle and its illustration in a membrane separation. *FEBS Letts.*, **21**, 20–33.

Wallach, D. F. H. and Schmidt-Ullrich, R. (1977). Isolation of plasma membrane vesicles from animal cells. *Methods Cell Biol.*, **15**, 235–276.

Walsh, F. S., Barber, B. H., and Crumpton, M. J. (1976). Preparation of inside-out vesicles of pig lymphocyte plasma membranes. *Biochemistry*, **15**, 3557–3563.

Walter, H. (1975). Partition of cells in two-polymer aqueous phases: A method for separating cells and for obtaining information on their surface properties. *Methods Cell Biol.*, **9**, 25–50.

Wang, Y. -J. and Mahler, H. R. (1976). Topography of the synaptosomal membrane. *J. Cell Biol.*, **71**, 639–658.

Warley, A. and Cook, G. M. W. (1976). Isolation of a Golgi-apparatus-enriched fraction from leukaemic cells. *Biochem. J.*, **156**, 245–251.

Warley, A. and Cook, G. M. W. (1973). The isolation and characterization of plasma membranes from normal and leukaemic cells of mice. *Biochim. Biophys. Acta*, **323**, 55–68.

Warren, L. and Glick, M. C. (1969). In K. Habel and N. Salzman (Eds.) *Fundamental Techniques in Virology*, pp. 66–71. Academic Press, New York.

Warren, L., Glick, M. C., and Nass, M. K. (1966). Membranes of animal cells. I. Methods of isolation of the surface membrane. *J. Cell Physiol.*, **68**, 269–288.

Weibel, E. R. (1969). Stereological principles for morphometry in electron microscopic cytology. *Int. Rev. Cytol.*, **26**, 235–302.

Wetzel, M. G. and Korn, E. D. (1969). Phagocytosis of latex beads by *Acanthamoeba castellanii* (NEFF). III. Isolation of the phagocytic vesicles and their membranes. *J. Cell Biol.*, **43**, 90–104.

Wiepjes, G. J. and Prop, F. J. A. (1970). Improved method for preparation of single-cell suspensions from mammary glands of adult virgin mouse. *Exp. Cell Res.*, **61**, 451–454.

Wilfong, R. F. and Neville, D. M., Jr. (1970). The isolation of a brush border membrane fraction from rat kidney. *J. Biol. Chem.*, **245**, 6106–6112.

Willingham, M. C., Ostlund, R. E., and Pastan, I. (1974). Myosin is a component of the cell surface of cultured cells. *Proc. Natl. Acad. Sci. USA*, **71**, 4144–4148.

Wisher, M. H. and Evans, W. H. (1975). Functional polarity of the rat hepatocyte surface membrane. Isolation and characterization of plasma–membrane subfractions from the blood–sinusoidal, bile–canalicular and contiguous surfaces of the hepatocyte. *Biochem. J.*, **146**, 375–388.

Wisher, M. H. and Evans, W. H. (1977). Preparation of plasma–membrane subfractions from isolated rat hepatocytes. *Biochem. J.*, **164**, 415–422.

Yamashita, K. and Field, J. B. (1974). Isolation of the plasma membrane from the thyroid. *Methods Enzymol.*, **31**, 144–149.

Zachowski, A. and Paraf, A. (1974). Use of concanavalin A polymer to isolate right-side-out vesicles of purified plasma membranes from eukaryotic cells. *Biochem. Biophys. Res. Commun.*, **57**, 787–792.

Zahler, W. L. and Doak, G. A. (1975). Isolation of the outer acrosomal membrane from bull sperm. *Biochim. Biophys. Acta*, **406**, 479–488.

Zucker-Franklin, D. (1968). Electron microscopic studies of human granulocytes: structural variations related to function. *Semin. Hematol.*, **5**, 109–133.

Index

Acetic acid, 91
Acetyl strophanthidin, 468
Acrolein, 253, 460
Actin binding protein, 514
Adherent cells, 249
Adjuvants, 30, 492
  Freund's, 32
  inorganic colloids, 31
Adriamycin, 455
Adsorption of antisera, 23, 198
Affinity chromatography, 76, 349, 368, 537
  activation of the matrix for coupling, 77
  buffers for elution, 91
Affinity constant,
  ammonium sulphate precipitation determination, 118
  functional, 115
  intrinsic, 112
  protein antigens, 117
Agarose beads, 64, 76, 77
Agglutination, 113, 139, 155, 348, 369
Alcohol dehydrogenase, 460
Allergic response, 295
Allyl alcohol, 460
Alumina, 31
Amino acid sequence, 9, 11
1-(4-Aminophenyl)-1,2-dicarba-*closo*-dodecaborane, 462
Ammonium sulphate precipation, 61, 118
Ampholytes, 70, 86
Anaesthesia, 49
Antibody (*see also* Immunoglobulin), 5
  as carrier of biological activity, 448
  bigamous binding, 117
  binding site, 7
  circulating, 296
  constant region, 7
  cooperative interactions, 119
  coupling, 190, 222, 246, 454

diversity, 9
drug complexes, 449, 450
Fab fragment, 406, 424, 466
$(Fab')_2$ fragment, 224, 456
fluorescent labelling, 190, 222
general properties, 5
half-life, 466
heavy chain, 5, 7
heterogeneity, 103
  clonal, 99
  delta functions, 108
  epitope, 98
  Gaussian distribution, 104
  restricted, 103
  Sips distribution, 104
homogeneous, 99
isoelectric focusing, 60
kappa chain, 5, 7
labels, 404
lambda chain, 5, 7
light chain, 5, 7
monogamous binding, 117
production, 11
purification, 59
structure, 3
tumour-specific, 449
usefulness to non-immunologists, 3
uses of, 14
variable region, 5, 7
Antigen, 14, 544
  cellular, 22, 415
  detection of, 97
  developmental, 299, 315, 419
  differentiation, 297, 313
  embryonic, 316, 419
  extracellular, 418
  histocompatibility, 411
  lipid, 28
  measurement by displacement assays, 108
  multivalent, 112

organelle, 316
organ specific, 299, 313
parasite, 486
plant, 298
plasma membrane, 544
pollen, 331
preparation of, 21
purification, 25
purity of, 26
Thy-1, 417
tumour, 17, 22, 449
teratoma, 421
trophoblast, 416
Antigen-antibody reaction, 97, 139, 163
  techniques used for visualization, 139, 238, 239
Antigen identification, 494
Antigenic silence, of trophoblast, 428
Antigenic variation, 486
  anti-idiotypic sera, 35, 474
Anti-immunoglobulin, 173, 407
Arsphenamine, 459
Ascites fluid, 49
ATPases, 540
Autoimmunity, 501
Automated radioimmunoassays, 182
Azobenzenearsonate, 59

B cell, 417
Babesia, 486, 489
Bacterial agglutination, 159
Bandeiraea simplicifolia lectin, 351, 357
Barbiturates, 470
Bauhinia purpurea lectin, 352
Bentonite, 33
Bleeding, 41
Bigamous, 117
Bio-gel®, 65, 69
Bladder, 533
Blood group substances, 368
Blotting techniques, 367
Bine-marrow de ived lymphocytes, 4
Bordetella pertussis, 31
Boron, 461
D,L-4-Boronophenylalanine, 462
Brain, 532
Buffers,
  acetate, 224
  affinity chromatography, 91
  barbital, 83, 146, 149
  bicarbonate, 90, 223
  borate, 90, 140

cacodylate, 222
carbonate, 90, 192, 223,
  coupling, 90, 192, 223, 258
  fixation, 222, 257
  glycine, HC1, 91
  immunediffusion, 143
  immunoelectronmicroscopy, 257
  immunoelectrophoresis, 149
  immunofluorescence, 192, 193, 210
  phosphate, 72, 143
  radioimmunoassay, 171, 178
  rocket immunoelectrophoresis, 152
  SDS electrophoresis, 45
  starch block electrophoresis, 83
  Tris-HC1, 72, 79

Calcium chloride, 51
Caps, 113, 371, 373
Carbodiimides, 29, 47, 259
Carcinoembryonic antigen, 410, 460
Cardiac puncture, 42, 43
Cardiolipin, 28
Carrier, 4
Castor bean lectin, 351, 356, 374, 382, 383
Cell,
  antigens, 22, 25, 415
  contact, 373
  disruption, 511
  fusion, 273, 275
  membrane, 24, 509
  receptors, 9, 389
  sorting, 212, 426
Central nervous system, 416
Chagas' disease, 501
Charcoal, 33
Chickens, 35, 42, 43
Chlorambucil, 450
Chloramine-T, 165
Chromatography,
  affinity, 73, 76, 368, 377, 537
  DEAE, 71, 193, 223
  gel filtration, 63, 80, 193, 223
  ion exchange, 71, 81, 193, 223
  lectin, 368, 377
  protein A, 73
Clonal heterogeneity, 99
Clonal restriction, 10
Clonal selection, 9, 274, 296
Cloning, 278, 283
Colloidal alum, 33
Colloidal gold, 234, 247, 261, 325

Column chromotography, 79
Combining site, 11
Complement, 35, 43
  fixation, 113
Concanavalin A, 350, 351, 374, 377, 382, 519
Conformational determinants, 21
Conjugated antigens, 28
Constant region, 10
Contamination markers, 520, 526
Cow, 74
Criteria of purity, 26
Cross-linking, 519
α-Crystallins, 418
β-Crystallins, 418
γ-Crystallins, 418
Cultured cells, 24
Cyanogen bromide, 76, 77, 89
Cytolipins, 28
Cytoskeleton, 326
Cytotoxicity, 409

Daunomycin, 455
Daunorubicin, 455
Deae, 71, 72, 193, 223
Delipidation, 51
Density perturbation, 535
Detergents, 377, 391, 519
Developmental antigens, 315, 419
Dextran, 64, 538
Dextran sulphate, 51
Diazo compound, 30, 77
Differentiation, 373
  antigens, 297
Diffusion-in-gel methods, 142, 298
Diisocyanates, 29, 246, 259
Digitoxin, 468
Digoxin, 464
Direct immunoelectronmicroscopy, 247
Direct haemagglutination, 156
Dogs, 74
Dolichos biflorus lectin, 357, 383
Domain, 7
Donkeys, 34
Double diffusion, 128, 142, 381
Doxorubicin, 455
Drug toxicity, 463
DTIC, 453

Ear bleeding, 42
Echidna, 74
Egg cells, 373

Electrophoresis, 67, 538
  immunoelectrophoresis, 147
  isoelectric focusing, 60, 84
  SDS-gel, 44
  starch block, 82
  zone, 68, 82
Electrophoretic mobility, 68
Elution buffers, 78, 91
Embryonic antigens, 316
Embryonic tissues, 370
Emulsification, 32
Enzymes, 323, 512, 457
Enzyme markers, 539, 541
Enzyme immunoassays (EIA), 179
Epitopes, 22
'Epitope' heterogeneity, 98
Equilibrium dialysis, 100
Erythrocytes, 156, 379, 407
Euglobulin precipitation, 63, 72
Expansion of cultures, 283
Exsanguination, 49
Extracellular antigens, 327, 418

Fab, 406, 424
  conjugates, 247
  half-life, 466
$(Fab')_2$, 224, 456
Fabulation, 490
Fat cells, 537
Ferritin, 234, 236, 246, 347, 373, 388, 405
Fetuin, 368
Fertilization, 373
Fibrinogen, 460
Fibronectin, 419
Fick's law, 125
FITC, 191
Fixatives, 221, 222, 257
Flow cytofluorometry, 212
  cytogram, 215
Fluorescein dyes, 190
Fluorescein isothiocyanate, 191, 322
Fluorescence activated cell sorter, 212, 278
Fluorescence
  quenching, 100
  enhancement, 100
  depolarization, 100
  microscopy, 326
Fluorescent compounds, 190, 405
Fluorochromes, 190
  conjugation to proteins, 192, 222
  degree of protein substitution, 195

structures, 191
stability of protein conjugates, 198
fluorescence characteristics, 199
Foetal calf serum, 285
Foeto-maternal relationships, 403, 428
α-Foetoprotein, 410
Forsmann antigen, 28
Freezing, 280
Freund's adjuvants, 32, 33, 40
Fusion, 281

Gamma (γ) chain, 5
Garden pea lectin, 351, 382
Gel electrophoresis, 385
Gel filtration, 63, 64, 80, 193, 223
Ghosts, 518
Glucose oxidase, 459
Glutaraldehyde, 246, 247, 251, 264, 519
Glycine-HCl buffer, 72, 79, 91
Glycolipids, 360
Glycophorin, 369
Glycoproteins, 347, 360, 385, 390
Glycosphingolipids, 28
Glycosyl transferase, 369
Goats, 34, 42, 74
Gold markers, 231, 234, 247, 261, 325, 377
Gorse seed lectin, 353
Grafts, 295
Grass pollen, 329, 331
Growth,
    cells, 278
    tumours, 284
Guanidine hydrochloride, 92, 377
Guinea pigs, 34, 42, 43, 74

H-2 system, 411
Haemagglutination, 155, 384
    direct, 156
    passive, 156
Haemocyanin, 234, 240, 247, 377, 405
Hamsters, 42
Handling of animals, 36
Hapten, 4, 28
HAT selection, 275
Helix pomatia haemagglutinin, 379
Hepatomas, 531
Heterokaryons, 275
Histocompatibility antigens, 411
Hormones, 403, 544
Hormone monitoring, 430
Horse gram lectin, 352

Horseradish peroxidase, 246, 405
Horses, 34
Horseshoe crab lectin, 353, 358
Host cell modification, 499
Human chorionic gonadotropin, 410
Human immunoglobulins, 6
Hybrid antibody, 249
Hybridomas, 473
Hypersensitive reactions, 295
Hypervariable region, 11
Hypoxanthine phosphoribosyl trans-
    ferase (HPRT), 276

IgA, 6, 75
IgG, 5, 35, 67, 71, 75, 246, 247, 254, 321
IgE, 6, 295, 331, 333
IgM, 5, 67, 71, 75
IgY, 35
Immune complexes, 501
Immune diffusion, 139, 142
Immunity against pathogens, 296
Immunization, 30, 36, 40, 49, 276, 419
Immunoxcytochemistry, 319
Immunodiffusion, 139
    radial, 127, 144
Immunoelectron microscopy, 233, 324
    cell preparation, 262
    indirect, 248
    markers, 236
Immunoelectrophoresis, 130, 139, 147
    rocket, 150
Immunofluorescence, 189, 323, 325
    direct, 217, 225
    indirect, 217, 225
    instrumentation, 202
    methodology, 217
    microscope, 206
    microphotometry, 210
    photomicography, 228
    specimen preparation, 220, 224
Immunoglobulin (Ig) (*see also* Anti-
    body), 5, 59
    binding to protein A, 73, 74
    binding site, 7
    constant region, 7
    diversity, 9
    Fab fragment, 406, 424, 466
    (Fab')$_2$ fragment, 224, 456
    gamma chain, 5
    general properties, 5
    genes, 11
    heavy chain, 5, 7

heterogeneity, 103
homogeneous, 99
isoelectric focusing, 60
kappa chain, 5, 7
lambda chain, 5, 7
light chain, 5, 7
purification, 59
structure, 3
variable region, 5, 7
Immunopathology, 501
Immunoprecipitation, 124, 139, 409
Immunoprophylaxis, 490
Infection, 286
Influenza virus, 369
Immunoradiometric assay, 182
Immunoprecipitation analysis, 307
Intestine, 532
Iodination, 388
Intracellular antigens, 324
Intracellular labelling, 251
Iodo-gen, 167, 388
Ion-exchange chromatography, 71, 81, 193, 223
Isolectric focusing, 60, 84
Isolectric point, 70

Japanese pagoda tree lectin, 352

Kappa chain, 5
Kidney, 531

Lactoperoxidase, 16, 167, 388, 459, 512
Lambda chain, 5
Langmuir adsorption isotherm, 102
Large animals, 42
Latex spheres, 234, 237, 247
Lead acetate, 237
Lectins, 306, 326, 347
cell binding, 379, 545
glycoprotein binding, 386
labelling, 387
purification, 380
receptors, 376
toxicity, 380
Leishmania, 489
Lentil lectin, 351, 355, 382
Lens culinaris lectin, 351, 355, 374, 382
Light chain, 5
Lima bean lectin, 352, 383
Limulus polyphemus lectin, 358, 382, 383
Lipid-containing sera, 43, 51
Lipids, 28

Lipoproteins, removal, 43, 51
Lissamine rhodamine, 191, 322
Lithium diiodosalicylate, 377
Liver, 531
Lotus tetragonolobus lectin, 352, 358, 383
Lung, 417
Ly antigen, 417
Lymphocytes, 4, 59, 225, 373, 524
bone-marrow derived, 4, 417
clonal restriction, 9
thymus derived, 4, 23

Mammary cell plasma membrane, 533
Mancini method, 127, 144, 306
Markers, 234, 245
conjugation of, 192, 246
of contamination, 543
Maturation of antibody response, 41
Membrane, 27, 360, 509
components, 378
glycoproteins, 368
isolation, 509
labelling, 16, 247, 545
vesiculation, 522
Metazoa, 489
Methotrexate, 457
Major histocompatibility complex antigens, 411
Mice, 34, 42, 43, 49, 74
Minor histocompatability antigens, 412
Mitogenic stimulation, 369
Mixed haemadsorption assay, 407
Molecular sieving, 69
Monoclonal antibody, 273, 473
Monogamous binding, 117
Monosaccharides, 348
Morphine, 469
Morphology, 520, 538
Mu (μ) chain, 5
Multiphor apparatus, 85
Murine immunoglobulins, 6
Murine leukaemia virus, 177, 181, 413
Muscle, 532
Mycobacteria, 32
Myeloma cell, 277
Myeloma proteins, 359
Myosin binding protein, 514

N-glycosidic linkages, 362
Non-specific absorption, 76
Nucleic acids, 29

Nylon fibres, 379

Oestrogens, 410
O-glycosidic linkages, 361
Orbital plexus, 43
Organ specificity of plant antigens, 313
Organelle antigens, 316
Osmium tetroxide, 253
Osmolarity, 253
Ouabain, 464, 468
Ouchterlony, 143, 298

Pancreas, 533
Parasites, 485
    acquisition of host characteristics, 487
    survival mechanisms, 486
Particulate markers, 234, 406
Partition techniques, 538
Patches, 371
Pea lectin, 355, 382
Peanut lectin, 351, 356
Peg, 275
Peptide hormones, 29
Percoll, 535
Period-specific antigens, 317
Peroxidase, 234, 245
Pevikon, 68
Phage, 116, 234
Phagocytosis, 519
Pharmacologic agents, 447
-*Phaseolus vulgaris* lectin, 357
p-Phenylenediamine mustard, 453
Phosopholipase C, 460
Phylogenetic distance, 35
Phytroalexins, 296
Phytohaemagglutinins (*see also* Lectins),
    348, 382
Plant virus, 234
Plasma membrane, 27, 360, 509
    components, 378
    glycoproteins, 368
    isolation, 495, 509
    labelling, 189, 247, 545
    markers, 520, 526
    vesiculation, 522
Plasmodium sp., 486, 488, 501
Pokeweed mitogen, 353, 359
Pollen-stigma interaction, 327
Polyacrylamide beads, 64, 78
Polyacrylamide gel electrophoresis, 7, 26,
    27, 33, 44, 70, 75, 517

stabilization with agarose, 46
Polyethylene glycol, 274
Polylysine, 327
Polyvinyl chloride microtitre plates, 367
Potassium chloride, 377
Potato starch, 68
Precipitation, *see* Precipitin
Precipitin reactions, 113, 121, 139
    equivalence zone, 123
    mancini technique, 127, 144
    prozone, 123, 124
    quantitative, 381
    radial, 127, 144
    ring test, 140
    soluble complexes, 123
Pregnancy-associated macroglobulin, 410
Primary immunization, 40
Pristane, 279
Protein-A, 74, 75, 407
Proteins, conjugation, 89, 192, 222, 258

Rabbits, 34, 42, 74
Radioallergosorbent test (RAST), 333
Radioimmunoassays, 163, 385, 410
Radiolabelling, 16, 165, 167, 388, 460,
    512
Ragweed pollen, 329
Rapid embedding, 264
Rate constant, 117
Rats, 34, 42, 43, 74
RB200SC, 191
Reaction between antigen and antibody,
    21, 97, 139, 163
Reactive groups, 77
Reaginic antibodies, 321
Red blood cells, 156, 379, 407
Red kidney bean lectin, 352, 357
Reproductive endocrinology, 430
Resins, 265
Rhodamine dyes, 190
Rikettsia, 489
Ring test, 140
Rocket immunoelectrophoresis (RIEP),
    150
    one-dimensional RIEP, 150
    two-dimensional RIEP, 153
Rod cells, 373
Rodents, 42

Salt precipitation, 61
Scanning electron microscope, 377

Scatchard equation (plot), 101, 120
Schistosoma, 486, 489
SDS-gel electrophoresis, *see* Sodium dodecylsulphate polyacrylamide gel electrophoresis
Second antibody, 173
Sendai virus, 274, 275
Sephadex®, 64, 69
Sepharose®, 64
    matrix for affinity chromatography, 73, 77, 89
Serodiagnosis, 496
Serum, 43, 69
    chicken, 43
    electrophoretic separation, 69
    preparation, 43, 44
    removal of lipoproteins, 51
Serum proteins, adsorbed onto cells, 24
Sheep, 34, 42, 74
Slime moulds, 370
Sodium dodecylsulphate polyacrylamide gel electrophoresis, 7, 17, 27, 44, 70, 309, 367, 512
    method, 44
Sodium sulphate precipitation, 61
Sodium thiocyanate, 91
Solid-phase radioimmunoassays, 180
Solid tissue labelling, 252
Somatic cell hybridization, 496
Sophora japonica agglutinin, 357
Soybean lectin, 352, 357, 383
Spectrin, 509
Sperm cells, 373
Spinal cord, 532
Staining of gel electropherograms, 47, 89
Starch block electrophoresis, 69
Steroid hormones, 29
Stilbene isothiocyanate, 322
Storage, frozen, 44
Sulphhydryl, 77
Surface-associated ligands, 545
Surface immunoglobulin, 417
Surface labelling, 16, 545
Surface markers, 22, 539

Temperature for immunoelectron microscopy procedures, 253
Teratoma-defined antigens, 421
Test bleeds, treatment of, 41, 42, 43
Tetrahymena, 490

Tetra methyl rhodamine isothiocyanate, 191, 322
Theileria, 489
Theta (θ) antigen (*see also* Thy-1 antigen), 22, 417
Thy-1 antigen, 22, 417
Thymidine kinase, 276
Thymocytes, 379
Thymus-derived lymphocytes (*see also* T lymphocytes), 4, 23, 417
T lymphocytes, 417
Thyroid, 533
Tissue culture vessels, 286
Tissue preparation, 320
Toluene-2,4 diisocyanate, 246, 259
Tooth germ, 419
Toxins, 457
    diptheria, 457
Transformed cells, 348
Transmission electron microscopy, 234
    fixation schedule for, 262
    O–T–O fixation for, 263
Transplantation, immunity and tolerance, 294
Tree pollen, 331
Tridacna maxima lectin, 382
Triaziquone, 454
Tritc, 191
Triton X-100, 178, 377, 519
Trophoblast, 413, 416
Trypanosoma, 488, 490
    defined antigens of, 499
Trypanosoma cruzi,
    preparation of plasma membrane, 495
Tumour antigens, 14
Tumour cells, 14, 17, 448, 515
    plasma membrane isolation, 515
Tumour specific antigens, 22

Ulex europaeus lectin, 358, 383
Uranyl acetate, 237
Urea, 92

Vaccination,
    target antigens for, 493
Vaccines,
    animal versus human, 492
Variable region of immunoglobulin molecule, 10
V_H, 10
Video intensification microscopy, 211

Viral infections, 25
Viruses, 237
  antigens, 14

Water in oil emulsions, 32
  preparation of, 33
Weeds, 331
Wheat, 353
Wheat germ agglutinin, 348, 358, 374,
  382, 385
Whole organisms as antigen, 22

Wistaria floribunda lectin, 352

m-Xylylene diisocyanate, 246

Zinc sulphate in immunoglobulin purification, 63
Zonal rotors, 535
Zone electrophoresis, 68
  on starch blocks, 82
  preparative, 82